Paediatric Emergencies

POSTGRADUATE PAEDIATRICS SERIES

under the General Editorship of

JOHN APLEY
CBE, MD, BS, FRCP

*Emeritus Consultant Paediatrician,
United Bristol Hospitals*

Paediatric Emergencies

EDITED BY J. A. BLACK MD, FRCP

Consultant Paediatrician, Children's Hospital, Sheffield
and
Jessop Hospital for Women, Sheffield

BUTTERWORTHS
London Boston
Sydney Wellington Durban Toronto

The Butterworth Group

United Kingdom London	**Butterworth & Co (Publishers) Ltd** 88 Kingsway, WC2B 6AB
Australia Sydney	**Butterworth Pty Ltd** 586 Pacific Highway, Chatswood NSW 2067 Also at Melbourne, Adelaide and Perth
Canada Toronto	**Butterworth & Co (Canada) Ltd** 2265 Midland Avenue Scarborough, Ontario, M1P 4S1
New Zealand Wellington	**Butterworths of New Zealand Ltd** T & W Young Building, 77–85 Customhouse Quay, 1 CPO Box 472
South Africa Durban	**Butterworth & Co (South Africa) (Pty) Ltd** 152–154 Gale Street
USA Boston	**Butterworth (Publishers) Inc** 10 Tower Office Park, Woburn, Mass. 01801

First published 1979

ISBN 0 407 00131 X

©Butterworth & Co. (Publishers) Ltd 1979

British Library Cataloguing in Publication Data

Paediatric emergencies.—(Postgraduate
paediatrics series).
1. Paediatric emergencies
I. Black, J A II. Series
618.9′2002′5   RJ370   78-41042

ISBN 0-407-00131-X

Printed in Great Britain by Page Bros (Norwich) Ltd

Contents

List of Contributors

E. H. Back, VRD, MB, BChir, FRCP
Consultant Paediatrician, Great Yarmouth and Waveney Health District; (formerly Professor of Paediatrics, University of the West Indies)

J. D. Baum, MA, MSc, MD, FRCP, DCH
Clinical Reader in Paediatrics, John Radcliffe Hospital, Oxford

Dion R. Bell, MB, ChB, FRCP, MFCM, DTM and H
Senior Lecturer in Tropical Medicine, Liverpool School of Tropical Medicine; Honorary Consultant Physician, Liverpool Area Health Authority (Teaching)

J. A. Black, MD, FRCP
Consultant Paediatrician, The Children's Hospital, Sheffield; and Jessop Hospital for Women, Sheffield

J. T. Buffin, FRCS, DLO
Consultant ENT Surgeon, Department of Communication, The Children's Hospital, Sheffield

Judith M. Chessells, MD, FRCP
Consultant Clinical Haematologist, The Hospital for Sick Children, Great Ormond Street, London

A. F. Conchie, MB, ChB, DCH, DA
Consultant Paediatrician, Doncaster Royal Infirmary and Worksop and Retford District

D. M. Danks, MD, FRACP
Professor of Paediatrics, University of Melbourne; Head of Genetics Research Unit, Royal Children's Hospital, Melbourne, Australia

R. C. W. Dinsdale, VRD, BChD, FDS, RCS(Eng)
Consultant Dental Surgeon to The Charles Clifford Dental Hospital, Sheffield Area Health Authority (Teaching); Honorary Clinical Lecturer in Dental Surgery, University of Sheffield

Carl Edmonds, MB, BS, MRCP, FRACP, MRCPsych; MANZCP
Consultant in Underwater Medicine to The Royal Australian Navy; Director, Diving Medical Centre, Mosman, Australia

J. C. Fallis, BA, MD, FRCS(C), FACS
Director, Emergency Medical Services, The Hospital for Sick Children, Toronto, Canada

D. N. Grant, MB, ChB, FRCS
Consultant Neurological Surgeon to the National Hospital for Nervous Diseases, London, and The Hospital for Sick Children, Great Ormond Street, London

B. Heyworth, MB, ChB, MRCP, DCH, D(Obs)RCOG, DTM & H (Liverpool)
Medical Superintendent, Mater Children's Hospital, South Brisbane, Australia. Formerly Senior Lecturer Tropical Paediatrics and Child Health, School of Tropical Medicine, University of Liverpool; Honorary Consultant Paediatrician, Infectious Diseases Department and Neonates Department, Fazakerley District Hospital, Liverpool, Merseyside Regional Health Authority

D. Anna Jarvis, MB, BS, FRCP(C)
Supervising Paediatrician, Emergency Department, Hospital for Sick Children, Toronto; Lecturer, Department of Paediatrics, University of Toronto, Canada

Elizabeth Lund, MB, BCh, BAO
Medical Officer in Newborn Nursery, Edendale Hospital, Pietermaritzburg, Natal, South Africa

Ian A. McKinlay, MB, ChB, MRCP, BSc, DCH
Consultant Paediatric Neurologist, Booth Hall Children's Hospital, Manchester

S. R. Meadow, MA, BM, BCh, FRCP, DCH, D(Obs), RCOG
Senior Lecturer, Department of Paediatrics and Child Health, University of Leeds; Honorary Consultant Paediatrician, Leeds Area Health Authority (Teaching)

R. W. S. Miller, FRCS(Ed), LRCP(Ed), LRFP and S(Glas)
Consultant Plastic Surgeon, Sheffield Area Health Authority
(Clinical)

A. D. Milner, MD, FRCP, DCH
Reader in Child Health, University of Nottingham; Honorary Consultant Paediatrician, Children's and City Hospitals, Nottingham

M. J. Noronha, FRCP(Ed), MRCP(Lond)
Consultant Paediatric Neurologist, Royal Manchester Children's
Hospital, Pendlebury, and Booth Hall Children's Hospital,
Manchester

J. R. Oakley, MB, ChB, DCH, MRCP
Clinical Co-ordinator, Multi-centre Post Neonatal Study, The Children's Hospital, Sheffield

Ian W. Pinkerton, TD, MB, ChB, FRFPS(Glas), MRCP(Ed)
Consultant Physician in Infectious Diseases, Ruchill Hospital, Glas-
gow; Honorary Lecturer in Infectious Diseases, University of
Glasgow

H. Alistair Reid, OBE, MD, FRCPE, FRACP, DTM and H
Head WHO Collaborative Centre for the Control of Antivenins;
Consultant Physician and Senior Lecturer, Liverpool School of
Tropical Medicine

Joan N. Scragg, MD(Cape Town), DCH, RCP and S (Eng)
Formerly Associate Professor, Department of Paediatrics and Child
Health, Faculty of Medicine, University of Natal, South Africa

Ian Shellshear, MB, BS(Qld), FRACP
T & G Building, Stanley Street, Townsville, Queensland, Australia;
Formerly Senior Registrar in Paediatrics, The Children's Hospital,
Sheffield

P. M. Smythe, MD(Camb), FRCP(Lond)
Formerly Professor and Head of the Department of Paediatrics and
Child Health, University of Natal, South Africa

Lewis Spitz, MB, ChB (Pretoria), FRCS(Ed)
Senior Consultant Paediatric Surgeon, The Children's Hospital,
Sheffield; Honorary Clinical Lecturer in Paediatric Surgery, Univer-
sity of Sheffield; Formerly Senior Paediatric Surgeon, Transvaal
Memorial Hospital for Children, and University of Witwatersrand,
Johannesburg, South Africa

J. Paget Stanfield, MD, FRCP, DCH
Senior Lecturer in International Child Health, Department of Child Health, University of Newcastle upon Tyne

A. Stanworth, MD, PhD, BSc, DOMS
Honorary Director of the University Department of Ophthalmology, University of Sheffield; Consultant Ophthalmic Surgeon, The Children's Hospital, Sheffield

F. G. Thorpe, MB, ChB, FRCPsych, DPM
Consultant in Children's Psychiatry, The Children's Hospital, Northern General Hospital and School Health Psychiatry Clinic, Sheffield; Medical Director, Department of Child Psychiatry (Shirle Hill), Nether Edge Hospital, Sheffield; Honorary Clinical Lecturer, University of Sheffield

Alan Usher, MB, BS, FRCPath, DMJ (Clin et Path)
Professor and Head of Department of Forensic Pathology, University of Sheffield

A. E. Walker, MD, MB, ChB, FRCP
Consultant Dermatologist, Royal Hospital, Chesterfield; Clinical Tutor, Chesterfield Postgraduate Centre

M. P. Ward, MA, MD, FRCS
Consultant Surgeon, St. Andrew's Hospital, London; Lecturer in Surgery, London Hospital Medical College

M. F. Whitfield, BSc, MB, ChB, MRCP, DCH, Dip(Obst) RCOG
Lecturer in Paediatrics, University of Sheffield

J. L. Wilkinson, MB, ChB, MRCP
Consultant Paediatric Cardiologist, Royal Liverpool Children's Hospital; Clinical Lecturer in Child Health, University of Liverpool

A. M. Wilson, MB, ChB, FFA, RCS, DObstRCOG
Head of Anaesthetic Service, Riyadh Military Hospital, Saudi Arabia

Wong Hock Boon, MBBS, FRCP(Ed), FRACP, FRCP(Glas), DCH, PJC, PPA
Professor of Paediatrics, Director of the School of Postgraduate Medical Studies, Faculty of Medicine, University of Singapore

Preface

An emergency can be defined as an acute illness in which lack of prompt and appropriate treatment may result in death, disability, or delayed recovery. In Europe and North America of all children admitted to hospital, 60 per cent are emergencies; in Africa and Asia this proportion is much higher.

Acute disease in children evolves more rapidly than in adults, but with correct treatment the child has a greater capacity for quick and complete recovery. Emergency treatment in the child must therefore be of a very high standard, and it is unfortunate that in most hospital services treatment of the emergency admission is in the hands of relatively junior staff, and the more experienced the clinician becomes, the less acute disease does he see. Normally, the Consultant or Specialist only becomes directly involved in emergency treatment when something goes wrong. It is for this reason that the management of the acutely ill child is seldom subjected to the same critical analysis as is that of the less acutely ill patient, and the traditions of emergency treatment are maintained at a sub-Consultant level, often with inadequate facilities. Thus the standard of emergency care in general paediatric departments tends to lag behind that of the more specialized units. In this book we have attempted to make available to the general paediatrician the practice of the best specialist units. With its emphasis on recognition of the emergency, we hope that this book will also be useful to those who are the first to see the acutely ill child, the family doctors, and the casualty officers. We have, where appropriate, attempted to describe the management of the emergency in sufficient detail to be of use to both medical and nursing staff.

We have included a section on diseases of the subtropics and tropics for a number of reasons, the most important being that rapid intercontinental travel makes it essential that the paediatrician should be able to recognize conditions which are not indigenous to his own country. Also, in many parts of the world, sick children are cared for by doctors without special training in paediatrics, and it seemed essential to combine in one volume the paediatric aspects of the more important diseases of the tropics and subtropics, and the management of those emergencies such as asthma, convulsions, etc. which the non-paediatrician would have to treat. A third consideration was that, with a few notable exceptions, textbooks of tropical medicine give inadequate attention to the treatment of the sick child, and, conversely, the general paediatric textbooks deal perfunctorily with tropical disease.

I would like to thank Dr John Apley for his invaluable support and advice in putting together this book, and to express my gratitude to my family, and particularly to my wife, for their tolerance of the piles of papers which threatened for a time to become a permanent feature of our home.

I would also like to thank Miss Joan Beynon for her help with correspondence, and Miss Eve Turner, Mrs Joyce Andrews, and Mrs Sandra Parfitt for their care and patience with the typing.

I am also indebted to all the numerous contributors for their help and for their hard work.

J. A. B.

Part I: Trauma, Accidents and Travel

Management of Acute Cardiorespiratory Collapse or Arrest

J. C. Fallis and D. Anna Jarvis

The diagrammatic scheme overleaf provides an easily memorized sequence for the management of acute cardiorespiratory failure.

We have given prominence to this table by placing it at the beginning of the book to emphasize that without the re-establishment of cardiorespiratory function in the desperately ill child, specific treatment related to the primary disease is ineffective.

This scheme supplies a framework of treatment which is common to any of the acute conditions associated with cardiorespiratory collapse which are described in the later chapters.

MANAGEMENT OF ACUTE CARDIORESPIRATORY COLLAPSE OR ARREST

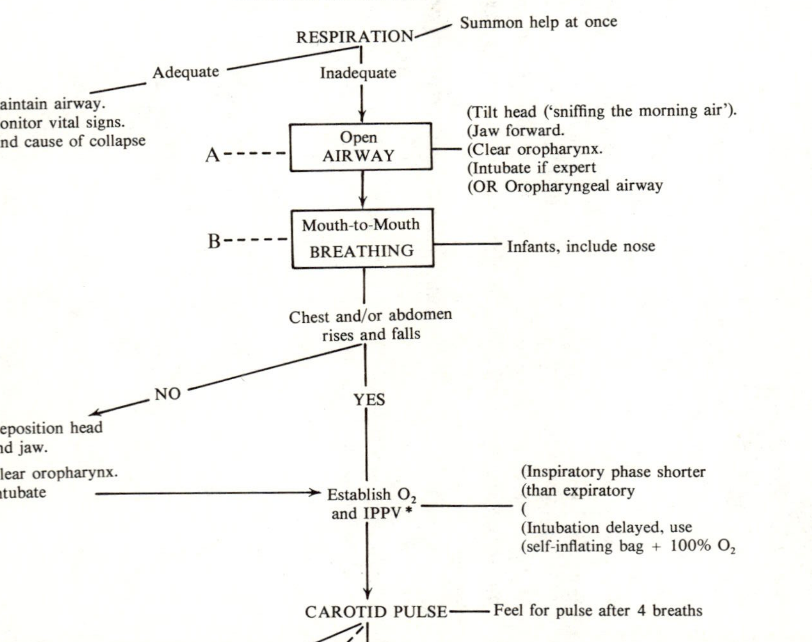

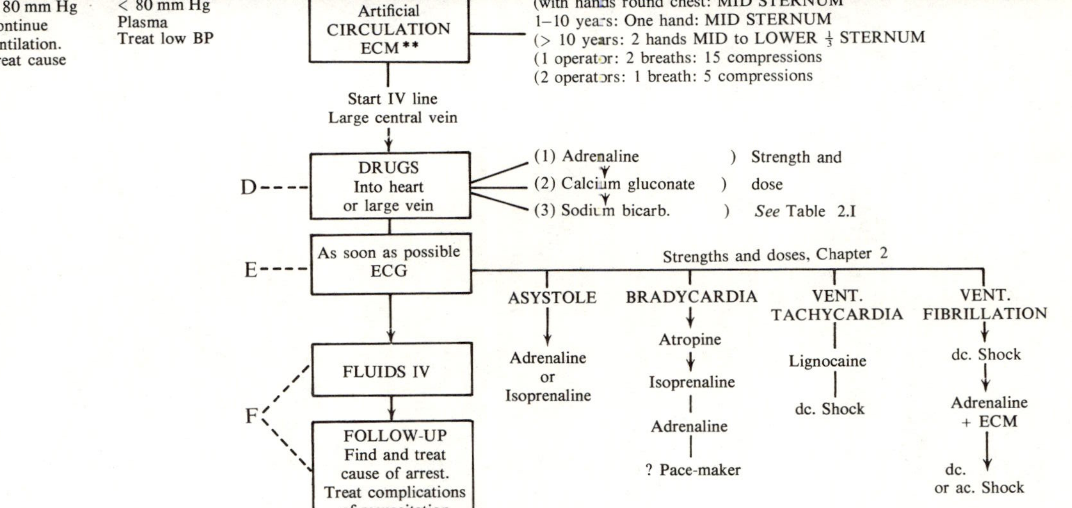

* Intermittent positive-pressure ventilation.

** External cardiac massage or compression

NOTES   (1) Resuscitation of the Newborn, *see* pages 599–606
         (2) Drugs in Resuscitation, *see* page 6
         (3) Use of Sympathomimetic Amines in Shock, *see* pages 115–119

CHAPTER 2

Drugs in Resuscitation: Cardiorespiratory Collapse/Arrest

A. M. Wilson

The doses given in the tables below have been set out in a simplified form so that they can be easily memorized for use without reference to a text, in an emergency. Alternatively, the Tables are suitable for conversion into wall charts in resuscitation rooms, operating theatres, or labour wards. For further details on dosages and methods of administration *see under the last column on the right in each table.*

TABLE 2.I
First line treatment

Drugs	Instructions	Age in years/Average weight for age in kg											Further details
		0–6/12/ 3.5–7	1/10	2/12	3/15	4/17	5/18	6/20	7/22	8/25	9/27	10*/30	
Adrenaline 1:1000 (0.1%) 1 ml = 1 mg Amps: 0.5 and 1.0 ml	IV or intracardiac over 1 min. Dilute 0.5 ml of 1:1000 into 10 ml to make 1:20 000. USE IN ASYSTOLE	1–2 ml	1–2 ml	2 ml	3 ml	4 ml	5 ml	6 ml	7 ml	8 ml	9 ml	10 ml	*See* pp. 112, 603
Calcium gluco- nate 10% (0.23 mmol Ca per 1 ml) Amps: 5 and 10 ml	IV or intra- cardiac. Over 1 min. USE IN ASYSTOLE OR RESPIRA- TORY ARREST	0.5 ml	1 ml	2 ml	3 ml	4 ml	5 ml	6 ml	7 ml	8 ml	9 ml	10 ml	*See* p. 303
Epinephrine *see* Adrenaline													
Sodium bicarbonate 7.5% (0.9 mmol per 1 ml) or 8.4% (1 mmol per 1 ml)	IV or intra-cardiac over 1–5 min. Give amount in columns × minutes of arrest. If not known assume	5 ml	10 ml	10 ml	15 ml	15 ml	20 ml	20 ml	20 ml	25 ml	25 ml	30 ml	*See* p. 303

TABLE 2.I (*continued*)

Drugs	Instructions	Age in years/Average weight for age in kg											Further details
		0–6/12/ 3.5–7	1/10	2/12	3/15	4/17	5/18	6/20	7/22	8/25	9/27	10*/30	
Difference in dosage be-tween these strengths is negligible, [1] Amps: 10 and 30 ml and 100-ml bags	3 min. USE IN ASYSTOLE OR RESPIRA-TORY ARREST												
Nikethamide Amps: 2 ml 25%	IV solution 25% dilute in to 10 ml. USE ONLY IN RESP. ARREST WHEN NO-ONE CAN INTUBATE	0.25–0.5 ml	1 ml	2 ml	3 ml	4 ml	5 ml	6 ml	7 ml	8 ml	9 ml	10 ml	
Intubation	External diameter of tube in mm	3 mm	3.5 mm	4 mm	4.5 mm	4.5 mm	4.5 mm	5 mm	5 mm	5.5 mm	6 mm	6.5 mm	Appendix 2.1

* Suitable starting doses for 10 years and above. [1] If using 5 per cent solution multiply these volumes by 1.7

TABLE 2.II
Second line treatment

Drugs	Instructions	Age in years/Average weight for age in kg											Further details
		0–6/12/ 3.5–7	1/10	2/12	3/15	4/17	5/18	6/20	7/22	8/25	9/27	10*/30	
Atropine	IV USE IN BRADY-CARDIA	0.1 mg	0.2 mg	0.3 mg	0.3 mg	0.3 mg	0.3 mg	0.6 mg	0.6 mg	0.6 mg	0.6 mg	0.6 mg	See p. 303
Isoprenaline Isoproterenol (Isuprel, Suscardia)	IV Dose to be used over 1 min. Continue till effective. Dilute 100 µg into 10 ml. USE IN ASYSTOLE OR PERSISTENT BRADYCARDIA	0.5 ml	1 ml	2 ml	3 ml	4 ml	5 ml	6 ml	7 ml	8 ml	9 ml	10 ml	See p. 303
Lignocaine Lidocaine (Xylocaine)	IV Use solution of 1 mg per 1 ml. Give at 1–2 mg per min. ARRHYTHMIAS	1 mg per kg	10 mg	10 mg	15 mg	15 mg	20 mg	20 mg	20 mg	25 mg	25 mg	30 mg	See p. 117

TABLE 2.II (*continued*)

Drugs	Instructions	Age in years/Average weight for age in kg											Further details
		0–6/12/ 3.5–7	1/10	2/12	3/15	4/17	5/18	6/20	7/22	8/25	9/27	10*/30	
Defibrillation for fibrillation or synchronized shock	Initial shock dc joules	5	10	20	30	40	50	60	70	80	90	100	*See* pp. 118, 291
ac for fibrillation only	Initial shock ac volts	12	25	50	75	100	125	150	175	200	225	250	*See* p. 118

* Suitable starting doses for 10 years and above

TABLE 2.III
Third line treatment

Drugs	Instructions	Age in years/Average weight for age in kg											Further details
		0–6/12/ 3.5–7	1/10	2/12	3/15	4/17	5/18	6/20	7/22	8/25	9/27	10*/30	
Aminophylline Amps: 250 mg in 10 ml 1 ml = 25 mg	IV over 30 min. USE IN STATUS ASTHMATICUS OR ANAPHY- LAXIS WITH BRONCHIAL SPASM	(3 mg/kg) 0.5 ml	1 ml	2 ml	3 ml	4 ml	5 ml	6 ml	7 ml	8 ml	9 ml	10 ml	See p. 254
Aramine (see Metaraminol)													
Dexamethasone (Decadron) Solution: 4 mg per 1 ml. 1 mg = 0.25 ml	IV PREVENTION OR TREATMENT OF CEREBRAL OEDEMA	2 mg	2 mg	2 mg	4 mg	4 mg	4 mg	8 mg	8 mg	8 mg	8 mg	10 mg	See p. 324
Diazepam (Valium) Amps: 10 mg in 2 ml. 1 mg = 0.2 ml	IV Over 2 min. DO NOT DILUTE. POST-HYPOXIC FITS	1 mg	1 mg	2 mg	3 mg	4 mg	5 mg	6 mg	7 mg	8 mg	9 mg	10 mg	See p. 318

TABLE 2.III (continued)

Drugs	Instructions	Age in years/Average weight for age in kg											Further details
		0–6/12/ 3.5–7	1/10	2/12	3/15	4/17	5/18	6/20	7/22	8/25	9/27	10*/30	
Frusemide Furosemide (Lasix) Amps: 20 mg in 2 ml 1 mg = 0.1 ml	IV PULMONARY OEDEMA OR RENAL SHUT-DOWN	(1 mg/kg) 5 mg	10 mg	10 mg	15 mg	15 mg	20 mg	20 mg	20 mg	25 mg	25 mg	30 mg	See p. 415
Hydrocortisone hemisuccinate vials: 100 mg and 500 mg	IV ANAPHYLAXIS OR ADRENAL FAILURE	25 mg[1]	25 mg[1]	25 mg[1]	50 mg[1]	50 mg[1]	50 mg[1]	100 mg	100 mg	100 mg	100 mg	100 mg	See pp. 114, 457
Mannitol 20% Bags 500 ml Warm to 60°C if crystals present, then cool to 37°C before giving. 20 g per 100 ml	IV 1–2 hours 20% solution CEREBRAL OEDEMA. ENSURE GOOD RENAL FUNCTION	5 g[1]	10 g[1]	10 g[1]	15 g[1]	15 g[1]	20 g[1]	20 g[1]	20 g[1]	25 g[1]	25 g[1]	30 g[1]	See pp. 315, 323

Metaraminol (Aramine)	IV Dilute 10 mg into 20 ml. ACUTE HYPO-TENSION	0.25 ml	0.5 ml	0.5 ml	0.5 ml	0.5 ml	0.5 ml	0.5 ml	1 ml	1 ml	1 ml	1 ml	*See* p. 116
			Doses are increments until effective										
Methoxamine (Vasoxine) Amps: 20 mg in 1 ml	IV Dilute 20 mg amp. into 20 ml. ACUTE HYPO-TENSION	0.25 ml	0.5 ml	0.5 ml	0.5 ml	0.5 ml	0.5 ml	0.5 ml	1 ml	1 ml	1 ml	1 ml	*See* p. 116
			Doses are increments until effective										
Paraldehyde Amps: 2, 5, and 10 ml	i.m. or IV[2] GLASS SYRINGE, POST-HYPOXIC FITS	0.25–0.5 ml	0.5–1 ml	1 ml	1.5 ml	2 ml	2.5 ml	3 ml	3.5 ml	4 ml	4.5 ml	5 ml	*See* p. 319
Valium (*see* Diazepam)													
Vasoxine Vasoxyl, (*see* Methoxamine)													

* Suitable starting doses for 10 years and above.
[1] If the required clinical response is not obtained, the doses can be repeated after 1 hour for hydrocortisone, and 2 hours for mannitol.
[2] Plastic syringe can be used if the injection is made within 30 minutes of drawing up the paraldehyce (*see also* page 319)

CHAPTER 3

Multiple Injuries

J. C. Fallis

Initial assessment

Nowhere is the accuracy of initial assessment more critical than in the management of the child with multiple injuries. The initial assessment establishes a therapeutic route which is only as correct as the assessment was accurate. Failure to recognize those injuries which may rapidly become life-threatening is an important cause of morbidity and mortality. Hence the physician who cares for those with multiple injuries must remain *serious-disease-conscious*. It matters little if the fracture of the clavicle or the metatarsal is not immediately detected. *But the child with a head injury which alone would not be lethal may die if a slowly expanding pneumothorax associated with it is overlooked.*

History

If a fraction of the effort expended in obtaining a history for a complicated medical illness were directed towards discovering, after major trauma, the details of the accident and the mechanism of injury, fewer important but initially obscure injuries would be missed. When an individual has landed on head or shoulder one must be alert to the possibility of an injured cervical spine. The head injury inadvertently inflicted by a golf club will rarely be associated with other major injuries. However, the child with a comparable head injury sustained when he was run over by a tractor, is likely to have other visceral injuries which pose a more serious threat to life than does the head injury.

Inspection, the basis of examination

The critically ill, seriously shocked or semicomatose child is usually too sick to make examination difficult through his unwillingness to cooperate. However, others, particularly the younger or frightened children, or those who are just ill behaved, cry while being examined or merely at the expectation of being examined. When a child will not co-operate it is necessary to obtain as much information as possible before causing any further discomfort. This is largely obtained by standing back and looking. Cardiorespiratory function can be evaluated, at least in general terms, by inspection alone, and the early manifestations of traumatic shock in the paediatric patient are all visible.

Adult hands are large and can hide much that is useful if they are applied too soon to the small child's body.

The first moments

The most important moments during the management of a multiple injury casualty are the first few after arrival in hospital. During this brief interval all injuries causing major physiological derangement must be detected and their effects countered. Although it is difficult to ignore the grossly displaced femoral fracture, the degloving injury of the foot, and the badly lacerated face, none of these will result in death. *The physician must single-mindedly focus on a sequence of priority items critical to survival.* He must complete a mental check list of vital functions before attending to items which are more obvious but have less influence on survival.

During these critical few minutes diagnosis merges with therapy. For example, respiration noted to be inadequate must be corrected while circulation is being evaluated. Priority assessment and resuscitation proceed simultaneously.

Critical assessment: the priority sequence

(1) Airway

(*a*) *Evidence of obstruction* Much is revealed about airway patency before palpation and auscultation. The gurgle or rattle of a partly obstructed airway is readily noted. Vigorous inspiratory effort serving only to suck in the abdomen, followed by abdominal protrusion as expiration is attempted, indicates complete obstruction.

(*b*) *Relief of obstruction*   Any degree of airway obstruction can be tolerated only briefly and must be corrected quickly while assessment is being completed. Extension of the head on the neck is often sufficient as this moves the mandible and tongue forward. Mechanical aspiration of saliva, vomitus or other liquid may be necessary and the physician may even have to remove solid foreign bodies from mouth or pharynx.

(*c*) *Position of the unconscious patient*   A comatose subject should be maintained in the semiprone position unless an endotracheal tube has been inserted. Although contraindicated in the presence of a cervical spine fracture and certain other injuries *the semiprone position permits ready drainage of oral secretions and vomitus, helps to keep the jaw and tongue forward, and can provide a safe airway indefinitely while comatose subjects are being transported.*

(*d*) *Artificial airway*   If a satisfactory airway has been obtained by simple measures it is often best to delay the insertion of an artificial airway, particularly if someone skilled at intubation is expected within minutes. Too few remember that an adequate airway, even one that will permit artificial ventilation can usually be maintained by proper head-positioning alone. However, tracheal intubation is indicated if there is coma from a head injury, or if artificial respiration will be needed for a prolonged period.

Although airway obstruction by a tongue which has fallen backwards can, theoretically, be dealt with by the insertion of an oropharyngeal airway most anaesthetists prefer the security of endotracheal intubation if artificial airway maintenance at any level is required. Oropharyngeal airways increase airway resistance; endotracheal tubes generally reduce it and offer the advantage of isolating the airway from the oesophagus.

Tracheal intubation for more than a few days was formerly an indication for tracheostomy. Latterly, nasotracheal intubation has been maintained for many days with few complications and has replaced tracheostomy in the majority of patients needing prolonged intubation. Emergency tracheostomy is now reserved for those situations in which facial or laryngeal trauma precludes the passage of a tube.

(*e*) *Gastric decompression*   In patients who are apt to vomit, gastric decompression should be maintained by means of a nasogastric tube. This applies particularly to children, in whom acute gastric dilatation is a very common complication of trauma to chest or abdomen. Any child with injuries which are multiple, involve chest or abdomen, or have produced peritoneal irritation to any degree, should have a nasogastric tube passed. In children who have impaired consciousness passage of the gastric tube should be preceded by tracheal intubation.

(f) *Airway obstruction in head injury is dangerous*   When a head injury is present even minor degrees of hypoxia or hypercapnia (hypercarbia) due to partial airway obstruction can cause sufficient increase in cerebral oedema that the patient may die who would otherwise have survived. For this reason airway maintenance and adequate ventilation is of critical importance in craniocerebral trauma. Airway obstruction is the leading cause of the respiratory failure seen from time to time following head injuries.

(g) *Diagnosis of airway obstruction in the apnoeic patient*   When the subject is apnoeic the diagnosis of airway obstruction will be made very quickly when positive-pressure insufflation is first attempted.

(h) *Oxygen*   Following major trauma oxygen therapy is indicated, particularly in the presence of a head injury.

(2) Breathing

(a) *Evaluation of respiratory function*   When the airway is open and oxygen is being given, adequacy of ventilation must be assessed. Looking and listening provide the initial evaluation, although arterial blood-gas analysis should be obtained as soon as possible in order to properly assess gas exchange. Before the blood-gas analysis becomes available ventilatory assistance is indicated unless the physician is absolutely confident that ventilation is adequate. This is of particular importance when there is a head injury.

(b) *Pneumothorax   After thoracic trauma grunting respirations usually signify pleural irritation and almost always indicate the presence of a pneumothorax or haemopneumothorax.* Immediate auscultation revealing decreased breath sounds on one side reinforces the diagnosis and the equipment needed for the closed insertion of a chest tube (thoracostomy) should be requested at once. The few moments needed for the preparation of the tray permit the initial assessment of the patient to be completed. With the child supine, the physician should quickly infiltrate the second or third interspace in the midclavicular line with local anaesthetic, taking care to avoid breast tissue and the internal mammary vessels. Local anaesthesia should be used even if the child is comatose so that the intrapleural air can be sucked back through the anaesthetic liquid remaining in the syringe. The bubbling produced is confirmation of the diagnosis. The tube is then inserted at the same site and connected either to an under-water seal or a one-way egress valve, (e.g. Heimlich valve). Evacuation of the pneumothorax is usually very rapid and almost immediately results in correction of the respiratory distress, cessation of the grunting, and restoration of air entry throughout. Suction applied to the tube will rarely be needed to empty the pleural space. *When a combination of several injuries includes a pneumothorax, and particularly when there has been cerebral trauma, there is no justification for waiting for radiographic confirmation of pneumothorax before treating it.* The first chest x-ray taken should be to show that the tube is properly located and the lung has expanded satisfactorily.

(*c*) *Ventilatory assistance*   Ventilatory assistance may be needed for any one of several reasons. Central depression of ventilation may result from direct brainstem or medullary damage or from the effects of increased intracranial pressure due to an intracranial clot or cerebral oedema. Advanced cerebral hypoxia from asphyxia or from hypovolaemic shock will also ultimately cause respiratory arrest as the patient reaches a terminal state.

Also, positive-pressure assisted ventilation (IPPV) is the treatment of choice for the paradoxical movement of a flail chest. This condition is not frequently seen in children in whom the chest wall is quite pliable and not prone to multiple fractures.

(3) Circulation

(*a*) *Evidence of shock*   Instant evaluation of circulation is reached by inspection. *Abnormal pallor and sweating in one who is prostrate after an accident are, for practical purposes, diagnostic of hypovolaemic shock.* This is particularly valid in children who usually show the pallor of shock long before tachycardia or hypotension are observed.

In children inadequate cerebral circulation secondary to hypovolaemia causes a characteristic type of behaviour. The confusion of a child fighting to pull the oxygen mask from his face or complaining bitterly of a bruised ankle when he has several other serious injuries, should not be interpreted as plain cussedness.

These are signs of cerebral hypoxia and signal the need for prompt action.

(b) *Blood for grouping and crossmatching, Hb and haematocrit (PCV)*   As this assessment is proceeding blood must be rapidly obtained for grouping and crossmatching, and determination of haemoglobin and haematocrit levels, although, if the haemorrhage is very recent, these may still be normal and serve only as a baseline.

(c) *Intravenous line*   A large bore venous cannula must be inserted in an arm vein, one in each arm if there is risk of major blood loss. The venous cannulae now available are designed for easy percutaneous introduction, and a cut-down is rarely needed.

(d) *Effects of cold-stored blood (see page 25)*   If a large transfusion volume is anticipated a blood-warming apparatus should be included in the infusion apparatus. The small blood volume of the child cools rapidly when mixed with cold bank blood and this has frequently resulted in cardiac arrhythmia and even arrest. A micropore filter (40 µm) should also be included in the line. It may reduce the incidence of subsequent pulmonary complications (shock lung).

(e) *Monitoring with ECG*   The leads from an electrocardiograph monitor with defibrillator should be attached to the patient as the venous infusions are being established.

(f) *Acid-base state*   When the arterial blood-gas analysis becomes available the degree of metabolic acidosis due to inadequate tissue perfusion can be estimated. In major trauma, arterial cannulation is desirable. This facilitates repeated sampling of arterial blood and provides a mechanism for continuous arterial-pressure monitoring.

(g) *External cardiac massage*   Finally, external cardiac compression to assist ineffective heart function is occasionally required. However, manual support for a heart which has suddenly failed because of advanced hypovolaemic shock must be combined with rapid blood-volume expansion, ventilatory assistance, and control of bleeding.

(4) Increased intracranial pressure (*see also* pages 314, 323)

There remains one more true emergency—increased intracranial pressure. Although acute extradural and subdural haematomata are not often part of the multi-injury complex, immediate operative treatment is required when they do occur. For this reason they must never go undetected.

(*a*) *Extradural and acute subdural haematoma*   History is the single most important feature in the diagnosis. The classic story is that of brief depression of consciousness after the accident, followed by gradual improvement, perhaps even to a normal state of alertness, followed by rapidly progressive deterioration of consciousness. Increased intracranial pressure must always be kept in mind as the course of events is not always that described above. A child may sustain seemingly minor head trauma, be only momentarily stunned, and then some hours later may develop the progressive drowsiness of an extradural haematoma. Similarly, when a subject is rendered deeply comatose in an accident, failure to improve can be at least partly due to an enlarging surface clot.

Gradual dilatation of one pupil and a decreasing responsiveness to light usually indicate an expanding clot over the ipsilateral hemisphere. This is a very important sign and, more consistently than any other, indicates the side of the haematoma. However it heralds advanced compression and is quickly followed by hypertension, bradycardia, and then respiratory depression due to brainstem ischaemia. Both pupils soon become fixed and dilated. Therefore accurate recording is important so that treatment which has been started when the pupils have become dilated can be directed towards the correct side without delay.

Papilloedema is a sign of increased intracranial pressure. However, with acutely raised tension, papilloedema seldom has time to develop. *In most instances of acutely enlarging intracranial clot the fundi are normal.*

(5) Exceptions to the sequence of priority

There are two exceptions to the above sequence of priorities which take precedence over all else.

(*a*) *An open chest wound must be closed.*

(*b*) *Major external haemorrhage must be controlled at once*   Usually either of these will have been accomplished by the first-aider, ambulance attendant, or receiving nurse. If not, the physician must take the necessary action immediately.

When the priority items of Airway, Breathing, Circulation, and Increased Intracranial Pressure have been assessed and managed appropriately, and resuscitation is proceeding, the physician can relax to some degree and complete his examination in a less hurried manner.

Completing the assessment

When the initial high-priority assessment has been completed, resuscitation is proceeding, and vital functions are stable, examination must be completed in detail. All parts of the body must be surveyed and all minor injuries itemized. Particular attention should be paid to abdomen and chest.

(*a*) *Haemorrhage into the abdomen*   Haemorrhage into the abdomen is the commonest cause of hypovolaemic shock in children. Although intraperitoneal bleeding is more common, extraperitoneal haemorrhage may be massive and is more difficult to assess. Acute gastric ileus is an almost constant manifestation of major trauma in children and gastric decompression by a nasogastric tube is usually necessary for satisfactory evaluation of the abdomen. For this reason it should be a routine measure.

(*b*) *Sequence of examination*   To ensure that no injuries are missed, it is useful to itemize them under four body zones— Head, Chest, Abdomen, and Extremities. However, two specific injury sites, *the cervical spine and the diaphragm, are frequently neglected until some time has elapsed*. As a result injuries to these structures may be diagnosed too late, with tragic results. Neither the neck nor the diaphragm is automatically included in any of the four body sections listed above. Each lies between two of the zones and is often remembered only as an afterthought. Hence the physician must look specifically for a fractured cervical spine and a ruptured diaphragm and he must do so early in order to avoid the complications which can occur if either is missed.

Investigation

(*a*) *Blood analysis*   Immediate tests necessary for the seriously-injured child include blood grouping and crossmatching, haemoglobin and haematocrit determination, blood acid-base and gas analysis, and urinalysis.

(*b*) *X-rays*   Radiographic examination follows—it must never replace, physical examination. X-rays of skull, cervical spine, chest, abdomen, and any extremities suspected to be injured can usually be obtained in the resuscitation room. *Cervical spine films, particularly the lateral, should be obtained in any child whose consciousness is impaired by a head injury; these must be reviewed before the manipulations needed to obtain skull x-rays are carried out.* Intravenous pyelography and catheter cystography are essential in the evaluation of the urinary tract. Other contrast studies (barium examinations, angiography, etc.) are occasionally required in the traumatized patient to identify specific lesions (e.g. renal artery tear). More sophisticated radiographic techniques such as tomography, including computerized tomography (CT scanner), are rarely indicated, although the potential of the latter in the identification of intracranial space-occupying lesions is becoming strikingly evident. Computerized tomography, and the 'CT scanner', will undoubtedly play an expanding role in emergency diagnosis as time passes in spite of the practical problems encountered when using it for a patient with multiple injuries and all the accompanying dressings, splints, tubes, and wires.

One must remember that emergency x-rays usually serve only to confirm clinical suspicions. It is the rare accident victim whose survival is determined by, or whose initial handling depends on, the immediate availability of x-ray studies, no matter how specialized or sophisticated.

(*c*) *Central venous catheter*   When massive fluid replacement is required, a central venous catheter may be useful. However, it is of less value in children than adults. Time should never be wasted in attempting to establish a central venous line in a child before all basic resuscitative measures have been carried out.

(*d*) *Arterial blood-gas analysis*   Arterial blood-gas studies are important in the assessment of cardiorespiratory function after trauma and are usually obtained by needle aspiration of an available artery (radial, temporal, femoral). More sophisticated techniques call for the insertion of an arterial line which facilitates monitoring of the arterial pressure and repeated sampling.

(*e*) *Confirmation of intraperitoneal bleeding*   Peritoneal aspiration or lavage is an important tool in the detection of intraperitoneal blood. The frequency with which it is used varies from centre to centre, but all agree that it has particular value in the child with multiple injuries or when there is an associated head injury making abdominal examination difficult.

(f) *Scanning and intracranial-pressure monitoring*   Although not as yet applicable in the emergency situation, intracranial-pressure monitors are being used in some specialized centres for continuous monitoring of pressure changes within the skull.

Although nuclear scanning has now been applied to many solid organs, particularly brain, lungs, and kidneys, indications for its use are infrequent in an emergency.

The variety and complexity of investigative techniques available are endless. However, the simplest are of greatest value immediately after major trauma. One must guard against becoming too dependent on tests and neglecting careful, repeated clinical assessment of the patient.

Hypovolaemic shock in children

Causes

In children severe shock is rarely due to injury of the limbs. The femoral shaft fracture which, in the 25-year-old, can cause enough bleeding into the thigh to produce the picture of shock, will rarely do so in the 8 or 10-year-old. A child may have no evident systemic signs even in the presence of bilateral femoral fractures. However, when signs of blood loss do appear in such a child, one must first look elsewhere for the cause, particularly towards the abdomen. Similarly, *the child who has a severe cerebral concussion and a fractured femur, who develops the picture of haemorrhagic shock, probably has a ruptured spleen.* Finally, in children as in adults, head injuries do not cause shock unless they are so serious that death is imminent.

Diagnosis

Compensatory vascular responses are so effective in the young child that a quarter or more of the circulating blood volume can be lost with little change in pulse rate or blood pressure. Progressive and very striking pallor and a cool damp skin, are the chief signs of hypovolaemic shock. Before the stage of hypotension and tachycardia, *a child who becomes increasingly pale and sweaty after trauma can, in most instances, be assumed to have lost at least a quarter of his estimated blood volume.*

An unusual and striking behaviour pattern is also noted as a result of the cerebral hypoxia of shock. A child in shock will fight the oxygen mask and is likely to complain constantly of some trivial bruise or scrape, while ignoring two or three major injuries.

As blood loss continues, tachycardia, hypotension, impaired consciousness, and a declining urinary output, will all occur. Nevertheless, the diagnosis of traumatic shock can be made before this stage if the history of trauma, the characteristic pallor and typical behaviour, are noted and their significance recognized.

Treatment

General aspects
Although the chief element in the management of traumatic shock is replacement of lost blood volume, other measures are important and easily neglected in the excitement of the moment.

  (i) External bleeding can usually be controlled by the application of simple pressure dressings. Operative management of internal haemorrhage is sometimes required before venous infusion can catch up with blood loss.

 (ii) Oxygen administration and the other elements of respiratory support have been previously discussed but are part and parcel of the total management of hypovolaemic shock.

(iii) Small children cool rapidly when exposed and tolerate poorly this accidental cooling. Hence there must be efforts to minimize heat loss.

(iv) Although splinting of fractures is not one of the immediate high-priority items it should be tended to when practicable. Persistent movement at a fracture site continues to cause pain, tissue damage, and increases blood loss.

 (v) Gentleness in handling is important and the injured child should not be jostled or moved more than is necessary. When resuscitation is complete and vital signs have been stabilized it is often beneficial to keep the patient a further half hour or so in the casualty department. During this period intravenous intake progresses and continued observation detects any delayed problems yet to be handled. In institutions where immediate transfer to intensive care or trauma-observation units is the practice this transfer must be done as gently as possible.

(vi) During the initial management the body weight must be obtained by asking patient or parents, by weighing him if this is possible, by consulting a weight for age chart (p. 741) or by guessing. This figure should be recorded and prominently displayed as it forms the basis for all infusion volumes and drug dosages to be administered subsequently.

Blood-volume expansion (*see also* page 101)

Transfusion   The single most important factor in survival is blood-volume expansion, large enough and soon enough. The choice of the ideal fluid for volume expansion remains an unsolved and controversial issue. In most centres a crystalloid such as lactate Ringer's solution or isotonic saline is used as the initial fluid until blood is available. Others will switch to a colloid solution such as plasma, plasma-protein fraction, serum albumin or dextran. At The Hospital for Sick Children, Toronto, it is usual to infuse lactate Ringer's solution while the blood grouping and crossmatching are carried out. A quick crossmatching can be finished in a little more than half an hour. If blood is needed sooner than this, group-specific but uncrossmatched blood can be obtained very quickly and in the rare critical situation group O Rhesus negative universal donor blood is given.

The ability of the child's vascular tree to compensate so effectively for quite large volume losses while maintaining an acceptable pulse rate and blood pressure has been emphasized. One must equate visible pallor after trauma in the younger child patient (i.e. under 10 or 11 years or older if physically small) with a blood loss of at least one-quarter the normal blood volume. *The normal blood volume should be estimated as approximately 75–85 ml per kg. One-quarter of this blood volume should be calculated and written down prominently.* This serves as an infusion unit and will be used throughout the resuscitation.

If the pallor of shock is noted, this unit of one-quarter blood volume should be infused rapidly as a bolus. One should then slow the infusion down to maintenance rate and take stock. If a degree of clinical shock persists a second such bolus is needed. If the clinical situation seems to have been corrected it is wise to slow the infusion to maintenance rates. Should subsequent deterioration occur the physician may more confidently infer that bleeding is continuing. If, on the other hand, the infusion is kept running briskly continued bleeding will be partially replaced, signs of shock will be delayed, and the need for surgical intervention may be obscured, with resulting delay.

Sites for IV infusion   Although the long saphenous veins are customary sites for infusions in children they are not recommended when there has been trauma to the trunk. *A deep liver laceration or a tear of the inferior vena cava or one of its major tributaries can provide a route by which fluid infused into an ankle vein merely increases the volume already extravasated into the abdomen.* For this reason there must be a large-bore cannula in at least one arm vein.

Effects of cold blood   A complication of massive transfusion seen occasionally in paediatric practice is cardiac arrythmia or arrest due to cold bank blood. The small blood volume of the child cools quickly even with small infusions if they are taken directly from the blood-bank refrigerator. For this reason a blood-warmer should be installed in the infusion apparatus when large intravenous volumes are required. The simplest consists of a coil included in the venous line and placed in a water bath at 40°C (104°F).

Autotransfusion   Rare instances occur in which rapid reinfusion of an accident victim's own blood (autotransfusion) is life-saving. Ingenious autotransfusion units are available for the purpose of reinfusing large amounts of blood which have accumulated within either abdomen or chest. However, the time required to prepare the apparatus and to obtain it from storage once the decision to use it has been reached detracts from its practical value. Nevertheless, even without such equipment, direct reinjection by syringe into a large venous cannula of blood collected in a sterile basin as it drained from a chest tube is feasible. In such cases an appropriate filter should be introduced into the venous line to remove the larger cell aggregates. In most instances autotransfusion will be a temporary measure designed to support circulation until surgical intervention can take place, and blood-bank resources can be mobilized.

The metabolic acidosis (*see also* page 123)

The acid-base changes resulting from inadequate tissue perfusion have serious effects. A respiratory alkalosis can result from the hyperventilation of excitement immediately after an accident. It is usually short-lived, of minor degree and rarely of clinical significance. Hyperventilation may also be caused by head injury.

On the other hand as tissue damage, blood loss, and shock develop, progressive and serious metabolic acidosis develops as a result of the accumulation of acid metabolites. Most subjects in established hypovolaemic shock have a metabolic acidosis which needs prompt treatment. For this reason immediate arterial sampling is important. However, even before the sample is obtained for analysis, and the base requirement calculated, definite shock from blood loss is an indication for a bolus of bicarbonate in order to begin the correction. Furthermore, restored tissue perfusion washes accumulated hydrogen ions from the previously ischaemic and acidotic tissues into the circulation and the resulting fall in arterial pH could cause sudden deterioration at a time when resuscitative measures are appearing to be effective. This potential danger can be countered by a dose of buffer given as soon as the venous infusions have been established and are running freely.

The total amount of bicarbonate required to correct the acidosis is calulated by the following formula.

Required sodium bicarbonate ($NaHCO_3$) in mmol =
Base deficit *or* Negative base excess ×
Bodyweight in kg × 0.3

Half the requirement should be given at once. More may be given in another thirty minutes but preferably after repeat arterial sampling and calculation of the acidosis. It is probably not necessary to give buffer when the H^+ concentration is less than 55 nmol per litre (pH over 7.25).

If no laboratory determination of base requirement is available a moderate base deficit (negative base excess) of 10 mmol per litre may be assumed and bicarbonate administered accordingly. This gives a dose of 3 mmol of bicarbonate per kg. Half of this can be given when the infusions have been established and should be repeated every 20 to 30 minutes during the period the child appears to remain in shock. Solutions of sodium bicarbonate of different strengths are available:

$$1 \text{ ml } 8.4\% \text{ NaHCO}_3 \text{ soln contains } 1 \text{ mmol NaHCO}_3$$
$$1 \text{ ml } 7.5\% \text{ NaHCO}_3 \text{ soln contains } 0.9 \text{ mmol NaHCO}_3$$

Continuing care

As time passes serial haemoglobin and haematocrit values help in judging the amount of haemodilution that has occurred and may indicate the need for further transfusion.

Urine output per catheter must be measured from the outset and provides an excellent continuing indication of fluid balance.

Trauma team: organization and duties

Smaller hospitals may have only two or three physicians in the building at any time and their ability to handle effectively the initial resuscitation of a seriously injured casualty will be greatly increased by pre-arranged protocols and routines. Larger institutions may have organized trauma teams on duty at all times. In the University Hospital where there is particular interest in trauma there may be full-time 'trauma fellows' who receive victims of trauma and carry out resuscitation and much of the definitive care.

The leader of the trauma team is usually a general surgeon. However, his speciality is of less importance than is his ability to co-ordinate and to generate co-operation among the various specialists and his willingness to accept the ultimate responsibility.

In sophisticated trauma units each member of the team has a well planned series of duties to be carried out, permitting resuscitation to proceed with a minimum of discussion and delay. The leader gives any orders necessary, supervises documentation, indicates further equipment or tests needed, and makes decisions relating to further therapy.

One example of the various ways in which duties may be assigned to members of a trauma team is shown (*Figure 3.1*).

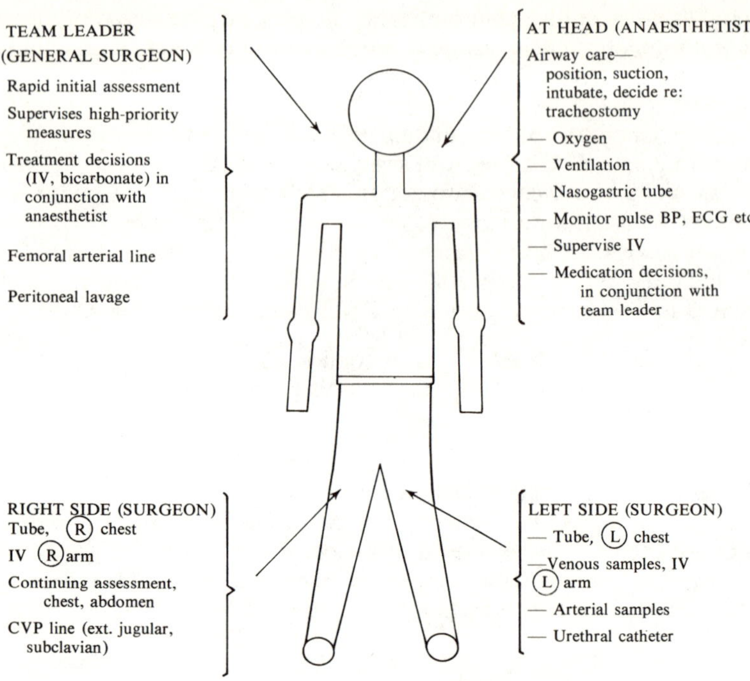

Figure 3.1. Trauma Team—duty assignments

Continuing evaluation

With the exception of those with serious head trauma, the majority of
accident victims who die do so because of haemorrhage into abdomen
or chest. Because of this, continuing assessment of trauma victims after
resuscitation and for the ensuing few days consists largely of repeated
examination of chest and abdomen.

Psychological trauma

Major and multiple injuries, unexpected hospitalization and surgery, all
have long-lasting emotional effects. Fractures unite, incisions heal,
wound scars improve in time. However, the psychological scarring is
deep-seated and persists for many years. What is most effective in
minimizing the psychological hurt is gentleness and kindness shown by
the nursing and medical staff from the moment of arrival. Painful

procedures should be carried out only if really necessary. On the other hand, it is not kindness to omit a test or procedure which is important, because of the discomfort which is associated with it.

The psychological effects of trauma are now sufficiently recognized and psychiatrists and psychologists are increasingly involved. It is hoped that this will become generally accepted in the future.

Parents

The parents of the injured child are too often forgotten. Parents should be kept completely informed from the beginning. Although one is loath to cause undue concern, it is wrong to give them a falsely optimistic prognosis. It is better to expect the worst than to be given falsely high hopes initially and then have them destroyed.

One must listen to and act upon concerns expressed by parents about their child. On occasion a parent will, through an increased sensitivity, recognize a change in colour, breathing, or facial expression, which heralds an impending complication, a change which might otherwise have gone unnoticed.

Although parents will need to be excluded from particularly complicated procedures, it is reassuring both for parents and child to permit them to be together as much as possible. Most parents have the strength to enable them to remain calm and supportive while with their child and they appreciate the opportunity to observe the repeated and meticulous examinations which are so often needed. Nothing is more reassuring for parents than to see their child's condition improving before their eyes as a result of careful assessment and appropriate therapy.

TABLE 3.I
Resuscitation room equipment

A.	Shock stretcher, adult size, with radiolucent litter-top.
	Anaesthetic machine.
	Oxygen, suction outlets.
	ECG monitor (with printout); defibrillator.
	X-ray viewing-box.

B.	Tongue blades	Auroscope
	Electric torches	Ophthalmoscope
	Stethoscopes	Reflex hammers
	Sphygmomanometers	

C.	Laryngoscope with 8-, 10-, and 12-cm blades (Welch-Allyn nos 1, 2, 3).
	Bronchoscopes, 3.5-, 4-, 5-mm sizes.
	Oropharyngeal airways, nos 00, 0, 1, 2, 3.

TABLE 3.I (*continued*)

      Endotracheal tubes, 3.0-mm to 9.0-mm sizes. Stylets.
      Nasogastric tubes, sizes 8 to 14 Fr.
      Tracheostomy tray with tracheostomy tubes—(Hollinger type) of sizes 0, 1, 2, 3, 4, and 5. Lengths vary, 33-mm (size 0), to 60-mm (size 5).

D.   Caps, masks, surgical gowns.
      Surgical gloves, gloves for rectal examinations.

E.   Sterile water, saline for irrigating wounds.
      Detergent, aqueous antiseptic.
      Syringes, needles, of all sizes.
      Bandages, dressings, sterile towels,—dressing trays.
      Laceration suture trays, variety of sutures.
      Minor surgical instruments.
      Venous cut-down trays.
      Chest tube trays. Chest tubes 12, 16, 20, 24 Fr., Stylets.
      Underwater bottle system or Heimlich valve.

F.   Venous cannulae, nos 16, 18, 20, 22.
      CVP line (radio-opaque catheter with stylet).
      Venous pressure manometer.
      Splints for restraining arms with infusions.
      Blood pump.
      Venous infusion lines, adult and infant (micro) drop sizes.
      Blood-warmer for IV line.
      Blood filter (maximum pore size 40 μm).

G.   Lumbar puncture trays.
      Urethral catheter trays.
      Catheters 8, 10, 12, 14 Fr. Straight and Foley.

TABLE 3.II
Infusion fluids

Isotonic saline (0.9% NaCl)
Lactate Ringer solution
0.45% Saline in 2.5% glucose
10% Glucose
Plasma (pooled or protein fraction)
Mannitol 50-ml vial of 25% ⎫
       500-ml bag of 20% ⎬ keep warm to prevent crystallization
     1000-ml bag of 10% ⎭

TABLE 3.III
Resuscitation drugs

Adrenaline	1:1000 in 1-ml amp. or 30-ml vial
Atropine	0.3 mg in 1-ml amp.
Calcium chloride	(10%) 1 g in 10-ml amp.
Calcium gluconate	(10%) in 10-ml amp.
Chlorpheniramine	10 mg in 1-ml amp.
Dexamethasone	8 mg in 2-ml vial
Diazepam *	10 mg in 2-ml amp.
Diazoxide	300 mg in 20-ml amp.
Digoxin	0.05 or 0.25 mg in 1-ml amp.
Frusemide (Furosemide)	20 mg in 2-ml amp.
Glucose	(50%) in 50-ml amp.
Hydralazine	20 mg in 1-ml amp.
Hydrocortisone sodium	100 mg, 250 mg, or 500 mg in 2-ml vial
Isoprenaline	0.2 mg in 1-ml amp.
Lignocaine	500 mg in 5-ml vial
Methoxamine	20 mg in 1-ml amp.
Morphine *	10 mg in 1-ml amp.
Pethidine *	50 mg in 1-ml amp.
Sodium bicarbonate	(7.5%) 44.6 mmol in 50-ml amp. or 8.4% containing 1 mmol of $NaHCO_3$ per 1 ml of solution
Sodium chloride	(0.9%) in 10-ml amp.
Sterile water	10-ml amp.
Theophylline	250 mg in 10-ml amp.
Thiopentone sodium	1-g bottle
Vitamin K, (phytomenadione)	5 mg in 1-ml amp.

* Kept locked up for security reasons

CHAPTER 4

Burns: Immediate Management

(*See also* Medical Emergencies Associated With Burns, p. 40)

R. W. S. Miller

A burn may be caused by any of the following, the severity depending upon the duration of contact and the area involved.

(*a*) *Dry Heat*	(i) Flash: a brief contact with a source of intense heat such as burning petrol, or an explosion.
	(ii) Flame.
	(iii) Direct contact with a hot object.
	(iv) Friction.
(*b*) *Wet Heat*	(i) Scald.
	(ii) Steam.
(*c*) *Chemical*	A chemical reaction generates heat.
(*d*) *Electrical*	(i) Local heat as from the firebar of an electric fire.
	(ii) Arcing which is an electric flash burn with contact completing the electric circuit. High local resistance produces localized deep burns.
	(iii) Tetanic spasm of nerves and muscles due to the passage of current prevents removal of the body from the electric source, while local heat produces the burn.
(*e*) *Ionizing*	Most forms of burn injury are obvious within seconds. Ionizing agents produce their effects in hours or days depending upon the dosage, and long-term effects may be manifested after years, e.g. sun, irradiation.
(*f*) *Combined Injuries*	

RECOGNITION

Without treatment the picture is one of 'shock' becoming progressively more severe. The pulse is thready and rapid, the skin cold and sweaty with little evidence of capillary filling. The breathing is at first rapid and shallow, but later becomes gasping. The urine flow is inadequate for the effective clearance of waste products. Initially the patient may be alert and apprehensive, but as shock progresses he becomes disturbed, noisy, disoriented and restless, complaining of thirst and cold.

MANAGEMENT

(1) Make certain that there is a clear airway. If in doubt call for immediate anaesthetic advice, and plan to perform a tracheostomy as soon as possible.

(2) Estimate the size of the burned area using Wallace's 'Rule of Nines' (*Figure 4.1*) as a rough guide, remembering that the palmar surface of the patient's hand is approximately 1 per cent of his total skin area. Compare the patient's hand with your own, and

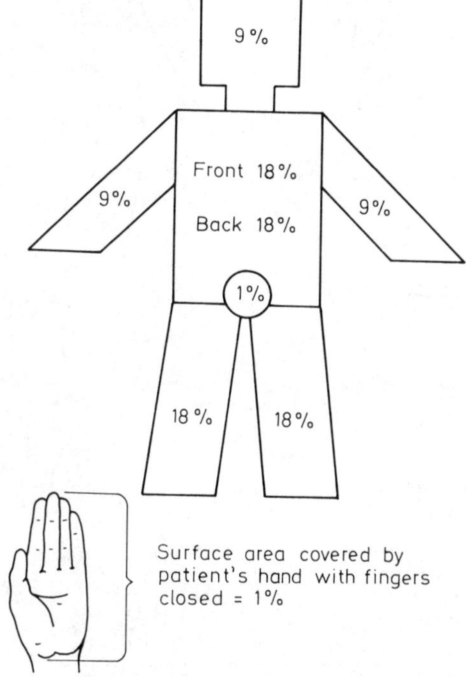

Figure 4.1. The 'Rule of Nines' assessment of burned area. For smaller areas a good guide is that the area covered by the patient's hand and fingers is 1 per cent of the body surface. (Muir and Barclay, 1974. Reproduced by kind permission)

roughly pat over the burned area to get an idea of the total extent (*Figure 4.1*). If the area is greater than 10 per cent in a child (excluding erythema) an intravenous infusion is necessary. Remember that there are variations in the area of skin on the head and legs depending upon the age of the child; the 'Rule of Nines' overestimates the area of the trunk and a more careful assessment of the area involved should be done when resuscitation has started using Lund and Browder's chart (*Figure 4.2*).

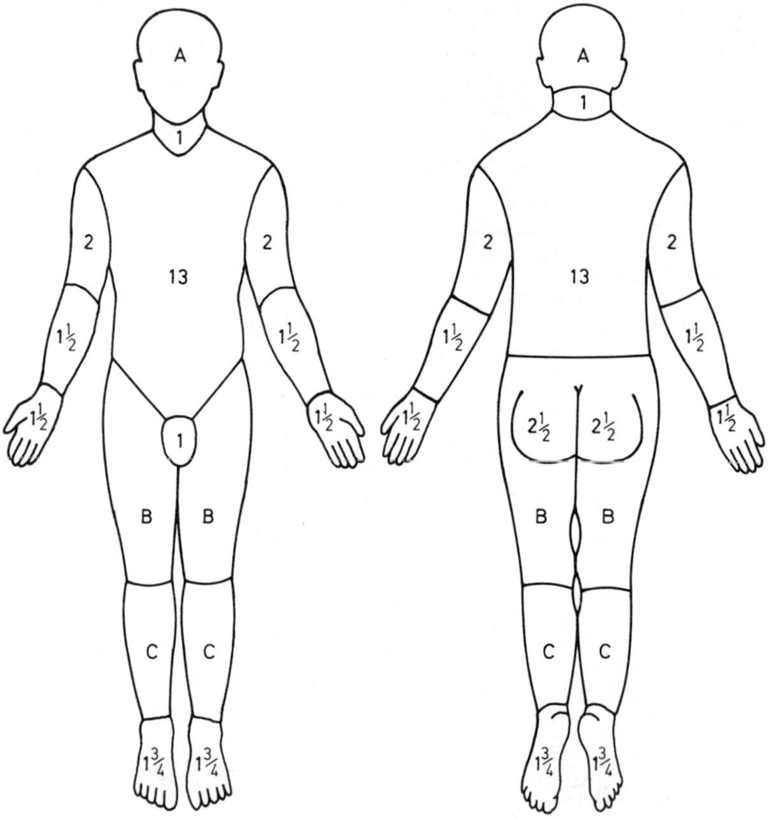

Relative percentage of areas affected by growth

Age in years	0	1	5	10	15.	Adult
A – ½ of head	9½	8½	6½	5½	4½	3½
B – ½ of one thigh	2¾	3¼	4	4¼	4½	4¾
C – ½ of one leg	2½	2½	2¾	3	3¼	3½

Figure 4.2. Chart for the accurate estimation of the area of burn. This can be used after resuscitation has been started. (Lund and Browder, 1944. Reproduced by kind permission)

If the area of the burn is greater than 10 per cent treat for shock.

(1) Set up a reliable intravenous drip using the largest possible size of cannula in an arm vein, securing it firmly. Use a vein beneath burned skin rather than one beneath unburned skin: no analgesics will be needed for a cut-down through burn eschar.

(2) Withdraw a sample of blood for:

> Haematocrit.
> Full blood count including platelets.
> Group and crossmatching.
> Plasma urea and electrolytes.

Remember to discard the first sample withdrawn through the cannula as it will be contaminated by the infusion fluid.

(3) Put up a bottle of plasma or a plasma-protein fraction (PPF).

(4) Obtain a history of the accident, and ascertain *the time when the accident occurred. The plan for fluid replacement is based on the time of the accident and not on the time of arrival in hospital.*

(5) Calculate the expected plasma requirement for each of 5 periods: 4 hours (*from the time of the accident*), 4 hours, 4 hours, 6 hours and 6 hours, using the formula devised by Muir and Barclay (1974).

$$\frac{\text{Total } \% \text{ area burned excluding erythema}}{2} \times \text{Wt of patient in kg} = \text{ml per period}$$

Give the plasma at a rate that will ensure that the whole of the first 4-hourly quota is given in the time remaining. (*See also* page 105 for further consideration of fluid requirement)

(6) If analgesia is required, and it rarely is once fluid is entering the circulation, give very small doses (0.1 mg–0.2 mg per kg) of morphine well diluted, intravenously. It will not be absorbed if given intramuscularly.

(7) If the burn is greater than 25 per cent insert a self-retaining catheter and lead it to a drainage bag via a burette so that the volume of urinary output can be measured hourly. (*See* Table A5.II for acceptable minimal hourly urine volumes.)

(8) When the result of the haematocrit is available calculate the volume of plasma deficit from the circulation assuming that no red cell loss has occurred by using the formula:

$$\text{Blood volume*} - \frac{\text{Blood volume} \times \text{Normal haematocrit}}{\text{Observed haematocrit}} = \text{Deficit in ml}$$

* (*see* Table 4.I)

Give the deficit as soon as possible in addition to planned volumes, in each 4-hour period. If the burn is greater than 10 per cent of the total skin area there will be red cell destruction requiring blood. Blood should be ordered; the volume necessary being 1 per cent of the normal blood volume for every 1 per cent of whole skin loss burn.

(9) Attend to the burn wound:

    (a) Assess the depth of involvement using a sterile needle. If sensation is present there will be partial skin loss only; if insensitive there is probably whole skin loss.

TABLE 4.I

Table of expected values (Muir and Barclay, 1974. Reproduced by kind permission)

Age	Wt in kg M. F.	Ht in cm M. F.	Haemato-crit M. F.	Haemo-globin % M. F.	Blood vol. in ml M. F.	Metabolic water req. ml/h. 1st 24 h	Minimum hourly urine vol. 1st 24 h
Birth	3·5	50	60	145	260	30	10
6/12	7	65	36	80	520	30	11
1	10	75	38	85	750	30	12
2	12·5	87	38	85	940	30	13
3	15	95	38	85	1120	35	14
4	17	103	39	88	1270	35	15
5	19	110	39	88	1420	40	16
6	22	116	40	90	1650	45	17
7	24	124	40	90	1800	50	18
8	26	130	40	90	1950	55	20
9	30	135	40	90	2250	55	22
10	32	140	40	90	2400	60	24
11	35	145	41 | 40	93 | 90	2620	65	26
12	40	150	42 | 40	96 | 90	3000	70	29
13	45	156	43 | 40	98 | 90	3370	75	32
14	50	160	44 | 40	100 | 90	3750	80	35
15	54 | 52	168 | 161	44 | 40	100 | 90	4050 | 3800	85	35
16	58 | 53	172 | 162	44 | 40	100 | 90	4350 | 4000	90	35
17	62 | 54	174 | 163	44 | 40	100 | 90	4650 | 4050	95	35
18	64 | 55	175 | 163	44 | 40	100 | 90	4800 | 4120	95	35
Adult	70 | 60	175 | 163	44 | 40	100 | 90	5000 | 4500	100	35

    (b) Apply dressings to all burned areas except the face and perineum, using an antibacterial tulle or cream, covered with gauze, Gamgee padding and a crêpe bandage. If the hands are burned they should be elevated.

(10) Prescribe antibiotics to prevent tetanus and staphylococcal infection. It is usual to use intramuscular benzylpenicillin for a limited period only.

(11) At the end of an hour reassess the patient's general condition. Estimate the fluid requirement for the next hour of the existing period and write it down on the fluid chart. Consider whether metabolic water requirements are best given orally or as additions to the intravenous regime.

(12) Write down all that has been done, recording details of haematocrit values and volumes of fluid given, together with the relevant clinical findings.

    If the burns involve certain special sites (*see below*) it is essential that the patient should be admitted to hospital; otherwise burns of less than 7 per cent can be sent home after dressings have been applied. (*See* page 45 for oral fluid requirements in burns of less than 10 per cent.)

Special sites

The eye

If there is any suspicion that the eye or the eyelid has been burned, the advice of an ophthalmic surgeon should be sought urgently. As a first-aid measure instill 0.9 per cent NaCl and 1 per cent atropine eyedrops. It is essential to keep the eye moist.

The face and neck

If the burns of the neck are deep, a tracheostomy is essential and should be done as soon as possible. When examining the patient it is necessary to look for evidence of burns of the tongue, singeing of the nasal hair or soot in the airway, redness of the throat or hoarseness. Obtain the advice of an ENT surgeon as to the best way to perform the tracheostomy. If the burn is not deep the child should be nursed on his back with his neck extended over a bolster.

The hands

The hand should be elevated. The nearest plastic surgery unit should be asked for advice about the future management.

Perineum

A burn of the perineum requires catheterization with a self-retaining catheter and sealed drainage.

SMOKE INHALATION: (*see also* page 41)
Any person who has been in a smoke-filled room even if they have no evidence of burns on the face or elsewhere should be admitted for close observation for a period of not less than 24 hours.

Quarter-hourly examination of chest, breathing and intercostal action should be made for at least 6 hours. A watch should be made for the onset of hoarseness. Should there be intercostal indrawing or a worsening of the hoarseness, tracheostomy and tracheal toilet is urgent.

OTHER MEASURES
    (a) The management of the burned child should be discussed with the parents, bringing them into the 'Treatment Team'. The treatment must be explained and the future outlook discussed. Parents may feel guilty about what has happened. This is manifested by questions about scarring, vision, speech, walking, etc., It is important to see both parents at the same time and to stress the importance of not looking for a scapegoat or finding someone to blame. The child needs their help during a long and painful illness as much as that of the medical and nursing staff. He must not be allowed to lose his trust in his parents. In some cases this talk will help to prevent the break-up of a family unit.

    (b) If the child's face is burned, it should be explained that the swelling will cause an alarming appearance for a day or two, but that the swelling will go down. This should also be explained to the child if old enough to understand.

    (c) If there is a special unit for the treatment of burns in the area, the transfer of the child by ambulance should be arranged, but only after an intravenous infusion has been set up and is seen to be running well. A badly-burned patient will travel well under these circumstances within 6 hours of the time of the injury.

A letter with the patient should include:
    (a) Type of accident and time when it occurred.
    (b) Time when the infusion was set up, and type of fluids being given.
    (c) Volume of fluid given in ml.
    (d) Haematocrit value on admission and any other results since.
    (e) The blood group, electrolyte and blood count results.
    (f) Urinary output since admission.
    (g) Dressings used, if any.
    (h) Name and address of the nearest relatives and their telephone number.

References

Lund, C. C. and Browder, N. C. (1944). The estimation of areas of burns. *Surgery, Gynec. Obstet.* **79**, 321

Muir, I. F. K. and Barclay, T. L. (1974). *Burns and Their Treatment.* 2nd edn. p. 33. London: Lloyd–Luke

CHAPTER 5

Medical Emergencies Associated with Burns

(See also Burns: Immediate Management, page 32)

J. A. Black

Medical complications usually arise after the initial period of resuscitation, but their prompt recognition and treatment have an important influence on survival in the severely burned child. Serious complications may be respiratory, neurological, septicaemic or renal.

Respiratory complications

Carbon monoxide (CO) poisoning

RECOGNITION
This is common in burns which have occurred in a confined space, and should be suspected in the presence of:
  (a) Mental confusion or unconsciousness if these are present on admission: other causes must of course be excluded (p. 43). The blood should be examined for carboxyhaemoglobin (HbCO); levels of less than 20 per cent are unlikely to cause significant symptoms.
  (b) Cherry-red lips: this is rarely obvious and may be masked by blackening of the lips by smoke, the presence of shock or hypoxia, or by skin pigmentation.

MANAGEMENT
  (a) If there is a clinical suspicion of CO poisoning, humidified 100 per cent oxygen should be given while laboratory confirmation (obtained by a sample from any available site) is awaited.
  (b) In severe cases, oxygen given in a hyperbaric chamber may be life-saving.

(c) There is no good evidence that the addition of CO_2 to the inspired oxygen is useful.

Inhalation of toxic gases (Mellins and Park, 1975)

The inhalation of combustion products such as sulphur and nitrogen oxides, hydrochloric acids (from polyvinylchloride) and aldehydes, is more likely to cause damage from an irritant effect than from the temperature of the gases. Recently, inhalation of hydrocyanic gas has been thought to be responsible for death in domestic fires involving plastic materials.

RECOGNITION

Symptoms of lower respiratory damage may not develop until 12 to 24 hours (occasionally as long as 2 to 3 days) after the incident. Early symptoms are: tachypnoea, cough, stridor, wheezing (bronchospasm), chest retraction and the coughing-up of mucus containing particles of carbon. Later, mucus plugs or casts of the bronchial epithelium may be coughed-up. In the early stages the chest x-ray shows few definite changes.

MANAGEMENT

(a) Humidified oxygen or an oxygen tent may be required.

(b) A broad-spectrum antibiotic such as gentamicin should be given; secondary infection with Gram-negative bacilli, particularly *Klebsiella*, is common.

(c) Repeated endotracheal suction by catheter may keep the upper airways clear. If this is not successful tracheostomy or intubation will be required. Occasionally bronchoscopic suction or lavage may be necessary, as in status asthmaticus (p. 252).

(d) Bronchodilator drugs, such as salbutamol, by aerosol, via a nasogastric tube or intravenously may relieve the bronchospasm.

(e) Corticosteroids: there is no clear evidence that high-dosage steroids are effective, but they should be tried (as in shock lung, *below*), if the child's condition is deteriorating from bronchial obstruction. However there is an additional risk of infection with candida.

(*f*) In severe cases, assisted ventilation with positive-end-expiratory-pressure (PEEP) may be required.

Shock lung

The aetiology of this condition is not well understood, but it should be suspected when respiratory difficulties develop at 18 to 36 hours after severe hypotension due to burn shock (or after severe haemorrhagic or septic shock), particularly in the absence of other factors such as the inhalation of toxic gases or fluid overload.

RECOGNITION
The initial symptoms are a loose cough, dyspnoea and sometimes the same type of expiratory grunt as in infants with Respiratory Distress Syndrome. There are high-pitched rhonchi and râles diffusely over both lung fields. The chest x-ray shows small areas of collapse or extensive fluffy shadows, mainly at the bases.

MANAGEMENT
The fluid intake must be carefully controlled to avoid hypovolaemia on one hand and fluid overload with pulmonary oedema on the other. Oxygen should be given to maintain a PaO_2 above 8.0 kPa (60 mm Hg); if this cannot be maintained without exceeding a 60 per cent inspired oxygen concentration, PEEP should be used. Antibiotics should be given until improvement in lung function has started.

The role of high dosage corticosteroids is as yet unclear but Sladen (1976) has shown that methylprednisolone sodium succinate (Solu-Medrone: *Upjohn*, Crawley, W. Sussex) given IV in a dose of 30 mg per kg every 6 hours for 48 hours has improved arterial oxygenation and hastened the clearing of the pulmonary oedema.

Pneumonia and tracheobronchitis

RECOGNITION
These complications are likely to develop after the 5th day in very severe burns; occasionally a subpleural abscess may rupture into the pleural cavity, causing an empyema (Monafo, 1971a). The chest x-ray may show pneumonic consolidation; intrapleural fluid suggests an empyema.

MANAGEMENT
The causative organism or organisms should be identified from sputum, aspirated tracheal secretions, or pleural aspiration. Antibiotics are given as indicated by the organisms and sensitivities.

Hyperventilation

RECOGNITION
(a) This may occur in severe burns without any obvious lung pathology and may be sufficient to cause a marked respiratory alkalosis.

(b) Hyperventilation is also seen in the metabolic acidosis produced by mafenide (Sulfamylon), owing to its inhibitory effect on the carbonic anhydrase of the renal tubules, causing renal bicarbonate loss.

MANAGEMENT

(a) Hyperventilation with respiratory alkalosis requires no treatment but care should be taken to avoid a metabolic alkalosis from hypokalaemia.

(b) A mafenide-induced metabolic acidosis may require correction if the hyperventilation is exhausting or distressing, or the acidosis is severe (standard bicarbonate < 10 mmol per litre). Occasionally it is necessary to change to another topical application.

Fluid overload

This is unlikely if one of the standard methods of fluid replacement is used (pp. 35–37).

RECOGNITION

The clinical picture is one of acute pulmonary oedema; the central venous pressure may be raised.

MANAGEMENT

If renal function is normal, diuresis can be rapidly induced by frusemide IV or i.m. (dose 1.0 mg per kg) or 20 per cent mannitol in a dose of 1 g per kg.

Neurological complications

Confusion

RECOGNITION

(a) In the early stages after a burn, confusion is likely to be due to hypoxia from hypotension and shock, or respiratory insufficiency; however the possibility of poisoning by carbon monoxide or cyanide (p.41), head injury, the effects of alcohol or other drugs, or postepileptic confusion should be considered.

(b) Confusion persisting or developing after the shock phase is usually due to unrecognized or inadequately treated hypoxia. Factors which may contribute are splinting of respiratory movement from burns of the chest wall or fractured ribs, unrecognized respiratory complications, and the enormously increased oxygen requirements in a severe burn.

(c) Confusion developing in the later stages of a burn may precede a fit and is likely to have the same causes (*see below*).

(d) Particularly if associated with a general clinical deterioration, septicaemia should also be considered (*see below*).

Fits

(a) *In the first 48 hours*

Present evidence suggests that these fits are usually due to cerebral oedema from water intoxication resulting from a combination of antidiuresis (ADH production from a painful burn) or hypervolaemia with 'pushing' water, other electrolyte-free fluids, or hypotonic electrolyte solutions (e.g. 0.18 per cent NaCl in 4 per cent glucose or sodium chloride–sodium bicarbonate mixture (p. 45) solution) by mouth. Hyperpyrexia may also occur separately or combined with water intoxication and may be the cause of the fit.

RECOGNITION

This type of fit usually occurs in young children with relatively small (<10 per cent) but painful burns or scalds in whom fluids are given orally, and takes the form of a generalized convulsion which may be preceded by confusion or drowsiness. A 'base-line' plasma sodium level is not always available, but at the time of the fit the plasma sodium level is likely to be <130 mmol per litre (sometimes 120 mmol per litre) and the urine is highly concentrated (high osmolality).

MANAGEMENT

It is important to find out whether the child has had any fits previously, particularly febrile convulsions, or is or has been on treatment for fits. If there is no history of previous fits, water intoxication is the most likely diagnosis, though a first febrile convulsion is a possibility if the child has developed a high temperature after the burn (*see below*) and the plasma sodium is > 130 mmol per litre.

(i) A lumbar puncture should NOT be done since it may precipitate 'coning' with medullary compression. It is important to realize that children may die from this cause immediately after a fit, or that it may cause sudden death without a preceding fit, even when a lumbar puncture has not been done.

(ii) Both skin and rectal temperatures should be measured. Shivering and vasoconstriction may cause a low skin temperature with a 'core' hyperpyrexia (Settle, 1974). If the rectal temperature is raised chlorpromazine should be given i.m. in a dose of 1 mg per kg in the first year, 10 mg at 1 year, 25 mg at 7 years, and a maximum of 50 mg at 14 years.

(iii) If the convulsion lasts longer than 10 minutes diazepam should be given IV or i.m. (p. 318); but the simultaneous use of chlorpromazine and diazepam should be avoided.

(iv) In the absence of clinical dehydration a forced diuresis with IV mannitol or urea should be induced, as for the treatment of cerebral oedema from other causes (p. 323).

(v) In the presence of hypotonic (hyponatraemic) dehydration the hyponatraemia should be corrected by IV 5 per cent sodium chloride solution (*see* page 132).

NOTE: Water intoxication from forcing low-electrolyte fluids is a preventable condition. For oral replacement a sodium chloride–sodium bicarbonate solution (Jackson, D. M. Personal Communication) should be used (5 g of sodium chloride and 4 g of sodium bicarbonate per litre of water; Na 133, Cl 85, HCO_3 48 mmol per litre). Acceptance is better if it is given chilled and flavoured with orange or other fruit juice; in borderline shock up to $1\frac{1}{2}$ times the normal maintenance requirement can be given during the first 24 hours but if shock is absent the normal maintenance requirement for age should be given (Table A3.I).

(b) Water intoxication after the first 2 days

RECOGNITION

This may occur in the presence of pre-existing hyponatraemia when additional electrolyte-free fluids are 'pushed' orally or when low-electrolyte solutions (e.g. 0.18 per cent NaCl in 4 per cent glucose) are given IV. Recently hyponatraemia has been caused by the removal of sodium from the burn surface by the application of topical silver nitrate but this application has been superseded by silver sulphadiazine which dose not cause hyponatraemia.

MANAGEMENT

The hyponatraemia may be corrected rapidly by IV 5 per cent sodium chloride (p. 132) or more slowly by changing the IV fluids to 0.9 per cent sodium chloride, and restricting the water intake.

(c) Other causes of fits which must be considered:

(i) A febrile convulsion in a child with a previous history of similar episodes.

(ii) Hypertensive encephalopathy: this is a recognized complication of burns, especially in children: it appears to be related to inadequate fluid replacement.

(iii) Fits in a known epileptic. The burn itself may have been caused by a fit. Anticonvulsant treatment may have been stopped after admission for the burn, or hyponatraemia and water intoxication may have lowered the threshold for fits, even with anticonvulsant treatment.

(iv) Local damage to the brain in deep burns of the scalp.

(v) Meningitis (*see* page 346).

(vi) Hypoglycaemia; this is only likely in severe hepatic failure due to hepatitis.

(vii) Hypocalcaemia is a rare complication (Monafo, 1971b).

(viii) Toxic absorption of locally applied drugs. This possibility should always be considered when any new topical application is used.

Septicaemia

RECOGNITION

This is unlikely to develop before the third day, and is more likely in extensive or deep burns or when the blood supply of a limb has been damaged.

Septicaemia should be suspected in the following circumstances:

(a) A sudden collapse or deterioration.

(b) A sudden rise, or a fall in temperature (to hypothermic levels).

(c) Sudden delirium with anxiety and trauma.

(d) Sudden oliguria.

(e) The development of ileus; other causes must also be considered, such as a peritonitis, acute gastrointestinal haemorrhage or hypokalaemia.

(*f*) With septicaemia from *Pseudomonas aeruginosa*, areas of necrosis of the skin develop in parts unaffected by the burn; the early lesion is a reddish-blue patch which rapidly becomes blueish-black and develops central necrosis with sloughing of the tissue.

(*g*) Also with pseudomonas septicaemia the urine may contain a green pigment (verdoglobin) which must be distinquished from the pyocyanin produced by the organism itself and which may be present in infected urine. Pyocyanin will fluoresce under ultraviolet light. For the identification of verdoglobin *see* Appendix 15.

MANAGEMENT

(*See* page 107 for septic shock).

Renal complications

Myoglobinuria and haemoglobinuria

Myoglobin, originating from damaged muscle, is usually excreted promptly, whereas the excretion of haemoglobin may be slightly delayed. Both myoglobinuria and haemoglobinuria may be associated with oliguria and the risk of renal 'shut-down'.

MANAGEMENT

Diuresis should be induced by mannitol given in a dose of 1 g per kg of a 20 per cent solution or with frusemide (p. 43). Repeated doses should not be given if there is no response to the first dose.

Renal failure or shut-down (*see* page 411).

Gastrointestinal haemorrhage

RECOGNITION

When sudden collapse with shock occurs the possibility of haemorrhage from an acute ulcer of the oesophagus, stomach or duodenum, small or large intestine must be considered. In oesophageal, gastric or duodenal bleeding there may be a haematemesis.

MANAGEMENT

A large transfusion of blood will be required (20 ml per kg) and a surgical opinion should be obtained urgently since a laparotomy may be needed to identify the bleeding point.

References

Mellins, R. B., Sungmin Park (1975). Respiratory complications of smoke inhalation in victims of fire. *J. Pediat.* **87**, 1.

Monafo, W. W. (1971a, b). *The Treatment of Burns*. St. Louis, U.S.A.: Warren H. Green Inc. (a) page 211: (b) page 64

Settle, J. A. D. (1974). *Burns: The First 48 Hours*. Smith & Nephew Pharmaceuticals Ltd., England.

Sladen, A. (1976). Methylprednisolone. Pharmacologic doses in shock lung syndrome. *J. thorac. cardiovasc. Surg.* **71**, 800.

CHAPTER 6

Drowning and Near-Drowning*

Carl Edmonds

Introduction

(Colebatch and Halmagyi, 1962; Harrison, 1975; Modell, 1971)

Drowning can be defined as the death of an air-breathing animal due to aspiration of fluid. This term has been used loosely to refer to incidents in which recovery occurs; however, the term 'near-drowning' is more appropriate for these cases.

The treatment at the scene of the accident is usually of little ultimate consequence in all accidents except drowning, but here it will often determine whether the child lives or dies. Important factors which influence this final outcome in near-drowning cases include the water temperature (and its combined effect on the diving reflex and hypothermia), and the general standard of first-aid and resuscitation training of the would-be rescuers.

Death may occur during or soon after aspiration of fluid, or after delayed complications. Whether the drowning occurs in sea or fresh water may have some influence on the prospects of recovery, and on the biochemical and pathological abnormalities of drowning. Other factors which influence prognosis include: the presence of chlorination and other chemicals and foreign bodies, the aspiration of stomach contents, the subsequent development of haemolysis, renal failure, pneumonitis, pneumonia, lung abscess, etc.

Near-Drowning

(Harrison, 1975; Edmonds, Lowry and Pennefather, 1976; Strauss, 1976)

* This chapter is revised and modified, with permission, from *Diving and Sub-aquatic Medicine,* 1976, by Edmonds, Lowry and Pennefather, published by the Diving Medical Centre, Mosman, Australia

Spectacular rescues have been performed on children who have been subjected to total submersion for extended periods of time. Case reports of submersion for 26, 30 and 40 minutes are in the medical literature, with many other similar cases known to clinicians experienced in this field. The explanations for such spectacular results include the following:

(a) The diving reflex is said to be well developed in small children. This reflex allows for bradycardia, oxygen conservation and a shunting of oxygenated blood to the vital organs, especially the heart and brain. The diving reflex is stimulated by the effect of cold water on the skin of the face and permits the prolonged submersion of many of the diving mammals; it is present at least in a rudimentary form in humans.

(b) Hypothermia is produced by both submersion in cold water and also by inhalation of cold water. In one Australian series the body temperature of near-drowned children averaged 31°C (88°F). The hypothermia is thought to act by protecting the central nervous system from the effects of hypoxia, to a variable degree. Because of the relatively increased surface area, hypothermia is more likely in the young.

(c) With laryngeal spasm, which is also probably more likely in children than adults, there is a reservoir of gas still retained within the lungs from which oxygen can be extracted and into which carbon dioxide can be discharged. The laryngeal spasm is often claimed to be the cause of the 'dry' drowning cases, in which fluid cannot be found in the lungs at autopsy. Even in cases in which fluid does enter the lungs, the effect of gravity makes it unlikely that a great deal of the gas will be replaced by fluid, unless the child's body is in the face-upwards, head-upwards position.

(d) Even with fluid in the lungs there is still some exchange of gases, both oxygen and carbon dioxide, between the blood stream and the alveolar contents.

The final outcome of the treatment of near-drowning in children, is unpredictable. Physical signs of decorticate rigidity, which would carry an ominous prognosis in adults, may be followed by recovery to apparent normality in young children. Alternatively, a good early response to treatment may be followed by severe cerebral dysfunction.

Clinical observations

(Fuller 1963; Griffin 1966; Modell 1971; Edmonds, Lowry and Pennefather, 1976)

SEQUENCE OF EVENTS BEFORE DEATH FROM DROWNING

(a) Initial submersion. This may be followed by immediate breath-holding. The duration of the breath-holding depends on several factors such as the general physical condition, exercise, previous hyperventilation, psychological reactions, etc. Swallowing water may reduce the desire to breathe, but will increase the subsequent tendency to vomit and aspirate the stomach contents.

(b) Water aspiration. Eventually hypercapnia or hypoxia compels inspiration. Laryngeal spasm may follow if aspiration occurs. While laryngospasm is maintained, the lungs may remain dry.

(c) Further breath-holding, hypoxia, impairment of consciousness and circulatory arrest may follow. It is thought that hypothermia due to immersion in cold water may give some protection from the effects of hypoxia.

(d) With loss of consciousness, passive flooding of the lungs may either precede or follow cerebral death.

(e) In a large series of cases of drowning and near-drowning the following observations were made:

    (i) Haemodilution did not occur in fresh- or salt-water drowning.

    (ii) Haemoglobinaemia and haemoglobinuria were rare.

    (iii) Ventricular fibrillation occurred once (fresh water).

    (iv) Metabolic acidosis was common.

    (v) Pulmonary oedema was common in fresh- and salt-water cases.

Clinical features in near-drowning

(a) Respiratory symptoms: dyspnoea; tachypnoea and cyanosis; retrosternal chest pain, increased during inspiration; blood-stained, frothy sputum; pulmonary crepitations and, occasionally, rhonchi. There is a decrease in the forced expiratory volume ($FEV_{1.0}$), vital capacity (VC), compliance and ventilation–perfusion ratio, and an increase in pulmonary-arterial pressure.

(b) Chest x-ray: this may show patchy opacities, varying in extent and distribution. Complications may include pneumonitis, pulmonary oedema, bronchopneumonia, pulmonary abscess and empyema.

(c) Central nervous symptoms: there may be impairment of consciousness, convulsions, and sequelae of focal cerebral damage, consistent with hypoxia and cerebral oedema.

(d) Pyrexia and rigors are common.

(e) Cardiovascular manifestations include tachycardia, hypotension and shock in severe cases, and various cardiac arrhythmias or arrest.

(f) Renal symptoms: there is oliguria, with increased specific gravity (in the case of salt-water drowning); occasional albuminuria, with or without haemoglobinuria; cyclindruria or haematuria. Acute tubular necrosis is an uncommon late complication.

(g) Biochemical and haematological findings include: decreased arterial oxygen with variable arterial carbon dioxide tensions; metabolic, and sometimes respiratory, acidosis; haemoconcentration; leucocytosis; increased lactic dehydrogenase; occasional azotaemia; laboratory evidence of haemolysis.

Usually, recovery from near-drowning is complete; however, residual neurological deficiencies may persist, in the form of personality disorders, mental impairment and/or extrapyramidal damage. These may be more common in warm-water drownings of children, as exemplified by the bath drownings of infants.

MANAGEMENT

(Modell, 1971; Harrison, 1975; Edmonds, Lowry and Pennefather, 1976; Strauss, 1976)

Treatment is to a large degree empirical, complemented by the patchy knowledge obtained from actual case reports. The efficacy of prompt initial measures in support of the respiratory and circulatory systems greatly influences the eventual outcome. Excellent results, without obvious neurological sequelae have resulted in children who have spent up to 40 minutes totally submerged, in cold water.

Treatment requires resuscitation, provision of oxygenated blood to the brain, management of respiratory and cardiovascular failure and, later, neurological and renal complications.

IMMEDIATE FIRST AID

(a) Respiration: the initial clearance of airway obstruction is followed by expired air resuscitation. The ventilation rate in children should be approximately 18–20 breaths per minute, with increased rate and decreased volume in infants. Attention is often misdirected to the copious quantities of blood-stained sputum exuding from the airways. Ventilation takes precedence over removal of this fluid.

(b) Circulation: if no pulse is detected, external cardiac massage should be performed at a rate of 80 to 100 strokes per minute or 100 to 120 per minute for infants. A good palpable pulse wave indicates that the correct technique is being used. Infants require 1.25 cm ($\frac{1}{2}$ in) compression with the tips of the fingers on the

sternum. Children up to 5 years require 2.5 cm (1 in) compression, with the heel of one hand.
(c) Transfer to hospital. An attempt should be made to remove the patient to a hospital once immediate resuscitative measures have been started. These should be continued until superseded by more efficient methods, which include the administration of 100 per cent oxygen, with or without positive-pressure respiration.

HOSPITAL TREATMENT
(a) Initial measures in hospital should consist of support of respiration and circulation. Oxygenation should precede intubation whenever possible to lessen the hazards associated with this technique in an hypoxic patient. In comatose patients early endotracheal intubation is indicated, with removal of stomach contents to prevent aspiration. In stuporous or delirious patients, intravenous relaxants may be needed. In any serious case, endotracheal intubation, intravenous infusion and bladder catheterization will be needed.
(b) Respiratory support may require positive-pressure respiration with 100 per cent oxygen. Several features of this positive pressure are important.
(i) The inflation pressure required is that which produces an acceptable arterial oxygen tension. This pressure overcomes increased elastic resistance and inflates atelectatic areas. Many automatic ventilators are pressure-limited and because compliance is reduced (so increasing inspiratory resistance), the inflation cycle may terminate before an effective volume of gas has entered the lungs. In these cases a hand-operated or controlled unit, or a volume-cycled automatic ventilator would appear to be preferable. Positive-end-expiratory pressure (PEEP) is recommended and used as a technique for increasing oxygenation and reducing pulmonary oedema, but at the risk of haemodynamic disturbances and pulmonary tissue damage. PEEP also reduces the degree of pulmonary shunting and allows the inspired oxygen concentration to be reduced. This is important as in severe cases ventilation may have to continue for several days.
(ii) Large volumes should be used to inflate as much lung as possible. Periodic hyperinflation is sometimes used to assist in the reinflation of atelectatic areas. The exact timing varies with the patient, but may involve one cycle every 10 to 60 minutes. PEEP is very effective in reducing atelectasis, and avoiding the need for periodic hyperinflations.

(iii) The respiratory rate should be relatively low, and of the order of 12 to 18 breaths per minute. The inspiratory phase when using intermittent positive pressures should be short in order to limit the impairment of venous return.

(iv) Good tracheobronchial toilet should be established, and the use of nebulized aerosols has been suggested. These may include ethyl alcohol (to suppress bubble formation associated with pulmonary oedema) or steroids.

(v) Systemic steroids reduce cerebral oedema and pneumonitis.

(vi) Broad-spectrum antibiotic cover is used to prevent or treat secondary infection of the lungs.

Respiratory stimulants are contra-indicated. Hyperbaric oxygenation and extracorporeal oxygenation have not received widespread acceptance in the treatment of near-drownings. If, however, extensive lung damage exists, survival may only be sustained with the use of a long-term pulmonary bypass technique. This may permit sufficient time for the lesions to heal.

(c) Circulatory support: this maintains adequate perfusion of vital tissues.

(i) External cardiac massage may be necessary until fibrillation or arrest are reversed.

(ii) An effective cardiac output is maintained by the correction of hypoxia, arrhythmias and failure.

(iii) The maintenance of an adequate circulatory blood volume is necessary. Central venous pressure (CVP) should be used to monitor the intravenous fluids used to treat haemoconcentration.

(iv) There is no clinical evidence to support the use of low-potassium solutions in fresh-water near-drowning, or low-sodium solutions for salt-water near-drowning. Lactate Ringer solution is probably a good initial choice, with further selection being based on individual assessment of the patient.

(v) Vasopressors and plasma expanders are not generally recommended; however, plasma (or plasma-protein fraction) or whole-blood transfusions (not exchanges) have been used when the CVP is low.

(d) Electrolyte disorders and renal function. Abnormalities are usually transitory, and little attention is necessary here. Metabolic acidosis (p. 123) should be treated by intravenous administration of bicarbonate. A good diuresis can be produced by the use of fluids and diuretics. Frusemide and ethacrynic acid have been recommended. This may be a valuable precaution if there is haemoglobinaemia.

(e) Adequate cerebral circulation and reduction of cerebral oedema may be obtained by steroids, osmotic diuretics or hypothermia.

GENERAL SUPPORTIVE PERIOD

This allows for the carrying out of clinical measurements. These include:

(a) The monitoring and recording of temperature, pulse and respiration, blood pressure, CVP, electrocardiogram, fluid balance, specific gravity or osmolality of urine and urinalysis.

(b) The detection of haemoglobinuria.

(c) Serial estimations of the following: arterial oxygen, carbon dioxide, H^+ concentration (pH), standard bicarbonate content, packed-cell volume, haemoglobin concentration, leucocyte count and serum haemoglobin and haptoglobin levels; serum specific gravity (or osmolality) and electrolyte levels especially those of sodium, potassium and chloride; plasma proteins, glucose, urea; urinary electrolyte levels; coagulation factors.

(d) Serial estimations of respiratory status by: chest x-ray; estimation of compliance or $FEV_{1.0}/VC$ in conscious patients.

(e) Assessment of central nervous system function, both clinically and by electroencephalography.

REHABILITATION

This includes physiotherapy and postural drainage until good respiratory function is achieved. Neurological assessment includes psychometric examinations, until a stable state is reached. If this is impaired, social and psychological support may be required for the patient, the parents and the siblings.

DEATH

Treatment depends on the severity of the condition and the response to resuscitative measures; these should be continued until unequivocal signs of death are present. These signs include:

(a) Nonactive electrocardiogram and electroencephalogram tracings.

(b) Segmented retinal vessels.

(c) Rigor mortis.

Unresponsive coma, areflexia, fixed dilated pupils or absent corneal reflexes are not in themselves diagnostic signs of death. If, however, they occur together with one or other of the above signs, they indicate an irreversible state of death. *Recovery has followed prolonged immersion with few sequelae. It is probable that many children have perished from premature termination of resuscitative measures.*

Prevention
(Harrison, 1975)

The prevention of the different types of accident will depend very much on the population being considered. Mothers should be present and vigilant at all times while the baby is bathing. This is also relevant to older children who have episodes of unconsciousness from any cause, commonly epilepsy. Bath accidents in older children are more likely to result from boisterous games and resultant head injuries. Where there are swimming pools, fish ponds or other water containers, there must be protective fences with self-locking gates with a child-proof lock, and at a height that will prevent young children from entry.

As the child becomes older he will be involved in more sporting activities which predispose to drowning accidents. The value of swimming training programmes and 'drown-proofing' techniques, cannot be overstressed. This is especially important in the countries where swimming is not a common social activity and therefore not frequently taught. While engaged in water sports and boating, life-jackets should be worn and should support the child's head well above the water level, if he does become immersed. The most important factor is adequate parental control and observation. Where a group of children are swimming together, many local authorities will insist upon experienced 'life-savers', trained in both aquatic skills and first aid. In most socially well-organized countries, instruction of school children, as well as their mothers and other adults, in the first-aid technique of mouth-to-mouth respiration is now available.

References

Colebatch, H. J. H. and Halmagyi, D. F. J. (1962). Reflex airway reaction to fluid aspiration. *J. appl. Physiol.* **17** (5), 787

Edmonds, C., Lowry, C. and Pennefather, J. (1976). *Diving and Subaquatic Medicine.* Mosman, Australia: Diving Medical Centre

Fuller, R. H. (1963). Drowning and the Post-Immersion Syndrome. *Milit. Med.* **128**, 22

Griffin, G. E. (1966). Near-drowning. Its pathophysiology and treatment in Man. *Milit. Med.* **131** (1), 12

Harrison, G. A. Ed. (1975). *Accident Prevention and Community First Aid.* Royal Australian College of Surgeons and the Faculty of Anaesthetists: Health Commission of New South Wales, Australia

    Brophy, T. The specific problems of cardiopulmonary resuscitation in infants and children, p. 168

Harrison, G. A. The incidence of deaths due to aquatic injuries in the community, p. 181

Dawson, G. Swimming pool deaths in Victoria, p. 204

Wright, R. Hospital therapy of near-drowning, p. 211

Kilham, H. Drowning in pre-school-age children, p. 217

Lah, F., Vonwiller, J. B. and Fisk, G. C. Children admitted to hospital after incidents of near-drowning, p. 221

Henry, F. J. Training of school children in cardiopulmonary resuscitation, p. 238

Modell, J. H. (1971). *The Pathophysiology and Treatment of Drowning and Near-Drowning*. Springfield, Illinois: Charles C. Thomas

Strauss, R. (1976). *Diving Medicine*. New York: Grune and Stratton

CHAPTER 7

Cold Injury

M. P. Ward

Environmental cold injury may be conveniently classified into:

General Accidental hypothermia or 'exposure'. This occurs in either wet and cold or dry and cold conditions. By definition, hypothermia occurs when the central core temperature falls below 35°C (95°F).

Local (a) Immersion Injury: when the tissues are at 0° to 15°C (32°–59°F) for long periods. (b) Frostbite: when the tissues are at 0°C (32°F)—that is in dry and cold conditions. More than one type of cold injury may occur at the same time in an individual (Ward, 1975).

Environmental hypothermia

With the increasing popularity of all forms of outdoor pursuits, especially mountain-walking and sailing, as a substitute for field games, the number of children and adolescents exposed to the risks of cold injury has greatly increased in the last few years.

About 40 per cent of victims of mountain accidents in the British Isles are under 21 years of age and a number suffer from hypothermia, apart from other injuries.

As a normal part of the 'character-building' process children are exhorted to exhaust themselves physically while playing games under controlled, though often atrocious conditions. In the natural environment such exhortation can lead to hypothermia and death, and should be avoided.

Children and adolescents at risk are those who run away from home and sleep out, and youths on mountain expeditions who are inadequately prepared, or are overtaken by very bad weather.

A. FACTORS IMPORTANT IN THE DEVELOPMENT OF HYPOTHERMIA

Fatigue

   (a) A recent illness may result in the unduly rapid onset of fatigue.
   (b) Inadequate food intake.
   (c) Changes in weather. The increased physical exertion necessary
       to walk into a gale-force wind may result in exhaustion and
       hypothermia.
   (d) Fear engendered by unfamiliar surroundings and changing
       weather conditions can precipitate exhaustion.
   (e) Adolescents may be unable to regulate energy output and have
       little in reserve. (In field games under controlled conditions these
       tendencies are no problem; in the mountains they can be
       disastrous)

Clothing

Insulation depends on the trapped still air in the clothes. External wind
removes the warmed microclimate of the body and the heat loss
increases dramatically.

As water is a good conductor of heat, water, either from outside as
rain or inside as sweat, will also cool the microclimate.

Internal garments, (i.e. shirt, sweater, vest,) should be kept dry and
protected from the wind. A water-repellent, moisture-permeable, wind-
proof anorak should be used.

Clothing should be put on and taken off as necessary to maintain an
equable body temperature and prevent sweating. Wind-proof and
water-proof clothing should be put on before the inner clothing has
become wet. Boots should fit well to prevent blisters. Mitts should be
used for the hands.

Heat loss from the head may be considerable and some form of
'Balaclava' should be worn.

B. ENVIRONMENTAL FACTORS

It is not always appreciated that the environmental temperature falls by
1.5°C (3°F) for every 300 metres (1000 feet) of ascent. Also a
combination of wind and low temperature has an extreme chilling
effect.

RECOGNITION

The individual often starts stumbling, and there is muscular inco-ordination and finally rigidity. Changes in mental outlook occur, with instability and non-co-operation, apathy, and confusion. Convulsions may occur followed by unconsciousness. Death has been reported within two to three hours of the onset of symptoms. However, 'dead' patients who are cold to the touch and apparently moribund, without respiration or pulse, have been known to recover.

MANAGEMENT

The commonsense precautions already outlined together with a balanced, sensible general outlook are necessary.

(a) *In the field*

It is better not to try to exercise the patient 'to come out' of hypothermia. He should be sheltered from the wind, while wet clothes are removed and replaced by dry ones. External heat is applied by huddling together. Hot fluids (+ glucose) should be given if possible. The patient must be insulated from the ground as well as the wind and placed in a bag of impermeable material to prevent further heat loss.

Heat loss from the lungs occurs in a hypothermic patient despite perfect insulation. Provision of heated humidified air to breathe abolishes this loss and provides a method of central rewarming. If oxygen is breathed through soda lime, the interaction of exhaled CO_2 and soda lime provides both heat and moisture for the patient. Portable equipment is available for first aid treatment in the field. (Lloyd, 1974).

(b) *In the hospital or the 'Centre'*

Central-core temperature should be measured with a low-temperature thermometer in the rectum.

Though the patient may appear dead, i.e. cold, pulseless and without respiration, recovery may still occur. The depressed respiration relates to low oxygen needs.

(c) *Hot bath treatment* (*Rapid rewarming*)
(Davies, 1975; Jackson, 1975),

The unconscious patient is immersed fully clothed in a bath at 45°C (113°F) (as hot as the hand can stand). The temperature of the water should be monitored. The risks of rapid rewarming are:

    (i) An 'after-drop' or fall in central-core temperature. Because of surface vasodilatation deep-core blood is further cooled as it enters the chilled superficial tissues.

(ii) Surface vasodilatation may exaggerate hypotension.

(iii) Exhaustion may result in loss of thermoregulation. Hot bath treatment in these cases may be contra-indicated. Once the patient has a regular heart beat and respiration, he is removed from the bath and placed flat under blankets in an air temperature of 36° to 40°C (97° to 104°F). An awkward movement or a poor carrying technique may further depress respiration.

Ideally all hypothermic patients should be air-lifted by helicopter to an Intensive Treatment Unit. Here facilities are available to monitor ECG, arterial pressure, plasma electrolytes, H^+ concentration (pH), pCO_2, pO_2 etc. The use of warmed IV fluids should be considered. Central warming through the airway should also be considered using an oxygen–helium mixture; alternatively a heart-lung machine could be used.

The airway must be kept clear but insertion of endotracheal tubes can cause reflex bradycardia and precipitate ventricular fibrillation, as can oesophageal thermistor probes.

Frostbite
(Ward, 1974)

This occurs in dry and cold conditions, i.e. at, or below 0°C (32°F) when the tissues freeze. It is common on exposed parts such as the nose, ears and cheeks, especially when there is a wind which lowers the effective skin temperature. Temperature variations may be considerable and individuals should dress for the temperature with which the part is likely to be in contact (e.g. while the ambient temperature may be many degrees above freezing, the feet in powder snow can be many degrees below freezing.)

Clothes and boots should fit well so as to prevent any constriction of the blood supply. Insulation must be adequate for the prevailing conditions.

PATHOPHYSIOLOGY
There are two main processes:

(a) Ice crystals form and enlarge in the extracellular fluid. The intracellular osmotic pressure rises, and enzyme mechanisms are disturbed, with resulting cell death.

(b) A vascular reaction occurs under the frozen tissue, with damage to the blood-vessel walls. Plasma leaks into the tissues, forming blisters. The remaining intravascular blood becomes more viscous (sludging). Thus end-arteries may get blocked with resulting tissue necrosis.

RECOGNITION

Frostnip

This produces reversible changes. The skin blanches and becomes numb with sudden cessation of cold and discomfort.

Superficial frostbite

Damage to the tissues occurs. The adjacent skin and subcutaneous tissue are involved but the part though white and frozen is soft and pliable when pressed. Blisters may form within 24 to 28 hours depending on the site of the injury. Then blister fluid is absorbed leaving a black carapace which is insensitive. In certain sites carapace formation may occur without blistering. There is associated oedema and within weeks a line of demarcation forms. Throbbing and aching may persist for weeks. If the contour of the blackened carapace corresponds to the original area then loss of tissue is unlikely.

Unlike that of arteriosclerosis, the dry gangrene of frostbite is normally superficial, being only a few millimetres thick.

Deep frostbite

This involves the deeper structure, bone, muscle, and tendons. The affected part is cold, feels 'solid' and unyielding, and is a mottled blue or grey. It may remain swollen for months, and blistering is not inevitable although it can take weeks to develop. Initially the part is painless, but abnormal sensation may be present.

As tendons are more resistant to cold injury than skin, the patient will be able to move his fingers and toes despite their gangrenous appearance. Thus even the most severely frostbitten patient can walk or move his fingers clumsily. Permanent loss of tissue is almost inevitable and this may be estimated from the loss of contour of the affected part.

Even with a diagnosis of deep frostbite a limb may return to normal over some months and amputation should never be carried out until a considerable period, say 6 to 9 months, has elapsed.

MANAGEMENT

Frostnip

This is the only form of frostbite that should be treated on the spot. Each person should watch for signs on the exposed portion of his companions. As soon as whitening of the skin occurs, a place sheltered from the wind should be found, and the affected part warmed. Once normal colour and consistency is obtained, normal working is resumed.

Frostbite

The affected part should NOT be rubbed with snow or the normal hand. It neither melts the ice crystals, nor increases the blood supply, but only breaks the skin and increases the chances of infection. All other forms of violent therapy are open to the same objections.

Rapid warming seems the most effective treatment. It has the advantage that it can be done in primitive conditions, once a tent or similar shelter has been reached, so shortening the time that the blood vessels remain frozen.

Once active rewarming has been started it seems doubtful if any other form of treatment is beneficial.

METHOD

A container with water at 43° to 44°C (111°F) should be used (measured by thermometer) as water that is too hot will damage the tissues. If a thermometer is not available the temperature should be assessed with the normal, unfrostbitten finger. It should not be too hot for comfort. If no container is available hot water poured over a towel or cloth wrapped around the part may be used. Warming should last for 20 minutes at a time. The temperature of the water should not fall below 42°C (108°F).

If rewarming by fluid is impossible, the part should be placed against a warm armpit or abdomen. It should never be placed by an open fire as it is partially anaesthetized and can be burnt without pain.

After rewarming, the part should be cleaned, and dirt removed gradually and gently. Blisters should be left as they form a covering.

Soft dry, absorbent dressings between the fingers and toes will prevent further damage. So long as the affected part is warm and does not get rubbed it may be kept exposed. Later, active exercises will be necessary to prevent joint stiffness.

Surgical intervention must be minimal; the blackened carapace will gradually separate without interference and efforts to hasten this separation are usually ill-advised and are likely to lead to infection and loss of tissue.

EVACUATION

Once the treatment of frostbite has started, the part should be protected from any mechanical injury, such as walking. Treatment should only be started at a camp from which evacuation by helicopter, car, porter, or animal is possible.

Damage to frostbitten tissue before treatment, can obviously occur, as in walking off a mountain. Yet in the mountain environment it may be quicker and safer for the frostbitten patient to reach a convenient place for evacuation by his own efforts before starting treatment.

Late effects

The skin may be scarred and hypersensitive, and the nails atrophied or deformed. Joint contractures may occur, and causalgia and hyperhidrosis have been reported.

In children, the epiphysis may be damaged leading to deformity in adult life. The distal phalanges and joints are most commonly involved. Later, surgery may be necessary to correct deformities (Bigelow and Ritchie, 1963).

Erosive lesions in the joints with secondary arthritic changes have been reported (Welch, Gormly and Lamb, 1974).

Hypothermia and frostbite

If these occur together the treatment of hypothermia should have priority as it is potentially lethal.

References

Bigelow, D. R. and Ritchie, G. W. (1963). The effect of frostbite in childhood. *J. Bone Jt. Surg.* **45B**, 122

Davies, L. W. (1975). The deep domestic bath treatment for advanced cases of hypothermia. In *Mountain Medicine and Physiology*. Eds C. Clarke, M. P. Ward, and E. S. William. Alpine Club

Jackson, J. A. (1975). Personal Communication

Lloyd, E. LL. and Frankland, J. C. (1974). Accidental hypothermia: central rewarming in the field. *Br. med. J.* **4**, 717

Ward, M. P. (1974). Frostbite. *Br. med. J.* **1**, 67

Ward, M. P. (1975). *Mountain Medicine. A Clinical Study of Cold and High Altitude.* St. Albans: Crosby Lockwood Staples

Welch, G. S. Gormly, P. J. and Lamb, D. W. (1974). Frostbite of the hands. *The Hand* **6**, 33

CHAPTER 8

Acute Poisoning

S. R. Meadow

Poisoning happens accidentally in or near the home. The child is usually under 5-years-old and typically is aged $1\frac{1}{2}$ to $3\frac{1}{2}$ years. Boys are involved more often than girls. In Britain suspected poisoning accounts for over a third of all childhood accidents and for over a fifth of all childhood medical admissions to hospital. Morbidity is low; only 10 per cent develop symptoms. There are about 20 to 25 deaths from poisoning each year in England and Wales (compared with 800 road accident deaths and 200 deaths by drowning), and in the United States the number of deaths is 1000 annually.

The substances ingested can be divided into three groups:

(a) Medical drugs (55%): about half of these are bought over the counter; the others are prescribed by a doctor.
(b) Household and garden products (25%).
(c) Berries and plants (20%).

Morbidity and mortality comes mainly from medicinal drug ingestion, especially from prescribed drugs. In the last 10 years salicylates, tricyclic antidepressants, iron and barbiturates have caused most of the deaths. In Britain fungi, berries and plants rarely cause serious symptoms and almost 'never' cause death.

The poisoning

Reported   The parent rushes to a hospital or the doctor with a toddler who has been found playing with a pile of tablets or sucking an emptied bottle of medicine. The child may have been seen to have a small amount of the substance in his mouth, but there is rarely any certainty about the amount he has swallowed, or indeed the amount to which he had access. The child is usually brought to the doctor, or he is telephoned, within an hour or two of the event.

Not reported   The poisoned child may be brought to the doctor ill but with no known history of poisoning. Therefore, in a child with unexplained symptoms poisoning must always be considered and the parents questioned closely about the availability and access to drugs and poisons in the home.

RECOGNITION

The following symptoms are particularly associated with poisoning:
  Drowsiness and loss of consciousness.
  Fits.
  Hyperventilation (salicylates).
  Bizarre motor disorders such as myoclonic jerks and tremors; extrapyramidal signs with antihistamines, phenothiazines and metoclopramide (Maxolon).
  Haematemesis with iron and salicylates.
  Ulcerated mouth with corrosives.
  Agitation, dilated pupils and hallucinations, with atropine-like agents.

IDENTIFICATION

Identification of the poison, prevention of its absorption, support of the patient and any specific therapy are all required immediately. They should take place concurrently and though they will now be dealt with in turn, the precise order of priorities will vary according to each situation.

(a) Has the child, in fact, ingested anything? It has been shown that up to half of all children presenting with 'accidental poisoning' have not actually swallowed anything. It is a poisoning scare rather than a poisoning ingestion. Therefore, a careful history is needed to discover whether anything has been taken. A straight abdominal x-ray may be helpful in identifying radio-opaque tablets.

(b) What has been ingested?

   (i) If the parents have not brought the container, they should be asked to fetch it; containers of drugs or household products will usually identify the substance.

   (ii) Identification charts and books, and a showcase container of common pills should be available for parents to identify. In addition, the *Monthly Index of Medical Specialities* (*MIMS*) gives a description of most drugs.

      If the child has eaten a berry or plant a sample should be obtained and identified using a book such as *Poisonous Plants and Fungi* (North, 1967)

   (iii) Tracing the source. If necessary the doctor, chemist, or shopkeeper who provided the substance should be questioned.

(iv) Poisons Information Centres (Table 8.I). These centres are an excellent source of information about the content and possible toxic effects of a large number of medicines, tablets and household products. In the United States, the regional poisons centre should be consulted. These centres are of little use in advising on direct management of an individual child, firstly because that depends on the actual situation, and secondly because the person giving the telephone advice will generally have much less clinical experience of poisoned children than the local clinicians.

TABLE 8.I
Telephone numbers of the Poisons Information
Centres in Britain and Ireland

Belfast	0232 40503
Cardiff	0222 33101
Dublin	0001 45588
Edinburgh	031-229 2477
Leeds	0532 32799
London	01-407 7600
Manchester	061-740 2254
Newcastle	0632 25131

(v) Laboratory detection. Identification of a poison, and sometimes the amount, (*see below*) may be possible in blood, urine or gastric aspirate. Some tests, such as Phenistix for salicylates, are simple; others are difficult. If the information is important the local laboratory should be consulted about the feasibility of an identification test. Usually the laboratory requires accurate information about the type of substance suspected.

(c) Type of product. Some drugs are marketed in different forms to give delayed absorption and effect. It is essential to identify 'sustained action', 'sustained release' or 'delayed action' preparations as their maximum effects may be expected 6 to 12 hours later.

(d) Does it matter? Reference to pharmacological books such as Martindale's *The Extra Pharmacopoeia* (1977) or a Poisons Information Centre will usually provide an answer. Information about the toxicity of commercial products is not always easily available. The toxicity grading of some commercial products is indicated in Table 8.II.

MANAGEMENT

Evacuation of stomach

In most situations the stomach should be emptied as speedily as possible by one of the two following methods.

Pharmacologically-induced emesis   This is effective in most children. Syrup of ipecacuanha (Ipecacuanha Paediatric Emetic Draught *B. P.C.*) (20 ml) is given with copious drinks of orange juice and water (THE FLUID EXTRACT OF IPECACUANHA SHOULD NEVER BE USED). If the child does not vomit within 20 minutes, the dose is repeated. If the child refuses to drink, a subcutaneous injection of apomorphine (0.1 mg per kg maximum dose) may be given, providing that the child is conscious. The gastric contents should be examined for the poison and retained for laboratory investigation if necessary.

Contra-indications to such emesis are:
(a) If there is *certainty* that an insignificant amount of poison has been swallowed or the toxicity of the substance is negligible. (*See* Table 8.II for non-toxic or slightly toxic substances.)
(b) If the poison was ingested more than 6 hours earlier (or up to 12 hours in the case of paraquat or massive doses of salicylate or iron).
(c) Caustics (strong acids, strong alkalis, bleach and phenols or cresols) since the risk of serious oesophagitis and perforation is increased.
(d) Hydrocarbons (paraffin, turpentine, petrol and some cleaning fluids). Aspiration of hydrocarbons is more likely to cause problems (from lipoid pneumonia) than is the hydrocarbon in the gut.
(e) Paraquat (Weedol and Gramoxone—*see* page 74).

Gastric lavage   This is used if emesis has failed or if the dose of a serious poison is so massive that emesis is unlikely to be completely effective, or if the child is unconscious. In the unconscious child it is performed by an anaesthetist using a cuffed endotracheal tube to prevent aspiration. A wide-bore (12 FG) soft rubber tube is used with the child tilted head-down on the left side. Suction apparatus should be available as aspiration into the bronchi commonly occurs. The lavage may be done with water, saline, bicarbonate or other additive according to the poison (a Poisons Information Centre or reference book will specify the best solution). Once in the stomach the tube can be used for administration of antidotes.

TABLE 8.II

Toxicity grading and probable lethal dose of commercial products

Grade 1 (practically non-toxic) Candles Chalk Cosmetics Crayons Fish bowl additives 'Lead' pencils Modelling clay Soaps Putty Toothpaste	Probable lethal dose: above 15 g per kg—more than 1140 ml	*Grade 3* (moderately toxic) Adhesives (rubber, linoleum, roofing, plastic cement) Antifreeze Bleach Brake fluids Cleaners (window, stain-removers) Disinfectants (bathroom, toilet, garbage-can) Indelible inks Lighter fuels Mothballs (most) Motor fuels Polishes (metal, wood, shoe, stove) Preservatives (brush, canvas, roof) Stain removers	0.5–5 g per kg—between 30 and 60 ml
Grade 2 (slightly toxic) Adhesives (most) Ballpoint pen inks Bubble-bath soaps Caps (toy pistol) Cigarettes or cigars Contraceptive pills Deodorants Deodorizers Detergents (most—not electric dishwasher) Fabric softeners Felt-tip markers Inks (most) Lubricating oils Perfumes and toilet water Shampoos Shaving creams	5–15 g per kg—between 60 and 1140 ml	*Grade 4* (very toxic) Ammonia Bleach—commercial Cresols (vaporizers) Degreasers (metal, etc.) Depilatories (some) Dishwasher granules—electric Disinfectants (acid, alkali, halogen, pine oil and phenolic types) Drain-cleaners (some) Dry-cleaner solvents (some)	50–500 g per kg—between 5 and 30 ml

Fire-extinguisher liquid
Leather dyes
Moth-repellents (naphthalene)
Petroleum products (most)
Radiator-cleaners
Rust-removers

Grade 5 (extremely toxic)
Drain- and sewer-cleaners (caustics)
Insecticides (some)
Fungicides (some)
Herbicides (some)
Rodenticides (some)

5–50 g per kg—between 7 drops and 5 ml

Full details are available in Gleason *et al.* (1969).

Purgation

This is likely to be most useful where emesis or lavage are contra-indicated. It may also be used with these measures if large quantities of a toxic substance have been taken. It is particularly indicated for the child who has taken sustained-release tablets. Oral magnesium sulphate, soap-and-water enemas and saline colonic wash-outs may be used individually or together according to the circumstances. Whole-gut irrigation may be needed for delayed-release tablets, paraquat and other very serious poisons. A stock solution for bowel irrigation should be kept:

$$\left.\begin{array}{l} \text{NaCl} \quad 6.14\,\text{g} \\ \text{KCl} \quad 0.75\,\text{g} \\ \text{NaHCO}_3 \quad 2.94\,\text{g} \end{array}\right\} \quad \text{in 1 litre distilled water (Na 137, K 10,} \\ \text{Cl 102, HCO}_3 \text{ 35 mmol per litre)}$$

The stock solution should be diluted 1:10 with water, warmed to 37°C (98.4°F) and delivered by gastric tube. If the child is below the age of two years, the solution should be run in at 20 ml per minute; if over two years, at 35 ml per minute. An infusion pump is useful to control the rate. Irrigation should be continued until clear fluid has been coming from the bowel for one hour; this is likely to be 2 to 3 hours after commencement.

General antidotes
Activated charcoal reduces the absorption of many chemicals. It should be given in the following circumstances:
  (a) If the child has had within the previous one hour:
        Salicylates
        Paracetamol (Panadol)
        Barbiturates
        Glutethimide (Doriden)
        Phenytoin (Epanutin)
        Phenothiazines (e.g. chlorpromazine)
        Tricyclic antidepressants (e.g. imipramine (Tofranil), amitriptyline (Tryptizol)
        Propantheline (Pro-Banthine)
        Phenylpropanolamine (Triominic, Triotussic, Eskornade)
        Chlorpheniramine (Piriton)
        Isoniazid
  (b) If the child has had very large quantities of any drug in the previous six hours and it is thought that quantities of the drug are still in the upper intestinal tract.
  (c) If the child has had within the previous six hours a drug which has an enterohepatic recirculation, (e.g. tricyclic antidepressants, glutethimide).

(d) If the child has had a sustained or delayed-release form of drug within the previous 24 hours

Repeated doses should be given to groups (b), (c) and (d). Charcoal adsorbs ipecacuanha, therefore it should be given *after* ipecacuanha-induced emesis.

Using these criteria about 1 in 8 poisoned children warrant the use of charcoal. Charcoal (*B.P.*) is difficult to mix. A convenient method is to mix 10 g of the powder into a slurry with 30 ml concentrated blackcurrant syrup (e.g. Ribena). Water is gradually added up to 120 ml. Although it looks unpleasant most children take it fairly easily. If the child vomits immediately afterwards, the dose is repeated.

Specific antidotes
  (a) Acids and alkalis are diluted by persuading the patient to drink milk or water.
  (b) Other antidotes are given if the situation warrants it and if advised by the Poisons Information Service or Pharmacopoeia. There are relatively few useful specific antidotes. (Iron and paraquat poisoning are considered below.)

Forced diuresis
If the drug is excreted by the kidneys, forced diuresis may be helpful, particularly for salicylates (*see below*) and barbiturates. In the very ill child, care must be taken to ensure that the large amount of intravenous fluid does not overload the circulation and create pulmonary oedema and heart failure. (*See also* Appendix 5: Urine Output in Acute Disease.)

Dialysis
The usefulness of either peritoneal dialysis or haemodialysis is limited. Most drugs are not removed effectively by peritoneal dialysis, and many are not removed by haemodialysis. In worrying cases of potentially severe poisoning, reference should be made to Table 8.III which gives a summary of those drugs which may be removed by haemodialysis, peritoneal dialysis or exchange transfusion. To justify dialysis it must be theoretically useful, and in the individual child it will be required because of the expected ineffectiveness of other methods of poison removal. Barbiturates, glutethimide and salicylates can be speedily removed by dialysis; iron and the tricyclic antidepressants cannot.

TABLE 8.III
Poisons that may be removed by haemodialysis include:

Alcohols:
  (primary): methyl (methanol); ethyl (ethanol);(tertiary): methylpentynol (Oblivon), ethchlorvynol (Arvynol)
Amanita phalloides (mushrooms)
Amphetamines
Aniline
Antibiotics: ampicillin, cephaloridine, chloramphenicol, cycloserine, kanamycin, neomycin, nitrofurantoin, penicillin, polymyxin, streptomycin, sulphonamides, tetracycline, vancomycin
Arsenic
Barbiturates
Boric acid
Bromides
Calcium
Carbon tetrachloride
Chloral hydrate
Chlorates
Chlorides
Chromic acid
Citrates
Cyclophosphamide
Dichloroethane
Dichromate (potassium salt)
Dichloralphenazone (Welldorm)
Ergotamine
Ethchlorvynol (Placidyl)
Ethinamate (Valmid)
Ethylene glycol
Eucalyptus oil
Fluorides

5-Fluorouracil
Gallamine triethiodide
Glutethimide (Doriden)
Isoniazid
Iodides
Iron (+ chelating agents)
Lead (+ chelating agents)
Lithium
Meprobamate
Mercury
Methaqualone (Melsedin and, with diphenhydramine, as Mandrax)
Methotrexate
Methyprylone (Noludar)
Monoamine-oxidase inhibitors: pargyline (Eutonyl), phenelzine (Nardil), tranylcypromine (Parnate)
Orphenadrine (Disipal)
Paracetamol
Paraldehyde
Phenacetin
Phenformin
Phenytoin(Epanutin)
Potassium
Primidone (Mysoline)
Quinidine
Quinine
Salicylates (aspirin; methyl salicylate)
Strontium
Strychnine
Thiocyanate (potassium salt)

Full details in *Dialysis of Poisons and Drugs* Schreiner, (1970)

TABLE 8.IV
Poisons that may be removed by peritoneal dialysis include:

Ethanol (ethyl alcohol), methanol (methyl alcohol) and other alcohols
Amphetamines
Bromide
Heavy metals
Isoniazid
Meprobamate
Primidone
Salicylate

Clearance of highly protein-bound drugs is increased by the addition of 5 per cent albumin to the dialysis fluid.

Full details in *Dialysis of Poisons and Drugs* Schreiner, (1970)

TABLE 8.V
Poisons that may be removed by exchange transfusion

This is technically difficult, but can be useful in small children for drugs that are strongly bound to plasma proteins or blood. It has been used successfully for poisoning with:

> Antihistamines
> Diphenoxylate (Lomotil)
> Heavy metals + chelating agent

In very small children, it may be easier than haemodialysis for the removal of:

> Alcohols
> Barbiturates
> Quinine

General aspects

SEVERE OR POTENTIALLY SEVERE POISONING

Resuscitation of the shocked or collapsed child is essential. An efficient intravenous line is needed, together with oxygen equipment, suction apparatus and ventilatory equipment should it be required. Close observation and skilled nursing are needed. If the child starts to have convulsions, paraldehyde (1 ml per year of age up to 7 ml maximum) is given by deep intramuscular injection. DIAZEPAM (VALIUM) SHOULD NOT BE USED BECAUSE OF ITS INTERACTION WITH CERTAIN POISONS AND THE POSSIBILITY OF RESPIRATORY ARREST. The child is observed in hospital for a minimum of 24 hours.

MILD OR DOUBTFUL POISONING

Having taken appropriate steps to identify and to remove a possible poison, the problem is whether it is necessary to observe the child any further. This will depend upon the likely amount of poison and its nature. If there is reasonable certainty that little or no toxic poison is inside the child, he may be allowed home, provided that the parent is informed of possible problems, is confident and knows where to bring the child for help in the event of trouble. If the child may have ingested a significant quantity of poison, he should be observed in hospital for 12 hours (or for 24 hours in the case of delayed-release tablets, or aspirin).

SUSPICIOUS CIRCUMSTANCES

(i) Deliberate poisoning by a parent is an occasional method of non-accidental injury (baby battering). Appropriate investigation and referral may be needed (*see* page 515).

(ii) Poisoning over the age of 5 years may not be accidental. Care must be taken to try to find out why the child over 5 years took the poison. All children over 10 years should be kept in hospital and seen by a child psychiatrist.

(iii) Repeated poisonings. Ten per cent of children who ingest poisons accidentally do so again. Referral to a health visitor or social worker for investigation of the home situation is likely to be needed.

(iv) Toxic drug effects. If the symptoms are not those expected from the dose and nature of a drug, the 'yellow card' notification of adverse drug effects should be sent to the Committee on Safety of Medicines.*

Particularly dangerous poisons

Some poisons are particularly dangerous to children because of their resistance to routine treatment or their widespread availability. Poisoning with paraquat, corrosives, iron, salicylates and the tricyclic antidepressants are considered below. Specific advice is given in each case which should be followed *in addition to* the general measures previously outlined.

Paraquat   This herbicide is marketed under different trade names (the 5 per cent product as Weedol, the 20 per cent as Gramoxone). Ingestion of large quantities is more likely from farm supplies rather than the weaker garden products; or it may be due to deliberate poisoning. Large quantities cause death in a few days from pulmonary oedema and haemorrhage, and by damage to the kidneys, liver and heart. Smaller doses may cause death later from progressive pulmonary fibrosis and respiratory failure. Therefore, the possible ingestion of even a small quantity must be taken seriously even though there may be no abnormal signs or symptoms at presentation or in the first 12 hours.

There is a useful qualitative test for paraquat in the urine (Widdop, 1976), but the laboratory will merely be able to specify its presence, and not the amount ingested.

Paraquat is absorbed very slowly from the gut, therefore every effort should be concentrated on its removal from the gut before it is absorbed. These efforts should be vigorous and prolonged. Thorough gastric lavage should be followed by purgation, or preferably whole-bowel irrigation (*see page 70*). This should be combined or followed by oral administration of 1% bentonite (*B.P.*) adsorbent. This is difficult to give and will almost certainly require a wide-bore gastric tube for

* Current address: Finsbury Square House, 33/37a Finsbury Square, London EC2B 2ZS

administration. *As bentonite requires 24 hours preparation it should be available ready-mixed in every casualty department or paediatric unit receiving poisoned children.* If whole-bowel irrigation is used, 250 ml of bentonite should be given initially and 250 ml at the conclusion, with the usual electrolyte solution in between. An intravenous line should be set up and a diuresis maintained to protect the kidneys. The child should be admitted for further care. Haemoperfusion through charcoal, or haemodialysis may be needed in the early treatment of severe cases, together with corticosteroids and immunosuppressive therapy.

Corrosives (*see also* ENT section, page 209)   The most important complication is severe oesophageal damage with subsequent stricture formation. The development of a stricture depends largely upon the depth of the oesophageal damage and the proportion of its circumference involved. Some of this information, but not all, can be obtained by oesophagoscopy, yet that procedure may itself carry the risk of perforation. In childhood many children feared to have swallowed corrosives will not actually have done so. If there is no oral-mucosal damage and there are no particular symptoms, serious mucosal damage of the oesophagus is unlikely but not impossible. However, in the presence of severe oral ulceration it is wisest to assume that similar damage exists in the oesophagus. Phenolic compounds such as cresols do not produce any pain initially. DO NOT EVACUATE THE STOMACH BY EMESIS OR LAVAGE. Copious fluids should be given.

(1) Hydrocortisone should be given parenterally for 24 to 48 hours; this may reduce oesophageal damage.
(2) A broad-spectrum antibiotic should be given parenterally.
(3) Consultation with a paediatric or thoracic surgeon should take place early. The role of oesophagoscopy is a contentious one. Many surgeons will prefer to perform it about a week after ingestion. Others may prefer early oesophagoscopy so that intraluminal splinting can be used if the depth and extent of the burn warrant it.

Iron   A simple ferricyanide test on the vomit or gastric aspirate will confirm the presence of iron. Most iron tablets are radio-opaque and can be seen on a straight abdominal x-ray. When large quantities are ingested necrosis of the gastrointestinal wall may occur. Initial symptoms are vomiting, haematemesis, melaena and shock, sometimes with severe abdominal pain.

The estimated lethal dose is about 300 mg of iron per 8 kg body weight (or 3 tablets per kg of the usual 300-mg ferrous sulphate tablet). Severity of poisoning is judged by the history, the clinical state and the serum iron level. A level of over 500 µg/100 ml in the first 6 hours after ingestion suggests serious poisoning. In severe poisoning, after evacua-

tion of the stomach, gastric lavage should be done with desferrioxamine
solution (2 g per litre), and 3 to 7 g in 50 to 100 ml of water is left in the
stomach. In addition 80 mg per kg is given by intravenous infusion over
an 8-hour period. Successful desferrioxamine therapy gives an orange-
brown colour to the urine. The child is admitted to hospital for further
care.

Salicylates   The products most commonly ingested are junior aspirin
(75-mg or 150-mg tablets) or standard aspirin tablets (300-mg). A
small dose of aspirin is absorbed rapidly and reaches a peak blood level
in 1 hour. Large doses produce peak levels at 4 to 6 hours. Methyl
salicylate, a major constituent of many linaments (e.g. oil of winter-
green) is absorbed more slowly.

Aspirin is excreted entirely in the urine and urine tests provide useful
confirmation of aspirin ingestion. It is also worth testing the vomit or
gastric aspirate for salicylate:

(a) Phenistix paper develops a brownish-purple colour (similar to
that from phenothiazines).
(b) Ferric chloride test. Ferric chloride (10 per cent) is added drop
by drop to the acidified urine. A purple colour indicates the
presence of salicylate. The somewhat similar colour (burgundy
red) produced by diacetic acid ('acetonuria') is reduced or
abolished by boiling before adding ferric chloride; a positive
'Acetest' is common in salicylate poisoning.

MANAGEMENT AND ASSESSMENT

All children believed to have ingested aspirin should be admitted for at
least 8 hours although the majority will require only one or two plasma
salicylate levels and a lot to drink.

Most children will have had their stomach evacuated within 24 hours
of ingestion, therefore, plasma levels should not rise further providing
that the evacuation has been thorough. The severity can be assessed by
a combination of clinical features and plasma level.

(a) Severe poisoning: coma, fits, collapse and hyperventilation.
(b) Moderate poisoning: hyperventilation and moderate
dehydration.
(c) Mild poisoning: no symptoms or mild hyperventilation.

Intravenous fluids should be given to any child with symptoms. Plasma
levels within 45 minutes of ingestion are likely to be unreliable, but
thereafter are most helpful.

(a) Plasma salicylate between 1 to 4 hours after ingestion.
at > 50 mg% IV fluids should be given.
at < 50 mg% copious oral fluids should be given.
A negative urine ferric chloride test more than one hour after

suspected ingestion makes salicylism unlikely. Plasma levels are retested 1 to 2 hours after starting fluids.

(b) Plasma salicylate level at or after 6 hours post-ingestion use Done's nomogram (*Figure 8.1*).

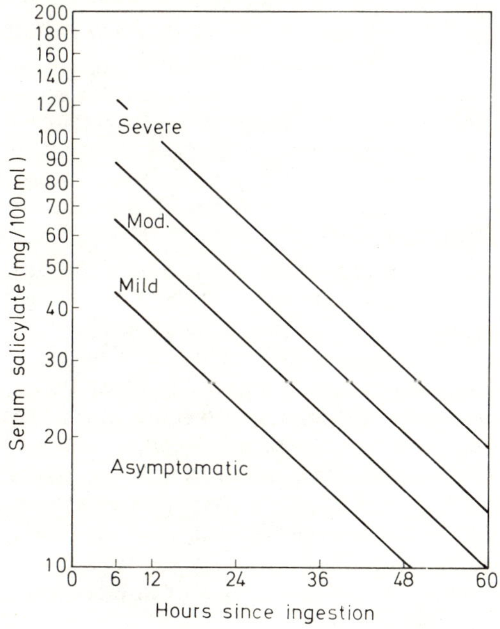

Figure 8.1. Done's nomogram. Relationship between serum salicylate and expected severity of poisoning following ingestion of a single dose of salicylate. (Done. 1960. Reproduced by kind permission)

> 100 mg per 100 ml, severe: intravenous fluids should be given.

80–100 mg per 100 ml, moderate: intravenous fluids should be given.

50–80 mg per 100 ml, no symptoms: oral fluids should be given.

(c) In all children with symptoms or a plasma level of > 50 mg per 100 ml: measure plasma urea, electrolytes, Astrup and glucose.

The young child who accidentally ingests aspirin or is given repeated doses is more likely to develop hyperglycaemia or occasionally hypoglycaemia and a metabolic acidosis rather than a respiratory alkalosis (which occurs in older children and adults). *It is dangerous to give insulin for the hyperglycaemia.*

Forced alkali diuresis is not generally required, but may be helpful in severe cases. Sodium bicarbonate is given intravenously in an initial dose of 3 mmol per kg followed by 1.5 mmol per kg 15, 30 and 45 minutes later. Additionally, in the first 8 hours, 5 per cent glucose + 35 mmol per litre $NaHCO_3$ and 20 mmol per litre KCl are given intravenously at a rate of 2000 ml per square metre. In the most severe cases peritoneal dialysis or haemodialysis may be helpful.

Tricyclic antidepressants   The danger of this poisoning is death from cardiac arrhythmia. The most usual drugs are imipramine and amitriptyline, which have been prescribed for a parent's depression or a child's bed-wetting. They are rapidly absorbed from the gut and metabolized in the liver. Because of their enterohepatic recirculation, oral charcoal is a particularly important part of general management (*see* page 70). Very little is free in the serum, or is excreted in the urine, which means that forced diuresis, dialysis and even exchange transfusion are ineffective.

The poisoned child rapidly shows the anticholinergic properties of the drug as well as some sympathomimetic features. Initial excitement and ataxia are followed by drowsiness and coma. Muscle-twitching and athetoid movements precede convulsions. Tendon reflexes are brisk and plantar responses extensor. The pupils are widely dilated and the mouth dry. Bowel sounds may be absent. In severe poisoning the main danger is from cardiac failure. Sinus tachycardia may precede a variety of dysrhythmias including bundle-branch block, ectopic beats, ventricular fibrillation and cardiac arrest. In addition or independently there may be profound hypotension.

MANAGEMENT

Many laboratories are able to identify these drugs in urine, but quantitative determinations are unreliable. A child believed to have ingested one of these drugs should be admitted as soon as general treatment has been completed. All should have a reliable intravenous line and a cardiac monitor. Sinus tachycardia does not require specific treatment, but ventricular dysrhythmia may require lignocaine hydrochloride 1 mg per kg intravenously, repeated as necessary, or even a cardiac pacemaker. For the unconscious child, equipment should be available for ventilation in the event of respiratory arrest.

References

Done, A. K. (1960). Salicylate intoxication. *Pediatrics* **26**, 800

Gellis, S. S. (Ed). (1976). Experimental treatment of corrosive esophageal burns. *Year Book of Pediatrics* p. 174. Chicago: Year Book Medical Publishers

Gleason, M. N., Gosselin, R. E., Hodge, H. C., Smith, P. R. (1969). *Clinical Toxicology of Commercial Products*. Baltimore: Williams & Wilkins Company
Lancet (1976). Paraquat poisoning. (Leading article). **(i)**, 1057
Martindale. (1977). *The Extra Pharmacopoeia* 27th edn. London: The Pharmaceutical Press
Monthly Index of Medical Specialities (MIMS). London: Haymarket Publishing Ltd.
North, P. (1967). *Poisonous Plants and Fungi*. London: Blandford Press
Pierce, A. W. (1974). Salicylate poisoning. *Pediatrics* **54**, 342
Schreiner, G. E. (1970). Dialysis of poisons and drugs. *Trans. Am. Soc. artif. internal Organs* **16**, 544
Widdop, B. (1976). Detection of paraquat in the urine. *Br. med. J.* **2**, 1135

ADDITIONAL READING
Poisoning in children. (1970). *Pediat. Clins. N. Am.* **17 (3)**
The management of accidental childhood poisoning. (1974). *Pediatrics*, **54**, 323
Aspirin and acetaminophen. (1977). *Pediatrics*, **62**, part 2

CHAPTER 9

Travel

A. F. Conchie

Motion or travel sickness

This can occur when travelling by land, sea or air. The young child is the usual sufferer, but infants can also be affected.

RECOGNITION

The major symptom is self-evident. Before vomiting the child sweats and appears pale. Older children may complain of nausea and upper abdominal pain.

MANAGEMENT

Travel sickness develops into an emergency when repeated vomiting leads to dehydration. Oral fluids are often retained better after a vomit. Plain water, boiled and cooled for the infant, should be given. Prevention is more effective than treating established travel sickness. Avoidance of a large meal before a journey, adequate fresh-air ventilation, games to occupy the attention, and on car trips, frequent stops, may help. Drugs are effective. Hyoscine hydrobromide in a dose of 0.15 mg to 0.3 mg or cyclizine 25 mg should be taken 30 to 60 minutes before starting the journey. (*See* Table 9.I for list of commonly used preparations).

Drug reactions

Hyoscine is available in proprietary travel sickness preparations. Accidental overdose can lead to tachycardia, flushed and dry skin, dilated pupils, and an acute confusional state with hallucinations. Mild symptoms can be treated expectantly but the acutely disturbed child requires hospital care.

Metoclopramide (Maxolon) is also an anti-emetic. In normal dosage in children it can cause severe dystonic spasms involving the head and neck and should be avoided for the prevention of travel sickness.

Travellers' diarrhoea

This is a common problem especially in countries where the hygiene is poor.

RECOGNITION
The diarrhoea may be accompanied or preceded by vomiting. The majority of episodes settle in one to three days. With those travelling in or who have been to the Middle or Far East, bacillary or amoebic dysentery, cholera and typhoid fever must be considered.

TABLE 9.I
Preparations used to prevent motion sickness

Approved name	Proprietary name
Cyclizine hydrochloride	Valoid (*Calmic*)
	Marzine (*Wellcome*)
Dimenhydrinate	Dramamine (*Searle*)
	Gravol (*Carter-Wallace*)
Hyoscine hydrobromide	Joy-Rides (*Stafford-Miller*)
	Quick Kwells (*Nicholas*)
	Sereen (*Boots*)
	Tranazine (*Wellcome*)
Meclozine hydrochloride	Sea-Legs (*Duncan Flockhart*)
Promethazine theoclate	Avomine (*May & Baker*)
Promethazine hydrochloride	Phenergan (*May & Baker*)
Chlorpheniramine	Piriton (*Allen & Hanburys*)

MANAGEMENT
The younger the child, the greater is the possibility of dehydration. If there is no vomiting, hydration can be maintained by giving water orally. This should be boiled and cooled for the infant, and also for the older child if the water supply is at all suspect. Vomiting usually settles within twenty-four hours, but small amounts of oral fluids may be given and retained while the child has this symptom.

In non-specific travellers' diarrhoea drugs are ineffective and therefore unnecessary. In particular clioquinol (Entero-Vioform) is contraindicated and there is no evidence that this drug or antibiotics are effective prophylactically in this condition.

D

Sleep disturbances

Many children have a sleep ritual. This often involves cuddling a particular blanket or toy. If this is not taken on a journey or is mislaid the child may have difficulty in getting to sleep. In addition travelling often causes a disturbance in the daily routine of a child so that he is not able to follow his usual pattern of sleeping.

RECOGNITION
The child with a sleep disturbance is usually fractious and may show signs of anxiety as well as having difficulty in falling to sleep.

MANAGEMENT
Parents should be advised to take any object associated with the child's sleep ritual with them when they go on a journey. If this is not done or the comfort object is mislaid it is worth trying to find a substitute. Effort should be made to make the child's routine as much as possible like that established at home. The problem is usually a temporary one but Chloral Mixture *B.P.C.,* 2.5 ml to 10 ml, according to age before bedtime for a few nights will help resolve the difficulty of getting to sleep. Dichloralphenazone Elixir *B.P.C.* (Welldorm) in a similar dosage is equally useful in this situation.

Emotional disturbances

Travelling may involve the child in having to contend with marked changes in his emotional as well as his physical environment. He may have to cope with unusual food, hotels in which the geography is unfamiliar and communication problems because of language differences. At the same time his parents may have similar anxieties and be preoccupied with their own problems associated with the journey.

RECOGNITION
The child may respond by displaying signs of anxiety with frequent and often prolonged outbursts of crying. He may become aggressive and rebellious or withdrawn and uncommunicative.

MANAGEMENT
Much can be done to avoid emotional problems if the parents have been advised of this possibility. The child, as far as possible, should be involved in planning and recognizing the difficulties, including emotional ones, that may arise during the course of the journey.

If the child's behaviour has become disturbed then a full explanation of the cause should be given to the parents. They should be reassured that with understanding and sympathetic handling the problem is usually a temporary one. Associated sleep disturbances can be helped with chloral or dichloralphenazone as suggested above.

Car travel

(a) *Heat exhaustion and heat stroke* (*See also* page 529)

These are likely to occur when a child, particularly an infant, is left in a closed car on a hot day. The higher the temperature and the greater the humidity, the greater is the probability of symptoms. The mildest form is heat exhaustion. Electrolytes and water are lost through sweating. The child is not in a situation to replace the water loss and so there is a tendency to develop hypertonic dehydration (*see* page 98).

RECOGNITION
The child appears flushed and irritable.

MANAGEMENT
Removal from the car, placing in a cool shaded area, and giving water by mouth overcome the problem.

In heatwaves the more severe condition of heat stroke may occur. (For the symptoms, signs and management *see* page 534) It should be noted that drugs of the hyoscine group given for the prevention of travel sickness may increase the risk of causing heatstroke by reducing sweating.

(b) *Carbon monoxide poisoning* (*See also* page 40)

Leaking and inefficient exhaust systems can cause carbon monoxide to seep into the travelling compartment of cars, and the problem is exaggerated if the ventilation system is poor and the windows are kept closed.

RECOGNITION
The severity of the symptoms depends upon the duration of exposure. The initial symptom is headache of which the older child may complain. Irritability and mental confusion may be followed by drowsiness.

MANAGEMENT
Once the condition is recognized the car should be stopped, the engine turned off and the occupants taken into the open air.

Aircraft travel

Food poisoning

With the catering techniques employed for aircraft travellers there is a possibility of food poisoning occurring during flight. The commonest agent responsible is staphylococcal enterotoxin.

RECOGNITION
Symptoms appear one to three hours after eating the contaminated food. Vomiting and abdominal pain are more prominent features than diarrhoea.

MANAGEMENT
The illness usually settles within a few hours. A careful watch should be kept for signs of dehydration and arrangements should be considered for the most severely affected to be given parenteral saline at the next airfield (*see also* page 95).

Sea travel

As in closed motor cars, the temperature and humidity in some cabins can be high and lead to heat exhaustion and even heat stroke (p. 532).

Part II: Shock and Dehydration States.

CHAPTER 10

Shock and Dehydration States

J. A. Black

Classification

The classification (Table 10.I) is based partly upon that of Hardaway (1968a). A standard plan of treatment is described for the management of isotonic dehydration. and is modified in other conditions associated with reversible shock. Refractory shock, which is usually combined with disseminated intravascular coagulation (DIC), requires special consideration (p. 482) apart from the treatment of shock.

TABLE 10.I
Clinical appearances and classification of shock

Clinical observations (vital signs)	*Early reversible shock (vasoconstriction)*		*Late reversible shock (capillary & venular dilatation)*	*Refractory shock (with DIC)*
	Mild	*Moderate*	*Severe*	*Very severe*
Skin colour	Pale	Grey	Mottled	Mottled skin, haemorrhages, oozing from puncture sites
Peripheral circulation (refilling of skin capillaries after light pressure)	Quick	Quick	Slow	Slow
Temperature of extremities (big toe and tip of nose)	Cool	Cool	Cold	Cold
Heart rate	Normal or slightly raised	Rapid	Very rapid	Very rapid
Blood pressure	Normal, or slightly high or low	Slightly low	Low	Very low
Mental state	Anxious	Restless	Confused or stuporous	Unresponsive

Recognition of shock and conditions leading to shock

The signs of established shock should be easily recognizable, whatever the initial diagnosis. The child is pale, anxious and restless, with a cold clammy skin and a rapid feeble pulse. The recognition of situations which may lead to shock (Table 10.II) and the avoidance of shock by appropriate treatment are equally important.

Comparison of fluid loss in shock from different causes

In order to establish a basis of comparison between the commoner causes of shock, these have been tabulated according to the degree of shock and the usual clinical estimates of fluid loss (Table 10.II).

TABLE 10.II
Degree of shock and fluid losses

	Mild	*Moderate*	*Severe*	*Very severe + DIC.*
Isotonic dehydration % loss of body weight mainly ECF*	5%	10%	15%	15% + other factors such as endotoxic shock
Loss per kg body weight	50 ml/kg	100 ml/kg	150 ml/kg	
Haemorrhage†				
% loss of blood volume	20%	30%	up to 50%	30–50% + other factors
Loss per kg body weight	15–20 ml/kg	25–30 ml/kg	30–40 ml/kg	
Plasma loss (Burns) % surface area burned	20%	40%	60%+	40–60%+, with other factors
Plasma replacement in first 24 hours** (2.5 ml per kg per 1% burn)	50 ml/kg	100 ml/kg	150 ml/kg	

* ECF = Extracellular fluid.
† Modified from *Table 7.2* Weil and Shubin (1967) and based upon blood volume of 8.5% of body weight, or 85 ml per kg
** Based on the 'Mount Vernon Formula', Muir and Barclay (1974). Plasma replacement continues at a slower rate up to 36 hours after the burn: metabolic water is given in addition (Table 4.I).

Common causes of shock in children

Although the common causes of shock are those given in Table 10.III, it should be remembered that there are many conditions, particularly those associated with severe hypoxia, in which shock develops in the absence of obvious losses from any of the body compartments. Shock in the newborn is easily missed and is commoner than is usually realized.

TABLE 10.III
Causes of shock in infants and children

	Type of shock	Cause	Fluid required	Other treatment
NEWBORN	Hypoxic	'Fetal distress', intrapartum hypoxia	10% glucose plasma,(*) $NaHCO_3$	Oxygen, IPPV(†)
	Haemorrhage	Acute bleeding from any cause	Plasma* → blood	Oxygen: correction of bleeding or coagulation disorder if present
	Endotoxic shock	Gram-negative septicaemia	Plasma*	Antibiotics, corticosteroids
	Isotonic dehydration (loss of ECF)	Gastroenteritis, intestinal obstruction, peritonitis, neonatal diabetes	0.9% NaCl in 5% glucose initially (omit glucose in diabetes)	According to diagnosis
	Hypoadrenal state (hyponatraemic dehydration)	Adrenal hyperplasia, hypoplasia, hypoaldosteronism	0.9% NaCl in 5% glucose	Salt-retaining steroids ± corticosteroids according to diagnosis
	Hypoadrenal state and haemorrhage	Bilateral adrenal haemorrhage	Plasma* → blood → 0.9% NaCl in 5% glucose	As above + antibiotics
INFANTS AND OLDER CHILDREN	Hypoxia	Cardiac arrest	IV $NaHCO_3$→ plasma*	ECM,** IPPV
	Haemorrhage	External or internal bleeding, acute haemolysis	Plasma* → blood	Oxygen: + treatment of primary condition
	Plasma loss ± blood	Burns, trauma, extensive urticaria	Plasma* ± blood	As above
	Isotonic dehydration (loss of ECF)	Gastroenteritis, diabetes mellitus, cholera, heat exhaustion, dengue haemorrhagic fever	0.9% NaCl in 5% glucose initially (omit glucose in diabetes)	As above
	Isotonic hypovolaemia due to acute oedema	Nephrotic syndrome ± hyponatraemia	Plasma* ± 0.9% NaCl in 5% glucose	Corticosteroids if responsive type
	Hypoadrenal state	Adrenal failure from any cause	0.9% NaCl in 5% glucose initially	Salt-retaining steroids ± corticosteroids according to diagnosis

TABLE 10.III (*continued*)

Type of shock	Cause	Fluid required	Other treatment
Endotoxic shock	Gram-negative septicaemia in burns, immunosuppression, meningococcal septicaemia	Plasma* initially	Antibiotics, high-dosage corticosteroids
Hypoxia + water depletion	Status asthmaticus, status epilepticus	0.18% NaCl in 4% glucose	Oxygen + treatment of primary condition
Acute poisoning	Salicylates, iron salts (commonly)	*See* pages 75–78	*See* pages 75–78

* Plasma is written for brevity; any other plasma expander would be suitable. Plasma–Protein Fraction (PPF) is replacing pooled plasma.
† IPPV = Intermittent Positive-Pressure Ventilation.
** ECM = External Cardiac Massage.

General principles in the management of shock

It is essential that an orderly sequence should be used in assessment and treatment:

History → Clinical examination → Recording vital signs + Initial investigations → Plan of treatment → Initial treatment → Reassessment of vital signs ± Repeat investigations → Adjustment of treatment.

History

Establish if possible:
(a) The primary condition causing the shock.
(b) The duration of the primary illness.
(c) The cause of shock; type of fluid lost and from which body compartment.
(d) Duration of shock.
(e) What drugs, antibiotics etc have been given previously; time, dose, route.

As a result:
(a) Instruct the nursing staff to prepare for any special investigation: (lumbar puncture, blood culture etc.) or drugs required.
(b) Especially at night or at week-ends, warn the laboratory staff about any investigations likely to be required.

Clinical examination

(a) Assess the degree of shock (Tables 10.I and II).
(b) Estimate the amount of fluid, blood and plasma to be replaced.
(c) Look for the cause of shock, i.e. the site from which fluid has been lost.
(d) Make a rapid clinical examination, with special reference to evidence of DIC, i.e. petechiae, skin, haemorrhages or oozing from previous puncture sites.

Recording of vital signs and base-line information

The following should be recorded in writing with *the date and time* when appropriate.

(a) Weight and length. Use these for surface-area calculations as required. If the child is too ill to be weighed, obtain the probable weight from a height-weight table (*see* Appendix 1).
(b) Skin colour of trunk and peripheries.
   Peripheral circulation (refilling after light pressure sufficient to blanch).
   Temperature of extremities (big toe and tip of nose) compared (by touch) with that of the trunk.
   Skin elasticity (turgor) (*see* Note 1).
   State of oral mucosa (moist or dry).
   Heart rate (at apex).
   Blood pressure (*see* Appendix 14 for BP by age).
   Respiration, rate and type.
(c) *In infants*, the state of the anterior fontanelle (*see* Note 2).
(d) The amount of urine passed or produced on catheterization before IV fluids: the urine should be tested according to the provisional diagnosis.

Notes

(1) Skin elasticity: a fold of skin is pinched between thumb and finger and is then released; normally it returns to its former state immediately. Two sites should always be used, preferably the chest wall in the mid-axillary line and the medial side of the thigh. The abdominal wall should not be used.
(2) Anterior fontanelle: this can give misleading information if used as the sole criterion of the degree of dehydration.
   (a) Many normal infants have such small fontanelles that it is impossible to judge depression, elevation or tension. In very wasted infants the fontanelle may be depressed in the absence of dehydration.
   (b) In meningitis, cerebral vein thrombosis or acute hydrocephalus

the fontanelle may be tense and bulging in the presence of severe dehydration.

Investigations

(a) In all children requiring IV fluids the plasma urea and electrolytes should be estimated.
(b) In severe shock, an Astrup (or equivalent method) of measurement of the acid-base state should be obtained.
(c) Blood gases should be measured in all cases with respiratory obstruction or insufficiency.
(d) In suspected DIC, *see* page 482.
(e) After blood loss or acute haemolysis, blood should be taken for Hb%, blood group and crossmatching.
(f) Urine: osmolality, specific gravity, or urea concentration in relation to blood urea are useful in assessing renal function (p. 413). The sodium level should be used in deciding whether the kidney is conserving or losing sodium. Specific tests are available in certain types of poisoning, e.g. salicylates.
(g) In acute poisoning the plasma levels of certain drugs can be estimated quickly as a guide to treatment, e.g. salicylates, barbiturates.
(h) Blood culture if endotoxic shock is suspected.
(i) A continuous recording of the ECG is important in the management of hyperkalaemia, and in poisoning with the tricyclic antidepressants (amitriptyline, imipramine).

Choice of intravenous fluids

There is considerable variation in the types of electrolyte solution used for resuscitation, repair and maintenance. Nomenclature is also confused; in general solutions are referred to here according to their actual composition (e.g. 0.9 per cent NaCl in 5 per cent glucose) or common usage (e.g. Lactate Ringer). Some descriptions are however so imprecise as to be dangerous ('normal saline', 'physiological saline'); 'glucose' is used throughout in preference to 'dextrose'.

Resuscitation fluids (*See* Appendix 6 for electrolyte content)

Any of those listed below will expand the intravascular compartment in hypovolaemia, but electrolyte solutions have a rather transient effect in counteracting hypovolaemia compared to blood, plasma or other plasma expanders. Nevertheless, electrolyte solutions are usually immediately available and can be used until a more appropriate substitute is obtained.

Suitable for resuscitation according to the requirements.

0.9 per cent (NaCl) in 5 per cent glucose.

0.9 per cent NaCl without glucose: indicated initially in diabetic ketoacidosis.

Lactate Ringer (Hartmann's solution is almost identical).

Plasma.

Dextran 110 (the most satisfactory molecular size for resuscitation).

Plasma-protein fraction (PPF) (this is replacing pooled plasma).

Blood.

Do NOT use:

0.18 per cent NaCl in 4 per cent glucose (too little sodium).

or Darrow's solution (too much potassium).

Repair fluids (*See* Appendix 6 for electrolyte content)

(a) For general purposes in isotonic dehydration with the necessity of supplying water in excess of sodium:

0.45 per cent NaCl in 2.5 per cent or 5 per cent glucose. For replacement of potassium 1 g of potassium chloride (13 mmol) is added to 500 ml (26 mmol per litre).

OR 0.18 per cent NaCl in 4 per cent glucose if water requirements are greater.

OR Darrow's solution (potassium 36 mmol per litre).

(b) For special situations, *see under* sections for hypotonic dehydration (p. 100), hypertonic dehydration (p. 98), protein-energy malnutrition (PEM) (p. 588).

(c) In conditions known to be associated with potassium depletion (diabetic ketoacidosis: long-continued gastroenteritis, diarrhoea in PEM), additional potassium should be added according to the estimated deficit (pp. 133, 590).

Maintenance fluids (*see* Appendix 6 for electrolyte content)

(a) For general purposes in short-term conditions of up to 3 to 4 days with no evidence of potassium depletion 0.18 per cent NaCl in 4 per cent glucose can be used.

(b) If potassium depletion is still present or probable, or continuing losses of potassium-containing fluid are occurring, or IV fluids are necessary for longer than 3 to 4 days, potassium supplements should be added to 0.18 per cent NaCl in 4 per cent glucose: the average maintenance requirement (in the absence of

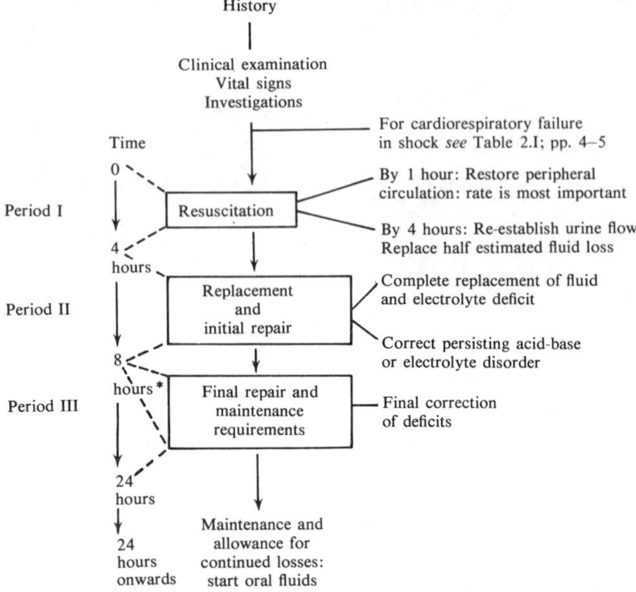

Figure 10.1. Standard plan of treatment (acute dehydration syndrome). This scheme is for use in dehydration and electrolyte disorders
* This can be varied to 9 hours (*see* page 97)

previous depletion or continuing losses) is 2 mmol per kg per day, normally supplied as a potassium chloride solution (a 10 per cent solution of potassium chloride contains 6.5 mmol of potassium in 5 ml)

OR Half-strength Hartmann's solution in 2.5 per cent glucose.

(c) For long-continued maintenance on IV fluids total parenteral feeding may be required (p. 751).

Acute dehydration syndromes

Dehydration is an inaccurate, but commonly used term and includes isotonic, hypertonic and hypotonic dehydration, according to the proportions of water and sodium lost and the resulting sodium level in the plasma and ECF (normal in isotonic, raised in hypertonic and low in hypotonic dehydration).

Accurate differentiation between these three conditions is important, since inappropriate treatment is either dangerous (fits in hypertonic dehydration) or ineffective (hypotonic dehydration).

TABLE 10.IV
Diagnosis of dehydration syndromes* (Table modified from Brusilow and Cooke, 1964)

	Isotonic (plasma Na normal)	*Hypertonic (plasma Na >150 mmol/l)*	*Hypotonic (plasma Na <130 mmol/l)*
Skin colour†	Grey	Grey	Grey
Temperature of extremities† (big toe and tip of nose)	Cold	Cold or hot	Cold
Skin elasticity (turgor)	Reduced	Thickened and rubbery	Much reduced
Fontanelle	Depressed	Depressed	Depressed
Heart rate	Rapid	Moderately rapid	Rapid
Blood pressure	Low	Moderately low	Very low
Mental state	Lethargic, confused or stuporous	Hyperirritability alternating with stupor	Coma

* Severe degree assumed for each syndrome
† Signs of shock

Isotonic dehydration (Normal plasma sodium level)

Isotonic dehydration occurs when there is an approximately equal deficit of water and sodium causing an initial contraction of the ECF followed by a relatively late reduction in plasma volume and reduction in glomerular filtration rate with raised urea and metabolic acidosis. Common causes in childhood are gastroenteritis, diabetes mellitus, intestinal obstruction, heat exhaustion, dengue haemorrhagic fever (p. 575).

RECOGNITION

Assessment of the degree of water and sodium deficit. The immediate pre-illness weight should give an accurate indication of actual weight loss, but this is seldom reliable, due to inaccurate recall and variation between different scales. A clinical assessment is preferable (Table 10.V).

MANAGEMENT
    (a) The decision to give oral or intravenous fluids is rarely a difficult one: all children assessed as having moderate or severe dehydration should have IV fluids. Mild cases (5 per cent weight loss or less) may tolerate oral fluids, but persistent refusal of feeds, vomiting or diarrhoea requires a change to the IV route.
    (b) Choice of fluids:
        (i) Oral treatment: a hypotonic solution of sodium and potassium chloride, sodium lactate or bicarbonate and glucose should be used at 100 to 150 ml per kg per day for 24 hours,

TABLE 10.V
Clinical assessment of isotonic dehydration *

| | Early reversible shock | | Late reversible shock | Refractory |
	Mild	Moderate	Severe	shock with DIC
Mucous membranes (mouth)	Dry	Very dry	Coated	
Skin elasticity† (turgor)	Normal,** or slightly reduced	Reduced	Much reduced	
Fontanelle†	Normal or slightly depressed	Depressed	Much depressed	
% loss of body weight	5%	10%	15%	
Deficit in ml/kg	50 ml	100 ml	150 ml	

* For other vital signs (peripheral circulation etc.) see Table 10.I
† Difficulties in assessing skin elasticity and fontanelle: see notes, page 91
** A change in facial appearance ('sunken eyes', 'eyes at the back of the head') can often only be appreciated by those familiar with the child's normal appearance

followed by half-strength milk feeds. (*See* page 401 for management of gastroenteritis with oral fluids)

(ii) Intravenous: initially 0.9 per cent NaCl in 5 per cent glucose should be used, except in severe shock, when plasma (or equivalent) should be used from the beginning. If shock is still present after 1 hour at an appropriate rate of 0.9 per cent NaCl in 5 per cent glucose, plasma should be substituted. If shock is still present after 4 hours of treatment, or no urine has been passed (confirm anuria by catheter or bladder puncture), the management and treatment require assessment and critical review. For repair solution, 0.45 per cent NaCl in 2.5 per cent glucose is the most useful. For maintenance: 0.18 per cent NaCl in 4 per cent glucose.

(c) Rate and volume of fluids (Table 10.VI).

(i) Oral (*see* page 402).

(ii) Intravenous.

Period I: (0–4 hours): During the first hour (0–1 hours) fluid should be given rapidly according to Table 10.VI; during the next 3 hours (1–4 hours) the rate is halved. Half the calculated deficit should be replaced during Period I (0–4 hours).

Period II: (4–9 hours): The remaining deficit should be replaced over the next 5 hours (4–9 hours). 0.9 per cent NaCl in 5 per cent should be continued or replaced by 0.45 per cent NaCl in 2.5 per cent according to plasma-sodium level and water requirement. Persisting metabolic acidosis or electrolyte disorder should be corrected.

Period III (9–24 hours): Maintenance rate should be started using maintenance fluid (normally 0.18 per cent NaCl in 4 per cent glucose). Further adjustments in electrolyte disorders, particularly potassium deficit, may be necessary in long-standing diarrhoea, diabetes mellitus and in protein-energy malnutrition.

After 24 hours: diluted oral feeds should be started and IV fluids proportionately reduced.

TABLE 10.VI
Isotonic dehydration: rate and volume of IV infusion

Severity % loss of body weight	Deficit	Period I		Period II 4–8 (or 9) hours	Period III 8 (or 9)–24 hours
		0–1 hours	1–4 hours		
Mild (5%)	50 ml/kg	10 ml/kg	20 ml/kg	25 ml/kg (4 hours)	100 ml/kg (16 hours)
		(10 ml/kg/h)	(6 ml/kg/h)	(6 ml/kg/h)	(6 ml/kg/h)
Moderate (10%)	100 ml/kg	20 ml/kg	30 ml/kg	50 ml/kg (5 hours)	90 ml/kg (15 hours)
		(20 ml/kg/h)	(10 ml/kg/h)	(10 ml/kg/h)	(6 ml/kg/h)
Severe (15%)	150 ml/kg	30–40 ml/kg	45 ml/kg	75 ml/kg (5 hours)	90 ml/kg (15 hours)
		(30–40 ml/ kg/h)	(15 ml/kg/h)	(15 ml/kg/h)	(6 ml/kg/h)

Note: Maintenance rates quoted are at 150 ml/kg, but will be less for older children (*see* Appendix 3, page 747)

EXAMPLE (*Figure 10.2*)

10-kg infant with 10% isotonic dehydration: plasma sodium normal, plasma urea 16 mmol/l (100 mg/100 ml), bicarbonate 17 mmol/l
Total deficit = 10kg × 10% = 1000 ml (100 ml/kg)

Period I: Replace half initial deficit (500 ml) over 4 hours
0–1 hours: 20 ml/kg/h = *200 ml over 1 hour*
1–4 hours: 10 ml/kg/h = *300 ml over 3 hours*
$\qquad\qquad\qquad = 100\ ml/h$

Fluid: 0.9% NaCl in 5% glucose:
(0.9% NaCl without glucose in diabetes mellitus)

Period II (4–9 hours): Replace remaining 500 ml over 5 hours
Rate: 10 ml/kg/h = *100 ml/h*
Fluid: 0.9% NaCl in 5% glucose; or 0.45% NaCl in 2.5% glucose if plasma sodium rises above 140 mmol/litre or water losses are excessive.

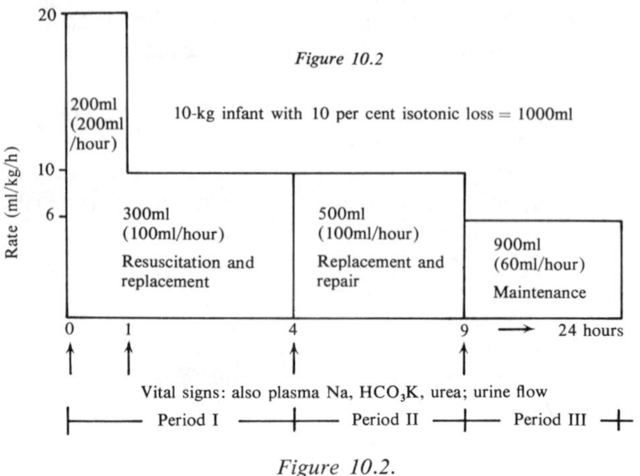

Figure 10.2.

Period III (9–24 hours): Volume 150 ml/kg/24 h
Rate: 6 ml/kg/h: 900 ml over 15 hours = *60 ml/h*
Fluid: 0.18% NaCl in 4% glucose

Hypertonic (hypernatraemic) dehydration (plasma sodium > 150 mmol per litre)

Hypertonic dehydration develops when there is a disproportionate loss of water compared to sodium, or less commonly, when a hypertonic sodium salt has been given. The increased osmolality of the plasma and ECF withdraws water from the brain cells (and other cells elsewhere) causing intracellular dehydration and shrinkage which may cause diffuse haemorrhage or bleeding from distorted dural sinuses. Fits occurring *before* treatment are usually due to one or other form of haemorrhage. Fits occurring *after* starting treatment are likely to be due to re-entry of water into the brain cells when the osmolality of the plasma and ECF is lowered. This is really a form of water-intoxication occurring at normal or supra-normal sodium levels. Plasma volume is maintained until a late stage and shock is only seen in severe cases.

Common causes in childhood are gastroenteritis with continued high sodium intake, hyperventilation, heat stroke, water deprivation, extensive burns; iatrogenic causes are the use of enemas containing hyperosmolar salts solution, 'Gastrografin' in radiology or in the treatment of meconium ileus, accidental salt poisoning (Saunders, Balfe and Laski, 1976).

RECOGNITION

The diagnosis should be considered in an infant with. any of the conditions given above and particularly in cases of diarrhoea and vomiting, in which the skin feels firm and rubbery, with alternating irritability and stupor or hyperventilation. A tense and bulging fontanelle may indicate intracranial haemorrhage (*see above*), or meningitis. Head retraction may occur without intracranial complications. In severe cases DIC may develop.

MANAGEMENT

Repeated estimations of the plasma sodium are essential and the level should not be allowed to fall more rapidly than 15 mmol per litre per day (Potter, 1973). There are numerous schemes of treatment, all having the object of lowering the plasma sodium sufficiently slowly to avoid fits.

Period I (0–4 hours)

(a) Severe shock and hypotension are rare, unless DIC is present, and therefore an initially rapid expansion of plasma volume is rarely necessary.

(b) In most cases an initial deficit of 50 ml per kg should be assumed; half of this deficit (25 ml per kg or 6 ml per kg per hour) should be replaced during the first four hours.

(c) Fluid: this is controversial. Plasma should be given, as above, in the first four hours if there is severe shock. Otherwise 0.9 per cent NaCl *without glucose* should be used. Either of these resuscitation fluids have a plasma-sodium concentration which is likely to be lower than that of the child's plasma sodium and ECF. Hyperglycaemia is common in the early stages; INSULIN SHOULD NEVER BE USED.

Period II (4–8 hours)

(a) Replace the remaining deficit of 25 ml per kg at the same rate as Period I (6 ml per kg per hour).

(b) Repeat the plasma-sodium level at the beginning of Period II and change to 0.45 per cent NaCl in 2.5 per cent glucose if the plasma sodium is < 150 mmol per litre.

Period III (8–24 hours)

Maintenance fluids should be used if the plasma-sodium level is < 150 mmol per litre; otherwise 0.45 per cent NaCl in 2.5 per cent glucose should be used as in Period II.

COMPLICATIONS

(a) Fits before intravenous treatment (*see* page 98). If the fontanelle is bulging or if there is head retraction, bilateral subdural taps should be done. A lumbar puncture should only be done if

the subdural taps show no fluid, there is a strong possibility of meningitis, and there is no papilloedema.
(b) Fits during IV treatment. These are difficult to control; phenobarbitone is usually useless and may depress respiration; diazepam IV (p. 318) should be used initially, followed by IV mannitol (p. 323) if the fits continue. Mannitol should only be used if there is already an adequate output of urine. Treatment with hypertonic saline may be tried, as for water intoxication (p. 130).
(c) Severe hypernatraemia due to salt poisoning (salt in place of sugar in the infant's feeds) may show higher plasma-sodium levels than are usually seen in hypernatraemia from other causes. Saunders, Balfe and Laski (1976) described an infant with a plasma sodium of 200 mmol per litre and suggested treatment with peritoneal dialysis, using a dialysis fluid with a sodium content of 140 mmol per litre and a glucose content of not more than 4.25 per cent (Dianeal, *Baxter-Travenol*).
(d) Disseminated intravascular coagulation (*see* page 482).

Hypotonic (hyponatraemic) dehydration (plasma sodium < 130 mmol per litre)

Hypotonic dehydration occurs when the loss of sodium is relatively greater than that of water.

RECOGNITION
Common causes in childhood are, hypoadrenal states, cystic fibrosis, and heat exhaustion.

Contraction of ECF and plasma volume quickly occurs and shock develops correspondingly early. It is important to determine whether the sodium is being lost or retained by the kidney; at a plasma level of <130 mmol per litre the sodium content of the urine should be <25 mmol per litre if the kidney is conserving sodium, whereas in renal salt-losing states the urine-sodium content will be >30 mmol per litre.

MANAGEMENT
(1) Salt-retaining steroids should be given if there is a possibility of adrenal insufficiency (p. 454).
(2) Fluids: vomiting and, to a lesser extent, diarrhoea are common and IV fluids should be given in all cases in which there is loss of skin elasticity or shock.
Period I (0–4 hours)
0–1 hours: if shock is present a 10 per cent deficit should be assumed and 0.9 per cent NaCl in 5 per cent glucose should be given at 20 ml per kg per hour.

1–4 hours: if shock persists, plasma should be given, otherwise 0.9 per cent NaCl in 5 per cent glucose should be continued at 10 ml per kg per hour.

Period II (4–9 hours)

If the plasma sodium is < 130 mmol per litre, 0.9 per cent NaCl in 5 per cent glucose should be continued: if the plasma sodium is normal, 0.45 per cent NaCl in 2.5 per cent glucose can be started. The rate should be 10 ml per kg per hour.

DO NOT GIVE POTASSIUM CONTAINING FLUIDS IF THERE IS ADRENAL INSUFFICIENCY.

Period III (9–24 hours)

If salt loss has been controlled and the sodium and water deficit have been replaced, maintenance fluids should be given at maintenance rates: for infants requiring 150 ml per kg per 24 hours this would be 6 ml per kg per hour.

Note: Hyponatraemia associated with *excess* water is considered under Water Intoxication (p. 130) and requires completely different treatment.

Acute loss of blood or plasma

Acute blood loss

RECOGNITION

If the source or site of the bleeding is obvious it may be possible to estimate the amount of blood lost, but this is rarely possible except at operation.

Symptoms depend upon the age of the child.

(a) Newborn (for causes in the newborn *see* page 652)

The site of the bleeding may not be obvious and haemorrhagic shock at delivery is easily mistaken for hypoxia. In haemorrhagic shock there is no apnoea but the respiration may be sighing, gasping or irregular, with hypothermia and feeble heart sounds. Tachycardia may change to bradycardia in extreme cases.

(b) Other age groups

Restlessness, anxiety, skin pallor and hypotension are the usual symptoms (*see also* Tables 10.I and 10.II for assessment of degree of shock and blood loss).

Acute blood loss may occur in the following conditions:

(i) External blood loss; trauma, damage to a major vessel.

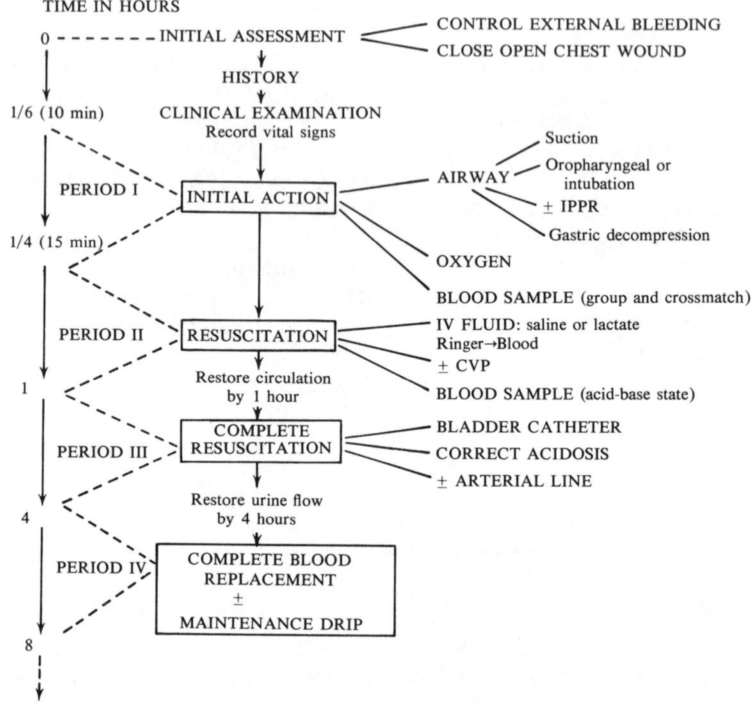

Figure 10.3

(ii) Bleeding into the intestinal tract (p. 398).

(iii) Bleeding into a closed cavity or organ; peritoneal, pleural, or pericardial cavities, wall of the intestine, skull, kidney, adrenal gland.

(iv) Bleeding into the tissues: multiple trauma, lungs, giant haemangioma, multiple haemorrhages in thrombocytopenia or DIC, retroperitoneal haemorrhage from any cause.

(v) Acute haemolysis, especially in glucose-6-phosphate dehydrogenase deficiency. (G-6PD deficiency).

MANAGEMENT

(1) Identify the site, source, and cause of the bleeding.

(2) Arrest obvious haemorrhage.

(3) Estimate the degree of shock and amount of blood lost (Tables 10.I, 10.II). *Figure 10.4* gives a semi-pictorial representation of the

blood volume at different ages, assuming one blood bottle contains 540 ml.

(4) Investigate the possibility, where appropriate, of a coagulation defect, thrombocytopenia or DIC (p. 482).

(5) Take blood for Hb%, haematocrit, blood grouping and crossmatching. If dextran is to be given blood *must* be taken beforehand.

(6) Record vital signs (Table 10.I, p. 87).

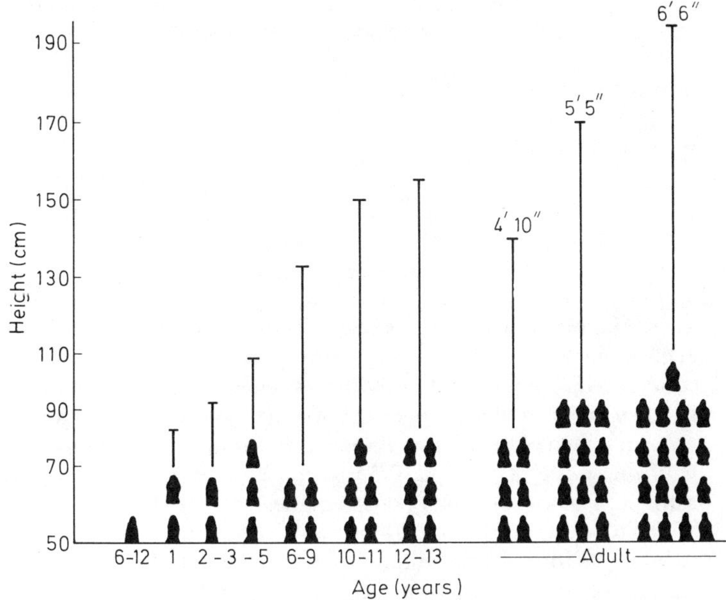

Figure 10.4. Variations in blood volume, measured in bottles, with age and size of patient. (London, 1968. Reproduced by kind permission)

(a) Severe blood loss: loss of 40 ml per kg or 40 to 50 per cent of blood volume. Children with severe thoracoabdominal injuries may require up to 300 per cent of their blood volume (Steward and Creighton, 1975); when using very large volumes of blood a central venous pressure (CVP) line should be used, and possible bleeding or coagulation disorders should be expected due to thrombocytopenia or reduction in the labile plasma factors V and VIII.

0–4 hours   During the first hour (0–1 hours) group O Rhesus negative blood may be given, setting up emergency and routine crossmatching at the same time, or blood of the patient's own group can be given after rapid blood grouping. Alternatively, the most quickly available plasma expander, 0.9 per cent NaCl in 5 per cent glucose, or lactate Ringer can be given. Crossmatching against blood of the appropriate group should also be set up.

Rate: 20 ml per kg per hour.

At 1 to 2 hours formally crossmatched blood should be available and should be given from 1 to 4 hours at half the initial rate (i.e. 10 ml per kg per hour).

4–8 hours   Blood should be continued at 10 ml per kg per hour until the estimated blood loss has been replaced and *shock has been relieved*.

Blood transfusion should be continued if:

   (i) Shock is still present.

   (ii) Blood loss is continuing.

   (iii) Operation is required within the next few hours.

   If the child's condition is satisfactory after replacement of blood loss, maintenance fluid should be started at maintenance rate if it is necessary to keep the drip going.

8–24 hours   Maintenance as required.

(b) Moderate blood loss: loss of 25 to 30 ml per kg or 20 to 30 per cent of blood volume. As for severe blood loss, but the initial resuscitation should be done with 0.9 per cent NaCl in 5 per cent glucose at 15 ml per kg per hour for the first hour, changing to crossmatched blood at 1 to 2 hours and continuing with blood at half the initial rate (i.e. 7.5 ml per kg per hour) until the estimated blood loss has been replaced.

(c) Slight blood loss: loss of 20 ml per kg or 20 per cent of blood volume; as for moderate blood loss, but the initial resuscitation should be done at the rate of 10 ml per kg per hour, and subsequently at 5 to 6 ml per kg per hour, until the estimated blood loss has been replaced.

Note: In acute haemolysis packed or sedimented cells should be used in place of whole blood.

EXAMPLE (*Figure 10.5*)

10-kg infant with moderate degree of blood loss; estimated blood loss of 25 ml per kg or 30 per cent of blood volume = 250 ml.

Acute plasma loss

RECOGNITION

Common causes in childhood are burns, extensive angio-oedema or

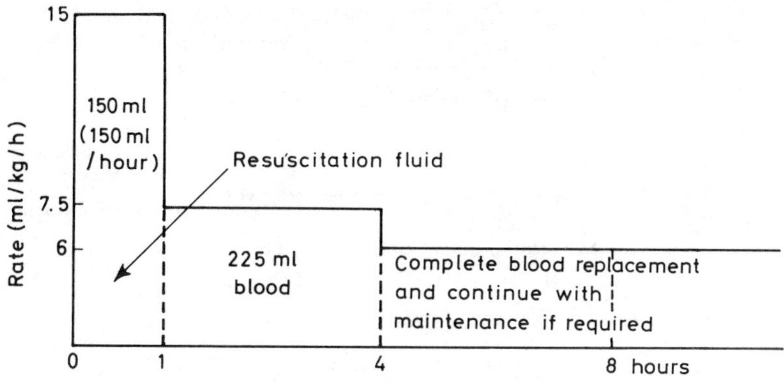

Figure 10.5

urticaria, sudden accumulation of protein-containing fluid in the peritoneal or pleural cavities, or into an oedematous or obstructed bowel.

MANAGEMENT

In the initial resuscitation, replacement of the lost plasma is of course
essential; but in burns, angio-oedema and urticaria, allowance must be
made for the return of the plasma to the circulation when the acute
episode is over.

Burns

For the general management *see* Chapter 4. For purposes of comparison with other forms of shock the resuscitation of a patient with an
extensive burn is described in the same terms as previously used.

This resuscitation scheme is based upon the Mount Vernon formula
(Muir and Barclay, 1974). Plasma is given in five blocks during *the first
24 hours* and one block from 24 to 36 hours; each block consists of the
same *volume* of fluid. The volume to be given during the *first 24 hours* is
calculated as follows:

$$\% \text{ burn} \times \text{body weight in kg} \times 2.5$$

that is, the volume during each block is

$$\frac{\% \text{ burn} \times \text{body weight in kg}}{2}$$

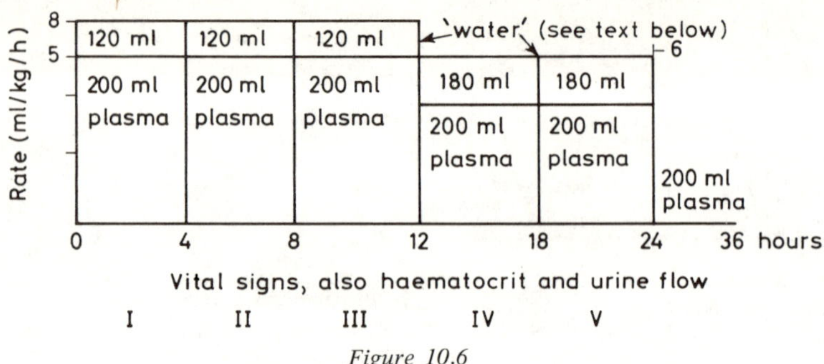

Figure 10.6

Water is given at the rate of 2–3 ml per kg per hour initially, as 5 per cent glucose, or 0.18 per cent NaCl in 4 per cent glucose. The exact amount of water and sodium given depends upon the type of local treatment. Exposure treatment causes considerable evaporative losses while silver nitrate causes large losses of sodium chloride, necessitating maintenance fluid with 0.45 per cent NaCl in 2.5 per cent glucose or 0.9 per cent NaCl in 5 per cent glucose. (*See* Table 4.I)

EXAMPLE (*Figure 10.6*)

10-kg infant with 40 per cent burns.
Plasma replacement during the first 24 hours will be:

$$40 \times 10 \times 2.5 = 1000 \text{ ml } (100 \text{ ml/kg})$$

or 200 ml per block period = 5 ml per kg per hour for the first 3 periods of 4 hours.

Acute angio-oedema and urticaria

    (i) Severe shock requires resuscitation with plasma at 10 to 20 ml per kg per hour for the first hour, followed by plasma at half the initial rate up to 4 hours.

    (ii) For anaphylactic shock, *see* page 111.
        For hereditary angio-oedema, *see* page 494.

Hypovolaemic shock in nephrotic syndrome

Shock in the nephrotic syndrome occurs in two situations:

    (i) A sudden accumulation of oedema with resulting isotonic expansion of the ECF and a corresponding reduction in the plasma volume. There is oliguria with a moderately raised blood urea.

(ii) Hypovolaemia with severe hyponatraemia, usually due to prolonged dietary restriction of sodium with the repeated use of
natriuretic (salt-losing) diuretics such as frusemide.

MANAGEMENT
(a) Sudden oedema. Plasma (or ideally salt-poor albumen) should
be given at 10 ml per kg per hour for up to 4 hours; the urinary
output should be carefully measured during this period. Concentrated solutions of plasma and albumen are potentially dangerous since they may cause left-ventricular failure, due to the rapid
re-entry of oedema fluid into the circulation. *Diuretics are
contra-indicated since they cause further reduction of plasma
volume.*
(b) Hyponatraemia. Diuretics are again contra-indicated; since
there is usually oedema, the sodium should be supplied in a small
volume as 5 per cent NaCl (page 132 for dose). Plasma may also
be required if the plasma albumen is very low, but salt-poor
albumen is obviously not indicated.

Endotoxic (Septic) shock

Shock may occur with a variety of bloodstream invasions (parasites,
fungi, rickettsiae, viruses as well as bacteria; but bacterial toxins are the
most important and frequent cause of shock. Gram-positive organisms
such as clostridia, staphylococci, streptococci and pneumococci can
occasionally cause shock (staphylococcal toxins can cause a fulminating diarrhoea) in various ways, but these organisms are readily elimi-
nated with antibiotics. Antibiotic treatment of Gram-negative organisms, particularly the bacilli, is much less effective and the shock is
difficult to reverse.

GRAM-NEGATIVE SEPTIC SHOCK
The usual causative organisms are: *E. coli, Klebsiella aerobacter,*
Proteus group, *Pseudomonas aeruginosa,* Bacteroides, and less commonly Serratia marcescens and related organisms. Though there is
some doubt as to the mechanism of shock production in meningococcal
septicaemia it should be treated in the same way as in shock due to
Gram-negative bacilli, as there is a high incidence of DIC in severe
cases. (Hardaway, 1968b).

RECOGNITION
(a) Newborn and young infants: *see* pages 633–634.
(b) All other age groups: initial symptoms may be high temperature,
rigors, hyperventilation, warm dry skin.

Late symptoms: vasoconstriction, peripheral cyanosis, hypotension, with evidence of DIC in severe cases.

(c) The diagnosis should be suspected if there is a sudden deterioration or change in the clinical condition in the following situations:

Burns.

Patients with indwelling bladder or intravenous catheters.

Immunosuppressed patients on treatment for leukaemia or malignant disease.

Children with other (often congenital) forms of immunological deficiencies.

Note: (a) A leucopenia may be secondary to the infection itself.

(b) Severely neutropenic individuals cannot make normal amounts of pus.

MANAGEMENT

(a) Any obvious source of infection such as an indwelling catheter should be removed and cultured. Adherent pus should be examined by Gram film.

(b) Other localized infection (abscess, cellulitis, osteitis, pneumonia, meningitis) should be sought.

(c) Blood, urine, sputum, CSF should be obtained and examined and cultured.

(d) Treatment of shock:

(i) IV fluids: 0.9 per cent NaCl in 5 per cent glucose should be used initially at the rate of 15 to 20 ml per kg per hour for $\frac{1}{2}$ to 1 hour followed by plasma at half the initial rate for the next 3 hours. Subsequent fluid therapy must be determined by the response to treatment.

(ii) Metabolic acidosis: if this persists after the initial resuscitation it should be corrected (p. 125).

(iii) Antibiotics: since it is not always certain whether the infection is due to a Gram-negative organism, the initial combination of antibiotics should have the widest possible spectrum and should be given intravenously. At the time of writing the most suitable initial combination is gentamicin with cephaloridine: alternatives to gentamicin are tobramycin, kanamycin and colistin; dosage may have to be adjusted when the blood urea is high or there is renal damage (for dosage *see* Appendix 10).

(iv) Corticosteroids: intravenous corticosteroids should be given using the following scheme:

Adults or children over 14 years initial dose: IV dexamethasone 40 mg (equivalents are methylprednisolone 200 mg or hydrocortisone 1200 mg).

Half the initial dose is given at 4 to 6-hour intervals. Treatment is stopped as soon as there is recovery from shock, but should not in any case be continued for longer than 48 hours.

Dosage for children:

(a) Scale down according to actual surface area:

e.g. dexamethasone 40 mg per 1.73 m^2 or 25 mg per m^2.

(b) 1 year 25% of ⎫
     5 year 40% of ⎬ adult dose (by surface area)
     7 year 50% of
    12 year 75% of ⎭

(c) Repeated clinical and haematological examinations should be made for DIC.

Common problems in the management of shock or dehydration

(a) The patient is still shocked 4 hours after starting appropriate intravenous treatment; the following should be considered:

  (i) Inadequate rate of transfusion initially or inadequate replacement of deficit.

  (ii) Inadequate allowance for continued losses; diarrhoea, vomiting, fluid loss from burn wounds, continued haemorrhage.

  (iii) Unrecognized complications: peritonitis, enclosed haemorrhage (within skull, pleura, pericardium, peritoneum, retroperitoneal tissues, kidney, adrenal); multipletissue haemorrhages, fat embolism (trauma).

  (iv) Failure to correct a severe or continued metabolic acidosis or electrolyte disorder.

  (v) Failure to recognize and treat appropriately the primary cause of shock, e.g. septicaemia, hypoxia, hypoadrenal state.

  (vi) Failure to recognize the water and electrolyte losses due to acute renal-tubular necrosis.

(b) Failure to pass urine 4 hours after starting appropriate intravenous treatment. The following should be considered:

  (i) Urine retained in bladder if a catheter has not been passed.

  (ii) Retention of urine in an uncatheterized bladder; due to clot, stone or crystals obstructing the bladder outlet; atonic bladder in deeply unconscious patients; unrecognized spinal damage.

  (iii) Blocked catheter.

(iv) Inadequate resuscitation (*see above*).

(v) Ruptured bladder or urethra.

(vi) Acute or chronic renal failure; pre-existing chronic renal disease.

(vii) Obstructive uropathy; bilateral renal calculi, uric-acid nephropathy during the initial treatment of acute leukaemia, pre-existing bilateral obstructive disease with exacerbation due to acute infection.

(c) Inadequate urine flow during or after resuscitation. The possibilities under (b) should also be considered; for actual urine flows as an indication of adequacy of resuscitation, definition of oliguria; *see* page 757.

References

Brusilow, S. W. and Cooke, R. E. (1964). Fluid therapy of diarrhoea and vomiting. *Pediat. Clins. N. Am.* **11 (4)**, 892

Hardaway, R. M. (1968a,b). *Clinical Management of Shock.* Chapter 4: (a) pp. 97–104, (b) p. 107. Springfield: Charles C. Thomas

London, P. S. (1968). Traumatic shock. *Br. J. Hosp. Med.* **1**, 313

Muir, I. F. K. and Barclay, T. L. (1974). *Burns and their Treatment*, 2nd edn. pp. 34–36. London: Lloyd-Luke

Potter, D. (1973). In *Pediatric Emergencies* Eds D. J. Pascoe and M. Grossman p. 193. Philadelphia: J. B. Lippincott

Saunders, N., Balfe, J. W., Laski, B. (1976). Severe salt poisoning in an infant. *J. Pediat.* **88**, 258

Steward, D. J. and Creighton, R. E. (1975). Anaesthetic management of the injured child. In *Care for the Injured Child*, pp. 29–30. Baltimore: Williams and Wilkins

Weil, M. H. and Shubin, H. (1967). *Diagnosis and Treatment of Shock.* Table 7.2, p. 118. Baltimore: Williams and Wilkins

CHAPTER 11

Anaphylactic Shock

J. A. Black

This is an extreme emergency in which immediate treatment can be life-saving. Early recognition and emergency treatment should be part of the training of all doctors and nurses. Appropriate drugs should be available on resuscitation trolleys and should be at hand in all situations where anaphylaxis could be expected.

No child should leave the premises until 30 minutes after *any* injection: children with known allergic conditions should be observed for longer.

In children the likely causes are:

(a) Penicillin and related drugs; by injection or orally.
(b) Diagnostic radiological investigations; angiography, intravenous pyelography, bronchography.
(c) Desensitization injection for asthma, hay fever.
(d) Local anaesthetics; also the IV anaesthetic alphaxalone (Althesin).
(e) Asparaginase or glutaminase injected IV in the treatment of leukaemia.
(f) Injection of immune sera: diphtheria, tetanus, etc.
(g) Blood or plasma expanders (especially dextran).
(h) Food allergies (e.g. milk, banana etc.).
(i) Insect stings: bees, wasps, hornets (*see* page 542).

RECOGNITION

(a) Early symptoms:
Apprehension, giddiness, sweating.
Itching, erythema, urticaria (local or general).
Nausea and vomiting, colic, diarrhoea.
Irritating cough.

(b) Potentially fatal symptoms:
Hypotension, circulatory failure, cardiac arrest.
Bronchial spasm.
Laryngeal oedema.

MANAGEMENT

(*a*) *During early symptoms*

(1) Stop the injection of the drug.
(2) If practicable, place a tourniquet, at a pressure sufficient to obstruct the venous return, just proximal to the site of injection and keep it in place for 20 to 30 minutes, and in any case until the acute symptoms of anaphylaxis have been relieved.
(3) Inject adrenaline (1 in 1000 $\equiv$ 0.1% $\equiv$ 1.0 mg in 1.0 ml) subcutaneously in a dose of 0.01 mg (0.01 ml) per kg (the maximum single dose is 0.5 mg $\equiv$ 0.5 ml); the site of injection should be vigorously massaged to prevent immobilization of the adrenaline at the site of injection by cutaneous vasoconstriction, with resultant delay in its action. If there is no improvement after 5 minutes, a second injection, in the same dosage, should be given. If necessary repeat injections can be given at intervals of 20 to 30 minutes, provided that there is no evidence of toxicity (palpitations, tachycardia, ventricular fibrillation, arrhythmia; *see* page 294 for treatment). Normally the maximum *total* dose should not exceed 0.5 mg (0.5 ml) unless the initial dose was 0.5 mg (0.5 ml), in which case a total dose of up to 1.0 mg (1.0 ml) may be used in children over 14 years.

(*b*) *Life-threatening symptoms* (*see* (b) *above*)

Give 1–3 as above.
(4) Maintain an adequate airway by suction, oropharyngeal airway, intubation $\pm$ IPPV, or tracheostomy, as indicated.
(5) Give oxygen as required, by the best available route.
(6) Give adrenaline IV.
   (i) Available solution: 1 in 1000 $\equiv$ 0.1% $\equiv$ 1 mg per 1.0 ml.
   (ii) *Diluted working solution:* dilute 0.5 mg (0.5 ml) in 10 ml of 5 per cent glucose in 0.9 per cent NaCl, giving a solution containing 0.05 mg (50 microgrammes) in 1.0 ml.
   (iii) Dose of diluted solution:
      0.05 mg (50 microgrammes) $\equiv$ 1.0 ml per year of age up to a maximum of 0.5 mg (500 microgrammes) = 10 ml.
   (iv) Rate of injection: give this dose over 10 minutes, preferably under visual ECG control, and stop if arrhythmia develops.

(v) Repeat injections.
The latent period between injection and effect is not more than 1 to 2 minutes, provided the venous return is adequate (massage towards the trunk may help, if an arm vein has been used) and the duration of action is between 5 and 20 minutes. It is therefore usually safe to repeat the original injection at least once after 20 minutes.

(vi) Intracardiac injection using the same dosage as for IV injection can be used if the patient is at the point of death and the venous return is clearly extremely slow.

(7) Set up an IV drip as a vehicle for drugs (*see below*) or plasma expander.

(a) If hypovolaemia is suspected, due to massive angio-oedema or urticaria, use any plasma expander, giving 20 ml per kg over 1 hour (*see also* page 93).

(b) For bronchial spasm, give aminophylline IV slowly over 30 minutes in a dose of 3 mg per kg (*see also* page 254).

(c) For persisting hypotension give metaraminol (Aramine (*Merck, Sharp & Dohme*)) IV, but DO NOT USE CONCURRENTLY WITH ADRENALINE OR UNTIL ALL ADRENALINE EFFECTS HAVE CEASED. Adrenaline and metaraminol are not interchangeable. Adrenaline has a specific anti-anaphylactic effect: metaraminol has a specific vasoconstrictor effect for hypotension. For method of use and dose of metaraminol *see* page 116. Metaraminol should be followed by, or given concurrently with, plasma expanders if shock is due to hypovolaemia.

(8) Give an antihistamine drug IV or i.m., according to the degree of urgency. The following antihistamine drugs are most commonly available for parenteral injection, and are given in order of preference.

(a) Mepyramine (Anthisan (*May & Baker*)).

(i) Available solution: 2-ml ampoules containing 2.5 per cent (25 mg in 1.0 ml).

(ii) The working solution is obtained by diluting the available solution to 10 times its original volume with sterile water for injection, giving a solution containing 2.5 mg in 1.0 ml.

(iii) Dose:
Up to 3 years: 6.25–12.5 mg.
3–7 years: 12.5–25 mg.
7–14 years: 25 mg.
Adult dose: 25–50 mg.

(iv) Rate of injection: give the required dose over 10 minutes.

(v) Repeat injection: *see below*.

OR
    (b) Chlorpheniramine, (Piriton (*Allen & Hanburys*)).
        (i) Available solution: ampoules containing 1% solution $\equiv$ 10 mg in 1.0 ml.
       (ii) Dilute as for mepyramine, giving a solution containing 1.0 mg in 1.0 ml.
      (iii) Dose: 0.25 mg per kg up to a maximum (adult) dose of 10 to 20 mg (not more than 40 mg over 24 hours).
      (iv) Rate of injection: as for mepyramine.
       (v) Repeat injection: *see below*.

OR
    (c) Promethazine (Phenergan (*May and Baker*)).
        (i) Available solution: 1-ml and 2-ml ampoules containing 2.5 per cent solution = 25 mg in 1.0 ml.
      (ii) Dilute as for mepyramine.
     (iii) Dose:
          Up to 1 year: 0.5 mg per kg.
          1–7 years: 5.0 mg.
          7–14 years: 10–25 mg.
          Adult dose: 25–50 mg.
      (iv) Rate of injection: as for mepyramine.
       (v) Repeat injection: *see below*.

(9) Give hydrocortisone (or equivalent) IV in a dose of 100 mg irrespective of age or size.

LATER MANAGEMENT:
    (a) If the response to treatment is slow, hydrocortisone should be continued by slow IV drip in a dose of 100 to 200 mg every 6 hours and the original antihistamines should be continued intramuscularly at 6 to 8-hour intervals; both drugs should be continued up to 48 hours.
    (b) In the long term, sensitive individuals should wear an information bracelet. If the risk of recurrence of anaphylaxis is great and unavoidable (e.g. insect stings), desensitization should be considered. Highly sensitive children at considerable risk should carry an inhaler containing adrenaline (p. 543) provided they clearly understand its use.

CHAPTER 12

Use of Sympathomimetic Amines in Hypotension and Shock

A. M. Wilson and J. A. Black

These drugs have an immediate but transient effect on the heart and circulation, and should ideally be used only when careful monitoring of their effect on the blood pressure and central venous pressure (CVP) is available. However it is appreciated that in sudden emergencies monitoring of the CVP is not always possible. With the exception of anaphylactic and possibly some cases of endotoxic (septic) shock, the shock usually encountered in children is likely to be due to or associated with hypovolaemia. Sympathomimetic amines it should be noted are *NO SUBSTITUTE* for the treatment of hypovolaemia but may be used in acute emergencies as a temporary measure before plasma volume can be restored.

In shock, delayed or erratic absorption of intramuscular or subcutaneous injections make the action of drugs unpredictable. The intravenous route ensures that the drug is completely absorbed and the effect can be assessed in a short time. For this reason, if vasoconstrictor drugs are to be used at all they should be given intravenously.

(a) Instructions for the use of these drugs should include:
    (i) The route of administration.
    (ii) The rate of administration.
    (iii) The exact amount of the drug in each individual dose.
    (iv) The maximum permissible total dose over a specified period.
    (v) Each dose should specify the amount of drug in mg or in microgrammes (written in full) with the volume in which this drug is contained in brackets.
    (vi) The strength of the diluted working solution should be stated in mg (or µg) per ml.
(b) Information about the drug.

The following must be written down and clearly understood:
  (i) Contra-indications.
  (ii) The latent period between IV injection and the expected effect.
  (iii) The usual duration of effect.
  (iv) Toxic effects which should be looked for, and treatment if necessary.

Predominantly vasoconstrictor drugs

Of these the most commonly used is metaraminol, but it should be clearly understood that vasoconstriction from its use may actually reduce the venous return and cardiac output unless plasma expanders are used within a few minutes of starting metaraminol. This drug should therefore be used to restore blood pressure in sudden life-threatening hypotension.

Use of metaraminol (Aramine *Merck, Sharp and Dohme*)

Contra-indications: Metaraminol should not be used concurrently with cyclopropane or halothane in which case methoxamine hydrochloride (Vasoxine, *Calmic*) should be used in the same dose as metaraminol. Neither drug should be used with monoamine oxidase inhibitors or if these have been used during the previous 2 weeks. Continuous monitoring of blood pressure, CVP and visual ECG recording should be used whenever possible.
  (a) Direct IV injection (metaraminol, methoxamine)
      (i) Available solution: 1-ml ampoules of 1 per cent = 10 mg in 1 ml (metaraminol or methoxamine) 10-ml vials of 1 per cent (metaraminol).
      (ii) Diluted working solution: dilute 1.0 ml in 20 ml of 5 per cent glucose or 0.9 per cent NaCl, giving a 0.05 per cent solution = 0.5 mg (500 microgrammes) in 1.0 ml.
      (iii) Latent period after IV injection: 1–2 minutes.
      (iv) Duration of effect: 20–60 minutes.
      (v) The initial dose is 0.25 mg = 250 microgrammes (0.5 ml) or 0.5 mg = 500 microgrammes (1.0 ml) according to the size of the child.
      (vi) Second dose: if there is no effect from the first dose, the same dose is repeated after 5 to 10 minutes.
      (vii) Further doses may be repeated at intervals of 20 minutes or longer, but if prolonged use is necessary, a continuous IV infusion should be used.

(b) Continuous IV infusion.
    (i) Available solution: concentration of 1 per cent = 10 mg in 1.0 ml.
    (ii) The working solution should be obtained by diluting 15 mg (1.5 ml) of the available solution in 500 ml of 5 per cent glucose or 0.9 per cent NaCl = 0.03 mg (30 microgrammes) in 1.0 ml.
    (iii) The diluted solution is given at a rate adjusted to maintain the blood pressure at the desired level.
    (iv) Stopping metaraminol: an infusion should not be stopped abruptly and the blood pressure should be continuously or repeatedly recorded for 2 to 3 hours after stopping the drug in order to detect any recurrence of hypotension.

Toxic effects:

Ventricular extrasystoles; sinus or ventricular tachycardia, cardiac arrhythmias, including ventricular fibrillation, excessive hypertension.

Treatment of arrhythmias

(a) Lignocaine hydrochloride may be used to abolish cardiac arrhythmias produced by sympathomimetic drugs. Special 'cardiac' solutions are available but in an emergency the local anaesthesia preparations may be used. *Plain* lignocaine, without adrenaline, must be used.

Dose: Available as 0.5 per cent (5 mg per ml) 1 per cent (10 mg per ml) and 2 per cent (20 mg per ml). Dilute to 1 mg per ml in 0.9 per cent NaCl and give 1 to 2 mg per min IV until the arrhythmia is brought under control (Wood-Smith, Vickers and Stewart, 1973).

Precaution: Lignocaine should be used with extreme care if the required dose approaches 3 mg per kg. Higher doses may be necessary but convulsions may be caused: the prodromal signs are twitching and restlessness.

(b) β-blocking drugs (β-receptor antagonist) such as practolol (Eraldin) may be more appropriate to overcome the effect of an overdose of a β-stimulating drug such as adrenaline and isoprenaline and metaraminol and methoxamine (Johnston, 1970).

Practolol (Eraldin) is available in 5-ml ampoules containing 10 ml (2 mg per ml).

Dose:

Under 5 years: 0.5 mg IV

Over 5 years: 1 mg IV and repeat after 10 minutes, up to a maximum of 10 mg.

ECG control of anti-arrhythmia drugs is essential.

Should ventricular extrasystoles proceed to ventricular tachycardia or ventricular fibrillation, defibrillation will be required. Defibrillation is likely to be successful only if the patient is well oxygenated by effective artificial ventilation, has a normal temperature, and a normal hydrogen-ion concentration. Sodium bicarbonate (8.4%) at a dose of 1 mmol per kg per minute of cariac arrest should be given while external cardiac massage (ECM) is performed. Efforts should be made to prevent cooling.

The contact parts of the defibrillator should be placed one on the front and one at the back of the chest to ensure that the current passes through the heart. After taking appropriate safety precautions a first shock may be given.

$$\left.\begin{array}{l} \text{dc JOULES} = \text{age in years} \times 10 \\ \text{ac VOLTS} = \text{age in years} \times 25 \end{array}\right\} \quad \text{for the first shock}$$

After an unsuccessful shock a further period of ECM is given before a stronger shock.

Predominantly vasodilator drugs

Isoprenaline (isoproterenol) is the most commonly used. This has a predominantly vasodilator effect on the peripheral circulation and has a stimulant effect on the myocardium. Its main use is to increase tissue perfusion when there is severe shut-down of the microcirculation. Uncontrolled vasodilation produces a catastrophic drop in central venous pressure and aggravates shock. Vasodilation should only be induced when one can titrate it against the central venous pressure and the vascular bed can be rapidly filled as it opens (Shandling, 1975). General opinion suggests that the greatest use of isoprenaline is in refractory endotoxic (septic) shock.

Use of Isoprenaline (Isuprel, Suscardia *Pharmax*)

Contra-indication: as for metaraminol.

Use continuous monitoring of blood pressure, CVP and visual ECG recording whenever possible.
Available solution: 2-ml ampoules of 1 in 1000 solution = 0.1 per cent = 1 mg in 1.0 ml.
  (a) For single injections IV, dilute 0.2 mg (200 microgrammes) = 0.2 ml in 20 ml of 5 per cent glucose or 0.9 per cent NaCl giving a solution of 0.01 mg (10 microgrammes) per 1.0 ml. Single dose: 10 microgrammes per year of age given over 3 minutes.

(b) For continuous infusion, 2 mg (2000 microgrammes) = 2 ml of available solution is diluted in 500 ml of IV solution, giving a working solution of 0.004 mg (4 microgrammes) in 1.0 ml. Rate of infusion: initially 0.05 microgrammes per kg per minute, increasing to a maximum of 0.5 microgrammes per kg per minute. (Grossman, 1973).
Toxic effects: Tachycardia, palpitations, cardiac arrhythmia, and ventricular fibrillation.
Treatment: As for metaraminol.

Dopamine (Intropin *Arnar-Stone*)

The use of this drug has been suggested for the treatment of shock and in low-output states. It stimulates myocardial contraction, produces vasoconstriction but causes coeliac, mesenteric and renal artery dilatation.

Dopamine is available in 5-ml ampoules containing 200 mg of dopamine hydrochloride (40 mg per ml).

Suggested dilution: transfer the contents of a 5-ml ampoule containing 200 mg of dopamine to 250 ml or 500 ml of any of the usual IV sodium chloride or glucose solutions (5 per cent glucose, 0.9 per cent NaCl in 5 per cent glucose, lactate Ringer) but it should not be added to sodium bicarbonate or other alkaline solutions.

These dilutions will produce the following concentrations:
250 ml dilution: 800 μg (microgrammes) per ml.
500 ml dilution: 400 μg (microgrammes) per ml.

Dopamine is given as an IV infusion at a rate of 5 to 10 μg per kg per minute controlled by the response of the blood pressure to treatment. An increase in urine flow indicates a favourable response.

Contra-indications

(a) Patients who are receiving treatment with monoamine oxidase inhibitors or who have received these drugs within the previous 2 weeks.
(b) In the presence of uncorrected arrhythmias or ventricular fibrillation.
(c) Concurrent use with cyclopropane or halothane.

References

Grossman, M. (1973). Septic shock. In *Pediatric Emergencies,* p. 240. Eds D. J. Pascoe and M. Grossman. Philadelphia: J. B. Lippincott

Johnston, M. (1970). Reflections on Beta-adrenergic blockade in anaesthetics. *Br. J. Anaesth.* **42**. 262

Shandling, B. (1975). Haemorrhage and shock. In *Care of the Injured Child.* p. 13. The Surgical Staff. the Hospital for Sick Children, Toronto: Baltimore: Williams and Wilkins

Wood-Smith, F. G.. Vickers. M. D. and Stewart. H. C. (1973). *Drugs in Anaesthetic Practice.* 4th edn. p. 238. London: Butterworths

Part III: Acidosis and Electrolyte Disorders

CHAPTER 13

Acidosis and Electrolyte Disorders

J. A. Black

Acidosis

An acidosis may require treatment as part of resuscitation in an acute emergency such as cardiorespiratory arrest, or in conditions of acid overload in metabolic disorders.

When an acidosis should be assumed or suspected

(a) A respiratory acidosis can be assumed in all cases of acutely developing respiratory insufficiency in which the pCO_2 has risen above normal. If there is accompanying hypoxia, there will be metabolic acidosis in addition. An acute respiratory acidosis can only be corrected by improved ventilation.

(b) A metabolic acidosis can be assumed to be present in all states of shock, cardiorespiratory arrest and hypoxia.

(c) A metabolic acidosis should be suspected when there is an increase in rate and depth of respiration without cardiac or pulmonary cause, or in the newborn, when the infant becomes lethargic in the absence of any demonstrable infection.

Acidosis in the acute emergency (a single reversible incident)

PATHOPHYSIOLOGY

(i) Complete cessation of all pulmonary gas exchange causes the H^+ concentration to rise at the rate of 10 to 12 nmol per litre per minute (a fall of 0.1 pH units), and the pCO_2 to rise at 2.6 kPa (20 mm Hg) per minute: oxygen stores are completely depleted by 3 to 4 minutes (Swyer, 1975).

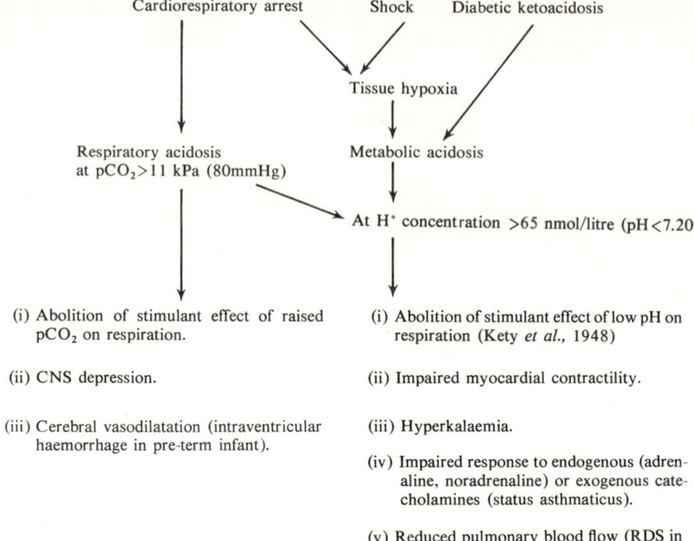

Figure 13.1. Acute acidosis

(ii) The results of an acutely developing acidosis are given in *Figure 13.1*; certain specific conditions are shown in brackets.

(iii) These disorders impair the response to resuscitation, but it is impossible to correct a progressively increasing respiratory or metabolic acidosis with the continued accumulation of hydrogen ion unless the primary condition is reversed at the same time.

(iv) It follows that the dose of alkali should be calculated to lower the H$^+$ concentration (raise the pH) to a level at which normal responses are restored. This is equivalent to an H$^+$ concentration of 50 to 55 nmol per litre (pH 7.25–7.30). Complete correction is unnecessary and may risk the production of a metabolic alkalosis when the primary condition is treated simultaneously.

THE CHOICE OF ALKALI IN AN ACUTE PROGRESSIVE ACIDOSIS

(i) Acute respiratory acidosis

Though Tham buffer has been recommended in acute respiratory acidosis, the amount of CO_2 which it can bind is trivial in the presence of a continuously rising pCO_2 without ventilation. There are additional difficulties in its use since the dose is difficult to calculate and the freshly prepared solution is unstable and must be used within a few hours of preparation. The solution may cause spasm of vein or artery, and tissue sloughing if there is extravasation. Side-effects include apnoea and hypoglycaemia which make it particularly unsuitable for use in the newborn. The advantage that an intracellular acidosis, as well as the extracellular acidosis, can be corrected is a largely theoretical one in an acute emergency. The use of Tham is not recommended. Sodium bicarbonate may be used to produce partial correction of a pure respiratory acidosis where the pH is at a lethal level (*see below*).

(*ii*) *Acute metabolic acidosis*

Sodium bicarbonate, lactate, citrate and occasionally acetate have been used for the correction of a metabolic acidosis. Apart from sodium bicarbonate, the other salts depend for their effect upon their conversion to sodium bicarbonate by the liver. Since in many acute emergencies there is an excess of lactate already and the metabolic functions of the liver may be impaired, the use of these salts is not recommended.

THE USE OF SODIUM BICARBONATE IN METABOLIC ACIDOSIS
Sodium bicarbonate itself has a number of disadvantages.

   (i) The commonly recommended 8.4 per cent solution, which conveniently contains 1 mmol of $NaHCO_3$ in each 1.0 ml of the solution, is a highly irritant solution which is hyperosmolar and which should be diluted before injection.

  (ii) The more stable emergency solutions of sodium bicarbonate (such as the 5 and 4 per cent solutions) are also highly irritant and hyperosmolar and should be diluted in an equal volume of 5 per cent or 10 per cent glucose: each injection should be given slowly over not less than one minute.

 (iii) The rapid injection of a large amount of hyperosmolar bicarbonate intravenously may cause a bolus of highly alkaline fluid to reach the myocardium or medullary centres, and the rapid increase in osmolality of the extracellular fluid (ECF) results in withdrawal of water from the brain, with a risk of intraventricular or diffuse haemorrhage, particularly in the pre-term infant.

     According to Finberg (1967) the maximum safe change in osmolality is 25 mosmol per kg of body water over 4 hours, but other data suggest that infants can tolerate smaller increases in osmolality over short periods; an IV injection of $NaHCO_3$ given over 5 minutes at a dose of 3 to 4 mmol per kg body weight will cause a rise of between 7.5 and 20 mosmol per kg body water

within 5 minutes of completing the injection (Siegel *et al.*, 1973; Baum and Roberton, 1975). A safe initial correction of an assumed base deficit of 5 mmol per litre in the absence of actual information on the acid-base states (*as in the apnoeic newborn infant*) would be 1.5 mmol per kg body weight of $NaHCO_3$ (1.5 ml per kg of 8.4 per cent $NaHCO_3$) given not faster than 1 mmol per minute (1 ml of 8.4 per cent $NaHCO_3$ per minute). *
To correct a known base deficit of 10 mmol per litre will require 3 ml of 8.4 per cent $NaHCO_3$ per kg body weight.
Examples:
(1) Newborn infant with birth weight 3.3 kg:

$$ECF = 3.3 \times 0.3 \text{ litres} = 1.0 \text{ litre}$$

Initial correction of assumed base deficit of 5 mmol per litre requires 5 mmol (5 ml 8.4 per cent $NaHCO_3$) or 1.5 ml per kg body weight.
(2) Pre-term infant with birth weight of 1.5 kg would require 2.0 to 2.5 ml of 8.4 per cent $NaHCO_3$.
(iv) The correction of a metabolic acidosis may cause coma from cerebral acidosis due to rapid transfer of CO_2 across blood-brain barrier, particularly in diabetic ketoacidosis (Ohman *et al.*, 1971).

CALCULATION OF THE DOSE OF SODIUM BICARBONATE IN METABOLIC ACIDOSIS

Since overcorrection results in a metabolic alkalosis, possibly with tetany, which is very difficult to reverse, it is better to undercorrect. This is achieved either by basing the calculation on a desired level of standard bicarbonate of 15 mmol per litre, or giving half of the amount calculated to produce complete correction. Most authorities base their calculation on the assumption that the injected bicarbonate is solely distributed within the extracellular fluid, which is probably correct in acute situations. Since the proportion of ECF to the body weight in the child is greater than in the adult the volume of ECF in the child is calculated as:

$$\text{Body weight in kg} \times 0.3 = \text{ECF in litres}$$
$$\text{(for adult or adolescents 0.2 is used)}$$

The number of mmols of bicarbonate required to produce the necessary correction is either:
(i) 15 minus actual standard $HCO_3 \times$ weight in kg $\times 0.3 =$ mmol of $NaHCO_3$ required: give the whole amount.

---

* It is recognized that in emergency conditions such a slow rate may not be practicable particularly if the operator has no skilled helper.

(ii) Base deficit × weight in kg × 0.3: give $\frac{1}{2}$ of the calculated amount initially.

NOTE: The notations upon which non-respiratory and respiratory deviations are frequently reported by laboratories are NOT in mmols or milliequivalents, and should NOT be used as a basis for calculation.

EMPIRICAL USE OF SODIUM BICARBONATE IN THE ACUTE EMERGENCY
Intravenous sodium bicarbonate can be given *without* previous estimation of the acid-base state in an acute emergency in which the diagnosis is known and when it can be assumed that a severe metabolic acidosis is present. For example: resuscitation of the severely hypoxic newborn infant (p. 599) or in cardiac arrest (p. 300). An empirical dose should not normally aim at a correction of more than 5 mmol per litre of base deficit (*see above* for effects on osmolality).

CALCULATION OF THE DOSE OF SODIUM BICARBONATE IN ACUTE RESPIRATORY ACIDOSIS.
This is not a common problem but may arise in sudden deterioration in

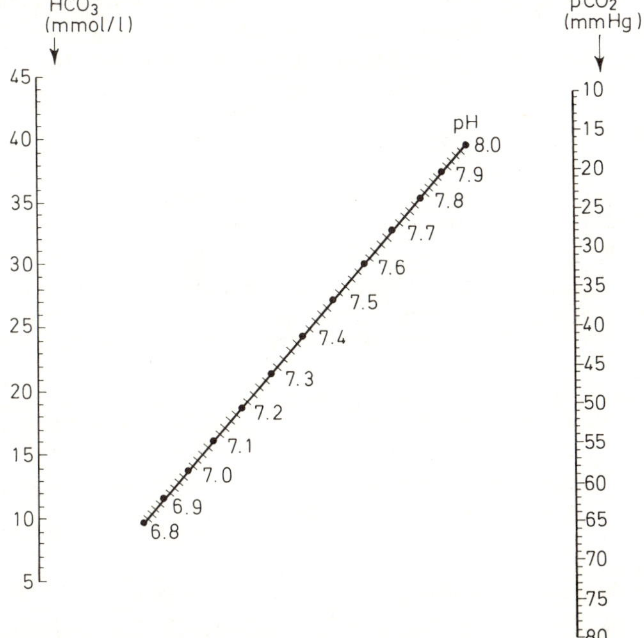

Figure 13.2. Nomogram by which the pCO_2 can be determined from the pH and the serum bicarbonate concentration (Goldberger, 1975d. Reproduced by kind permission)

respiratory distress syndrome in the pre-term infant. In most cardiorespiratory emergencies there is a coexistent metabolic acidosis due to
tissue hypoxia. However the situation may arise in which the high
pCO_2 has caused a potentially lethal H^+ concentration (>95 nmol per
litre, <7.00 pH) which requires correction. Goldberger (1975d) suggests the following calculation, using the nomogram (*Figure 13.2*) to
determine the plasma-bicarbonate concentration which would be present if the H^+ concentration were lowered to 65 nmol per litre (pH raised
to 7.20) and the pCO_2 remained unchanged. If the actual standard
bicarbonate level is known, the calculation becomes:

$$\text{Desired std } HCO_3 \text{ (from nomogram) minus actual std } HCO_3$$
$$\times \text{ weight in kg} \times 0.3 = \text{mmol of } NaHCO_3 \text{ required}$$

Goldberger warns that this correction should be done cautiously and
therefore it is best to aim at a H^+ concentration of 65 nmol per litre (pH
7.20) since a sudden reduction in pCO_2 after improved ventilation may
leave a residual metabolic alkalosis.

Acidosis in renal disease or metabolic disorders

Symptoms may arise quite suddenly as a result of a slowly developing
metabolic acidosis.

In the newborn: a metabolic acidosis may be seen in the following
conditions:

(i) LATE METABOLIC ACIDOSIS OF NUTRITIONAL (ACID OVER-LOAD)
ORIGIN

This is usually seen in the smaller pre-term infant below 1.5 kg on or
after the 3rd day of life when the protein intake has built up. In the
infant fed with modified cow's milk formulae (protein content adjusted
to that of human milk) or human milk, the acidosis is less common and
less marked. In general the less mature the infant the more severe the
acidosis.

RECOGNITION

The infant shows an unsatisfactory weight gain in spite of an apparently
adequate intake and becomes lethargic with a greyish pallor or apnoeic
attacks. In the more severe cases there is vomiting and loss of weight.
Hyperventilation is very rarely seen.

MANAGEMENT

(a) Estimation of the acid-base state is required, apart from the
necessity of excluding infection: respiratory compensation is
unusual (hence the absence of hyperventilation) and the pCO_2 is
usually normal.

(b) Additional sodium bicarbonate should be added to the feeds in divided doses (the total 24-hour requirement divided equally between the feeds) and adjusted to maintain a blood H^+ concentration between 45 and 50 nmol per litre (pH 7.30–7.35). To avoid the danger of overcorrection it is best to start with a dose of 2 to 3 mmol per kg of sodium bicarbonate per 24 hours. Increase the dose every 3 to 4 days until the required correction has been achieved.

> Example: 1.5-kg infant with base deficit of 10 mmol per litre will require $1.5 \times 10 \times 0.3 = 4.5$ mmol of $NaHCO_3$ (3 mmol per kg).

A hypertonic solution should not be used: the 8.4 per cent solution containing 1 mmol per 1.0 ml of solution can be diluted 1 in 4 giving a 2.1 per cent solution containing 1 mmol per 4 ml.

(c) Duration of treatment is variable, but may be required for 3 to 6 weeks.

(ii) RENAL HYPOPLASIA

RECOGNITION
If the infant is mature, hyperventilation with increased respiration rate may become obvious during the first week or later, depending upon the degree of renal insufficiency, due to a slowly developing metabolic acidosis with a markedly raised blood urea, usually in the region of 33 mmol per litre (200 mg%). When the acidosis has been corrected an IVP will confirm the diagnosis.

MANAGEMENT
The metabolic acidosis can be treated in the same way as in the late metabolic acidosis of the pre-term infant. Additional water may be required between feeds and a milk formula having a protein content similar to that of human milk should be used. The prognosis is variable: many children no longer require treatment with alkali during their phase of active growth.

(iii) INBORN ERRORS OF METABOLISM (*see also* Chapter 8)

RECOGNITION
A metabolic acidosis is common to many inborn errors of metabolism: symptoms of respiratory compensation are variable; other symptoms are: failure to thrive, vomiting, dehydration, apnoeic attacks.

MANAGEMENT
The relevant diagnostic tests and dietary management are discussed in Chapter 87 (p. 699).

(iv) NEONATAL DIABETES MELLITUS:
See page 443.

Water intoxication

Symptoms rarely occur at plasma levels above 120 mmol per litre except in the recovery phase of hypertonic dehydration (p. 98). However the *rate* at which the plasma sodium falls may also determine whether symptoms occur. The actual symptoms of water intoxication are due to cerebral oedema, which results from an imbalance between the osmolality of the brain cells and that of the ECF. This imbalance develops when the osmolality (mainly the plasma-sodium level) of the ECF falls rapidly, due to the addition of water in the presence of a pre-existing hyponatraemia, or less often with a previously normal plasma-sodium level. When the reduction of osmolality occurs so quickly that readjustment of osmolality between cells and ECF cannot take place, the brain cells remain in a relatively hyperosmolar state and water moves into the cerebral tissue, causing cerebral oedema with obliteration of the lateral ventricles and flattening of the sulci and, finally, evidence of raised intracranial pressure.

Water intoxication may occur in the following circumstances:
(a) With normal renal function:
    (i) Excessive (compulsive) drinking of water faster than it can be excreted. This is a rare condition in children (Linshaw, Hipp and Grustein, 1974) and symptoms of water intoxication from this cause have not been described in children, but hyponatraemia and fits have been observed during oral rehydration with water (Dugan and Holliday, 1967).
    (ii) As a result of the excessive use in hyponatraemic states of IV solutions which are initially hypotonic or which become so when the glucose is used up by the tissues. Examples of such solutions are 0.18 per cent NaCl in 4 per cent glucose, or 5 per cent glucose. The pre-existing hyponatraemia may be due to adrenocortical insufficiency, cystic fibrosis (excessive sodium losses in the sweat), heat exhaustion (p. 532), increased sodium losses through the surface of burns treated with silver nitrate (p. 45), or sodium depletion due to a prolonged salt-poor diet.
    (iii) The use and retention of water or hypotonic enemas in Hirschprung's disease.
    (iv) In the newborn, excessive water absorption through the respiratory tract during mechanical ventilation.
(b) With normal renal function but excessive (inappropriate) antidiuretic hormone (ADH) production. This may occur in:
    (i) Post-operative states when there is retention of water in excess of sodium: this may be accentuated by the use of hypotonic solutions IV or when water or other hypotonic fluids are 'pushed' by mouth postoperatively.
    (ii) After trauma: as above.

(iii) In small but painful burns or scalds in children in whom oral water or sodium-free fluids have been given in excess of the temporarily-reduced urinary output.

(c) Reduced or absent renal function.

Excessive water or hypotonic fluids given by any route to induce a diuresis may cause water intoxication if there is severe chronic glomerular disease, bilateral obstructive disease, acute renal 'shut-down', or during the transient anuria or oliguria of acute nephritis.

RECOGNITION

(a) The symptoms are diverse but usually include the following:

(i) Early symptoms which are probably due to disturbance of function from oedema. Generalized fits; sometimes preceded by other cerebral symptoms, but in infants and small children often without warning.

Lethargy, stupor, hallucinations, disorientation, irritability. Muscular weakness or twitching.

(ii) Late symptoms, due to raised intracranial pressure.

Vomiting.

Symptoms of medullary compression or decerebrate rigidity from 'coning' (p. 359). These may occur before a lumbar puncture or may develop after one.

(b) (i) Papilloedema and a tense or bulging fontanelle are inconstant signs, possibly because (in contrast to hydrocephalus) compression of the lateral ventricles allows considerable swelling to occur before the actual intracranial pressure rises.

(ii) Oedema or skin oedema (finger-printing) may be present if there is a chronic water over-load.

(c) The urine.

(i) With water over-load and normal renal function and no ADH production there will be a high flow of urine of low osmolality ($<$250 mosmol per litre) and a specific gravity (sp.gr.) of $<$1008. The sodium concentration is usually low ($<$20 mmol per litre) except in salt-losing states when it is disproportionately high in relation to the low plasma level.

(ii) With inappropriate ADH secretion the urine flow is low with an osmolality of $>$450 mosmol per litre, a sp. gr. of $>$1014 and a sodium content of $>$20 mmol per litre.

(iii) In renal failure, there is a small flow of urine of fixed osmolality (300–350 mosmol per litre) and a sp. gr. of 1010.

MANAGEMENT

(a) Water overload without cerebral symptoms. Water should be witheld for 24 hours. The plasma-sodium concentration and urinary output should be carefully checked.

(b) Cerebral symptoms, especially fits.

(i) The amount of sodium required to raise the plasma sodium level by 10 mmol per litre is 6 ml of 5 per cent NaCl per kg of body weight. Goldberger (1975b) advises giving $\frac{1}{4}$ of this amount (1.5 ml per kg) over one hour: the patient is then observed for half an hour and a further $\frac{1}{4}$ (1.5 ml per kg) given over another hour. If the symptoms are not completely relieved the remaining 3 ml per kg should be given slowly over the rest of the 24 hours.

(ii) In the presence of inappropriate ADH production in the absence of sodium depletion and normal renal function, IV mannitol will overcome the antidiuresis (*see* page 415 for dose). This method is especially applicable to small children with burns (p. 43).

(c) In the presence of known sodium depletion, and particularly where there is evidence of shock, dehydration or hypovolaemia, the amount of sodium required for replacement can be calculated from the following formula, which assumes the total body water (TBW) to be 0.70 litres per kg of body weight.

$Na = Na_d$ minus $Na_e \times TBW$

Na = number of mmol of sodium required.

Na_e = existing plasma-sodium concentration in mmol per litre.

Na_d = desired plasma-sodium concentrate in mmol per litre.

TBW = weight in kg $\times$ 0.70.

Note:

(1) 5 per cent NaCl contains 855 mmol of sodium per litre.
 3 per cent NaCl contains 513 mmol of sodium per litre.

(2) Interpretation of plasma-sodium levels.

(a) If the anion gap is <9 mmol per litre, laboratory error should be considered. The normal anion gap is usually somewhat less than 16 mmol (Goldberger, 1975a).

(b) Hyperlipidaemia, hyperglycaemia, hyperproteinaemia and uraemia may each cause an apparent hyponatraemia (Goldberger, 1975c, i).

(i) The plasma-sodium concentration decreases by 1.6 mmol per litre for each 5.5 mmol per litre (100 mg%) increase in plasma glucose above the normal level of 5.5 mmol per litre (100 mg%).

(ii) An exact calculation of the effect of a high plasma

urea or the plasma-sodium level is not possible, nevertheless there is a dilutional effect on the ECF which must be taken into account.

(iii) In hyperlipidaemia and hyperproteinaemia the chemically-estimated plasma sodium may be as much as 20 per cent below its true value. In hyperlipidaemia the chylomicrons can be separated by ultracentrifugation.

Hypokalaemia and potassium depletion

The correlation between the plasma level of potassium and body (intracellular) stores is poor, and normal or high plasma potassium levels may occur in haemoconcentration or metabolic acidosis in the presence of a depletion of total body stores.

A low plasma potassium (<3.5 mmol per litre) invariably indicates depletion, except in hypokalaemic periodic paralysis. For brevity hypokalaemia will be used as synonymous with potassium depletion.

Hypokalaemia should be suspected in the following situations

In some conditions the causes may be multiple:
(a) Renal losses.
  (i) Metabolic disorders from any cause.
  (ii) Prolonged use of high-dosage corticosteroids.
  (iii) Potassium-losing diuretics such as the thiazides, frusemide, ethacrynic acid.
  (iv) Potassium-losing states: the distal-tubular type of renal acidosis, recovery (polyuric) phase of acute tubular necrosis, cystinosis.
  (v) Metabolic response to trauma.
  (vi) A persisting metabolic alkalosis from any cause.
  (vii) Primary aldosteronism (rare) or secondary aldosteronism.
(b) Gastrointestinal losses.
  (i) Persisting vomiting, as in pyloric stenosis.
  (ii) Continuous aspiration from the gastrointestinal tract.
  (iii) Intestinal fistula.
  (iv) Acute gastroenteritis.
  (v) Chronic diarrhoea.
(c) Inadequate intake: starvation, undernutrition, persistent vomiting.

RECOGNITION
In all conditions likely to be associated with hypokalaemia the plasma

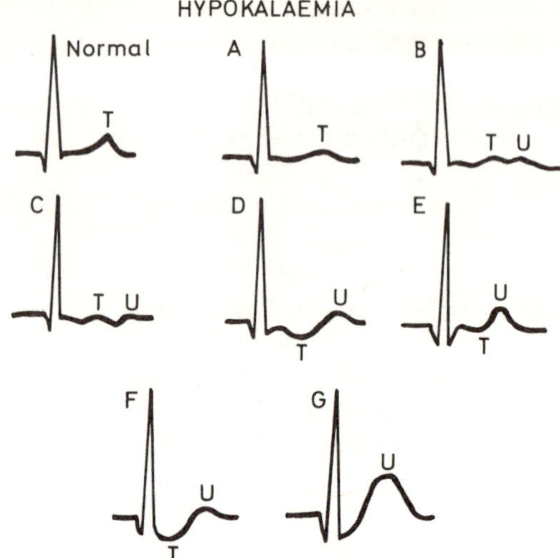

Figure 13.3. Electrocardiographic patterns of hypokalaemia. (Goldberger, 1975f. Reproduced by kind permission)

(1) Lowering and broadening of the T wave (A). The Q–T interval is also slightly prolonged. Such a pattern may occur when the serum potassium is merely at a low normal level, for example, 3.5 mmol/l(mEq/l).
(2) Low, broad T waves with a double summit, due to superimposition of the U wave on the T (B). The Q–T interval may appear markedly prolonged in such cases. However, the prolongation may be more apparent than real because it may be difficult to determine where the T ends and the U begins. As a consequence, the Q–U interval, rather than the Q–T interval, is often measured.
(3) Downward T waves and prominent U waves (D, E, F). Such a pattern is best seen in precordial leads such as V_1 through V_4, which overlie the right ventricle and thus have an rS or RS pattern.
(4) Depression of the RS–T segment and slight lengthening of the Q–T interval (D, E). The RS–T may be slightly depressed, or may show several small undulations (C). D, E, F, G, show more marked RS–T deviations. These RS–T segments have a sagging appearance, characteristic of hypokalaemia.
(5) Increase in P wave amplitudes, and widening of the QRS interval.
(6) Numerous arrhythmias, including sinus bradycaridia, prolonged P–R interval. Wenckebach type of A–V block, paroxysmal atrial tachycardia with A–V block (PAT with block). Arrhythmias due to digitalis toxicity may be precipitated or worsened.

potassium and ECG should be recorded frequently, or the ECG should be continuously visible.

Symptoms which suggest hypokalaemia are:

(a) Lassitude, anorexia, abdominal distension, or ileus.

(b) Muscle weakness, beginning in the legs and later involving the respiratory muscles, does not usually develop until the plasma level is 2.5 mmol per litre or lower.

(c) Cardiac arrhythmias include sinus bradycardia, prolonged P–R interval, A-V block, paroxysmal atrial tachycardia with A-V block. (Goldberger, 1975f).

(d) The ECG changes do not correlate with plasma levels. The usual abnormalities are shown in *Figure 13.3.*

MANAGEMENT

(a) IV potassium salts should NEVER be given in the following circumstances:

   (i) The plasma level is >5.5 mmol per litre.

   (ii) If there is oliguria from any causc.

   (iii) In untreated adrenal failure.

(b) Whenever possible, potassium salts should be given *orally*.

(c) Estimation of the deficit; this is somewhat empirical and cannot be judged from the plasma level but many studies have indicated the likely deficits:

   (i) In the commoner dehydration states the deficits vary according to the type of dehydration.

TABLE 13.I

Deficits of water and potassium in moderately severe dehydration (From Winters, 1968)

	Water ml per kg	Potassium mmol per kg
Hypertonic	120–170	2–5
Isotonic	100–150	7–11
Hypotonic	40–80	10–14

   (ii) In diabetic ketoacidosis the deficit is usually of the order of 4 to 7 mmol per kg.

(d) Replacement: this should normally be at the rate of 3 mmol per kg (2 mmol per kg under 1 year) per 24 hours. Potassium chloride is normally used but in renal-tubular acidosis potassium citrate should be substituted.

   (i) Oral route: a 7.45 per cent potassium chloride solution contains 1 mmol of potassium in 1.0 ml of solution. Other alternatives are potassium chloride effervescent tablets (Sando-K tablets contain 12 mmol of potassium and 8 mmol of chloride; Kloral tablets contain 6.7 mmol of potassium and 6.7 mmol of chloride; potassium chloride slow tablets (Leo K, Slow-K tablets) contain 8 mmol of potassium and chloride in a slow-release base).

   (ii) IV solutions should not contain >40 mmol of potassium per litre; a standard solution is potassium chloride and dextrose (glucose) which contains 5 per cent glucose and 40 mmol per litre of potassium chloride. A useful solution can also be made up by adding an ampoule of 2 mmol (0.15 g of potassium chloride) in 5 ml to each 100 ml of IV fluid, giving a final concentration of 20 mmol per litre. The original IV solution must of course contain no potassium.

(iii) In severe undernutrition, as in protein-energy malnutrition (p. 590) large amounts may be required to replenish the deficit but it is safer to give the replacement at the normal rate but to continue for longer, rather than to increase the actual amount given in each 24 hours.

Hyperkalaemia

(*See also* Acute Renal Failure, page 416)

The clinical manifestations of hyperkalaemia, such as cardiac arrhythmias, or less commonly muscular weakness and paraesthesiae, are rare, and should not occur if the clinician is aware of the commoner situations associated with hyperkalaemia and takes appropriate action before the plasma potassium reaches a critical level.

Causes of hyperkalaemia

Hyperkalaemia can be expected in situations where the renal excretion of potassium is less than that entering the extracellular fluid (ECF), whether this is from tissue breakdown or from exogenous sources. Reduced renal excretion may be due to acute renal failure or to oliguria in shock or dehydration states.

Contributory conditions which may accentuate or accelerate hyperkalaemia are:

(a) Metabolic acidosis.
(b) Cellular breakdown in trauma, burns, operation, haemolysis, infection, severe hypoxia and acute starvation.
(c) Potassium salts given inadvertently or as part of treatment.
    (i) Orally. Fruit drinks: 'Imperial Drink' (contains potassium citrate), potassium salts given to alkalinize the urine, drugs containing potassium (1 mega unit of potassium penicillin contains 1.7 mmol of potassium).
    (ii) Parenteral injections: penicillin (as above), stored blood especially if >5-days-old, plasma.
    (iii) Potassium salts given too rapidly IV or in the presence of renal disease, oliguria or acidosis (*see* Appendix 6 for potassium preparation for IV use).
(d) Adrenocortical failure with mineralocorticoid or aldosterone deficiency: in practice this may occur in any of the forms of acute adrenal failure in infancy or childhood (p. 451).
(e) The use of potassium-sparing diuretics (spironolactone, triamterene) in oedematous patients with renal disease or in patients

receiving other diuretics (thiazides, frusemide, ethacrynic acid) with potassium supplements. (Cannon, 1973).

RECOGNITION

(a) Falsely high values may be due to haemolysed blood samples which are particularly common in capillary blood which has been obtained with difficulty. The laboratory should always indicate when the plasma or serum is sufficiently haemolysed to give a misleadingly high result.

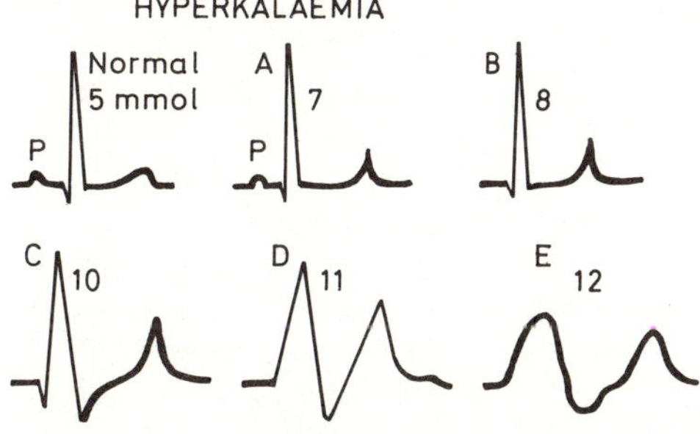

Figure 13.4. Electrocardiographic patterns of hyperkalaemia. (Goldberger, 1975e. Reproduced by kind permission)

At a concentration of approximately 6 to 7 mmol/l(mEq/l) tall peaked T waves with a narrow base and a normal or decreased Q–T occur (A).

At approximately 8 mmol/l(mEq/l) the P waves may disappear or wander in and out of the QRS (B).

At approximately 10 mmol/l(mEq/l) wide, aberrant QRS complexes appear (C).

At approximately 11 mmol/l(mEq/l) biphasic deflections, caused by a fusion of the QRS complex, RS–T segment and the T wave, appear (D).

At 12 mmol/l(mEq/l) (or even at a lower concentration of 10 mmol/l(mEq/l), ventricular fibrillation and cardiac standstill and death may occur (E).

(b) In the immediate neonatal period (3 days) the plasma potassium may be as high as 8 mmol per litre in normal infants.

(c) In all conditions in which hyperkalaemia can be expected, plasma potassium levels and ECG should be recorded at frequent intervals, or the ECG should be continuously visible.

(d) The onset of a cardiac arrhythmia (sinus bradycardia, first-degree A-V block, nodal or idioventricular rhythm, ventricular tachycardia) in circumstances in which hyperkalaemia can be expected, requires urgent treatment to be started (*see below*) to reduce the plasma-potassium level, without waiting for laboratory confirmation. Once an arrhythmia has become established the characteristics of hyperkalaemia (*Figure 13.4*) may not be easy to identify in the ECG.

(e) The ECG changes correlate reasonably well with the plasma-potassium level (*Figure 13.4*).

(f) Less common symptoms are paraesthesiae, and ascending paralysis.

MANAGEMENT
(a) In readily reversible conditions such as diabetic ketoacidosis or adrenocortical insufficiency, treatment of the primary condition will reduce the level of plasma potassium.
(b) Immediate treatment is required in the presence of:
  (i) ECG changes such as disappearance of the P wave and widening of the QRS.
  (ii) Cardiac arrhythmias associated with hyperkalaemia.
  (iii) A plasma level of >8.0 mmol per litre in the presence of renal impairment causing oliguria, which is not due to dehydration or hypovolaemia.
(c) Treatment should be given in the following order:
(1) Stop all sources of additional potassium.
(2) Inject IV 0.5 ml per kg of 10 per cent calcium gluconate over 2 to 4 minutes with ECG control. Use a single dose only. This provides temporary protection of the cardiac conduction system, and does not change the level of plasma potassium.
(3) Give $NaHCO_3$ IV in a dose of 2.5 mmol per kg over 30 to 60 minutes. This should also be given as a single dose. Further doses of $NaHCO_3$ should only be given after measurement of the acid-base state.
(4) Give insulin (soluble/regular or monocomponent equivalent such as Actrapid MC) with 10 per cent glucose in a dose of 40 ml per kg; this is followed by insulin in the proportion of 1 unit subcutaneously for every 3 g of glucose (= every 30 ml of 10 per cent glucose).
NOTE: None of these measures will *remove* potassium from the body: (3) and (4) reverse the release of intracellular potassium.
(d) In the presence of established renal failure with no possibility of increasing renal excretion, potassium can be removed from the body by ion-exchange resins in the sodium phase (Resonium-A, Kayexalate) in a dose of 1 to 1.25 g per kg per 24 hours, in divided doses 1 to 4 times daily up to a maximum dose of 60 g. The resin can be given orally (preferably by gastric tube) in 150 to 200 ml of water, or less for small children. Rectally, the resin can be given as an enema in a proportion of 30 g to 200 ml of water. The enema should be heated to body temperature and retained for 4 to 10 hours, and is then followed by a 'cleansing' enema. Resin therapy can be stopped when the plasma potassium reaches 4 to 5 mmol per litre. Loss of calcium and

magnesium can occur with prolonged use of the resin and plasma levels of these ions should be checked. (Goldberger, 1975e).

NOTE:

(i) 1 g of resin binds approximately 1 mmol of potassium ion.

(ii) The effect of resin treatment is slow and no effect may be seen for 24 hours.

(e) If the plasma potassium cannot be kept <7 mmol per litre in the anuric or persistently oliguric patient, peritoneal dialysis (in small children) or haemodialysis may be required.

Hypocalcaemia

Symptoms of hypocalcaemia are unlikely at calcium levels of >1.9 mmol per litre (3.8 mEq per litre = 7.5 mg%).*

ECG changes of hypocalcaemia: prolongation of the Q–T interval with normal RS–T segment and normal T waves. ECG changes are difficult to interpret in the newborn.

The newborn

In the newborn, hypocalcaemia should be suspected in any infant with jitteriness, hyperirritability or fits for which no cause (hypoxia, hypoglycaemia, meningitis, cerebral haemorrhage) can be found.

Hypocalcaemia is relatively common in the newborn infant: hypomagnesaemia (p. 145) may accompany hypocalcaemia and in these circumstances the hypocalcaemia is resistant to the usual treatment but corrects itself or responds to treatment if the hypomagnesaemia is corrected first. For this reason, in the newborn, a request should always be made for estimation of both calcium and magnesium and laboratories serving neonatal, medical and surgical units should routinely report both ions even if one (usually calcium) is requested.

In many newborns hypocalcaemia is transient and asymptomatic and the calcium level returns to normal when the infant recovers from an episode of acute illness, (e.g. severe hypoxia). Symptoms of hypocalcaemia in the newborn are usually non-specific and should only be attributed to hypocalcaemia after exclusion of other conditions (*see below*). There is no evidence that transient hypocalcaemia, whether symptomatic or not, causes cerebral damage, but persisting untreated or unrecognized hypocalcaemia is associated with mental retardation

---

* For calcium 1.0 mg per 100 ml (mg%) = 0.5 mEq per litre = 0.25 mmol per litre.

and it is therefore important to distinguish between transient and persisting hypocalcaemia.

CAUSES OF HYPOCALCAEMIA
    (a) Transient
        (i) Onset during the first 48 to 72 hours of life. This is seen in the infants of low birth-weight, and especially in pre-term infants with respiratory distress syndrome, and also after birth hypoxia. The hypocalcaemia of the infant of the diabetic mother usually occurs *after* the first 48 to 72 hours. In none of these conditions does the hypocalcaemia last for more than 2 to 3 days and it is frequently asymptomatic.
        (ii) During or immediately after exchange transfusion with citrated blood.
        (iii) Between the 4th and 8th days of life (the exact time of onset depending upon the type of feeding schedule) in infants fed on unmodified (high-phosphate) cow's milk. Symptoms rarely last longer than the 3 to 4 days even if untreated. Infants fed on human milk or modified (low-phosphate) cow's milk do not develop this form of hypocalcaemia.
        (iv) At the end of the first week up till the third week. Transient hypoparathyroidism may occur due to maternal hyperparathyroidism, whether primary or secondary.
    (b) Persisting
        (i) Severe vitamin-D deficiency in the mother, with resulting neonatal rickets, may cause hypocalcaemia with an onset at the 7th day onwards (Ford *et al.*, 1973), which persists if untreated.
        (ii) Idiopathic hypoparathyroidism and the 3–4th pharyngeal pouch syndrome (Taitz–DiGeorge syndrome) may cause symptomatic hypocalcaemia as early as the first week, or not until the age of a few months.
        (iii) Hypocalcaemia may be secondary to persisting hypomagnesaemia from any cause (*see* page 145).

RECOGNITION
    (a) Symptoms which can be attributable to hypocalcaemia are:
        (i) Clonic fits: focal, unilateral or generalized. The affected side may alternate. Tonic fits are rarely due to hypocalcaemia.
        (ii) Hyperirritability, 'jitteriness' (repetitive jerking of the limbs either spontaneously or in response to any sort of stimulus, including loud noises).
        (iii) Increased muscle tone.

(iv) Generalized oedema; rare (Benson and Parsons, 1964).

(v) Cardiac failure; rare (Troughton and Singh, 1972).

NOTE: The absence or presence of Chvostek's sign is of no significance in the newborn.

(b) Confirmation that hypocalcaemia is the cause of the symptoms

Since all the above symptoms can be due to other more serious causes the diagnosis of symptomatic hypocalcaemia is one of exclusion and IV calcium gluconate should NOT be used as a therapeutic test (*see below*).

(i) Fits. It is necessary to exclude hypoglycaemia, meningitis, intracranial haemorrhage, posthypoxic states and hypomagnesaemia. In continuous or very frequent fits pyridoxine dependence must also be considered (p. 689).

(ii) Hyperirritability and 'jitteriness'. These occur in hypoglycaemia, posthypoxic states and in hypomagnesaemia.

(iii) Increased tone is more likely in hypocalcaemia or hypomagnesaemia, and hypotonia in hypoglycaemia. The distinction is not a reliable one and increased tone alone is more likely to be due to one of the conditions given in (i) above.

(iv) Oedema and cardiac failure. Hypocalcaemia should only be considered when all the commoner causes have been excluded. A coexistent hypomagnesaemia may potentiate the effect of digoxin, as in potassium depletion (Chiswick, 1972).

(c) Diagnostic levels of plasma calcium

In the newborn it is unlikely that levels above 1.9 mmol per litre (3.8 mEq per litre = 7.5 mg%) would cause symptoms though it must be recognized that the total plasma calcium gives no good indication of the level of ionized calcium, which is really responsible for the symptoms.

MANAGEMENT

(a) Asymptomatic

Even if hypocalcaemia, when discovered, appears to be asymptomatic repeated plasma-calcium levels should be done until the level has returned to normal. If this is not done, a persisting and potentially damaging hypocalcaemia will be missed.

(b) Symptomatic

(i) In all cases, the milk should be changed to a low-phosphate milk (human or a modified cow's milk). Oral calcium supplements should be given (*see below*).

(ii) If fits are recurrent and severe an attempt should be made to control them with diazepam or phenobarbitone (p. 689) rather than with IV calcium gluconate, except in cases when conventional anticonvulsant treatment fails.

(c) Oral preparations available.

  (i) Calcium gluconate 10%: this is the same preparation as is used IV; dose 15 ml (1.5 g) three or four times daily. 1.5 g of calcium gluconate contains 3.3 mmol (6.6 mEq) of calcium.

  (ii) Calcium lactate as a 6 per cent suspension; dose 300 mg (5 ml) three or four times daily. 300 mg contains 2.0 mmol (4.0 mEq) of calcium.

  (iii) Calcium gluconagalactogluconate syrup (Calcium-Sandoz); dose 5 ml four to six times daily. 5 ml contains 2.7 mmol (5.4 mEq) of calcium.

  (iv) Calcium chloride (*see below*).

Oral preparations of calcium should be used for all cases of symptomatic hypocalcaemia, except those with severe, very frequent, or continuous fits. The plasma level should be estimated after 12 to 24 hours on treatment, and earlier if necessary, and again 2 to 3 days after stopping treatment. If the hypocalcaemia is thought to be of the transient type, treatment is rarely necessary for longer than 3 to 4 days but it is necessary to demonstrate that a normal level can be maintained after stopping treatment.

(d) Magnesium sulphate in the treatment of hypocalcaemic fits due to high-phosphatc load (4th to 8th day). Turncr, Cockburn and Forfar (1977) have suggested that even in the absence of symptomatically low levels of plasma magnesium, i.m. magnesium sulphate solution may be more effective than either phenobarbitone or oral calcium salts. They used 0.2 ml per kg of a 50 per cent solution of magnesium sulphate in two (rarely three) doses at 12-hourly intervals (*see* page 146 for technique of injection).

(e) The indications for Vitamin D.

  (i) Confirmed neonatal rickets.

  (ii) Persisting hypocalcaemia which cannot be controlled by oral calcium salts.

DOSE. Initially 1000 units (as calciferol) daily; the plasma-calcium level should be estimated weekly. Large dose of vitamin-D preparations given i.m. are not recommended because of the danger of hypercalcaemia.

NOTE: Hypoparathyroidism should be treated with one of the newly available compounds, 1,25,dihydrocholecalciferol $(1,25\text{-}(OH)_2D_3)$ or $1,\alpha$-hydroxycholecalciferol $(1\alpha(OH)D_3)$.

(f) Drugs contra-indicated.
   (i) Injections of parathyroid hormone are of more use diag-
        nostically than therapeutically since resistance soon devel-
        ops if repeated doses are given.
   (ii) Intravenous 10 per cent calcium gluconate; this is contra-
        indicated in all except the very rare cases of continuous or
        repeated hypocalcaemic fits, which are resistant to diaze-
        pam or phenobarbitone. If it must be given, a dose of 1.0 ml
        per kg should be used at each injection and given at the rate
        of 1 ml per minute, monitoring with ECG or stethoscope at
        the apex. The injection should be stopped if there is any
        slowing. The effect of intravenous calcium on the heart is
        said to be potentiated by digoxin and by hypokalaemia.

        The reasons against the use of IV calcium gluconate are
        that it is rarely indicated urgently and there is a danger of
        cardiac arrest; also leakage outside a vein causes severe
        tissue necrosis and calcification. Its effect is extremely brief
        and it is unnecessary in most cases of transient hypocalcae-
        mia and is ineffective in persisting cases.
   (iii) Calcium chloride: there is a risk of gastric perforation, and
        if given for more than 3 to 4 days a severe metabolic
        acidosis may result, particularly in pre-term infants.

Hypocalcaemia in the older child

Hypocalcaemia is relatively uncommon but should be considered as a
possible cause of fits in the following situations:
   (a) In Asian children, particularly if there is clinical evidence of
        rickets, but even in its absence.
   (b) Children with known renal insufficiency, particularly if alkalis
        have been given.
   (c) In children who are dwarfed and mentally retarded (hypopara-
        thyroidism, pseudohypoparathyroidism).
   (d) Any child with cataracts.
   (e) Children with heart disease and recurrent infections (3rd and 4th
        branchial arch, Taitz–DiGeorge syndrome).
Hypocalcaemia as a cause of tetanic manifestations such as carpopedal spasms, painful muscle cramps and paraesthesiae round the
mouth and in the fingers and toes, is relatively rare in childhood and is
likely to be accompanied by clinical evidence which may point to the
primary cause (*see above*). With increasing age the incidence of fits
decreases and that of tetany increases. In adolescent girls hyperventilation tetany may occur with a respiratory alkalosis and a normal plasma
calcium.

MANAGEMENT

In the older child the danger of extravasation of calcium gluconate outside the vein is small and there may be an indication for its use in continued or repeated hypocalcaemic fits or tetany until other and slower forms of treatment have taken effect (*see* page 143 for precaution with IV injection). The maximum single dose at any age is 10 ml of the 10 per cent solution.

On a long-term basis, treatment depends upon the primary cause.

Hypercalcaemia

Hypercalcaemia is usually defined as a plasma-calcium level of >2.8 mmol per litre (5.5 mEq per litre = 11.0 mg per 100 ml (mg%)).

ECG changes in hypercalcaemia: shortening of the Q–T interval with rounded T waves and normal RS–T segments. Incomplete or complete A–V block or cardiac arrest may occur at levels of 4.5 mmol per litre (9.0 mEq per litre = 18.0 mg per 100 ml (mg%). (Goldberger, 1975g)

This is a rare emergency in childhood. Nevertheless levels of 3.8 mmol per litre (7.5 mEq per litre = 15 mg per 100 ml (mg%)) or higher carry a risk of renal damage and are seen in severe overdosage with vitamin D preparations and occasionally in severe idiopathic hypercalcaemia.

RECOGNITION

In infants and children the usual symptoms are: muscular hypotonia, vomiting, thirst, polyuria and constipation. In long-standing severe hypercalcaemia band-keratopathy may be present and nephrocalcinosis may be visible on a plain film of the abdomen. In vitamin-D overdosage the long bones may show bands of increased density at the metaphysis with an area of reduced density just proximally. In idiopathic hypercalcaemia similar bands of increased density occur at the metaphyses but without the area of decreased density; in some cases there is also increased bone density in the supra-orbital region and in the base of the skull.

MANAGEMENT

Treatment is indicated when the plasma-calcium level is >3.8 mmol per litre (>15 mg per 100 ml), in the presence of severe symptoms such as vomiting, coma, or with a rising blood urea or oliguria.

    (a) Isotonic saline intravenously is said to be useful in a hypercalcaemic crisis but should be used with care because glomerular filtration may be impaired and there is therefore a risk of circulatory overload.

(b) Large doses of corticosteroids will reduce hypercalcaemia in vitamin-D poisoning and in idiopathic hypercalcaemia but not in hyperparathyroidism.

(c) Calcitonin (Calcitare, porcine, Calsynar and Miacalcic salmon). Preparations are available for subcutaneous or i.m. injection (160 International Units (iu.) per vial) to be made up to 1 or 2 ml with the gelatine diluent and, for IV use (50 International Units per vial), supplied with saline acetate diluent. The recommended dose is 4 to 8 units per kg daily intramuscularly; by the intravenous route 15 to 35 iu. have been given in a single dose to adults. Salmon calcitonin may be effective where the porcine preparation has failed; the maximum dose is 0.05 to 0.1 ml (5–10 iu.) per kg i.m. daily. Salmon calcitonin can also be given intravenously (*Drug and Therapeutics Bulletin*, 1975).

Hypomagnesaemia

Symptoms of hypomagnesaemia are unlikely to develop unless the plasma level is <0.5 mmol per litre (1.0 mEq per litre = 1.2 mg%), ECG changes are rarely specific and are particularly difficult to interpret in the newborn.

The newborn

In this age group hypomagnesaemia may accompany hypocalcaemia, and when this occurs the hypocalcaemia is resistant to treatment with calcium salts or vitamin D. Correction of the hypomagnesaemia corrects the hypocalcaemia or renders it responsive to treatment. Isolated hypomagnesaemia is uncommon and is usually transient and asymptomatic.

CAUSES OF HYPOMAGNESAEMIA

(a) Any of the usual causes of transient hypocalcaemia may cause hypomagnesaemia also.

(b) Maternal magnesium depletion from malabsorption may produce symptomatic hypocalcaemia-hypomagnesaemia (Davis, Harvey and Yu, 1965).

(c) A specific disorder of magnesium absorption (Strømme *et al.*, 1969; Nordio *et al.*, 1971) may cause symptomatic hypocalcaemia-hypomagnesaemia in the neonatal period, but more commonly at the age of a few months.

For magnesium 1.0 mg per 100 ml (mg%) = 0.8 mEq per litre = 0.4 mmol per litre. Normal levels: 0.75–1.25 mmol per litre (1.5–2.5 mEq per litre = 1.8–3.0 mg per 100 ml (mg%).

RECOGNITION

It is usually impossible to distinguish, in this age group, on the basis of symptoms, between hypocalcaemia and hypomagnesaemia. Hypomagnesaemia should always be considered when hypocalcaemia is resistant to treatment, or in the investigation of hyperirritability or fits in which óther causes have been excluded.

MANAGEMENT

Symptoms may be more severe and fits may be more frequent in hypocalcaemia-hypomagnesaemia than in isolated hypocalcaemia. Symptoms which are due to hypomagnesaemia will be completely relieved by magnesium salts, IV, i.m., or orally, according to the degree of urgency.

(a) Intravenous route

This should only be necessary when rapid relief of continuous or repeated fits is required, or when other routes are not practicable. A 1 per cent solution of magnesium sulphate should be used (0.04 mmol = 0.08 mEq per ml), in a dose of 0.25 to 0.5 mmol (0.5–1.0 mEq) in 6 to 10 ml at a rate of not more than 1 ml per minute, using ECG controls since IV magnesium salts have similar effects on the heart to calcium salts, and should NEVER be injected rapidly: if practicable the blood pressure should be checked during and after the injection since magnesium salts cause hypotension.

(b) Intramuscular route

This is the usual route for the relief of acute symptoms, or when there is a possibility of failure of absorption from the gastrointestinal tract. The preparation normally used is a 50 per cent solution of magnesium sulphate, given at 12-hourly intervals in a dose of 0.2 to 0.5 mmol (0.4–1.0 mEq) or 0.1 to 0.25 ml per kg. In transient hypomagnesaemia or in the treatment of phosphate-load hypocalcaemia (Turner, Cockburn and Forfar, 1977) two or occasionally three doses are adequate. Magnesium sulphate is a highly irritant solution and should be injected deep into the muscles of the mid-thigh. In very small infants a more dilute solution (25 or 12.5 per cent) may be preferable.

(c) Oral route

This is used in all non-urgent cases. The following preparations are available.
   (i) Magnesium sulphate can usually be tolerated in therapeutic amounts without producing diarrhoea, but should be diluted to 25 or 12.5 per cent before use.

Dose: 0.25 to 1.0 mmol (0.5–2.0 mEq) of magnesium (0.125–0.5 ml) per kg of 50 per cent solution, in divided doses.

(ii) If there has been recent diarrhoea, or large amounts are required to maintain magnesium balance or replace a large deficit, magnesium hydroxide (milk of magnesia) may be better tolerated than magnesium sulphate. The standard magnesium hydroxide preparation contains 8 per cent of magnesium hydroxide, or 6.8 mmol (13.6 mEq) in 5 ml.

Dose: 1 to 2 ml three times daily initially.

(iii) Other preparations available are magnesium citrate, lactate, gluconate and glycerophosphate.

Hypomagnesaemia in the older child

(a) Infancy

Hypomagnesaemia, with or without hypocalcaemia may develop after extensive resection of the small intestine, and also in the various forms of cirrhosis in infancy (Kaya and Özsoylu, 1972). In the rare, proba bly genetically-determined form of magnesium malabsorption (Strømme *et al.*, 1969; Nordio *et al.*, 1971) hypocalcaemia-hypomagnesaemic fits usually occur at the age of a few months but occasionally as early as 2 weeks.

(b) Other age groups

Hypomagnesaemia has occasionally been found to accompany hypocalcaemia in most of the conditions in which hypocalcaemia occurs. Probably the most important type of hypomagnesaemia occurs with the severe magnesium depletion seen in protein-energy malnutrition (protein-calorie malnutrition), (p. 590); in such cases hypocalcaemia is uncommon.

RECOGNITION
Recurrent fits are the commonest presenting symptom, but, particularly in the older child, hyperirritability, carpopedal spasms, increased muscle tone, increased tendon reflexes and coarse tremors may occur. Symptoms are unlikely above a level of 0.5 mmol per litre (1 mEq per litre = 1.2 mg per 100 ml (mg%)).

MANAGEMENT
Treatment is as for the neonatal period. In the magnesium malabsorption syndrome much larger quantities than usual are required to maintain a normal or near normal level of plasma magnesium and a total daily intake (not per kg) of 10 to 15 mmol (20–30 mEq) may be

required even in small children or infants: treatment has to be maintained indefinitely.

In protein-energy malnutrition the acute symptoms may be relieved by i.m. magnesium sulphate (*see above*), followed by oral treatment until repletion has occurred (*see* page 590).

Hypermagnesaemia

Hypermagnesaemia exists at >1.25 mmol per litre (2.5 mEq per litre = 3.0 mg%).

ECG changes: prolonged P–R interval, prolonged QRS interval, tall T-waves, various degrees of A-V block or ventricular premature contractions. (Goldberger, 1975h)

The newborn

(a) In infants born after a hypoxic delivery a transient and symptomless hypermagnesaemia may occur but requires no treatment.

(b) Treatment of toxaemia in the mother by injection of magnesium sulphate just before delivery may cause symptomatic hypermagnesaemia in the newborn, with drowsiness, hypotonia and respiratory paralysis (Brady and Williams, 1967; Lipsitz and English, 1967).

In the older child

(a) In renal failure symptomatic hypermagnesaemia may occur after the IV injection of magnesium sulphate to control hypertensive episodes.

(b) Magnesium sulphate enemas in Hirschsprung's disease have caused hypermagnesaemia from retention of the enema fluid.

(c) Magnesium sulphate purgative or the use of magnesium-containing antacids in renal failure have also caused symptomatic hypermagnesaemia.

RECOGNITION

Hypermagnesaemia should be considered when drowsiness or muscle weakness develops in any of the situations described above.

Clinically the progression of symptomatology is given in Table 13.II.

For magnesium 1.0 mg per 100 ml (mg%) = 0.8 mEq per litre = 0.4 mmol per litre
Normal levels: 0.75–1.25 mmol per litre (1.5–2.5 mEq per litre = 1.8–3.0 mg per 100 ml (mg%).

TABLE 13.II

Symptoms of hypermagnesaemia in relation to plasma level. (After Goldberger, 1975h. Reproduced by kind permission.)

Symptom	Plasma levels		
	mg per 100 ml (*mg%*)	*mmol per litre*	*mEq per litre*
Hypotension, peripheral vasodilation	3.6–6.0	1.5–2.5	3.0–5.0
Drowsiness	6.0–8.5	2.5–3.5	5.0–7.0
Loss of tendon reflexes	8.5	3.5	7.0
Depression of respiration	12.0	5.0	10.0
Coma	14.0–18.0	6.0–7.5	12.0–15.0
Cardiac arrest	18.0–24.0	7.5–10.0	15.0–20.0

MANAGEMENT

(a) In the newborn, weakness or incipient paralysis of the respiratory muscles may require an exchange transfusion and assisted ventilation.

(b) In the older child the plasma magnesium level may be lowered by increasing the fluid intake provided that renal function is normal.

(c) IV calcium gluconate has been suggested as an antagonist to the acute effect of magnesium on the heart.

(d) At any age respiratory weakness due to hypermagnesaemia may require mechanical ventilation, and other symptoms of acute intoxication (Table 13.II) with ECG changes may require peritoneal dialysis or exchange transfusion, according to the age of the child.

References

Baum, J. D. and Roberton, N. R. C. (1975). Immediate effects of alkaline infusion in infants with respiratory distress syndrome. *J. Pediat.* **87**, 255

Benson, P. F. and Parsons, V. (1964). Hereditary hypoparathyroidism presenting with oedema in the neonatal period. *Q. J. Med.* **33**, 197

Brady, J. P. and Williams, H. C. (1967). Magnesium intoxication in a premature infant. *Pediatrics*, **40**, 100

Cannon, P. J. (1973). Diuretic therapy in patients with renal disease. In *The Body Fluids in Pediatrics*, pp. 514–517. Ed. R. W. Winters. Boston: Little, Brown and Company

Chiswick, M. L. (1972). Heart failure and neonatal hypocalcaemia. *Br. med. J.* **4**, 364

Davis, J. A., Harvey, D. R. and Yu, J. S. (1965). Neonatal fits associated with hypomagnesaemia. *Archs Dis. Childh.* **40**, 286

Drug and Therapeutics Bulletin (1975). Salmon calcitonin (Calsynar, Miacalcic). **13**, 89

Dugan, S. and Holliday, M. A. (1967). Water intoxication in two infants following the voluntary ingestion of excessive fluids. *Pediatrics* **39**, 418

Finberg, L. (1967). Dangers to infants caused by changes in osmolal concentration. *Pediatrics* **40**, 1031

Ford, J. A., Davidson, D. C., McIntosh, W. B., Fyfe, W. M. and Dunnigan, M. G. (1973). Neonatal rickets in Asian immigrant population. *Br. med. J.* **3**, 211

Goldberger, E. (1975). *A Primer of Water, Electrolyte and Acid-base Syndromes*, 5th ed. Pages: (a) 18, (b) 77, (c) 141–142, (d) 187, 220–221, 244, (e) 348–349, (f) 387–388, (g) 445, 448, (h) 469–471, (i) 587–592. Philadelphia: Lea and Febiger

Kaya, G. and Özsoylu, S. (1972). Serum magnesium levels in children with cirrhosis. *Acta Paediat. Scand.* **61**, 442

Kety, S. S., Polis, B. D., Nadler, C. S. and Schmidt, C. F. (1948). The blood flow and oxygen consumption of the human brain in diabetic ketoacidosis and coma. *J. clin. Invest.* **27**, 500

Linshaw, M. A., Hipp, T. and Gruskin, A. (1974). Infantile psychogenic water-drinking. *J. Pediat.* **85**, 520

Lipsitz, P. J. and English, I. C. (1967). Hypermagnesaemia in the newborn infant. *Pediatrics* **40**, 865

Nordio, S., Donath, A., Macagno, F. and Gatti, R. (1971). Chronic hypomagnesaemia with magnesium-dependent hypocalecaemia. *Acta Paediat. Scand.* **60**, 441

Ohman, J. L. jun., Marliss, E. B., Aoki, T. T., Munichoodapa, C. S., Khanna, V. V. and Kozak, G. P. (1971). The cerebrospinal fluid in diabetic ketoacidosis. *New Engl. J. Med.* **284**, 283

Siegel, S. R., Phelps, D. L., Leake, R. D. and Oh, W. (1973). The effects of rapid infusion of hypertonic sodium bicarbonate in infants with respiratory distress. *Pediatrics*, **51**, 651

Strømme, J. H., Nesbakken, R., Normann, T., Skjörten, Skyberg, D. and Johannessen, B. (1969). Familial hypomagnesaemia. *Acta Paediat. Scand.* **58**, 433

Swyer, P. R. (1975). *The Intensive Care of the Newly Born*. p. 36. Basle: S. Karger

Troughton, O. and Singh, S. P. (1977). Heart failure and neonatal hypocalcaemia. *Br. med. J.* **4**, 76

Turner, T. L., Cockburn, F. and Forfar, J. O. (1977). Magnesium therapy in neonatal tetany. *Lancet* (i), 283

Winters, R. W. (1968). Disorders of electrolyte and acid-base metabolism. In *Pediatrics* 14th edn. Ed. H. L. Barnett. Englewood Cliffs, New Jersey Appleton-Century-Crofts

Part IV: Emergencies Involving Face and Neck

CHAPTER 14

Emergencies Involving the Eyes

A. Stanworth

Except in the neonatal period, ophthalmic emergencies are little different in children from those in young adults as far as immediate management is concerned, though the long-term results may be influenced by any interruption of the development of vision and binocular coordination in a child. Any situation therefore which calls for prolonged covering of an eye or any possibility of interference with vision, however minor, should be referred to an ophthalmic surgeon promptly after immediate treatment has been given.

Mechanical trauma

Orbit

(a) Orbital haemorrhage

RECOGNITION
The common black eye will usually resolve without treatment, the haemorrhage being subcutaneous and largely in front of the orbital septum, but haemorrhage inside the orbit itself may produce proptosis and intereference with ocular movements, giving double vision. Even so, orbital haemorrhage rarely leads to any long-term ill-effects.

MANAGEMENT
No specific treatment is required; it is usual to cover with a light pad or shade. Admission for observation is advised if the intra-orbital pressure is obviously high. It is important to exclude orbital fracture and ocular injuries.

(b) *Orbital fracture*

RECOGNITION

Fracture of the floor of the orbit may lead to depression of the bone and trapping of orbital tissue and extra-ocular muscles in the fracture line. This 'blow-out' fracture can be produced by relatively minor trauma even in the absence of much bruising, and if untreated is likely to lead to permanent interference with ocular movement and troublesome diplopia.

It is important to remember the possibility of this condition after any blunt trauma to the orbit; diplopia should be asked about, ocular movements examined and the lids separated if they are closed by the swelling, so as to permit proper examination. Radiography is essential if there is any doubt; the fracture may not be shown by straight radiographs but may require tomography.

MANAGEMENT

Treatment is not an emergency, the ocular movements being observed for a few days before deciding whether or not exploration and repositioning of the orbital contents and support of the orbital floor by a silicone implant is necessary.

(c) *Penetrating wounds of the orbit*

RECOGNITION

These can injure the extra-ocular muscles, the nerves supplying the muscles, blood vessels and even the optic nerve if the penetration is to the apex of the orbit.

MANAGEMENT

No treatment should be given other than a simple pad, and referral to an ophthalmic surgeon; in particular, protruding foreign bodies should not be removed in the casualty department since this may produce unnecessary trauma and haemorrhage.

Lids

Trauma

RECOGNITION

Trauma to the lids is usually obvious but the possibility of additional injury to the eye, orbit and head must be remembered.

MANAGEMENT

Blunt trauma without rupture of the skin or conjunctiva, leading to bruising will resolve without treatment. Wounds of the lid heal well if adequately sutured with preservation of as much injured tissue as possible. Involvement of the lid margin needs very careful suturing with fine sutures to restore the margin and is best done by an ophthalmologist; the margin is sutured first with a fine suture which slightly everts the wound edges, using the grey line which runs between the lash line and the openings of the tarsal glands as a landmark. The main substance of the lid is then sutured in layers from back to front using buried absorbable sutures for the deep layers and fine silk for the skin.

Lacrimal involvement in trauma

RECOGNITION

Any laceration at the inner end of the lower lid should be carefully examined to assess the possibility of canaliculus damage. A lacrimal probe passed through the lower canaliculus after dilating the punctum with a dilator will demonstrate whether or not the canaliculus is involved; this manoeuvre is best carried out by an ophthalmologist since false passages are easily produced.

MANAGEMENT

A torn lower canaliculus can be repaired around a nylon thread introduced through the upper canaliculus and sac and left in place for some weeks.

Conjunctiva

The conjunctiva heals remarkably well and small lacerations of 3 mm or so can be left without stitching. Larger gaping lacerations require stitching with fine catgut.

FOREIGN BODIES

These can usually be lifted off with a moist swab but if embedded may require to be picked up with fine forceps and snipped off leaving a small hole in the conjunctiva which easily heals without a suture. Foreign bodies can be easily missed in the upper fornix but treatment can be delayed until they are seen by an ophthalmic surgeon.

SUBCONJUNCTIVAL HAEMORRHAGE

This produces a localized red patch which obscures the vascular markings. No treatment is needed.

Cornea

(*a*) *Corneal abrasions*

RECOGNITION
These can be delineated by fluorescein drops which stain the loss of
surface a bright green colour.

MANAGEMENT
Small abrasions will normally heal rapidly if given antibiotic drops (e.g.
chloramphenicol) to prevent secondary infection. Large abrasions may
need the addition of a short-acting mydriatic such as cyclopentolate; a
light pad may make the patient more comfortable but does not accelerate healing.

(b) Foreign bodies

These may be gently wiped off with a moist piece of cotton wool; if
embedded they are best removed by someone with experience of this
manoeuvre, using a fine needle so as to minimize trauma, followed by
antibiotic drops; if a large abrasion remains, mydriatic drops such as
cyclopentolate or homatropine are needed.

(c) Corneal lacerations

These will need expert treatment; if gaping, they may require suturing
even if they do not penetrate the full thickness of the cornea.

Perforating wounds of the globe

RECOGNITION
*After injuries to the lids and surface of the eye a careful examination
should be made for evidence of perforating wounds.* These may include
obvious lacerations of the cornea and sclera, protrusion of the iris
through the cornea (the iris always appearing black), or protrusion of
the ciliary body or choroid through the sclera; a hole may be visible in
the iris—it is best seen by using an ophthalmoscope and noting that red
light is reflected back from the fundus through the hole in the same
manner as it is through the pupil. The pupil may be distorted. Blood
may be seen on the iris or in the anterior chamber; blood in the vitreous
may appear as opacities or prevent a view of the fundus. A foreign body,
if large, may be seen inside the eye but most foreign bodies are too small
or too obscured to be visible.

MANAGEMENT
Any suspected perforating wound should be treated by no more than a
simple pad to protect the eye, prevention of the child rubbing the eye,
keeping the child at rest, and *referring immediately to an ophthalmic
department.*

Non-perforating injury to the globe

RECOGNITION
Contusions involving the interior of the eye may produce haemorrhage into the anterior chamber (hyphaema), distortion of the pupil, tears in the iris, vitreous haemorrhage, and injury to the choroid and retina.

MANAGEMENT
Any evidence of these conditions requires admission of the patient to an ophthalmic department.

Chemical and thermal injury

RECOGNITION
Such injury is usually obvious from the history, swelling of the lids, congestion of the conjunctiva, and opacity of the cornea. The severity of the injury may be underestimated if the blood vessels of the conjunctiva have been destroyed, leading to a white appearance rath·r than to congestion; the extent of the damage to the cornea can be shown by staining with fluorescein drops which will stain loss of surface a green colour.

MANAGEMENT
Immediate treatment is vital. Copious irrigation with any bland fluid that is available should be started at once, and kept up for at least 10 minutes. The fluid used for irrigation is of little consequence; saline is as good as any and water can be used if saline is not available. The volume of the fluid used is more important than its nature. Any obvious pieces of foreign matter such as lime can be removed with moist cotton wool or a swab, but force to do this should not be exerted. Meanwhile arrangements should be made for treatment in an ophthalmic department since thorough cleansing of the burnt area requires skilled nursing and even general anaesthesia. The installation of wide-spectrum antibiotic drops is worthwhile if there is any delay.

Acute inflammation

Orbital cellulitis

RECOGNITION
Infection entering the orbit from the nasal sinuses or blood-stream may produce signs of cellulitis, with swelling, redness, and closure of the

lids, pain and tenderness, and pyrexia; the orbital pressure may reach such a degree as to obstruct circulation and so lead to visual loss, though this is rare in children. A superficially similar condition without the hyperpyrexia and tenderness may follow haemorrhage into an orbital neoplasm.

MANAGEMENT
Wide spectrum systemic antibiotics are indicated, and admission to an ophthalmic department.

Acute dacryocystitis

RECOGNITION
In infancy this is a rare complication of congenital blockage of the naso-lacrimal duct, giving rise to tenderness and swelling at the inner canthus.

MANAGEMENT
A systemic antibiotic will be necessary in the severe cases, with subsequent treatment of the underlying cause by probing.

Styes and inflamed tarsal cysts

RECOGNITION
These produce localized tender swellings on the margin (styes) or in the substance (tarsal cyst) of the lids.

MANAGEMENT
Antibiotic drops or ointment hourly are usually sufficient to control the acute attack.

Rapid onset of lid swelling

This may be due to one of the preceding infections, to allergies to drops or ointments or associated with generalized allergies, or to bee or wasp stings. The management is that appropriate to the cause.

Acute conjunctivitis

RECOGNITION
This is characterized by redness and discharge; it is uncomfortable but not very painful. Most cases will respond well to cleansing of the eye with moist cotton wool to remove discharge, together with antibiotic drops in frequencies varying from every few minutes in the acute type of

gonococcal ophthalmia neonatorum to every 2 hours in the less acute inflammations. Padding of the eye is contra-indicated. Severe ophthalmia neonatorum should be seen by an ophthalmologist and transferred to an ophthalmic department if necessary (*see* page 629 for antibiotic treatment); i.m. benzyl penicillin should always be given in addition to local treatment.

Corneal ulceration related to acute conjunctivitis

RECOGNITION

This may follow or accompany acute conjunctivitis; the redness is more marked around the edge of cornea, the condition is painful, and discharge is produced only by the accompanying conjunctival irritation. Vision will be blurred unless the ulcer is confined to the periphery of the cornea. Pyogenic corneal infections usually produce obvious opacity in the cornea, but herpes simplex infections may be difficult to see without the instillation of fluorescein drops; the primary infection with herpes simplex often shows as punctate corneal staining points, but secondary infections may show the typical dendritic figure. *Fluorescein drops should be used in any eye in which corneal ulcer is a possibility*. Treatment is by an ophthalmic surgeon with atropine and appropriate antibiotic drops for pyogenic infections or idoxuridine drops for herpes simplex infection. Steroid drops should NOT be used.

Infantile glaucoma (Buphthalmos)

RECOGNITION

The condition may be already present at birth but more commonly becomes obvious at the age of a few months. Infantile glaucoma may lead to an increased size of the eye with stretching of the cornea and rupture of the corneal endothelium. This can give rise to corneal oedema and is a cause of red irritable eyes with photophobia and watering. Discharge is not a feature. The eye may not be so obviously enlarged as to attract attention unless the possibility is considered.

MANAGEMENT

Treatment to lower the intra-ocular pressure is urgent, as prolonged pressure for more than a few days will lead to permanent visual loss.

Acute iridocyclitis

RECOGNITION

This is not common in children; subacute iridocyclitis may be seen in association with Still's disease (juvenile rheumatoid arthritis). The disease produces a painful eye with circumcorneal injection, variable diminution in vision, and usually an irregular small pupil. This latter sign indicates that atropine drops can be given four-hourly, but an ophthalmic assessment is urgent. Do NOT use steroid drops unless it is certain that there is no corneal ulceration from herpes simplex infection.

Sudden loss of vision

Sudden loss of vision is not common without obvious evidence of ophthalmic disease. Chronic and even congenital diseases affecting mainly or entirely one eye may present as sudden loss of vision since the early stages of visual loss may not be noticed by the patient. Hysteria may also have to be considered (p. 508).

RETINAL DETACHMENT
This may occur apparently spontaneously as a result of congenital or old inflammatory defects in the retina; it may also follow blunt trauma to the head or any trauma to the eye after an interval of days, weeks or months. Operation is urgent unless the detachment is of long standing.

CHRONIC IRIDOCYCLITIS
As in Still's disease this leads to vitreous opacities and fairly rapid loss of vision in some patients. The fundus may be difficult to see.

PAPILLOEDEMA
In its early stages this does not cause more than transient episodes of blurring of vision, but when prolonged may lead to visual loss and secondary optic atrophy.

Double vision

A squint leading to double vision is not usually an emergency but the sudden onset of 6th nerve palsy may herald a blocked valve in hydrocephalus or other cause of acutely raised intracranial pressure.

Neonatal emergencies

OPHTHALMIA NEONATORUM
This is dealt with under conjunctivitis (*see above; also see under* Acute Infection in the Newborn, p. 629).

WATERING OF THE EYES
This is due to lacrimal blockage and is not usually obvious in the first two or three weeks since tear production is low, but it may be the basis of chronic redness and discharge in infancy, requiring antibiotic drops three times daily, repeated digital pressure over the lacrimal sac to try to empty it into the nose, and probing of the lacrimal ducts at the age of 4 to 6 months if the condition does not settle.

CORNEAL OPACITY
This may be due to:
(a) Infantile glaucoma (*see above*).
(b) Rupture of the posterior layers of the cornea during birth particularly after the use of forceps; this produces corneal oedema which gradually subsides over a few days but may leave marked astigmatism and interference with vision; no treatment is indicated in the acute stage but the potential visual loss needs ophthalmic management.
(c) One of the mucopolysaccharidoses.
(d) A developmental anomaly of the anterior eyeball.
All require an ophthalmic opinion.

LARGE EYES
An obviously large eye may be due to infantile glaucoma (*see above*), a congenitally-large cornea without glaucoma (megalocornea), or a congenital anomaly of the anterior eyeball. Only infantile glaucoma requires immediate treatment.

CHAPTER 15

Emergencies Involving the Face and Neck

R. C. W. Dinsdale

Traumatic injuries of the head, face and neck
(*See also* sections on Acute Neurosurgical Emergencies; Ear, Nose and Throat; and Eye Injury)

In all cases presenting for treatment, it should be remembered that:
- (a) *Urgent* neurosurgical intervention has priority over other injuries.
- (b) The injury may be non-accidental.
- (c) Even if a particular accident does not present as an emergency, accurate assessment and treatment may be essential to prevent permanent disability.

On arrival at the accident and emergency department

As soon as it is safe to do so, an unconscious patient should be transferred to an Intensive Treatment Unit.
(1) Immediately review the patient and ensure that:
- (a) The mouth and pharynx are clear of blood and foreign bodies.
- (b) Aspiration of blood is not taking place. This is best achieved by placing the patient on the right side. Insert an oral airway if required.
- (c) A note is made of the size, response to light, and position of each pupil.
- (d) An assessment is made of the degree of shock by reference to the blood pressure, pulse and respiration rates. The accessory muscles of respiration are used both in the 'air hunger' which follows acute blood loss and also when the airway is partly obstructed.
- (e) The site of an accessible vein for infusion is marked or noted.

(f) Heat loss is reduced to a minimum; a metal foil blanket is ideal, but make sure that the face, neck and upper thorax are visible.

(2) Each case should now be formally written up and the notes should include:

(a) An account of the circumstances of the injury. This should record the time, place, and cause of accident, if known, with a clear description, including the duration of any episode of loss of consciousness.

(b) The medical history (especially of any bleeding tendency) should be obtained from the parents or guardian if they are with the child, *or a note made to do this when they arrive.*

(c) The result of symptomatic enquiry (if the level of consciousness permits). A direct enquiry of a small confused and crying child with a severe injury is unlikely to be helpful, but when possible, it is advisable to concentrate upon changes of sight (loss of vision, or double vision) and changes in hearing.

(d) Clinical examination should be carried out systematically to discover injury to:

  (i) the skull (acute brain injury);
 (ii) the eyes and ears;
(iii) the maxillary complex, malar, nasal bones, and palate;
(iv) the mandible, the lower facial tissues and neck;
 (v) other regions, particularly bleeding into the thorax (page 17); peritoneal cavity, pelvis and tissues surrounding the long bones.

The nature and consequences of these injuries are now considered in turn:

The skull (acute head injury)

This is dealt with more fully under 'Acute Neurosurgical Emergencies' (p. 307). The most important conditions to consider are:

(a) Destructive injury to the brain which may be indicated by limb weakness, hemiparesis or irregularity of the pulse (p. 309).

(b) Deterioration of consciousness due to continuing intracranial bleeding, extradural haemorrhage, or traumatic cerebral oedema (p. 307).

The eyes and ears

(a) 'Blow-out' fractures with depression of the orbital floor are easily missed and are disfiguring if not properly treated (p. 154).

(b) Penetrating injuries of the cornea, orbit and globe are also serious and should be looked for carefully (p. 156).

(c) Direct injury to the nose or ear including the mastoid area require careful assessment by an ENT surgeon (p. 208).

The maxillary complex including the malar, nasal bones, and palate

The maxillary complex may be detached from the skull by fracture of its thin, leaf-like plates of bone. The detached portion as a whole, or in pieces, may be driven backwards and downwards towards the sphenoid body, taking the nasal bones, palate, alveolar process and attached soft tissues with it. A common single 'piece' injury consists of an infracture of the malar bone, with the occasional involvement of the structures in the orbit. Detached teeth may be inhaled and will require removal by bronchoscopy (*see* Ear, Nose and Throat section, page 207). *A radiograph of the chest should be requested if teeth are found to be missing.*

The possible effects of this type of injury are:

(a) The nasopharyngeal airway may be narrowed or completely obliterated by this displacement of the bony complex.

(b) As a consequence, there is a reduction in the alternative (oral) airway by encroachment upon the tongue space.

(c) The brisk bleeding from torn blood vessels in the nasal and pharyngeal region into the tissues and pharynx, and the impaired efficiency of the muscles of the nasopharyngeal sphincter due to displacement of the palate are both likely to cause further obstruction of the airway.

(d) Where the fractures extend into bony fissures and across foramina, important structures may be damaged by direct compression and tearing, or, indirectly, from the pressure from clotted blood. These structures may include:

   (i) The olfactory nerve and dura mater by involvement of the cribriform plate.

   (ii) The optic and ophthalmic nerves, retinal artery and other structures in the foramen lacerum.

   (iii) The chorda tympani nerve as it leaves the temporal bone.

   (iv) The maxillary division of the 5th nerve as it passes through the foramen rotundum and its branch in the infra-orbital canal.

A penetrating injury of the palate caused by a fall on to pointed objects is more common in children than adults and an ENT or plastic surgical opinion should be obtained (p. 208).

The mandible, the lower facial tissues and the neck

The mandible, to a large extent, protects the tongue, hyoid bone and larynx from direct injury, and involvement of these structures in the absence of damage to the mandible is unusual, the exception being strangulation. In most fractures of the mandible in the child, there is little displacement, but where a segment carrying the musculature attached to the genial process is detached, control of the tongue can be lost with obstruction of the airway, especially when the patient is supine.

The airway may also be at risk from swelling of the soft tissues under the tongue and in the laryngeal region, in particular, after an attempt at strangulation. If larger vessels are ruptured in the neck or floor of mouth, a haematoma may cause a similar embarrassment. The lip may be insensitive if the inferior dental nerve has been damaged, and rarely, the tongue, if the lingual nerve is involved.

An indirect fracture of one or both mandibular condyles at the neck may follow a blow or fall on to the chin.

The examination of the mid-face, mandible and neck

(a) GENERAL
Engorgement of the neck veins with use of the accessory muscles of respiration suggests a possible obstruction of the airway. There may also be stridor if there is laryngeal involvement.

(b) EXTRA-ORAL EXAMINATION
(1) The facial contour, despite swelling, may be changed following the set-back of the bony complex with a widening in the malar area, depending upon the direction of impact (seldom exactly mid-line). Downward displacement will produce an apparent lengthening of the face, and the mouth may be propped open upon the maxillary molar teeth. A similar appearance may result from a bilateral fracture of the mandibular condyles with shortening of the ascending ramus.

The systematic examination should look specifically for:
  (i) A leak of cerebrospinal fluid from the ear or nose. In the nose this may be difficult to see because of mixture with blood, or because the fluid is lost as a postnasal drip.
  (ii) Bleeding from the ear, nose or mouth, also the presence of clotted blood.
  (iii) The presence and distribution of subconjunctival haemorrhage. This examination may not be possible due to extensive soft-tissue swelling, and this fact *should be recorded* so that there is a reminder in the notes to do it later (eye examination, p. 156).
(2) It is important to remember that, as time passes from the moment of injury, the mid-face tissues swell quickly and the presence of a step or gap that would indicate a fracture is often difficult to detect by

palpation. The extent of swelling which could mask a considerable displacement must therefore be taken into account.

Examination is best carried out standing behind the patient and 'crawling' with the fingers around the orbital margins and nasal bones feeling for defects and comparing left with right. The less-obviously injured parts should be examined first so that the child, if conscious, may gain confidence from this selective approach. It is normally possible to feel the uninjured heads of the condyles on jaw movement and the whole of the lower border of the mandible. The presence of surgical (interstitial) emphysema and its distribution, especially any extension into the cervical and mediastinal areas, should be noted.

(c) INTRA-ORAL EXAMINATION

The facial soft tissues and lips may be torn from the underlying bone of the jaws in falls, particularly from bicycles, horses or moving vehicles. Impacted material from the ground may be present. In road-traffic accidents, non-radio-opaque foreign bodies such as wood, plastic, or glass may be in the tissues. Fractures of the underlying bone will be seen through the wound. With closed fractures, the presence of an ecchymosis into the soft tissues on the alveolus or in the floor of the mouth, will prompt a search for an underlying fracture. The teeth should be checked, looking especially in either jaw for groups of loose teeth attached to the alveolar process (in the younger child a detached segment may contain the forming permanent teeth). A search should be made for loose tooth fragments in open wounds. If empty sockets are present, the missing teeth may still be in the mouth, lying in the sulcus or under the tongue and obscured by blood. A tooth lying in the pharynx will be difficult or impossible to see, *therefore a request for airway radiographs should state that teeth are missing; a dislodged tooth may be seen on a chest radiograph* (*see* Ear, Nose and Throat section, page 210).

(d) RADIOGRAPHIC EXAMINATION

If radiographs can be obtained, two views (plain film) at least should be requested and should include preferably an occipitomental and lateral view of the skull and jaws. Fractures of the facial bones are difficult to diagnose and an expert opinion on the films should be obtained before discharge.

Management of injuries to the mid-face, mandible and neck

It is important to ensure that *further* episodes of airway obstruction do not occur, particularly where there has been an earlier loss of consciousness through obstruction, throttling or injury to the brain.

The prognosis may be changed from complete recovery to one of permanent brain injury through hypoxia. The same effect may also result from a second episode of obstruction in the presence of a continuous severe blood loss, particularly in the small (under 2 years of age) child with relatively small blood volume.

IMMEDIATE ACTION

(a) A regular routine of observation *in a good light* should be established to detect and treat:
  (i) changes in the level of consciousness (*see* Acute Head Injuries, page 309).
  (ii) changes in the adequacy of the airway.
  Whenever there is a possibility of obstruction to the airway and especially in mandibular fractures, a suture of 2/0 black silk should be passed as far back as possible through the dorsum of the tongue. The thread should be long enough to be secured to the chest.
  In the deeply unconscious patient or where a downward displacement of the maxillary complex has occurred, an oral airway should be inserted. The passage of an orotracheal tube in a severely injured child is not easy, but is life-saving if it can be managed. If these measures do not ensure an adequate airway, a tracheostomy must be carried out immediately (*see* page 221).

(b) The position of the patient should be reviewed from time to time, not only from the point of view of airway maintenance, but also in relation to continuing blood loss. It is difficult to detect postnasal or pharyngeal bleeding into the respiratory tract especially where the cough or swallowing reflex is impaired. An adequate aspiration routine should be established.
  Continued nasal haemorrhage demands treatment and a pack of ribbon gauze should be inserted. The time of insertion should be recorded with an instruction in the notes that it *should be removed* or replaced within 24 hours (*see also* page 213).

(c) It is wise at this stage to set up an IV line before collapse of the veins in shock makes this difficult.

(d) Where a cerebrospinal fluid leak is suspected, ampicillin should be given intramuscularly or intravenously in a dose of 150 mg per kg per 24 hours for 7 to 10 days. Ampicillin should also be considered in extensive open fractures of the facial bones, or where the viability of soft tissue is in doubt.

MEDIUM-TERM MEASURES

In the first twenty-four hours

    (a) If a tracheostomy has been necessary, a regular nursing routine of observation should be established.

    (b) If an anaesthetic is to be given to cover some other urgent surgical procedure, the opportunity should be taken to secure and tie the accessible bleeding vessels in the soft tissues to reduce total blood loss. Care should be taken to avoid the inclusion of the larger sensory nerves in the forceps. An effort should be made to obtain coverage of exposed bone, preserving as much soft tissue as possible. Quite large sections of jaw with teeth attached and teeth inside will survive.

    (c) Tetanus toxoid should be given if the wound is open or contaminated.

    (d) Provided that the airway is clear and haemorrhage is under control, all other maxillofacial procedures can be deferred, if necessary for several days, but should be planned at the earliest opportunity as part of the overall surgical management.

MISTAKES IN MANAGEMENT

    (a) In the early stages of any head, face or neck injury:
        (i) Drugs which depress the central nervous system and the respiratory centre in particular should NOT be used.
        (ii) A general anaesthetic should be avoided except to cover a life-saving operation such as tracheostomy.

    (b) Any solution containing adrenaline or noradrenaline should not be injected, particularly if it is possible that a general anaesthetic might be required later. A preparation containing 3 per cent prilocaine with felypressin would be acceptable for local analgesia.

    (c) The manipulation of loose fragments is unwise, as this can cause further bleeding. (However, if a dental or maxillofacial specialist is available, a severe continuous haemorrhage can sometimes be controlled by the stabilization of the larger fragments.)

    (d) A repair of a penetrating injury of the palate should not be undertaken until an ENT or plastic surgical opinion has been obtained.

CHAPTER 16

Dental Emergencies

R. C. W. Dinsdale

Oral haemorrhage

Primary haemorrhage, and traumatic post-extraction

In the normal child, persistent haemorrhage from a tooth socket after a dental extraction or a traumatic incident, is uncommon. The occasional dental case may present as a true emergency, which must be distinguished from the emotionally-charged minor problem that arises from time to time in all accident and emergency departments.

RECOGNITION

In the immediate period, the emphasis should be upon control by local measures, having secured a clear account of the current episode, concentrating upon:

(a) *The history*

The following questions will help with the diagnosis and subsequently with assessment of suitability for anaesthesia.

   (i) Where and when were the extractions carried out?

  (ii) Why? For drainage of an abscess, or as a routine part of a treatment plan. The hyperaemia of acutely inflamed tissue may be a factor in continued haemorrhage.

 (iii) Were any tablets taken for pain before or since the extraction, in particular those containing aspirin or narcotic drugs?

 (iv) Which method of anaesthesia was used?

  (v) How many deciduous and, more important, permanent teeth were removed (the latter will have a larger root surface area with a greater potential for blood loss)?

 (vi) Has the bleeding ever stopped?

(vii) Has the patient been rinsing excessively?
(viii) Has the patient been overactive, restless or crying?
(ix) What measures have already been tried?
(x) Was there a period of reduced fluid intake on account of toothache before the extraction?
(xi) Have there been any previous episodes of post-extraction dental bleeding, of spontaneous nasal bleeding or bruising, or is there any known family history of a bleeding or coagulation disorder?

(b) Examination

THE PALLOR OF A CHILD WITH A STOMACH FULL OF SWALLOWED BLOOD MUST NOT BE CONFUSED WITH THE PALLOR ASSOCIATED WITH EXCESSIVE BLOOD LOSS.

Therefore, an assessment of blood loss and degree of dehydration should be made. This should include recording of blood pressure, pulse and respiration rates, making an allowance for the effects of apprehension.

Account should be taken of the rate of blood loss and this must be considered in relation to the blood volume and age of the child (*see* page 103).

The Local Examination should be carried out in a good light, in the following manner.

Using a small swab applied gently and intermittently to the bleeding site and an aspirator fitted with a small tip (a large aspirator with a vigorous sucking action is frightening) the following observations should be made:

(a) Is there bleeding from one or more than one socket?
(b) Is there evidence of local trauma? A forceps laceration should be obvious; these are less easily seen on the lingual side of the lower teeth.
(c) Is any unsupported tissue present which can be moved by cheek or tongue?
(d) Is there evidence of an ecchymosis or haematoma by extension from the extraction site into adjacent tissues. The presence of a large haematoma may be the first manifestation of a previously unsuspected bleeding diathesis in a young child.
(e) Have the sockets already been sutured?

From these observations and the history, an estimate of total and continuing rate of blood loss into the mouth or tissues should be made.

It should also be possible to suggest a likely cause for the bleeding, usually due to local factors, but impairment of platelet function from aspirin intake must also be considered, particularly in the absence of any previous personal or family history of bleeding.

MANAGEMENT

Immediate

As an interim measure, the patient should be encouraged to close lightly on a small swab trimmed to cover the tooth socket and to fit between adjacent teeth.

Provided that the bleeding is not copious and the cardiovascular system is stable, treatment may then be deferred for up to two hours until the services of a dental surgeon can be obtained.

If this is not feasible, the following routine should be followed:
  (i) Smear a little lignocaine surface-anaesthetic paste on to the mucous membrane on either side of the socket—a small pledget of cotton wool may be tolerated.
 (ii) One minute later, using a short fine needle, inject 0.5 ml 3 per cent prilocaine with felypressin under the lax mucosa on either side of the tooth socket.

In the small child, or where co-operation is not forthcoming, the administration of a general anaesthetic in order to place the sutures accurately, must be considered. Intubation is essential because of the risk of a sudden reflux of swallowed blood from the stomach. The opportunity can also be taken to gain access to a vein for any subsequent infusion that may be needed.
(iii) It should now be possible to place one or two across-the-socket sutures using 3/0 black silk or catgut on a curved 22 mm, preferably reverse-cutting, needle. If catgut is used, it should be 'triple'-tied.
(iv) A second tailored swab, of a height just greater than the crown of the extracted tooth, can then be placed over the newly stabilized socket and left in place for 15 minutes.
 (v) Now remove the swab and wait. If there is no fresh bleeding after a further 15 minutes, it can be assumed that a stable clot has formed.

Continued bleeding

The site should be re-examined carefully and the placement of further sutures (possibly under a general anaesthetic) should be considered.

If the bleeding is from *more than one* tooth socket and sutures have failed to control it, a systemic cause should be suspected. Should facilities for the assay of clotting factors and study of platelet function not be immediately available, the injection of hydrocortisone 100 mg or dexamethasone phosphate 4 mg IV may be tried. If effective, the bleeding will stop spontaneously in approximately half an hour. These drugs appear to reduce capillary permeability (Robson and Duthie, 1952) and enhance platelet activity. The short-lived elevation of the serum-cortisol level will not interfere with subsequent coagulation studies.

IMPORTANT NOTE.
Intramuscular injections should be avoided until the presence of a coagulation disorder has been excluded.

Recurrent haemorrhage

Infection of the soft-tissue wound in the mouth is the most usual cause. The bleeding is brisk and *difficult* to control, the tissues being swollen and friable. Several episodes of bleeding may have occurred before referral, with considerable blood loss, and the patient may also be dehydrated.

MANAGEMENT
    (a) A dental specialist should be called immediately.
    (b) A transfusion with whole blood may be required to treat shock and anaemia, and to cover the further blood loss that will occur during treatment.
    (c) A general anaesthetic is often necessary to provide the best conditions for a detailed examination. This should be given by an experienced anaesthetist who will take into account the state of the cardiovascular system and previous drug therapy.
    (d) A series of sutures, taking deep bites of tissue, should be inserted across the socket and the adjacent soft tissues undersewn. A specific bleeding point may be secured with a fine artery forceps and tied off. Exuberant granulation tissue should also be removed at this stage and an impression taken for the construction of a splint.
    (e) An antibiotic, preferably benzylpenicillin should be given.

Spontaneous haemorrhage

Spontaneous haemorrhage from the gums or continued haemorrhage from some trivial injury, for example an accidental bite of the tongue or cheek or frenal tear, is unusual in the normal child, and a systemic cause, or non-accidental injury, must be suspected. An abnormal tendency to bleed may be revealed at the time of eruption or when the change from the deciduous to the permanent dentition is taking place.

The deciduous teeth will be loose and there is often a hyperaemia at the point of attachment. Spontaneous bleeding from the gums will most often be associated with a severe anaemia, leukaemia or similar blood disorder, and it may also occur during the treatment of some of these conditions with chemotherapeutic agents.

Suspicion that a blood disorder is present will be supported by the presence of small petechial haemorrhages on the soft palate and cheeks, especially if there is bruising elsewhere on the body.

MANAGEMENT

In post-extraction dental haemorrhage, the emphasis is upon control by local means, whereas the successful management of this type of bleeding lies more upon the correct diagnosis and treatment of the underlying disorder, e.g. infusion of blood and the administration of concentrates of factors VIII or IX appropriate to the diagnosis.

In such cases a haematologist should be consulted and the services of an experienced dental surgeon obtained. Should this not be feasible, the case should be considered for transfer to the nearest centre known to provide such a service.

Local treatment must be co-ordinated with general treatment. The local measures will include suturing to stabilize soft tissue, *removal of loose teeth* and *excision* of soft tissue where necessary. Occasionally splints may be specially constructed to fit over and protect exposed sites from trauma until healing can take place. An antibiotic will be required, especially for those cases on immunosuppressive or chemotherapeutic drugs.

Traumatic injuries to the teeth

While accidental damage to the teeth cannot be regarded as life-threatening, doctors in accident and emergency departments are frequently asked by anxious parents to provide advice and treatment. These injuries may be broadly classified as follows:

Direct damage to crown, pulp or root.

Avulsion, with or without attached alveolar bone.

Indirect damage to the developing tooth (resulting in enamel hypoplasia or root dilaceration).

(For general reference: Andreason, 1972).

Direct damage to crown, pulp or root

It is customary to describe injuries to the teeth numerically (Ellis, 1960).

Class I   Traumatized tooth. No crown or root fracture.
Class II   A fracture confined to the enamel or including both
enamel and dentine but not exposing the pulp.
Class III   A fracture involving enamel with pulp *visible* through a
thin layer of dentine.
Class IV   A fracture involving enamel, dentine and exposing the
pulp.
Class V   A fracture involving dentine, cementum and pulp (root
fracture).

MANAGEMENT

All patients with a history of trauma to the teeth should be seen by a
dental surgeon even if no obvious injury has been sustained. In Class I
injuries tooth pulp may degenerate gradually and regular examination
is required to detect change and start treatment. Radiographs will
exclude in particular Class V (root fracture) injuries and damage to
adjacent and opposing teeth.

Class I, II and V injuries require no immediate treatment. Class III
and IV injuries require treatment within 24 hours to offer the best
prospect of retaining the vitality of the pulp tissue. This is important if
the root is still forming. If possible, a dental surgeon should be called to
these cases as materials are now available to provide immediate protection to the exposed pulp tissue (Watkins and Andlaw, 1977).

Avulsion

Replantation may be tried. The chances of a successful result are
reduced if:
(a) More than two hours have elapsed since the tooth was lost.
(b) The root surface has been allowed to dry out.
(c) The root cementum has been damaged by instrumentation or
excessive handling.
(d) The root is not fully formed.

MANAGEMENT

If a dental surgeon is not available:
(1) Immerse the tooth in sterile normal saline immediately.
(2) Smear a little lignocaine surface-anaesthetic paste onto the mucous
membrane on either side of the socket—a small pledget of cotton
wool may be tolerated.
(3) One minute later, using a short fine needle, inject 0.5 ml 3 per cent
prilocaine with felypressin into the lax tissues on either side of the
socket.
(4) Completely aspirate the blood clot and irrigate with normal saline
until the socket is clean.

(5) Reinsert the tooth and hold it in place for at least 10 minutes. Many teeth will stay in place even if protruding slightly from the socket. It will usually be possible to realign the tooth by orthodontic means at a later date.
(6) An antibiotic preferably benzylpenicillin in standard dose should be given.
(7) Tetanus toxoid should be given.
(8) Refer to dental surgeon preferably within 24 hours. An assessment can then be made as to whether to proceed with treatment which may include stabilization, or to remove the tooth and compensate for the loss in some other way.

Indirect damage to developing teeth, enamel hypoplasia and root dilaceration

Both types of injury may follow from the impaction of the root of a deciduous incisor tooth into the follicle of the permanent successor. The permanent central incisor is unfortunately the tooth most frequently involved.

MANAGEMENT

Depending upon a number of factors, including the age of the child, it will occasionally be possible, after extracting the impacted tooth, to reposition the displaced permanent crown by pressure through the buccal plate of bone. This will give the dentine papilla a chance to continue the process of root formation in reasonable alignment and so reduce the degree of dilaceration.

References

Andreason, J. O. (1972). *Traumatic Injuries to the Teeth*. Copenhagen: Munksgaard
Ellis, R. G. (1960). *The Classification and Treatment of Injuries to the Teeth of Children*. 4th edn. Chicago: Yearbook Publishers Inc.
Robson, H. N. and Duthie, J. J. R. (1952). Further observations on capillary resistance and adrenocortical activity. *Br. med. J.* (i), 994
Watkins, J. J. and Andlaw, R. J. (1977). Restoration of fractured incisors with an ultraviolet light polymerized composite resin. *Br. dent. J.* **142**, 249

CHAPTER 17

Acute Swellings of the Face

R. C. W. Dinsdale

Causes

A rapidly enlarging swelling of the facial and intra-oral tissues, including the floor of the mouth and the tongue, is usually caused by an acute spreading infection, but may occasionally have an allergic or urticarial basis as in bee or wasp stings. The recognition and management of the latter and of the rare hereditary angio-oedema which can arise unexpectedly from a minor injury, an injection, or surgery, are discussed on pages 542 and 494.

The patient may also present with extensive swelling resulting from accidental or non-accidental injury, or following dental or surgical treatment. The swelling may be caused by the products of injury, infection, or the accumulation of blood in the tissues. A haematoma which can develop after the injection of a local anaesthetic, may form rapidly and result in an urgent referral to hospital. Occasionally the development of a large haematoma is the first manifestation of a previously unsuspected bleeding diathesis in a young child.

The management of a swelling arising from accidental injury is dealt with in the section on Traumatic Injuries to the Head, Face and Neck (pp. 162–168).

Facial swelling due to a severe haematoma

MANAGEMENT
(1) If the airway is thought to be at risk, admit the patient.
(2) Assess the effect of blood loss into the tissues upon the cardiovascular system.
(3) Prescribe an antibiotic in standard dose, avoiding the intramuscular route.

(4) If a disorder of coagulation is thought to be present, a haematolo-
    gist should be consulted as soon as possible.

COMPLICATIONS
It should be remembered that death has resulted from all of the acute
swellings described, from:
  (a) Obstruction of the airway due to an extension of swelling into the
      lax tissues around the larynx.
  (b) An acute pulmonary oedema from a secondary chest infection or
      as part of an acute anaphylactic response.
  (c) A cavernous sinus thrombosis by the extension of an acute
      infection via the communicating veins.
  (d) The development of a septicaemia.

Acute infections of the face

With modern antibiotic therapy, infections of the facial tissues rarely
become emergencies. A rapid spread in the healthy child is unusual but
in a malnourished child cancrum oris and acute osteomyelitis of the
facial bones from secondary invasion can follow a viral infection such
as measles. The association of an acute infective process with diabetes
and with genetically determined disorders such as the Wiskott–Aldrich
syndrome and the use of immunosuppressive drugs, should not be
overlooked.
    It should be remembered that whatever the origin of the organism,
whether dental, from the skin surface or tonsil, a lymphatic gland in the
drainage area may break down, the resulting swelling being the *chief
presenting feature* of the case.
    In the differential diagnosis of acute infective swellings in the
cervical and submandibular region, acute parotitis and the submandibular adenitis of infancy must be considered.
The commonest sources of organisms are the teeth (and supporting
structures) and the skin surface.

CAUSES

(a) Dental disease

Extension by direct spread usually occurs:
  (i) through the alveolar process from the root of a tooth in which the
      pulp has become necrotic and infected from caries, or due to the
      effects of injury.
  (ii) from an infection of the soft tissues around the crown of an
      erupting tooth.
From the maxillary teeth the spread may be upwards into the lip and

G

between the muscles of facial expression to involve the lax tissues in the infra-orbital region or posteriorly to the infratemporal fossa. From the mandible the spread may be downward to include the floor of the mouth, the submandibular spaces and, posteriorly to involve the cervical spaces. The skin over a large abscess may rupture spontaneously leading to the development of a chronic dentocutaneous sinus.

(b) Skin surface

In children the usual portal of entry is via an infected lesion at the ala of the nose and the angle of the mouth; an abscess or cellulitis may result. There is a small risk of cavernous sinus thrombosis if the swelling occurs in the area of the upper lip, inner canthus or the nose.

The lymphatic gland anterior to the facial artery as it passes over the mandible is often enlarged and may be confused with a swelling of dental origin.

ASSESSMENT

(a) It is important at the outset to determine whether access to the mouth and throat will be possible if an anaesthetic is required. Four observations are important:

    (i) Can the mouth be opened? Trismus from pain is usually dental, but acute tonsillar infections and parotitis can also be responsible.

    (ii) Are the tissues in the floor of the mouth and around the base of the tongue swollen?

    (iii) Is the tongue fixed or elevated?

    (iv) Is there evidence of airway obstruction?

(b) In pyogenic infections, it is important to distinguish between a cellulitis alone and a cellulitis with abscess formation. An abscess is present if fluctuation can be elicited. However, the swelling may be too tense and too painful to obtain this sign. The presence of a soft, exquisitely tender spot is sufficient evidence of pus formation and will indicate a suitable point for drainage.

MANAGEMENT

(a) A child with a rapidly enlarging inflammatory swelling of the face or neck, who is pyrexial and ill, should be admitted for observation, especially if the airway is considered to be at risk.

(b) Surgical intervention will often be necessary. The anaesthetist should be informed in good time as these cases carry a high risk of an airway complication.

(c) An incision along the line of a natural skin crease should be made to drain an established abscess. At this time it is preferable to *extract* the causative tooth if the swelling is of dental origin; the pus can be sent for culture.

(d) Where there is no evidence of pus formation, no attempt at surgical decompression of a brawny swelling should be undertaken. Until there are positive signs of localization of pus, management should concentrate on antibiotic therapy and preservation of the airway, if necessary by tracheostomy (Holland, 1975).

(e) Where there is toxaemia with an elevated temperature suggesting septicaemia or there is a possibility of sub-acute bacterial endocarditis (in a child with a cardiac lesion), blood should be taken for culture *before* an antibiotic is given.

Provided that the patient is not sensitive to penicillin, this is the antibiotic of choice. If oral penicillin has already been started, this should be supplemented by an intramuscular injection, with the addition of cloxacillin when there is reason to suspect a resistant staphylococcal infection. No change should be made with this regime until the results of culture and sensitivity tests are available.

Where the patient is known to have had a sensitivity reaction to penicillin, the choice is more difficult for there is no one antibiotic as effective as penicillin. *See* Appendix 9 for choice of other antibiotics.

(*c*) *Complications*

(i) An obstruction of the airway should not be allowed to develop; an early tracheostomy is essential.

(ii) Dehydration should be corrected by IV fluids (p. 95).

(iii) Hyperpyrexia should be treated by cooling.

(iv) At the earliest sign of a possible cavernous sinus thrombosis, anticoagulant and parenteral antibiotic therapy should be started.

References

Holland, C. S. (1975). The management of Ludwig's angina. *Br. J. Oral Surg.* **13**, 153

Part V: Intensive Treatment and Emergency Anaesthesia

CHAPTER 18

An Intensive Treatment Unit for Children

A. M. Wilson

Organization

An intensive treatment unit is a meeting point in the hospital for many disciplines. Usually the beds are undesignated, thus allowing any doctor to admit to the unit. Nevertheless there must be one person in charge to co-ordinate the functions of the unit. He does not look after the patients but is in administrative charge. It is important to understand his function in order to achieve the best use from an Intensive Treatment Unit.

Functions of the administrative leader
(a) Decisions on admission and discharge policy. He will make these in consultation with all staff, medical and nursing, and adjust the work load of the unit to the facilities available.
(b) Decisions on operational policies. Although many individuals are admitting patients there must be standard routines. These, for example the use of recording charts, may be peculiar only to the unit.
(c) Liaison with nursing, radiology and laboratory staff.
(d) Support for unit nursing and junior staff.
(e) Availability for consultation on any of the above points. If of appropriate speciality, offering of specialist opinion.
(f) Training of nursing and junior staff in new techniques, and new equipment, and in resuscitation.
(g) Co-ordination of the purchase and use of equipment.
(h) Supervision of emergency services for the remainder of the hospital.

(i) Involvement in any major accident plan.
The administrative leader need not be involved in the practical management of each patient, but acts as co-ordinator. To be able to do this he will:
   (a) Follow the progress of each child.
   (b) Ensure equipment is being used correctly and to maximum advantage.
   (c) Attempt to co-ordinate treatment if more than one firm is involved.
   (d) Ensure that the whole aspect of the child's care is being considered.
   (e) Ensure that the case notes are adequate to achieve continuity of care during staff changeover.
   (f) Ensure that instructions to nursing staff are of correct standard.
It is therefore important that medical staff admitting patients to an intensive care unit should keep the consultant in charge informed, as only in this way can the unit be run efficiently.

Any physician or surgeon admitting a child under this system retains independent medical care of the patient but must sacrifice some control of the technical and practical management. In return his patient receives more intensive nursing and medical observation. Where conditions are likely to change suddenly this is of the utmost value and the I.T.U. staff will independently start resuscitative or restorative measures by virtue of having the medical staff immediately available, and uncommitted to out-patient sessions, etc. No I.T.U. will work effectively without rules but the final result will depend upon the personalities of the co-ordinator and the admitting consultants. Fortunately, most children's hospitals and units are sufficiently small for friendly relationships to rule the organization. Under these conditions the level of treatment actually given by the I.T.U. staff, e.g. the duty anaesthetists, will vary according to work load and individual abilities and enthusiasms. The overriding principle must be communication so that each member of the therapeutic team knows exactly what he is expected to do and not to do.

Suggested rules for practical administration

   (a) Patients remain under the primary care of the admitting consultant.
   (b) Emergency treatment will be undertaken by unit staff and the admitting firm is to be informed as soon as possible.
   (c) No treatment to be changed by anyone without informing the house officer of the admitting firm.
   (d) All changes of condition to be recorded in the case-notes.

(e) All changes of treatment, including the reason for such change, to be recorded.

(f) On no account will any verbal message be accepted.

(g) All settings of apparatus, drip rates, ventilators and monitor alarm limits to be recorded.

(h) Only I.T.U. standard records to be kept.

(i) On admission to the I.T.U. each child's notes must contain a summary indicating:
> Diagnosis, provisional if necessary.
> Reason for I.T.U. admission, e.g. nursing, monitoring, etc.
> Indications for change of treatment.
> Likely course of progress.
> Destination on discharge.

(j) Everything done to a child must be prescribed. This includes:
> Diet
> IV therapy
> Oxygen therapy
> Physiotherapy
> Drug therapy
> Monitoring (type and alarm limits)
> Humidification
> Turning

The above suggests a rigid approach which is necessary when so many are working in one area. However it is equally necessary to be flexible, especially when dealing with children.

Parents must be considered as patients of the intensive care unit when their child is admitted. They need support and explanation. A booklet or leaflet outlining the function of the unit is useful especially when a child is admitted as an emergency rather than postoperatively (when explanation and a visit to the unit is possible beforehand). Toys also should be welcomed, even a favourite cuddly toy which looks bacteriologically suspect. The child has lived with this animal for a long time and its psychological benefits outweigh any danger. We have on occasion autoclaved a teddy-bear but do not recommend it.

Indications for admission to an intensive treatment unit

No rigid criteria can be applied as the size of the unit will determine what type of cases shall be admitted. The ability of other wards of the hospital to handle very ill children will affect the case load of an I.T.U. The unit should not be used merely for any child with a problem out of the ordinary. This approach is self-defeating as the unit becomes full and either unable to take severely ill patients or is forced to discharge the patient unnecessarily admitted. The admission of a child to I.T.U. is traumatic to the parents and should be used like any drug, i.e. prescribed only when genuinely indicated.

The indications for admission include:

(a) Support of depressed vital function of:
- (i) Respiratory system.
- (ii) Cardiovascular system.
- (iii) Renal system.
- (iv) Central nervous system.

(b) Where special equipment is, or may be, necessary.
- (i) Respiratory: ventilation, intubation, inhalation therapy, blood-gas analysis,
- (ii) Cardiovascular: intra-arterial monitoring, automatic infusion control, implanted pacemaker.
- (iii) Renal dialysis.
- (iv) Exchange transfusion.

(c) When a sudden change in condition is anticipated or possible.
- (i) Respiratory system: this is especially applicable to respiratory obstruction where intervention may be necessary, or to postoperative cases where respiratory failure may occur with tiring or the necessary use of analgesics.
- (ii) Cardiovascular system: after cardiac operations when the haemodynamic state is changing rapidly, or in acute blood loss. Where diffuse intravascular coagulation is a possibility.
- (iii) Poisoning: where changes in level of consciousness, respiratory depression, or cardiac abnormalities are expected. When the drug cannot be identified, or the nature of its action is unknown a child should be admitted to an I.T.U.

  When changes are expected it is always better to transfer a child early; this can then take place in a planned, unhurried manner, and thereafter the child is near the equipment and staff which may be required. This avoids emergency intervention under unsuitable conditions.

(d) When special skills may be necessary.

The I.T.U. offers the opportunity for a concentration of monitoring both by nursing staff and by machine. The high nurse–patient ratio allows nurses to observe and record at very frequent intervals, even continuously if necessary. Monitoring by machine permits a number of advantages which become more apparent the smaller the patient. Machine-monitoring of basic vital signs such as temperature, pulse, pulse rate, ECG, rate and depth of respiration, can be performed without handling the child. This is important in small or premature babies who do not tolerate handling well. If they are being nursed in an incubator any intrusion in it for observations causes the incubator atmosphere to return to that of room air within 30 seconds. There is thus a fall in oxygen concentration and humidity, and a loss of heat. These intrusions can be kept to a necessary minimum by mechanical and electronic monitoring. If records are to be kept they must be accurate. A machine-monitor is capable of counting rapid pulse and respiratory rates with a greater accuracy than a human observer. Lastly, automatic monitoring can be set to give an alarm if pre-set limits are exceeded, and so allow continuous rather than intermittent observation.

Such monitoring is best carried out in an I.T.U. as the maximum use of these machines can only be achieved by those with experience. The introduction of an automatic monitor into a ward should not be seen as a substitute for adequate nursing care. These machines assist nursing care and do not replace it.

Within the limits of an I.T.U. it is possible for some nurses to be trained to undertake duties outside their normal range, such as intravenous injections. Children who must receive such treatment frequently may do so in an I.T.U.

(e) When uncommon procedures are to be performed. It is logical to concentrate uncommon procedures in an I.T.U. so that the staff can gain sufficient experience to become expert. These uncommon procedures include:

    (i) Intravenous nutrition. This requires strict attention to long-catheter central-vein systems, and to asepsis of the IV liquids.

    (ii) Exchange transfusion. Babies undergoing this procedure require temperature control, pulse and ECG monitoring. Since these are available, with control of inspired oxygen and humidity in addition, the I.T.U. is well equipped to handle exchange transfusions.

    (iii) Peritoneal dialysis. The above equally applies.

(f) When frequent alteration of treatment is likely. The staff in an I.T.U. will always include a high proportion of trained nurses who are able to administer drugs as soon as required. In addition an I.T.U. will carry a more comprehensive stock of drugs ready for use.

(g) When medical and nursing procedures are very time-consuming. It is difficult to make time for patients who require a lot of attention on a general ward when there are others requiring treatment. An I.T.U. can more easily adjust work load to its staff to accommodate this problem.

Attention to the child as well as the disease

An intensive treatment unit is so named because it provides care in addition to treatment. The child with the disease must not be forgotten, and tender loving care is part of the treatment. I.T.U. nurses are encouraged to nurse, and play with, the children. It is sometimes necessary to cuddle a child for a long period, for example where extubation is followed by residual stridor made worse by restlessness due to respiratory difficulty. This treatment does not look like intensive care but it may be the soothing care needed to avoid re-intubation. Visiting is encouraged for short but frequent periods and this precludes the wearing of overshoes, masks and gowns which are frightening to a child.

Care after the acute emergency

Children frequently recover quickly, resulting in an apparently well child remaining in I.T.U. Patients should not be discharged too quickly, in case of relapse. Having to be re-admitted to I.T.U. is very frightening for the child, and worrying for his parents. It upsets the morale of the unit staff and loses the confidence of the rest of the hospital. Also, and very important, I.T.U. nursing is very wearing with many disappointments. Being able to talk to and play with a cured child is therapy for the staff.

Ethical problems of turning off a ventilator
(*See also* section on cardiac arrest p. 303).

The decision to stop ventilator treatment when there are still signs of life, but when disease or accident have produced severe cerebral damage is always difficult. It must rest only with the consultant in charge of the patient but he will wish to consult with others concerned in the treatment, and with the family. There is much talk about consultation and collective decisions but someone has to take the action, and the responsibility. Some guidance to be used in coming to this most arduous decision is given below.

    (a) The consultant must be certain that all possible forms of treatment have been tried.

    (b) He must be certain that an adequate time has elapsed since the accident or disease for a steady state to have been reached. There are many reports of unexpected recovery after severe damage, but, in fact, this is rare. Nevertheless, the possibility must be considered.

    (c) The consultant must feel that no survival is possible off the ventilator. If survival without the ventilator is possible, but with impaired cerebral function, the problem for the doctor is resolved. Ventilation may then be stopped and the child allowed to take his chance as a self-supporting if not self-sufficient individual.

(d) The consultant must further feel that survival on the ventilator will *never* result in conscious awareness. There is no objective test to ascertain whether this last point holds true. Use must be made of clinical observations, experience of similar cases, and investigations.

Clinical observations

(a) No sign of conscious awareness.

(b) No response to a normally painful stimulus.

(c) Loss of all pupillary reflexes.

(d) Loss of control of *more than one* of the body's internal servo-systems.

    (i) No respiration in the presence of an elevated pCO_2 and normal hydrogen ion level.
    No response to chemical respiratory stimulants.

    (ii) Highly variable pulse rate.

    (iii) Labile blood pressure for no cause.

    (iv) Loss of temperature control.

    (v) Unexplained electrolyte disturbance.

INVESTIGATIONS THAT MAY BE OF HELP

(a) Cerebral angiogram
Where cerebral oedema had complicated a head injury or hypoxic episode, this investigation may show that there is no return of cerebral blood flow. If this is absent no recovery is possible.

(b) Electroencephalography
This is considered a necessary investigation in some countries before a ventilator may be turned off. It must be *performed* under ideal conditions by an expert to be reliable. If there is no activity at normal body temperature and in the absence of any drugs this may be conclusive of brain death. It has been recommended that no action should be taken until two, or three, such EEGs have been taken at 24-hour intervals.

The overriding statement must always be: if in doubt wait.

Whoever makes the decision must consider the parents. It is not fair to their future life to give parents this decision to make but many will wish to participate, and may even ask for ventilation to be stopped. Others seem to prefer to be told some such formula as 'We will have to try him without the ventilator', and later to be told that the attempt has failed. Parents must always be told explicity or implicitly that such a course is indicated.

The nursing staff on an I.T.U. will have spent day and night working for the child and a sudden reversal from full treatment to abandonment can leave them hurt and confused. The sister-in-charge must be involved in the decision with full explanation so that she can support her nurses in their understanding of the situation.

With the ever present risk of litigation only a consultant may actually switch off a ventilator. This can never be a delegated duty. He must record accurately why the action was taken and personally certify death.

CHAPTER 19

Emergency Anaesthesia

A. M. Wilson

All children undergoing anaesthesia must be considered at some small, but definite, risk, although the normal child does not present an increased anaesthetic risk over adults. Where the preoperative preparation must be reduced, as for emergency anaesthesia, this risk will be increased. Before anaesthesia the resident should take a brief history and make a short examination with emphasis on points of importance to the anaesthetist. Ideally, the anaesthetist will do this for himself or repeat it. The resident should, however, consider these points in his clerking of the patient as some findings may suggest further investigations or alter the management, such as requiring the child to be admitted. This history-taking and examination (*see* Table 19.I and page 197) is designed to find any points that may result in anaesthetic difficulty, or increased anaesthetic risk.

These can be elicited by a few questions and a brief examination and occasionally also by investigation.

The history will often be included in the admission of the patient but where this is obvious, as in the case of a limb fracture, the following questions must be asked specifically:

(*a*) *Was the child well until this present illness?*

(*b*) *Was there any sign of cough or cold?*
The presence of even mild upper respiratory disease, especially nasal discharge increases the risk of laryngeal obstruction during induction and awakening, and also the risk of postoperative bronchopneumonia. Any sign of a cough or cold should cause the child to be admitted following an emergency anaesthetic and treated with chest physiotherapy.

TABLE 19.I
Cases of risk

Mechanical

Poor airway:	Facial abnormality
	Restricted neck movement
	Restricted jaw movement
	Large tongue
	Loose teeth, or dental bridges
	Enormous tonsils
	Blocked nose
	Pharyngeal infection
	Known laryngeal abnormality
	Airway narrowing due to infection
Full stomach	

Intercurrent illness

Respiratory infection
Asthma
Cardiac abnormalities
Anaemia
Renal disease
Electrolyte disturbance
Jaundice
Hypovolaemia

Drug therapy

Steroids
Diabetes mellitus
Cardiac glycosides (digoxin usually)

Untoward reactions

Pseudocholinesterase deficiency
Malignant hyperpyrexia
Hypersensitivity to anaesthetic agents
Porphyria

(c) *Does the child suffer from asthma or have any other allergic
disease, e.g. eczema?*
Some anaesthetic drugs, e.g. curare, cause histamine release and are
better avoided. Some induction agents have a higher incidence of
hypersensitivity response which may be increased in patients already
showing such reactions.

(d) *Is there any history of previous heart or chest disease?*
Particularly, one is looking for a history of congenital cardiac abnormality, especially a shunt which may reverse with the alteration of
intrathoracic pressure during anaesthesia. Any patient in whom there is

such a history must be admitted to hospital so that anaesthesia can be performed in a theatre fully equipped for cardiac resuscitation by competent personnel. Antibiotic treatment should be started to prevent sub-acute bacterial endocarditis whenever there is a risk of bacteraemia occurring during the procedure, e.g. dental extraction, abscess incision.

(e) *Is there any current renal disease?*

The patient with chronic renal disease may have electrolyte disturbances. Such disturbances, particularly of intra- to extracellular potassium balance can cause difficulty with some muscle relaxants, e.g. suxamethonium.

(f) *Is there any history of jaundice or hepatitis?*

Although many anaesthetic drugs are metabolized by the liver, it is rare for liver disease unless severe, to have a prolonged effect. Where liver disease exists, barbiturates should be given sparingly or avoided, and this includes thiopentone. Liver disease is an absolute contra-indication to the use of fluothane and trichlorethylene. In obstructive jaundice opiates should be avoided because of their effect on the sphincter of Oddi. In active hepatitis (suspected or proved serum hepatitis B) it is best to avoid contact with the patient's blood samples and to warn anaesthetic and laboratory staff similarly.

(g) *What drugs is the patient taking or has taken in the last year?*

Children are prescribed few drugs that affect or may interact with anaesthesia. Nevertheless there are a few receiving tranquillizers and cardiac glycosides, and this question must be asked.

   (i) Corticosteroids

   A number of children receive steroids, particularly for asthma and eczema. Anaesthesia and operation stimulate an increase in the output of endogenous steroids. If this response has been reduced by atrophy due to exogenous steroids there will be no increase in the level of circulating steroids, with the risk of hypotension and 'adrenal crisis'. This is most likely to occur just before anaesthesia and in the postoperative period. Most emergency conditions involve a strong emotional stimulus, so the steroid requirement will be very high. Under ideal conditions adrenocortical function could be tested by giving artificial ACTH (the synacthen test) and increased steroids only given if the response is diminished. Under emergency conditions it is best to err on the safe side and where there is any doubt, even if the last course of steroids was up to nine months ago, to give hydrocortisone over the period of the operation and for the next day. For a standard course of steroid cover *see* page 458. There is probably no harm in such a short course and it avoids the risk of an unnoticed hypotensive episode during the night after the operation.

(ii) Cardiac glycosides (digoxin etc.)
Children taking these drugs must be admitted and fully monitored with an ECG during the operation.

(iii) Insulin in diabetes mellitus (*see also* page 439).
Patients with diabetes mellitus present little anaesthetic difficulty, but the anaesthetic and operation upset the control of the diabetes, partly by requiring starvation and partly because the stress of the procedure results in changing insulin requirements.

If the patient is controlled by oral hypoglycaemic drugs or by diet alone (unlikely in children), the hypoglycaemic drug is omitted until the patient is able to take food again. In the more usual case where the diabetic child is taking insulin it is more difficult.

The aim of management is to be as simple as possible. For emergency surgery there is not time to stabilize the diabetes on soluble insulin. Enquiry must be made as to the time of the last dose and the type of insulin. A 5 per cent glucose drip is set up to prevent the risk of hypoglycaemia, and kept running during the operation. The greater risk is that of hypoglycaemia. Stabilization can be attempted after the operation when the ability to take food returns.

(h) Has he attended hospital previously?

Any disease may be of importance to the anaesthetist. A child with porphyria is equally likely to break a limb as a normal child and his disease may go unmentioned in a busy casualty department when the diagnosis of the injury is so obvious. An induction dose of thiopentone can be fatal in such a case.

(i) Has he been given an anaesthetic previously?

This is most important as it may reveal previous anaesthetic problems. Parents and children rarely know details, only that there was difficulty. This is usually a problem related only to that anaesthetic but should suggest a search of any previous case-notes. Important points to record are difficulty in breathing, prolonged awakening, a transfer to an Intensive Treatment Unit, or admission after a day-case booking. If there has been any problem one should ask whether a card or identity disc was issued. If the rest of the family were investigated, it is important to obtain further details. Certain units have a specific interest in one disease and this may be a useful clue.

All intravenous induction agents have on occasion caused hypersensitivity reactions. In the absence of the case-notes, questioning may elicit a comment made by a previous anaesthetist.

Adverse reactions may occur with any agent and local anaesthetics should be remembered. Lignocaine, especially in excessive dosage, may cause epileptiform seizures requiring control by intravenous thiopentone. The addition of adrenaline to local anaesthetic solution can cause fainting in susceptible individuals.

(j) *Is there a family history of anaesthetic difficulties?*
There are a few familial conditions causing anaesthetic problems.

Malignant hyperpyrexia

RECOGNITION
The incidence of this condition is 1:60 000 anaesthetics but where a parent or grandparent suffered an attack the risk for children is greatly increased. It is possible that some cases described as 'ether convulsions' and 'atropine convulsions' were malignant hyperpyrexia. This can be lethal and is recognized by the difficulty in achieving relaxation and efficient ventilation at the beginning of an anaesthetic. Shortly afterwards the patient is noticed to be very hot. The cause is an enzyme-uncoupling which allows metabolism to proceed unrestrained, resulting in stiff muscles and the production of heat. The temperature can rise 4°C (8°F) in 10 minutes and this can be fatal if unchecked. Numerous drugs act as a trigger; halothane, suxamethonium and nitrous oxide have all been implicated. There is no certain blood test for this condition, but a raised serum creatine phosphokinase is suggestive, though false positives and negatives occur. A muscle biopsy is the definitive test but takes a long time and can be performed only in certain centres.

MANAGEMENT
   (a) Preventive
       Where possible only thiopentone and oxygen should be used. No pre-medication should be given as some of these, e.g. diazepam, have caused temperature rise.
   (b) Emergency
       If the condition is suspected under anaesthesia, due to poor relaxation, cyanosis in the presence of adequate volumes of oxygen, or a hot patient, action must be prompt.

(1) All anaesthetic agents are withdrawn and ventilation continued with oxygen alone.

(2) Large doses of steroids are given, e.g. 4 mg dexamethasone intravenously.

(3) Cooling is started. Cooling children is easier than cooling adults with their relatively large surface area. A water blanket above and below is most effective, otherwise ice bags packed into groins, axillae and around the neck may be used. The temperature should be measured continuously in the nasopharynx by an electric thermometer.

(4) An arterial sample of blood should be taken for analysis of acid-base state to allow control of the metabolic acidosis which always occurs.

(5) If resuscitation is successful the patient should be transferred to an Intensive Treatment Unit for temperature monitoring, as the rise in temperature can recur.

Pseudocholinesterase deficiency

This is seen in 1 in 2000 anaesthetics and is due to an inability to break down the normally short-acting muscle relaxant suxamethonium. There may be an absolute absence or reduction in the amount of pseudocholinesterase, or an abnormal enzyme. This difference can be demonstrated by laboratory test but the effect is the same.

RECOGNITION

After a dose of relaxant for intubation, to achieve muscular relaxation for a manipulation, or to allow closure of a tight abdomen, the respiration instead of returning to normal after 5 to 7 minutes, fails to return and depending on the pseudocholinesterase level may take up to 48 hours to return. This is an acutely embarrassing situation but not dangerous in a well-equipped hospital. When suspected, confirmation is by:

(i) Nerve stimulator to demonstrate complete neuromuscular blockade.

(ii) An enzyme test on the blood.

MANAGEMENT

Treatment remains with the anaesthetist in continuing ventilation of the sedated patient. As it is transmitted as a Mendelian dominant other members of the family should be investigated later. If the diagnosis is confirmed the parents should receive genetic counselling and an identification card or disc should be issued.

(k) When did he last eat or drink?

This is the most important question of interest to an anaesthetist. The patient with a full stomach may vomit and inhale the vomitus, causing respiratory obstruction, bronchopneumonia, or the acid-inhalation syndrome. In fact, the stomach is never empty and the risk of vomiting during induction is always a possibility. For medico-legal reasons it is often assumed that the stomach will be empty by four hours after the last meal and it is customary to wait this time before anaesthesia. There are many factors which delay gastric emptying and may apply to emergency conditions. Pain, shock, hypotension and fear reduce gastric motility. If the child has eaten, especially a fatty meal, just before an injury this will further delay emptying. Therefore, enquiry must be made of the interval between the last meal and the accident.

When a patient is known to have a full stomach the operation should be delayed for some hours or done under local anaesthesia. When this is not possible precautions must be taken to prevent inhalation of vomited or regurgitated material. The anaesthetist may choose to induce anaesthesia on the side with head-down tilt or he may prefer to use Sellick's manoeuvre. For this manoeuvre help may be required and everyone should know how to perform it. The aim is to press the cricoid cartilage, the only complete tracheal ring, back on to the oesophagus, so compressing it against the cervical vertebral bodies. To do this the cricoid is identified with an index finger and steadied between middle finger and thumb. As soon as anaesthesia is induced pressure is applied with all three digits and only released when the anaesthetist is satisfied that the endotracheal tube is correctly placed. If vomiting occurs, prompt tipping may prevent inhalation. Small children can be elevated by the legs and held upside down if necessary.

Acid-inhalation syndrome

The gravest risk is that of acid-inhalation syndrome. Small quantities of strong acid, H^+ concentration > 100 nmol per litre (pH 4.0 or less), when inhaled cause severe bronchospasm, cyanosis, and increased pulmonary secretion, and can be fatal. The treatment should be immediate artificial ventilation with oxygen, support of the circulation with IV fluid, isoprenaline if necessary, and IV steroids. Bronchoscopy may be useful but bronchial lavage is now thought not to be of use. Inhalation of larger quantities of partly solid material requires immediate bronchoscopy to recover as much as possible to limit lobular collapse. This should be followed by antibiotics and vigorous physiotherapy.

Examination of the patient for emergency anaesthesia

Examination before anaesthesia starts with a quick look at the shape of the head, face and neck, and the colour of the mucous membranes. Difficulty in fitting an anaesthetic mask, indicating the need to intubate, will be found if there is severe facial asymmetry, either general or due to local disease. Intubation problems will occur if the jaw is small, and this should be examined in a profile view. Difficulty in maintaining an airway may occur if there is a large tongue, as found in Down's syndrome, if there is pharyngeal swelling or enormous tonsils or even just a blocked nose. In addition head and neck movements should be tested as restriction of head extension may reduce the laryngoscopic view so preventing easy intubation. The child should be asked to open his mouth wide so that the teeth can be examined for any likely to be dislodged. If any are obviously loose a note should be made so that there is no doubt later.

Routine examination of heart and lungs will show up any obvious disorders. If possible, the weight of the child should be recorded.

INVESTIGATIONS

Chest x-ray and an Hb estimation should be performed in an emergency if the history and examination suggest the necessity. Pallor, unexplained by recent blood loss, would suggest a haemoglobin estimation. An arbitrary level of 10 g per 100 ml is accepted as that below which anaesthesia for *routine* surgery should not be performed.

FITNESS FOR ANAESTHESIA

The final decision must rest with the anaesthetist concerned but it will often fall to the resident in an emergency to decide this in order to make the arrangements for anaesthesia and operation. A general rule is as follows: 'In the absence of obvious disease of the cardiorespiratory, renal or hepatic systems a patient whose exercise tolerance is equal to or approaches that of his peers in size should be considered fit for anaesthetic.'

It remains only to communicate these findings to the anaesthetist as concisely as possible.

Administration of emergency anaesthesia

It is unlikely that the paediatric resident will be asked to give an anaesthetic without having received special training. In circumstances in which this is required each doctor should learn a simple safe anaesthetic technique, understanding the dangers and difficulties. The description suggested below would be suitable for children of two years upwards for manipulation of fractures, incision of abscesses or even, if circumstances require, emergency abdominal surgery. It must be emphasized that the doctor who has not received postgraduate training in anaesthesia should only attempt anaesthesia *if there is no-one else available.*

(a) PRE-OPERATION ASSESSMENT

The doctor should decline all small patients and babies, and any whose history and examination reveal serious abnormality because of the risk to these patients of unskilled anaesthesia. The child should be known to have been starved for four hours. It is most dangerous to anaesthetize a hypovolaemic patient; blood or fluid loss should have been replaced before induction.

(b) PRE-ANAESTHESIA CHECK

All doctors should be sufficiently familiar with the standard Boyle's anaesthetic apparatus to be able to use it to give oxygen by positive pressure ventilation.

(i) The machine should be checked to ensure that there are two cylinders containing oxygen and two of nitrous oxide.

(ii) The anaesthetic circuit, bag, tube, valve and mask should be checked by occluding the outlet with a thumb, inflating the bag with gas and then compressing it to demonstrate the ability to produce positive pressure.

(iii) The expiratory valve is left wide open.

(iv) A laryngoscope and suitable sized endotracheal tube must be available.

(c) ADMINISTRATION OF ANAESTHESIA

The principal points are:

(i) Only 33 per cent oxygen or more should be used.

(ii) A clear airway must be maintained at all times.

(iii) A slightly too deep anaesthetic is safer than a slightly too light anaesthetic.

(iv) A minimum number of alterations and adjustments should be made.

(v) Atropine should be given to all patients during the anaesthetic, either 0.3 to 0.6 mg i.m. one hour before or 0.2 to 0.4 mg IV just before induction.

(vi) The child is placed on the left side on a level table.

(vii) The position of the table-tilting control is checked.

(viii) A working suction unit must be available.

(ix) The oxygen is turned on at 3 litres per minute, nitrous oxide at 6 litres per minute and halothane (Fluothane) at $\frac{1}{2}$ per cent.

(x) While talking to the child, gradually approach his face with the mask, encouraging him until the mask can be applied to the face. When the mask is applied lightly to the face the reservoir bag can be seen moving showing respiration without obstruction. This should be monitored continuously, as should the pulse.

(xi) The concentration of halothane is increased by $\frac{1}{2}$ per cent steps up to 3 per cent.

(xii) If the respiration becomes obstructed, the chin is held forward.

(xiii) If laryngeal stridor develops the halothane is decreased to 1 per cent and the concentration gradually increased again.

(xiv) When there is steady unobstructed respiration at 3 per cent halothane the patient can, if necessary, be turned onto the back or the operation commenced.

(xv) When the operation has started, if there is no response to surgical stimuli, the halothane concentration is reduced to $1\frac{1}{2}$ per cent and maintained at this level for the whole operation.

(xvi) Maintaining the airway may be made easier by the introduction of an oropharyngeal airway. If possible this should only be done when adequate anaesthesia has been attained. It should pass over the tongue to avoid oral damage.

(xvii) At the end of the operation the anaesthetic is continued until the child is turned onto the side again. The halothane and the nitrous oxide are then turned off. Oxygen is then given at 5 litres per minute.

(xviii) It is essential to remain with the child until the child wakes.

What can go wrong?

(a) VOMITING AT INDUCTION AND AWAKENING

If vomiting occurs during induction the table is immediately tilted head-down and oxygen is given. The mouth and pharynx must be sucked out. In this position inhalation is most unlikely. When the vomiting stops anaesthesia is continued. Vomiting during emergence is less dangerous, and providing the child is on the side and being given oxygen it is unlikely to cause difficulty; however, the suction unit should be immediately available.

(b) LARYNGEAL STRIDOR DURING INDUCTION

This is due to secretions irritating the vocal chords. At the first sign of this the halothane concentration is reduced by 1 per cent and the nitrous

oxide is turned off. As the stridor decreases the halothane is increased
again by two steps before reintroducing nitrous oxide. The too-early
introduction of an airway is a likely cause of stridor; if so, it should be
removed.

(c) CESSATION OF RESPIRATION DUE TO HALOTHANE

The halothane is turned off, the expiratory valve is screwed down a
little, and respiration controlled by squeezing the bag rhythmically
until respiration returns. The halothane is then re-started at a lower
concentration than before, after opening the expiratory valve.

(d) CARDIAC ARREST

This is most unlikely in the absence of previous hypoxia. An overdose
of halothane will first cause respiratory arrest and if this is treated
correctly cardiac arrest will not occur.

If cardiac arrest does occur, the surgeon is immediately informed,
the oxygen is turned on fully, the anaesthetic agents are turned off and
manual ventilation is started to ensure an adequate volume of oxygen
with each breath. The surgeon should immediately start external
cardiac massage by pressing regularly on the mid-sternum (p. 303). An
intravenous drip should be set up with 8.4 per cent sodium bicarbonate
(1 ml contains 1 mmol) and a dose of 1 ml per kg per minute of arrest
should be given. If the pulse was properly monitored and the arrest, due
to anaesthetic causes, was noticed immediately, withdrawal of anaesthesia and prompt external cardiac massage should result in a rapid
return of heart beat.

Part VI: Respiratory Tract Emergencies

CHAPTER 20

Ear, Nose and Throat Emergencies

J. T. Buffin

Accidents

FOREIGN BODIES

Ear and nose

RECOGNITION
They are often inserted deliberately by the child or his friends (though
the episode may be forgotten) and they are therefore usually smooth
and may be easily visible.

MANAGEMENT
Ideally they should be removed at a specialist clinic since removal is
rarely urgent. A hook or ring probe may be used in the ear, passing the
instrument beyond the foreign body (FB) and rolling it out. In the nose
and occasionally in the ear, the foreign body may be grasped with
dressing forceps. It is often helpful to lock the FB in the nasal vestibule
by pressing a finger in the groove at the side of the nose and then
'milking' it out.

Pharynx

RECOGNITION
Fish bones or other sharp objects may stick in the pharynx causing
dysphagia and pain on swallowing. Older children can localize the site
of impaction quite accurately.

MANAGEMENT
A good light and a spatula are essential; impaction is commonest at the

lower pole of the tonsil and posterior third of the tongue; the back of the tongue can be seen with a laryngeal mirror.

Occasionally, direct removal using forceps and a mirror is possible but commonly a general anaesthetic is necessary.

Oesophagus

RECOGNITION

FBs stick in the oesophagus because of their size or because of their sharp edges. At the narrowest site, the cricopharyngeal sphincter, there is acute discomfort and profuse salivation. Lower down, symptoms are less dramatic though there will be a moderate or complete dysphagia.

MANAGEMENT

At the cricopharyngeal level the diagnosis is usually obvious from the history, and urgent removal under general anaesthetic is necessary; preliminary radiography is unnecessary and causes delay. Lower down, smooth objects such as coins can be identified and localized by a plain radiograph; removal is rarely so urgent since the symptoms are not severe and quite large objects can sometimes pass the cardiac sphincter and continue on through the gastrointestinal tract. Sharp or impacted FBs require urgent removal because of the risk of perforation and mediastinitis. Oesophagoscopy and the removal of such objects may be difficult and is best done by an expert.

Larynx (*See also* Upper Airway Obstruction, page 217).

RECOGNITION

There is usually a history of cough or choking followed by inspiratory stridor which may be very severe. In the absence of an adequate history a diagnosis of 'Croup' or laryngotracheobronchitis may be made which may cause serious or even fatal delay in the removal of the obstruction.

MANAGEMENT

Under general anaesthetic the pharynx and larynx should be examined and the FB removed. If the patient is desperately ill, with oedema of the larynx or vocal chords, subsequent endotracheal intubation may be necessary.

Bronchus

RECOGNITION

There is frequently a history of choking with cyanosis during a meal, while sucking a sweet, or eating peanuts. Dislodged teeth may be inhaled into the bronchus in facial injury (*see* section on Traumatic Injury of Head, Face and Neck, p. 164). Relief of symptoms may indicate that the FB has been coughed up and swallowed or that it has passed through the larynx and is lodged in a bronchus, most commonly the right main bronchus. An FB in the bronchus may produce an expiratory wheeze or whistling on expiration which may be mistaken for asthma. Symptoms are often minimal.

MANAGEMENT
If a bronchial FB is suspected a chest radiograph should be taken *in full inspiration and full expiration*; the FB may occlude one of the bronchi completely, causing collapse of one lobe (commonly the right-middle lobe) or may cause a valvular obstruction with overdistension of the affected lobe which is particularly obvious on the expiratory film. The majority of inhaled FBs are not radio-opaque.

Bronchoscopic removal by an expert under general anaesthesia is essential.

LOCAL TRAUMA

The Ear

Acute trauma

RECOGNITION
The injury to the ear, the meatus or the tympanic membrane itself is usually obvious, with pain and bleeding.

MANAGEMENT
The meatus is filled with blood which is best left untouched because of the risk of introducing infection. Analgesics and systemic antibiotics should be given. Later referral to an ENT unit is advisable. More serious injuries with vertigo or facial palsy require immediate transfer to a specialist unit.

Otitic barotrauma

A difference in pressure between the air on either side of the tympanic membrane may cause pain and deafness or even rupture, with bleeding and tinnitus.

RECOGNITION
Sudden pressure changes are due to: a box on the ear, explosion, diving or falling into water, or sudden decompression accidents in aircraft.

Slower pressure changes occur in aircraft during take-off and descent and are especially likely when the Eustachian tube is blocked by an acute or chronic catarrhal condition. Again, pain and deafness result with occasional rupture if the tympanic membrane has been previously damaged or perforated.

MANAGEMENT
If rupture occurs, secondary infection is likely and should be prevented by antibiotics.

The Nose

RECOGNITION
The history of injury is obvious. Fracture of the nasal bones is rare in young children but common in older ones. Displacement of the nasal bones is apparent unless obscured by bruising. X-rays of the nose have limited value except as medico-legal evidence. Submucosal haematoma of the nasal septum may also occur and cause considerable obstruction. There is a risk of infection of the haematoma with abscess formation and also of necrosis of fragments of cartilage with subsequent deformity.

MANAGEMENT
Manipulation and reduction of the displaced nasal bone fragments must be completed within three weeks of the accident.

Reduction of displaced septum or cartilages must await resolution of the haematoma. For a haematoma of the septum antibiotic cover should be started immediately and the clot should be drained by a curved incision anteriorly and inferiorly on the septal mucosa: unattached fragments of cartilage should be removed.

Pharynx and palate

RECOGNITION
Laceration may result when a stick, or some similar sharp object in the mouth is pushed into the palate while running and falling. Occasionally the soft palate may be perforated completely and partially detached from the bony palate. Deeper injuries may involve the region of the great vessels at the base of the skull.

MANAGEMENT
The area heals rapidly, usually without any intervention. Indications for surgery are continued bleeding, possible presence of the lacerating agent in the wound, and extreme detachment of the soft palate. Exposure under general anaesthesia will be required.

INSECT STINGS

RECOGNITION
A bee or wasp sting in the mouth may produce rapidly extending oedema involving the supraglottic region, with severe airway obstruction.

MANAGEMENT
  (i) Assessment of degree of obstruction and maintenance of airway (*see* page 219).
  (ii) Prevention of further oedema. *See also under* Venomous Bites and Stings (p. 542) and Anaphylactic Shock (p. 111).
Drugs which are of use are, in order of potency and speed of action:
  Adrenaline 1:1000
  Hydrocortisone   Doses in section on Anaphylactic Shock (p. 112)
  Antihistamine drugs
Antibiotics should also be given.

SWALLOWED CORROSIVES
(*see also under* Acute Poisoning, page 75)

As with other poisons one must know exactly what has been swallowed, how much, and how long ago.

RECOGNITION
The history is usually self-evident: burns round the mouth, face and neck and inside the mouth are likely, but the oesophagus may be burned without lesions in the mouth. Pain is usually present except with phenolic compounds such as cresols (e.g. vaporizers): salivation is usually marked. Oedema of the pharynx may occur, spreading to cause laryngeal obstruction. When there has been vomiting, there is the possibility of inhaled corrosive with lower-respiratory obstruction. In severe cases there may be perforation of oesophagus or stomach within a short time.

MANAGEMENT
(*i*) *Local*

As soon as the child's general condition permits, a nasogastric tube should be passed under general anaesthesia: this allows nasogastric feeding and will prevent complete occlusion of the lumen of the oesophagus by adhesion. Where respiratory obstruction is present, a tracheostomy should be performed. The nasogastric tube is retained for three weeks.

H

(ii) General

Antibiotics: a wide-spectrum antibiotic such as ampicillin should be given parenterally and later down the nasogastric tube. Corticosteroids i.m. or IV (hydrocortisone, 25 mg 6-hourly) should be continued for three weeks.

MAJOR TRAUMA TO HEAD AND NECK

This is considered in detail under Emergencies Involving the Face and Neck (pp. 162–168). However, the following additional points are of particular importance.

  (a) Haemorrhage from major arteries in the facial region may show itself as epistaxis: local pressure may stop the bleeding but surgical haemostasis may be required.

  (b) Direct injury to the larynx may fracture the cartilage. Crepitus should be looked for by palpation of the larynx; there may be excessive bruising of the neck or surgical emphysema of the neck. Exploration of this area is for the specialist.

  (c) Local haematoma causing airway obstruction may necessitate tracheostomy.

  (d) Dislodged teeth may be inhaled: they can usually be identified on a chest radiograph and should be removed by bronchoscopy.

  (e) Torn mucosal lining of the airway may cause air to track into the mediastinum with resulting pneumothorax.

  (f) Loss of cerebrospinal fluid (CSF) from the nose or ears implies a fracture of the skull and tear of the meninges. Close observation in hospital is required and the opinion of a neurosurgeon should be obtained. When CSF leaks from the ear the lesion is usually self-sealing.

  (g) All patients with craniofacial injuries who have a facial palsy or weakness should be seen by an otologist.

Symptomatic emergencies

It is important that the parents' anxieties should be appreciated and allayed as far as possible. This will reduce the child's anxiety and increase co-operation.

PAINFUL CONDITIONS

Earache

Infants cannot complain of earache but they may scream, rub their ears or bang their head. The ears of an infant (or non-communicating child) who appears to be in pain should always be examined. Otitis media should be suspected in a child who has had a cold and wakes screaming during the night.

Apart from otitis media, tonsillitis, oral infection, or disease in the teeth especially in the lower jaw may all cause pain referred to the ear.

(i) Otitis media

RECOGNITION

In actual inflammation of the middle ear the tympanic membrane may show appearances ranging from slight indrawing, with congestion of vessels, to a grossly distended bulging membrane.

MANAGEMENT

Simple analgesics may be necessary: antibiotics should be given, either penicillin, ampicillin or amoxycillin. In most cases oral treatment is adequate but an inadequate response within 24 hours suggests a failure of the oral route and intramuscular benzylpenicillin should be started. Myringotomy is very rarely needed.

Note: Haemophilus influenzae is a common infecting organism under the age of 5 years and in such children ampicillin or amoxycillin should be the first choice (Bass *et al.*, 1967).

(ii) Acute mastoiditis

RECOGNITION AND MANAGEMENT

There is evidence of otitis media, and in addition pain and tenderness over the mastoid bone which must be distinguished from painful deep cervical lymph nodes. In late cases the child will be very ill and there will be redness and oedema or even fluctuation over the mastoid region. Full doses of antibiotics should be given immediately. Cortical mastoidectomy will be indicated for most patients.

(iii) Furunculosis of the external meatus

RECOGNITION

This is a very painful condition. The swelling of the ear canal sometimes spreads behind the ear, with redness and oedema over the mastoid region. The pre-auricular gland is sometimes enlarged and tender. The characteristic finding is acute pain on touching or attempting to move the pinna or on introducing an aural speculum into the meatus. The distinction from mastoiditis is not always easy: radiography may show loss of definition in the mastoid air cells in mastoiditis. In difficult cases the opinion of an otologist should be obtained.

MANAGEMENT
The infecting organism is invariably a staphylococcus. Antibiotics may
be withheld if the diagnosis is certain and the infection is localized. A
wick soaked in glycerine and ichthyol will reduce the pain. Analgesics
and local heat are also helpful.

Painful throat conditions

Tonsillitis

This is the most likely cause of pain on swallowing.

RECOGNITION
The red fauces and tonsils are easily recognized; an exudate does not
necessarily indicate a bacterial infection and may occur in glandular
fever or other viral infections.

MANAGEMENT
Viral infection should be treated symptomatically, while clear-cut
bacterial infection will respond to penicillin, ampicillin or amoxycillin;
a throat swab should be taken if antibiotics are to be used.

BLEEDING

The nose

RECOGNITION
Normally this is obvious, but it may not be obvious when the blood is
swallowed. The first sign of trouble may be vomiting of blood.

(*i*) *Local causes*   Physical agents, trauma (picking or rubbing the
nose) coughing and sneezing. Drying of the nasal mucosa produces
crusts whose separation causes bleeding: this is sometimes aggravated
by central heating. Congestion occurs in colds, chronic sinusitis and
allergic rhinitis.

(*ii*) *Vascular abnormalities*   Haemangioma of the face involving the
nose may bleed heavily; occasionally a capillary abnormality may be
the cause. Hereditary telangiectasia should also be considered.

(*iii*) *Disorders of haemostasis*   Normally there will be other evidence
of blood disorder, such as petechiae or bruising. Epistaxis may be the
presenting symptom in idiopathic thrombocytopenic purpura or other
causes of thrombocytopenia, including leukaemia. Coagulation disorders such as haemophilia rarely cause epistaxis unless as a result of
direct trauma.

MANAGEMENT

(*i*) *Assessment of blood loss*   A description should be obtained: 'steady drip', 'continuous stream', 'constant ooze', etc. It is also important to discover whether bleeding is still continuing, and to ask if there have been previous episodes, and if so how many, at what intervals and how long ago was the last one. This will give some idea of an anaemia present before the epistaxis. The pulse rate and blood pressure must be recorded at regular intervals if there is evidence of shock.

(*ii*) *Estimation*   A base-line haemoglobin estimation should be obtained.

(*iii*) *Transfusion*   If transfusion may be required, blood is taken for grouping and crossmatching at the same time as the Hb estimation.

(*iv*) *Local treatment*   The local lesion is usually a single point on the antero-inferior part of the septum. Suction may be necessary to obtain a clear view of the bleeding point. Local pressure can be applied to the side of the nose which is bleeding, close to the face and pressing on to the nasal floor as well as the septum. The child's own thumb can be used to apply this pressure. If local pressure fails or bleeding recurs whenever pressure is released or if a blood disorder is suspected, packing the nose will be necessary. In a child 1 to 2.5-cm ($\frac{1}{2}-1$-inch) ribbon gauze lubricated with glycerine or liquid paraffin should be used (or Bismuth Iodoform Paraffin Paste—BIPP). Gauze impregnated with a vasoconstrictor can be used, but with care, since considerable absorption may occur, with systemic effects.

As a preliminary to cauterization, ribbon gauze soaked in a mixture of 5 ml of 10 per cent cocaine with 2 to 3 drops of 1:1000 adrenaline is used to produce anaesthesia and vasoconstriction.

Packing the nose is unpleasant and must be done firmly, packing on to the floor of the nose first and folding the gauze on itself in layers until the roof of the nose is reached. The pack is retained by an adhesive dressing on the nostril. In small or frightened children, packing should be done under general anaesthesia. If bleeding persists in spite of packing the nasal cavity, the nasopharynx may also be packed. Various methods are available: using an inflatable balloon catheter of the Foley type or a gauze swab secured by thread stays passing through the nasal columella. If bleeding persists in spite of these measures, division of the external carotid artery or the anterior ethmoid artery in the orbit will be necessary unless the haemorrhage is accepted as the terminal phase of malignant disease or leukaemia.

The throat

RECOGNITION

Bleeding from a tonsillar vessel occurs sometimes in acute tonsillitis but rarely requires treatment. Postoperative bleeding after tonsillectomy usually occurs within the first few hours after surgery and is the responsibility of the surgeon. Secondary haemorrhage, after return home, is due to infection and may occur from several days, up to three weeks, after operation.

MANAGEMENT

Secondary haemorrhage: the child should be readmitted to hospital and observed. Mild sedation and antibiotics should be given. The occasional case in which bleeding does not settle will require examination under general anaesthesia and diathermy coagulation.

The ear

Bleeding from the ear generally induces a disproportionate amount of parental anxiety: blood loss is usually trivial.

RECOGNITION

Traumatic laceration may be obvious. Spontaneous bleeding followed by a purulent discharge may occur after rupture of the drum in otitis media and is normally preceded by the characteristic pain; however this may not have been recognized in the young child. In influenza epidemics blisters containing blood or blood-stained serum are sometimes found on the tympanic membrane; a small amount of bleeding occurs if these blisters rupture. In chronic otitis media brief episodes of bleeding may occur.

MANAGEMENT

For lacerations, *see under* Trauma. Bleeding from the other causes described above requires treatment of the primary condition though the bullous influenzal condition needs no specific treatment; however if this diagnosis is uncertain it is safer to treat as for acute otitis media.

ACUTE LOSS OF FUNCTION

The ear

RECOGNITION

Acute loss of function in the ear may be indicated by one or more of the following: deafness, vertigo, facial paralysis.

MANAGEMENT

None of these symptoms constitute a threat to life but all require prompt referral to a specialist.

The nose

RECOGNITION

The two important symptoms are anosmia and inability to breathe through the nose. Anosmia as an acutely presenting symptom must be extremely rare.

Nasal Obstruction in the Newborn (*see* page 650)

Acute dysphagia

For oesophageal atresia and tracheo-oesophageal fistula in the newborn *see* page 278.

Dysphagia is a rare cause of urgent trouble in children except as a result of an impacted foreign body (*see* page 206) or from food impacted above a stricture due to previous surgery, or trauma, or stricture at the lower end of the oesophagus in hiatus hernia.

RECOGNITION

In the older child, food impaction causes sudden difficulty in swallowing; treatment is the same as for a foreign body.

Aphonia

Loss of voice may develop suddenly as a result of acute laryngitis or extreme over-use of the voice from shouting, singing or screaming. In older children hysterical aphonia may occur.

RECOGNITION

The circumstances in which aphonia occurs are usually obvious. In the newborn, lack of cry may be due to paralysis of the vocal chords from birth trauma; this is usually unilateral; bilateral cord paralysis presents severe inspiratory stridor.

MANAGEMENT

Aphonia alone is not an emergency but accompanying inspiratory stridor from inflammation in the young child ('croup', epiglottitis, laryngotracheobronchitis) or bilateral cord paralysis in the newborn may require urgent relief by tracheostomy. Hysterical aphonia requires prompt attention since the longer it is allowed to persist the more difficult is its cure.

Reference

Bass, J. W., Cohen, S. H., Corless, J. D. and Mamunes, P. (1967). Ampicillin compared with other anti-microbials in acute otitis media. *J. Am. med. Ass.* **202**, 697

CHAPTER 21

Upper Airway Obstruction

(For Stridor in the Newborn *see* page 647 and for Nasal Obstruction in the Newborn *see* page 650)

A. D. Milner and J. T. Buffin

Obstruction to the upper airway is a potential threat to cerebral function and to life. Relief of the obstruction may in some circumstances have to precede an exact diagnosis. The younger the child, the narrower the air passages and the greater the risk of obstruction.

Acute onset of inspiratory stridor

The differential diagnosis is often difficult owing to lack of accurate history, but the following should be considered.

Foreign body

The possibility of a foreign body impacted in the larynx should always be considered in any small child with suddenly developing inspiratory stridor, particularly if there was no preceding upper-respiratory infection. Many small children, too young to express themselves clearly, are left to eat unattended and may inhale a peanut, bone, or toy. Animal bones and metal objects should be visible in a good lateral radiograph of the neck. A foreign body should be discovered at laryngoscopy which should always precede intubation or tracheostomy for relief of laryngeal obstruction.

Acute laryngotracheobronchitis ('croup')* (Table 21.I).

This is the commonest cause of acute inspiratory stridor and is due to a

* Croup is such an imprecise term as to be dangerous: it is better to describe the degree and site of obstruction.

viral infection, usually the para-influenza virus. It is a potentially fatal condition because the inflammatory oedema causes an increase in airflow resistance; this resistance is greater on inspiration than on expiration, owing to dynamic factors (*Figure 25.2*). Initially there is hyperventilation but as obstruction progresses hypoxia and hypercapnia (raised pCO_2) occur due to the fall in alveolar ventilation. The more distressed the child, the greater the dynamic constriction of the larynx on inspiration.

RECOGNITION

There is usually a one- or two-day history of coryza and cough. Inspiratory stridor usually develops first at night, and if mild is only present when the child is upset and hyperventilating. As the condition progresses persistent inspiratory stridor develops, followed by cyanosis on breathing air and eventually impaired consciousness. This progressive obstruction is relatively uncommon and the majority of such cases can be managed at home. However, in a small proportion the laryngeal

TABLE 21.I

Differential diagnosis of acute inspiratory stridor due to infection (After Russell, 1971. Reproduced by kind permission)

	Viral laryngotracheobronchitis	*H. Influenzae epiglottitis*
Age	Usually under 3 years	Usually over 3 years including adults
Sex	Boys >girls	Boys >girls
Preceding coryza	Most cases	One-quarter of cases
Onset	Gradual, usually over several days	Rapid, often over only a few hours
Hoarseness	Variable	Usually severe
Dysphagia	Absent or mild	Usually severe, may be drooling
Fever	Absent in 50%	Present, often severe
'Toxic' symptoms	Mild	Severe
Nasopharyngeal findings	Hyperaemia and oedema. Epiglottis may be red, never cherry-red	Pharyngeal oedema: cherry-red epiglottis
Chest findings	Usually rhonchi	Seldom rhonchi
White blood corpuscles	Normal until bacterial superinfection occurs	Marked neutrophil polymorphonuclear leucocytosis
Microbiology	Nil, virus or virus plus secondary invaders	*H. influenzae* type B from nasopharynx or blood
Treatment	Symptomatic, seldom tracheostomy	Ampicillin or chloramphenicol. Intubation or tracheostomy often necessary

obstruction becomes severe. The trachea and bronchi become partly obstructed by thick secretions, causing expiratory stridor and coarse rhonchi in the lung fields.

The indications for admission of a child with inspiratory stridor of recent onset are:

(a) Any child under 1 year.
(b) Suspected foreign body in the larynx.
(c) Failure to improve in humidification at home.
(d) Progressively increasing stridor and recession.
(e) Symptoms suggestive of epiglottitis (*see below*).

Acute epiglottitis (Table 21.I)

RECOGNITION

This is an acute septicaemia usually due to *Haemophilus influenzae* type B, and is one of the most acute emergencies in paediatrics. The child is flushed and pyrexial with a short history, commonly only a few hours. Often the child can only breathe by leaning forward. The voice may be muffled rather than hoarse and there may be salivation due to dysphagia. The swollen, red epiglottis can sometimes be easily seen in the pharynx, but a difficult examination with a spatula may precipitate respiratory arrest and should not be done in an acutely obstructed child. A lateral radiograph of the neck may show the swollen epiglottis as a soft-tissue shadow.

Diphtheria (*See* page 224)

This is now rare in Britain; there is usually a gradual onset with severe constitutional disturbance and induration of the neck.

MANAGEMENT OF ACUTE LARYNGOTRACHEOBRONCHITIS AND ACUTE EPIGLOTTITIS

Observations indicating the site and degree of obstruction

(*a*) *Stridor*   This is produced by the passage of air through an abnormally narrowed or partly obstructed airway.

   (i) Absence of stridor may be due to an almost complete obstruction (e.g. laryngeal stenosis in the newborn).
   (ii) Inspiratory stridor indicates obstruction in the upper airway.
   (iii) Hoarse voice or cry indicates involvement of the vocal chords.
   (iv) Expiratory stridor indicates bronchial or bronchiolar obstruction.
   (v) Inspiratory and expiratory (to-and-fro) stridor indicates tracheal obstruction.

(*b*) *Use of the accessory muscles of respiration*   Dilatation of the alae nasi does not necessarily indicate obstruction, since it occurs in lobar pneumonia. Contraction of the sternomastoids, and in older children the fixing of the arms to use the pectoral muscles, indicates a severe degree of obstruction.

(*c*) *In-drawing or recession*   The amount of in-drawing or recession is assessed by the degree of sucking in of the suprasternal, supraclavicular, subcostal or epigastric regions and the intercostal spaces, lower ribs or sternum.

(*d*) *Colour*   Pallor indicates hypoxia, and greyish cyanosis requires urgent intervention.

(*e*) *Restlessness and anxiety (Apart from the initial anxiety of admission to hospital)*   These indicate hypoxia.

(*f*) *Impaired consciousness (Apart from sleep from exhaustion)*   This is often preceded by confusion or disorientation and is an indication for urgent intervention.

(*g*) *Pulse rate*   A rising pulse rate is due to exhaustion or to hypoxia.

(*h*) *Other danger signs*
    (i) Reduction in loudness of stridor, with diminution of air-entry (compared to previous observation) indicates exhaustion or increased obstruction, rather than improvement.
    (ii) Reduction in the respiration rate may indicate deterioration, especially if the rhythm is irregular.

General measures

(*a*) *Oxygen*

Cyanosis in air is an indication for intubation or tracheostomy. Oxygen can be given while preparations are made to relieve the obstruction.

(*b*) *Humidity*

This has been traditionally used in the treatment of laryngotracheobronchitis, but there is no evidence that the standard cold mist alters the course of the disease or has much effect on the relative humidity within the larynx. A mist which is dense enough to be effective makes observation in the tent difficult.

(c) *Antibiotics*

In epiglottitis or suspected epiglottitis a blood culture should be taken and ampicillin should be given parenterally, preferably IV (400 mg per kg per 24 hours), for at least 48 hours, followed by oral ampicillin in the same dosage, or alternatively, chloramphenicol (50 mg per kg per 24 hours) may be given in the same way as for ampicillin.

(d) *Steroids*

There is no convincing evidence of the value of steroids in laryngotracheobronchitis, but their use may reduce the oedema after extubation. Hydrocortisone (100–200 mg, 6-hourly), should be given IV in all cases of epiglottitis, whether intubated or not.

Intubation or tracheostomy

Approximately 1 per cent of children in hospital with acute laryngotracheobronchitis, but 40 to 60 per cent of those with epiglottitis, require intubation or tracheostomy. In epiglottitis the obstruction will be completely relieved on bypassing the larynx, but this is not necessarily the case in laryngotracheobronchitis, in which thick secretions or crusts may obstruct the trachea or larger bronchi. In laryngotracheobronchitis it may be necessary to remove these secretions through a tracheostomy, or by passing a bronchoscope.

  (a) The decision to bypass the obstruction must be made on clinical grounds and is indicated as soon as there is evidence of exhaustion or deterioration in the level of consciousness. Intubation is preferable if done by a skilled anaesthetist; a clumsy and unsuccessful attempt at intubation may precipitate complete obstruction and respiratory arrest.

  (b) Minor manipulation, such as moving the child on to a trolley or theatre table may precipitate respiratory arrest, and examination of the pharynx or laryngoscopy should NOT be done in a severely obstructed child, unless intubation or tracheostomy can be done immediately. A doctor able to intubate (with laryngoscope and tubes) should accompany the child to theatre for intubation only or tracheostomy. The child with epiglottitis who is able to breathe only by leaning forward should NOT be made to lie flat on the trolley or in bed since this may worsen the obstruction.

  (c) Facilities for a tracheostomy must be immediately available when intubation is attempted.

  (d) An emergency tracheostomy is better than a failed intubation. Indication for tracheostomy as opposed to intubation:

(a) Failed intubation or broncoscopy. (b) Clinical indications that intubation will be exceptionally difficult, or impossible.

(e) *Technique of tracheostomy* (*see also* page 341) for tracheostomy in neonatal tetanus). The child should be lying supine on a firm surface with a support under the shoulders to extend the neck. A vertical incision is made from the laryngeal prominence to just above the sternal notch. The stoma should be formed just above the thyroid isthmus. In desperate cases a thyrotomy may be performed through an opening made in the cricothyroid membrane which is subcutaneous and easily palpable. The trachea is opened with a vertical incision, but the cricothyroid membrane requires a horizontal incision. A metal or plastic tube is inserted, the choice depending upon availability and the possibility of subsequent mechanical ventilation.

Difficulties may be encountered, especially in the asphyxiated child:

(a) The veins are distended.
(b) The left innominate vein may lie above the suprasternal notch.
(c) A communicating vessel between the anterior jugular veins may cause a lot of bleeding.
(d) In a low tracheostomy the dome of the pleura comes to the level of the first rib and the pleura may be torn.

COMPLICATIONS

Pneumothorax or interstitial (surgical) emphysema may develop. Air may be removed from the pleural cavity by continuous or repeated aspiration.

Alternatives to tracheostomy or intubation

(a) A life-saving alternative is cannulation of the trachea with a needle: in a small child the needle used for transfusion sets will allow sufficient oxygen to preserve life until a definitive procedure can be done.
(b) Intermittent positive-pressure breathing with nebulized adrenaline. Some centres in the U.S.A. have claimed excellent results in laryngotracheobronchitis with nebulized adrenaline (1 in 1000) delivered by face mask and triggered by the child's inspiratory efforts (Adair, 1971). The child initially fights the treatment but apparently obtains considerable benefit. This method requires further evaluation; there is evidence that the benefit from adrenaline lasts for less than 30 minutes, and although this treatment

may be useful in the management of in-patients it should not be used in out-patients. It should not be used in epiglottitis.

References

Adair, J. C. (1971). Ten years experience with intermittent positive-pressure breathing in the treatment of acute laryngotracheobronchitis. *Anaesth. Analg.* **50**, 649

Russell, G. (1971). Childhood Croup. *Practitioner* **206**, 781

CHAPTER 22

Diphtheria

B. Heyworth

The severity of diphtheria varies with the type of organism, mitis being least, intermedius the next, and gravis usually the most severe. The site and extent of the infection and immunity of the patient are also important. As regards toxicity, pharyngeal infection is usually the most severe, laryngeal infection less and nasal least. Conjunctival lesions, with palpebral inflammation, oedema and some membrane formation and cutaneous lesions of the external auditory meatus or vulvo-vagina are usually associated with little toxaemia, but can give rise to complications. Other superficial fissures or impetiginous lesions may contain virulent diphtheria strains, as does the typical circumscribed, punched-out skin ulcer with an undermined, thickened edge and greyish membranous base, the so-called desert or veldt sore. This too may be associated with toxaemia and gives rise to the later complications of diphtheria. Age affects mortality and morbidity by its effect on the site and extent of infection (e.g. laryngeal infection is worse in infants; pharyngeal infection occurs less frequently in those under six years of age but has a higher mortality). In some temperate countries diphtheria is now rare, but is still imported. In some tropical countries it has been said to be rare but is now being increasingly reported, while in others it occurs frequently all the year round.

Diphtheria may cause four emergencies:
(a) Laryngeal obstruction.
(b) Haemorrhagic and severe toxic pharyngeal diphtheria.
(c) Cardiovascular involvement.
(d) Paralysis.

Laryngeal diphtheria

This usually presents early in children but in adults it occurs 1 to 2 weeks after the onset, by extension from the pharynx. Especially in the tropics, it may be associated with mitis infections. It is worse in patients under 3 years of age.

RECOGNITION OF SYMPTOMS

These are gradual in onset and initially 'dry', so differing from croup or measles. There is a change in voice and cry. A croupy cough 'like the bark of a distant young dog', progresses to stridor. The child loses appetite and develops fever, usually slight (37°–38°C; 98.6°–100.4°F).

Signs   Tachypnoea and increasing dyspnoea develop with suprasternal, epigastric, subcostal and intercostal recession and the use of accessory muscles. Restlessness, a weak rapid pulse, rising blood pressure and cyanosis indicate severe respiratory failure with hypoxia and hypercapnia.

IMMEDIATE TREATMENT

Tracheostomy should be done preferably *before* signs of respiratory failure are present. Antitoxin and benzylpenicillin are given (*see below*).

OTHER COMPLICATIONS

Secondary bronchopneumonia occurs in laryngeal and pharyngeal diphtheria in children. Continued fever, rising pulse and BP in a restless child after tracheostomy with an adequate tube, indicate extension of the membrane to the lower respiratory tract. This is grave, but repeated aspiration, humidification and physiotherapy may allow expectoration of the bronchial cast and recovery.

Toxaemia is less than in pharyngeal diphtheria, paralysis is rare and heart failure occurs late or secondary to pulmonary pathology.

Haemorrhagic diphtheria

This occurs early, mainly in children.

RECOGNITION

(a) Severe toxaemia, restlessness or apathy, usually with obvious nasopharyngeal diphtheria.
(b) A thin, usually blood-discoloured membrane on the tonsils and throat is associated with marked oedema and lymphadenopathy, the 'bull-neck' appearance.
(c) Petechiae and small ecchymoses, particularly over pressure points and bony prominences. Epistaxis and occasionally mucosal bleeding may occur.

Most children die from toxaemia. Many of those who recover will suffer severe myocardial damage in the second and third week and almost all survivors suffer paralysis. The mortality is over 80 per cent without early antitoxin treatment.

MANAGEMENT
Antitoxin ⎱
Penicillin ⎰ *See below*

Cardiovascular complications

These may present early or late.

(*a*) *Peripheral circulatory failure*

This usually occurs in the first few days of illness in a severely toxic child.

RECOGNITION
The signs are hypotension, tachycardia, pallor, apathy and often hypothermia. Vomiting may occur and may be persistent. There may be little cardiac enlargement but the heart sounds are faint and the ECG usually shows low voltage QRS complexes, with flattened or inverted T waves, prolonged or depressed S-T segment and sometimes conduction defects. Nevertheless the ECG is sometimes entirely normal.

MANAGEMENT
Rest is essential. Attempts to treat 'shock' with corticosteroids have not been encouraging but they may help with conduction defects. ECG monitoring should be continuous if possible. Intravenous fluids may precipitate heart failure.

The use of an α-blocker, such as phenoxybenzamine, may be helpful but careful monitoring of the central venous pressure is essential and its use in diphtheria has not been reported.

(*b*) *Late cardiovascular complications*

These occur in the second or third week in about 10 per cent of cases with a mortality of about 60 per cent.

RECOGNITION
Many ECG abnormalities occur, not always with clinical manifestations. Serious heart disease is due to myocardial damage with conduction defects. Right- or left-sided failure can occur, sometimes together. Almost all cardiac arrythmias have been described and repeated exami-

nation is necessary to detect arrythmia early. Serial chest x-rays will detect early cardiomegaly and a raised serum aspartate aminotransferase is suspicious. Continuous ECG monitoring avoids disturbing the child. The following arrythmias are associated with a bad prognosis.

(a) Atrial fibrillation and flutter. These are unusual.

(b) Complete heart block.

(c) Bundle-branch block, right, left or alternating, in combination with A-V dissociation or nodal rhythm.

(d) Ventricular paroxysmal tachycardia leading to ventricular fibrillation.

Mural endocarditis can occur and give rise to emboli and hemiplegia. Valvular endocarditis and pericarditis are rare.

MANAGEMENT

Rest.

Digitalization at the first sign of heart failure.

The treatment of cardiac arrythmias is conventional.

Digitalization has been carried out prophylactically but may unnecessarily complicate the picture and is of unproved value.

Paralysis

(*a*) *Palatal paralyses* Can occur in the first week with severe pharyngeal diphtheria, probably by direct spread of toxin. It is not itself usually serious but may indicate serious disease and future complications.

(*b*) *Other paralysis* Normally occurs 3 to 5 weeks after the onset of the disease, in about 20 per cent of cases of pharyngeal diphtheria, less commonly in laryngeal and nasal disease. In about 10 per cent of cases it is severe and in about 3 per cent it is fatal. Most affected are children between 2 and 10 years. Emergencies occur due to paralysis of the *pharynx and larynx, intercostals and diaphragm.*

RECOGNITION

For the presentation of symptoms and signs *see* Poliomyelitis (p. 330).

MANAGEMENT

As there is usually a combination of swallowing and respiratory difficulty, the best treatment is probably tracheostomy with or without intermittent positive-pressure ventilation. Paralysis may last a few days or a few weeks. Although recovery is usually complete, paralysis may cause an increased mortality during the 6th to 9th week of the disease. Other paralyses occur but do not cause emergencies.

Drug therapy

ANTITOXIN

Before antitoxin was used the overall mortality in diphtheria was about 20 per cent. It is now less than 10 per cent even when antitoxin is not given until the 4th day or later. The dose of antitoxin does not vary with age, but with site, extent and toxicity. The following is a suggested regime (*Table 22.I*).

TABLE 22.I

Site	Toxicity	Dose (units)	Route
Nasal	Usually slight	2–10 000	i.m.
Faucial	Usually moderate	10–30 000	i.m.
Laryngeal with respiratory symptoms	Usually slight	30–50 000	i.m. or IV
{ Nasopharyngeal { Faucial-nasopharyngeal }	Usually severe	50–100 000	IV

Before giving diphtheria antitoxin, sensitivity testing must be done. The method varies. Some suggest that 0.1 ml intradermally of a 1:1000 solution will give a positive wheal of 1 cm ($\frac{1}{2}$ in) or more 20 minutes later. Or 1 drop of a 1:10 solution can be instilled into the lower conjunctival sac and will give rise to conjunctivitis and lacrimation 20 minutes later in a sensitized patient. Such symptoms can then be treated with adrenaline drops. Others believe that a subcutaneous injection of 0.2 ml of 1:10 solution of antitoxin given 2 hours before therapy is a more sensitive test of hypersensitivity than an intradermal injection. About 1 hour before giving *IV* therapy it is also suggested that about 10 000 units be given i.m. and any reaction observed. Adrenaline should, of course, be immediately available and may be incorporated into the IV antiserum therapy.

PENICILLIN

This is the antibiotic of choice. The usual dose is 300 to 600 mg (500 000–1 million units) of benzylpenicillin 6-hourly for 7 to 10 days. Soluble penicillin can be replaced by procaine penicillin after the initial toxic symptoms have subsided or where toxicity is slight. Erythromycin is best reserved for carriers.

General references

Krugman, S. and Ward, R. (1973). *Infectious Diseases of Children and Adults*. 5th edn. p. 13. St. Louis: Mosby

Martindale's Extra Pharmacopoeia (1977). 27th edn. Diphtheria Antitoxin, p. 1613.
   London: Pharmaceutical Press
Morgan, B. C. (1963). Cardiac complications of diphtheria. *Pediatrics* **32**, 549

Treatment of cardiac complications
Textbook of Medical Treatment (1971). 12th edn. Eds. S. Alstead, A. G. MacGregor
   and R. H. Girdwood. p. 120. Edinburgh: Churchill Livingstone

CHAPTER 23

Haemoptysis

J. A. Black

Haemoptysis is an unusual symptom in childhood, perhaps because sputum is usually swallowed by infants and small children. Though frightening to the parents, haemoptysis in a child rarely constitutes an emergency though it may draw attention to a serious, possibly urgent, underlying condition.

The newborn

RECOGNITION

The important causes of haemoptysis in this age group are:

(a) *Massive pulmonary haemorrhage* (p. 272)

The diagnosis is usually obvious since acute dyspnoea develops, with fine rales all over the chest with large amounts of bright red frothy blood coming up from the trachea. Radiography shows patchy infiltration of both lung fields. Small-for-dates and pre-term infants are more likely to be affected.

(b) *Fulminating staphylococcal pneumonia*

The symptoms are similar to those in (a), but physical and radiological signs may not show the same degree of symmetry. The possibility of staphylococcal pneumonia should be considered when pulmonary haemorrhage occurs in a previously well term infant.

(c) *Intrathoracic gastrogenous cyst*

Symptoms usually develop shortly after birth with dyspnoea or difficulty with feeding. Erosion of the cyst into a bronchus or pulmonary vessel causes repeated severe haemoptysis which can prove fatal.

Radiography shows a rounded solid area in the chest and vertebral abnormalities may be present at the same level.

MANAGEMENT
(*a*) *Massive pulmonary haemorrhage*

Frequently progress is so rapid that little investigation or treatment is possible. However, when time permits, coagulation defects and thrombocytopenia should be looked for and any abnormality promptly corrected (p. 482). Antibiotics (*see* (*b*)) should also be given intravenously or intramuscularly if staphylococcal pneumonia cannot be excluded.

(*b*) *Staphylococcal pneumonia*

Cloxacillin and gentamicin should be given intramuscularly.

(*c*) *Gastrogenous cyst*

If the diagnosis is suspected and the infant is fit enough, pulmonary arteriography should be performed; this shows that the cyst does not have a pulmonary blood supply (Chang *et al.*, 1976). In an emergency, a thoracotomy should be done without previous arteriography.

After the neonatal period

Haemoptysis is rare and in many instances the cause is trivial.

RECOGNITION
(*a*) *Minor causes*

Small streaks of blood may be coughed up after severe coughing fits in whooping cough, or in acute tonsillitis, due to bleeding from the inflamed tonsil.

(*b*) *Major diseases*

(*i*) *Lobar pneumonia*   Still occurs, with an acute onset, high temperature, and signs of lobar consolidation. The characteristic rusty brown sputum is sometimes seen.

(*ii*) *Inhaled foreign body*   May cause haemoptysis: for diagnostic features *see* page 206.

(*iii*) *Sickle cell anaemia*   The possibility should be considered in any child of African descent (p. 471).

(*iv*) *Bronchiectasis*   The previous history and physical and radiological findings are usually characteristic.

(*v*) *Cystic fibrosis*   This is usually a late symptom in older children who have severe pulmonary disease. The diagnosis is invariably already known.

(*vi*) *Pulmonary haemosiderosis*   This is a rare condition in which haemoptysis occurs with attacks of dyspnoea, wheezing, fever, and tachycardia. Radiographic findings are variable but may show diffuse changes.

MANAGEMENT
(*a*) *Minor causes*

No treatment of the actual haemoptysis is necessary; but reassurance of the parents is required since they may have fears of pulmonary tuberculosis; a normal chest x-ray is usually convincing.

(*b*) *Major diseases*

No treatment is normally required for the haemoptysis, but the underlying condition should be treated.

References

Chang, S. H., Morrison, L., Shafner, L. and Crowe, J. E. (1976). Intrathoracic gastrogenic cysts and haemoptysis. *J. Pediat.* **88**, 594

CHAPTER 24

Acute Respiratory Failure

A. M. Wilson

Acute respiratory failure is life-threatening. Action is required within minutes to prevent brain damage and death. A person can survive total apnoea or anoxia for a time due to the oxygen 'stored' in the pulmonary alveoli and in the blood. An adult consumes about one sixth of his body stores of oxygen in one minute while a neonate consumes just under one-third in the same time. *The smaller the child the more rapid must be the relief of respiratory failure.*

Respiratory failure, like cardiac arrest, may be due to many causes (*see* Table 24.I) but the dire effects make treatment of the signs more urgent than making a diagnosis. In respiratory failure treatment will often precede diagnosis. Set out in *Figure 24.1* is a scheme suggesting the urgent approach to the treatment of respiratory failure from any cause. This is preceded by some definitions, and succeeded by notes referred to in the scheme (p. 235).

Acute respiratory failure should be suspected or anticipated in the presence of severe dyspnoea, stridor or wheezing. The contraction of the sternomastoids and in-drawing of the suprasternal notch are important signs of inspiratory difficulty *and an almost silent chest may indicate severe obstruction. Cyanosis suggests a serious situation but the absence of cyanosis is compatible with severe hypoxia. Anxiety, pallor and restlessness indicate hypoxia which requires urgent relief.*

Definitions

(a) Respiratory arrest

There is no respiratory effort and therefore no mechanical exchange of gas between the lungs and the atmosphere. The patient becomes cyanosed due to hypoxia and the pCO_2 level of the blood rises steadily. Survival is dependent on the 'stored oxygen'. This is an absolute, easily

MANAGEMENT OF ACUTE RESPIRATORY FAILURE

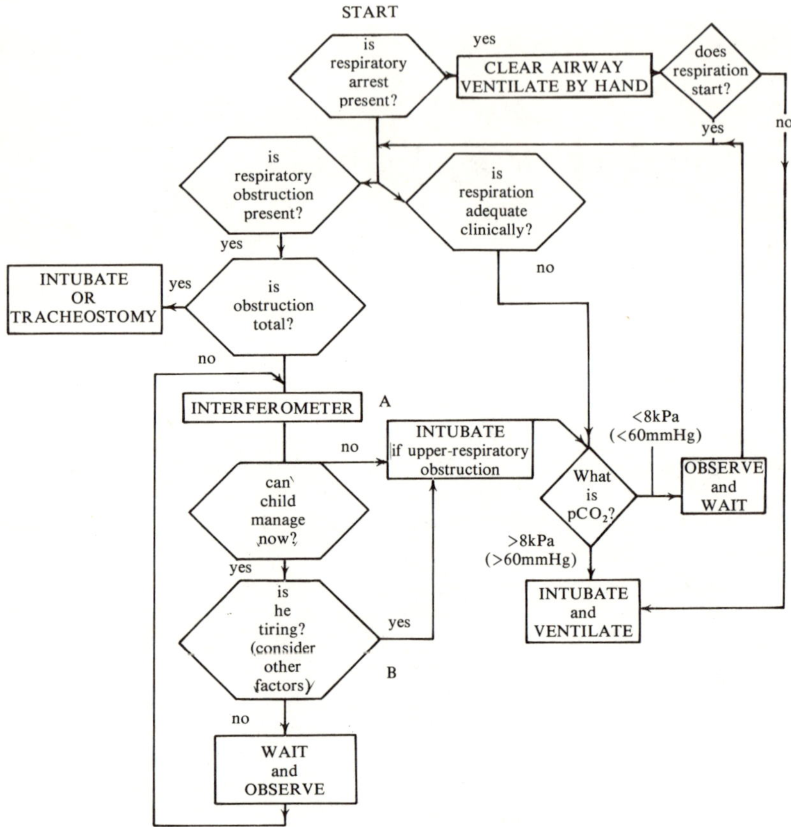

Figure 24.1. Scheme for management of acute respiratory failure. A *and* B *refer to text*
(p. 235)

diagnosable state. The patient needs both maintenance of the airway
and ventilation.

(b) Respiratory failure

Respiratory activity is present but is ineffective. This is divisible for
diagnostic and therapeutic purposes into:

(i) Inadequacy failure   Here there is no obstruction of the airway and
gas exchange is reduced by the depression of some part of the respira-

tory system, neural or muscular. It is difficult to assess clinically the degree of respiratory depression. It can be measured by the level of arterial pCO_2. A capillary pCO_2 may be used if the peripheral circulation is unimpaired. The normal value is 5.3 kPa (40 mm Hg). A value of 8.0 kPa (60 mm Hg) represents 50 per cent depression and is a strong indication for artificial ventilation.

(*ii*) *Obstructive failure*   There is noisy respiration and obvious respiratory difficulty. Noise will be absent if the obstruction is total which will result very rapidly in respiratory arrest. Respiratory effort is seen in in-drawing of the thoracic wall and the use of accessory muscles. The child may sit up or clutch objects in an effort to breathe. This patient requires relief, either medical or surgical, of the obstruction. It is important to realize that *there is no test* to determine the degree of obstruction or the moment to intervene. This must be a clinical judgement based on the observations below. The point of intervention will be before an element of inadequacy is overlaid on the obstruction.

A INTERFEROMETER (*See Figure 24.1*)

This is a set of signs to aid the clinical decision when to intervene and intubate a child to overcome an upper respiratory obstruction. These include:

Both inspiratory and expiratory stridor—a grave sign indicating severe obstruction.

Cyanosis. This indicates some inadequacy and also the possibility of pneumonic involvement.

Increasing loss of awareness. This is suggestive of hypoxia.

Failure to take food and drink. This suggests that the respiratory effort is totally absorbing the child's capabilities.

A rising pulse rate.

Obvious tiring, especially with inability to sleep.

A rising pCO_2. This is a *too-late* sign.

A rising pCO_2 shows that inadequacy of ventilation has occurred. In acute respiratory obstructive disease in children the pCO_2 remains at near normal levels even in the presence of cyanosis. A high pCO_2 means that the child is severely ill and close to respiratory, and possibly cardiac, arrest.

B (*See Figure 24.1*)

The above list of signs cannot give an absolute answer. The significance

of the observations will be affected by other factors. These include:
Length of history. If respiratory obstruction has lasted for many
    hours with no improvement intubation may be preferred.
Time of day
Availability of staff
Availability of ancillary services
Consideration of the last three factors may suggest a planned
intubation at the end of the day rather than risk an emergency proce-
dure at night when x-ray and laboratory services are at a minimum.

TABLE 24.I
Causes of acute respiratory failure in children

Respiratory arrest and inadequacy failure (pCO_2 *is diagnostic*)	*Obstructive failure* (*No test of severity*)
Cerebral	ANY LEVEL
Coma from any cause	
Head injury	FOREIGN BODY
Poisoning	
Anaesthesia	Epiglottis
Meningitis or encephalitis	Acute epiglottitis
Tumour	
	Larynx
Spinal cord	Laryngeal spasm
Cervical cord injury	Laryngeal oedema
Poliomyelitis	Laryngeal trauma, e.g. anaesthesia
Tetanus	
	Acute laryngitis
Neural	Acute laryngotracheobronchitis
Polyneuritis (Guillain-Barré)	
	Small airways
Neuromuscular junction	Acute bronchiolitis
Myasthenia gravis	Asthma
Anaesthetic relaxants	Pulmonary oedema
	Inhalation of liquids and drowning
Musculoskeletal	
Flail chest injury	Pleura
Porphyria	Tension pneumothorax

Not easily classifiable (pCO_2 level depends on many aspects of the illness) Pneumothorax Pleural effusion Pulmonary collapse Pneumonia

Management of acute respiratory failure

RESPIRATORY ARREST AND INADEQUACY

(a) ENSURING A CLEAR AIRWAY

The patient should be placed on the side, usually the right. This allows secretions, vomit and blood to drain away from the larynx and encourages the jaw and tongue to fall forwards. The jaw is held forward by pressing from behind the angle of the mandible. In small children 'holding the jaw up' by pressing below the chin causes obstruction by raising the tongue against the palate. The mouth should be inspected for any debris including dislodged teeth. Such debris can be cleared with a finger or by suction. Respiratory efforts should be watched to see if they return or are obstructed.

(b) ARTIFICIAL VENTILATION

If respiratory arrest is present, artificial ventilation should be started. In hospital it should always be possible to perform this with oxygen from an anaesthetic or resuscitation circuit, or with air from an 'Ambu' or similar self-inflating bag.

However, it may be necessary to perform expired air resuscitation by mouth-to-mouth or mouth-to-tube. All doctors should make themselves familiar with the equipment available locally. The principles are the same for all equipment. Artificial ventilation is most easily performed with the patient supine, after ensuring a clear airway.

(i) Bag and mask

The mask is applied over the mouth and nose and held with the left hand with 3rd, 4th and 5th fingers under the mandibular ramus. This hand also extends the head to maintain a clear airway. The use of a rubber or plastic airway passed over the tongue may help in this. The bag of the apparatus is squeezed regularly to inflate the lungs. The rate of inflation should be approximately 32 minus age in years respirations per minute in children. The depth, determined by the amount of squeeze, should be observed by watching the chest to limit the expansion to the expected normal range. A baby only needs 20 to 40 ml of air per breath and overinflation can produce pneumothorax. Ventilation will have to be continued until spontaneous respiration returns, or in its absence until the child can be intubated and ventilated by machine.

(ii) Mouth-to-mouth (expired air) resuscitation

Expired air resuscitation relies on the 14.5 per cent oxygen in the expired breath being sufficient to sustain life in an apnoeic patient.

Mouth-to-mouth ventilation is performed after clearing the airway of debris. The head is held extended using the fingers of one hand to occlude the nostrils and the fingers of the other to pinch the cheeks to hold the mouth open. In this position the lips are applied to the patient's lips and a breath whose size will depend upon that of the child is forcibly exhaled. Removing the face well away allows expiration. This is repeated at the appropriate rate. The use of a barrier is more pleasant. This may be a porous plastic sheet designed for the purpose or even a pocket handkerchief.

Tubes such as a double-ended or a Brook airway make the process more efficient and acceptable. These are placed over the tongue into the pharynx. With these the mouth and nose are occluded to prevent escape of gas.

(iii) Endotracheal intubation

Endotracheal intubation should be within the scope of all doctors. A laryngoscope is used to visualize the larynx. In an emergency with anoxia and loss of tone this is relatively easy. With the head extended on the neck, as for producing a clear airway, the curved laryngoscope blade is introduced over the tongue and slid back until its blade tip comes to lie in the fossa between the tongue and epiglottis (*Figure 24.2a,b*). When the laryngoscope is correctly placed, traction in the direction of the handle (arrowed) will make the laryngeal opening

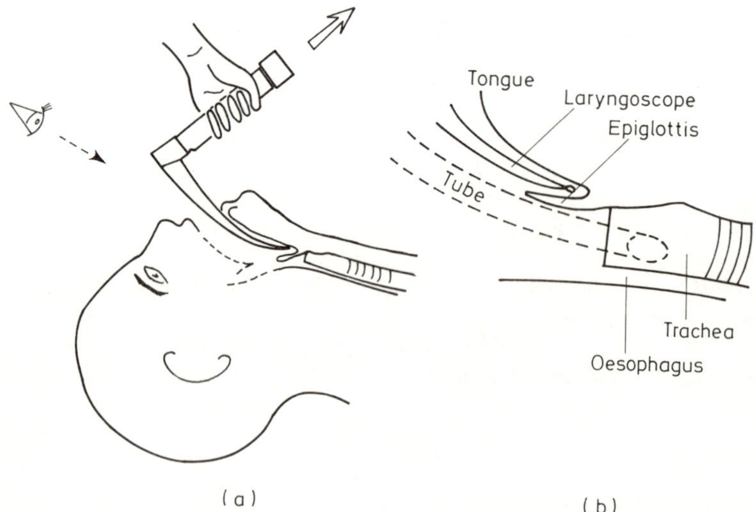

Figure 24.2a, b. Laryngoscopy using the curved-bladed laryngoscope

visible. Choosing a tube of the correct size and length can be difficult in an emergency. The sizes of tube most likely to be suitable at various ages are shown in Appendix 21. These refer to children with no abnormality, and it may be found that the recommended size will not pass through the cords. An endotracheal tube should never be forced into position, and if there is difficulty a smaller one should be tried so that a loose fit is obtained. Care must be taken not to advance the tube into a main bronchus. Normally the end of the tube should be passed 2 to 3 cm (~1 in) past the cords, but where an obstruction is present the tube should be advanced until the obstruction is relieved. In all cases the tube should be firmly fixed to prevent any further movement. In children under six months the use of the straight-bladed laryngoscope is easier; it is passed over the tongue into the lower pharynx. While looking down the laryngoscope, it is withdrawn slowly until the larynx comes into view (*Figure 24.3a,b,c*). This is preferred because the large floppy epiglottis obscures the view of the larynx when the curved-blade

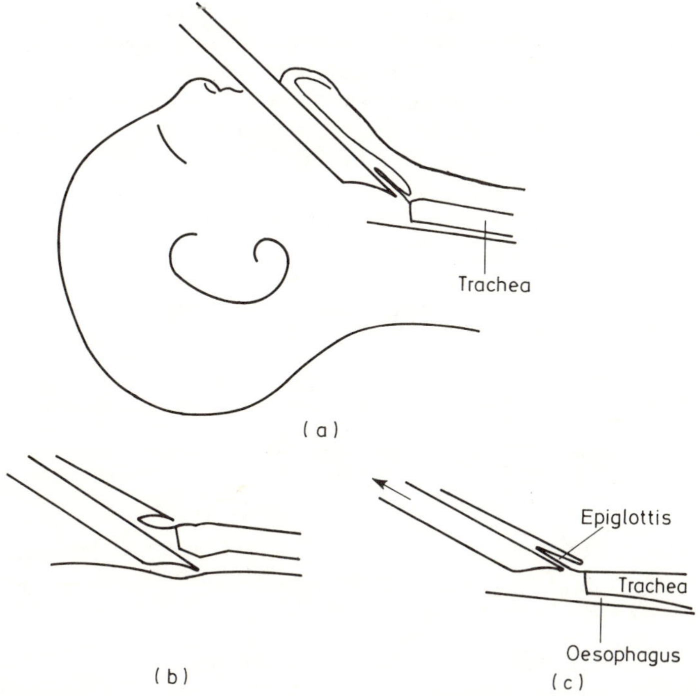

Figure 24.3a, b, c. Laryngoscopy using the straight-bladed laryngoscope (for children under the age of six months)

technique is used. After intubation, artificial ventilation may be continued with the resuscitation circuit connected directly to the tube. There must be some form of escape valve in the circuit as direct connection of oxygen to an intubated patient can be fatal.

(c) CONDITIONS REQUIRING SPECIFIC TREATMENT

(i) Tetanus

The spasms not only fail to produce adequate ventilation but obstruct ventilatory treatment. These patients need paralysis and heavy sedation in an intensive treatment unit. There are often sympathetic activity episodes with wide variations in pulse and blood pressure. These may require sympathetic blocker therapy. (For treatment of tetanus *see* Chapters 33–35).

(ii) Myasthenia gravis

Respiratory crises may be precipitated by failure to take treatment, by overtreatment or intercurrent infection. Emergency treatment is edrophonium chloride 0.5 to 1 mg IV or i.m. as a test. If this is successful neostigmine 0.04 mg per kg may be given for more prolonged action. The patient should be treated where there are facilities for artificial ventilation if there is no response to treatment, or in the case of a neostigmine crisis which requires withdrawal of treatment.

(*iii*) Patients who have received non-depolarising anaesthetic relaxants e.g. curare, pancuronium, or alcuronium may show prolonged or renewed effect after return from the operating theatre. The initial treatment is neostigmine 0.04 mg per kg IV with atropine 0.2 to 0.6 mg IV to counteract the cardiac-slowing effect of neostigmine.

OBSTRUCTIVE FAILURE
(*See under* Upper Airway Obstruction and Respiratory Emergencies)

COMPLICATIONS OF INTUBATION AND VENTILATION
(*See also* under IPPV treatment with tracheostomy in neonatal tetanus, page 341, and Upper Airway Obstruction, page 222)

The following list outlines many of the possible complications of intubation and ventilation therapy. It must be remembered that intubation removes the protective function of the nose in warming and humidifying the inspired gases, and of the cough in removing secretions or foreign material. It also removes the ability of the child to cry and attract attention. The psychological trauma of intubation must be remembered. The intubated child must never be left alone if he is confined to bed.

Dangers of intubation

(*a*) *Obstruction*

    (i) Tube obstruction due to:
      kinking;
      movement in trachea;
      secretions and crusting;
      dislodgement.
    (ii) Bronchial obstruction due to above causes and unilateral bronchial intubation.

(*b*) *Damage to structures involved in intubation*

    (i) During insertion of the tube—damage to:
      lips;
      teeth;
      frenulum of tongue;
      pillars of fauces;
      posterior pharyngeal wall;
      larynx.
    (ii) Structures on which the tube and allied apparatus rests and in which pressure necrosis is possible.
      Skin of face and head;
      Upper lip;
      Nasal septum;
      Pharynx;
      Vocal cords and arytenoids;
      Subglottic region, especially cricoid ring;
      Tracheal mucosa.

(*c*) *As a consequence of sedation*

    Corneal damage (open eyes);
    Pressure sores;
    Intestinal ileus;
    Dehydration;
    Constipation.

(*d*) *As a consequence of by-passing the nose and larynx*

    Tracheal dehydration and crusting of secretions;

I

Loss of tracheal ciliary action;
Entry of infection;
Inability to cough effectively.

(e) Added dangers of ventilator treatment

Failure of the machine;
Accidental disconnection;
Pneumothorax or pneumomediastinum;
Hyper- or hypoventilation;
Oxygen toxicity;
Results of using neuromuscular blocking drugs;
Alteration of intrathoracic pressures.

Tube obstruction

Tube obstruction is a common complication. The breathing of dry gas, especially when using high oxygen concentration rapidly stops ciliary action in the tracheal mucosa in the region of the end of the tube. This results in interruption of the normal upward sweep, and a build-up of secretions. This gradually encroaches on the lumen of the tube eventually blocking it. If allowed to dry, these secretions become crusted and may be impossible to remove.

PREVENTION
Warmed gas (34–37°C; 93–98.4°F) should be used fully saturated with water vapour from a suitable humidifier; also a regular and effective suction technique. Children who have been intubated for respiratory infections produce much secretion, and suction must be done frequently if necessary every quarter of an hour. This may be assisted by the instillation of 0.1 ml to 1 ml of saline into the tube before suction. Instillation is additional to humidification and cannot replace it.

RECOGNITION
If a tube becomes totally obstructed the child will become very restless, with intercostal and suprasternal in-drawing and increasing cyanosis. It is essential to listen to the open end of the tube and if there is no movement of air not to waste time trying to suck out the tube, but PULL IT OUT. *The child with respiratory obstruction and no tube stands a chance. The child with a blocked tube stands no chance.*

Although the accumulation of secretions is the most common cause of obstruction, if the child is restless or if the ventilator pressure is high it is necessary to look for mechanical obstruction due to kinking or the rotation of the bevel of the tube against the tracheal wall. Both sides of the chest must be examined with a stethoscope to exclude a main bronchus intubation due to too long a tube. To confirm that the breath sounds are equal it is necessary to listen in the axillae to reduce the effect of tracheal noise.

Damage during insertion of the tube

(a) TECHNIQUE
Damage can be minimized by careful intubation technique, but also by avoiding intubation at the last minute. If a child is expected to become worse a consultation should be requested with the department responsible for intubation as early as possible. This allows planning and if necessary moving the child to an ITU while still fit for transfer. When the morbidity of intubation is very low it is better to intubate earlier under ideal conditions. It should be remembered that intubation is an operation and may require anaesthesia; therefore a consent form should be completed.

(b) SIZE OF TUBE
The longer the tube is left in position the more likely is there a complication due to pressure. Avoidance of these complications starts with the selection of the correct size tube for diameter and length (*see* Appendix 21). It is usual in children to use an uncuffed tube of such a size that there is a small leak of air between the tube and trachea.

(c) FIXATION
Adequate fixation is essential both to prevent dislodgement and also repeated movement between tube and mucous membranes. Nasotracheal tubes should be fixed to lie just clear of the nasal septum. Necrosis in this region is the commonest complication of long-term intubation and is easily avoided. Occasionally the adhesive plaster used for holding the tube causes a reaction of the underlying skin. This has been a factor in changing to a tracheostomy, and is more likely in the hot humid atmosphere of an incubator.

(d) DAMAGE FROM TOO LARGE TUBES OR TUBES OF UNSUITABLE MATERIAL
Laryngeal trauma will occur if too large a tube or one of unsuitable material is used for too long. Red rubber tubes should only be used for operations. Pressure necrosis of the vocal cords with subsequent granuloma formation may occur. This is more likely if there has been continuous movement due to insecure fixation. The most serious complication is subglottic stenosis. In children the cricoid ring is the

narrowest part of the upper airway. Selection of too large a tube may result in oedema, or even necrosis with fibrosis at this site. This may appear as inspiratory stridor immediately after extubation and requires immediate re-intubation; however this complication may develop as long as three months later. A fibrous stenosis can also occur at the site of the tube end due to the repeated movement of an inadequately sedated patient.

(e) SUCTION OF THE TUBE

Care must be taken when suctioning the tube and trachea not to use too large a catheter. The catheter should be about one-third of the diameter of the lumen. A larger catheter will subject the lung to negative pressure, with possible collapse. The suction catheter should not project more than $\frac{1}{2}$ cm ($\frac{1}{4}$ in) beyond the tube, for routine suction. When stiff catheters are necessary for sucking small tubes, greater projection will result in the taking of 'suction biopsies' of the tracheal mucosa. Suction technique must be aseptic and gentle.

(f) SEDATION

Although children tolerate both intubation and ventilation remarkably well and quickly, a period of sedation is always necessary. During this period of immobility, which may include paralysis by neuromuscular blocking drugs, further protective reflexes are abolished. These patients need full neurosurgical nursing including eye and mouth toilet, regular turning, treatment of pressure areas and routine physiotherapy.

(g) INTRAVENOUS LINE

All intubated patients must have an IV line for drug therapy and to maintain hydration. Oral intake will cease for at least twelve hours and dehydration increases tracheal crusting. Immediately after intubation gastric emptying ceases and a nasogastric tube must be passed. This is allowed to drain freely to prevent gastric dilatation due to air swallowing. As it is difficult to ensure a high-roughage diet for patients on ventilators attention must be paid to the prevention of constipation.

(h) MECHANICAL FAILURES

A patient receiving artificial ventilation runs the risk of intubation complications and, in addition, those of the machine. All machines must be expected to fail. Nursing instructions should include details of the action to be taken in such event. There must be a separate method of ventilating by hand immediately available. If there is any doubt about the machine's function the rule is 'Disconnect the ventilator and ventilate by hand using the simplest circuit while the problem is diagnosed'. Pneumothorax is more common with artificial ventilation and cannot be clinically diagnosed with certainty. If pneumothorax is suspected in a patient on a ventilator an x-ray should be taken. If this is not possible and there are signs of ventilating difficulty, rising ventilator pressure, uneven chest movement, unexplained cyanosis, and tracheal deviation, a needle should be inserted into the pleura in the mid-axillary line. If there is no air leak this should be repeated on the opposite side, and followed by a chest drain if necessary.

(i) HYPERVENTILATION AND HYPOVENTILATION

Most patients are moderately hyperventilated to assist in the control of spontaneous respiratory efforts. Restlessness suggests hypoventilation which is frequently due to leaks in the circuit or accidental alteration of the ventilator controls. A check for leaks should be made at every joint *especially* at any restrained with sticky tape.

(j) OXYGEN TOXICITY

Pulmonary oxygen toxicity can occur whenever the inspired oxygen is above 20 per cent, given enough time. Care should be taken to ensure that the prescribed concentration is maintained as there is always a tendency to increase it 'just to be safe'.

(k) HYPOVOLAEMIA

Artificial ventilation raises the mean intrathoracic pressure to a positive value. This can embarrass the venous return to the heart, causing hypotension. Patients on ventilators must have their fluid balance monitored as they tolerate hypovolaemia badly.

It will be seen that the dangers of intubation and ventilation are many. These procedures should only be practised when there are adequate staff and facilities. Only under these conditions and with meticulous attention to detail can good results be obtained.

CHAPTER 25

Respiratory Emergencies

A. D. Milner

Respiratory disorders are the commonest cause for admission to paediatric medical wards. The aim of paediatric respiratory emergency care is to prevent or overcome respiratory failure. Respiratory failure should be suspected when there is difficulty in breathing (evidence of obstruction or weakness of respiratory effort) with cyanosis or clinical evidence of hypoxia without cyanosis (pallor, anxiety or restlessness).

Respiratory failure

This is present when:
 (a) The arterial carbon dioxide tension ($PaCO_2$) is greater than 7.7 kPa ($>$50 mm Hg).
 (b) The arterial oxygen tension (PaO_2) is less than 8 kPa ($<$60 mm Hg) when breathing air.
or (c) Both (a) and (b) are present.

MECHANISMS

(a) *Low alveolar oxygen concentration despite adequate alveolar ventilation*

This occurs when the inspired air contains too little oxygen and usually too much carbon dioxide. It occurs only too frequently in intubated children who are breathing spontaneously through systems with large dead spaces and insufficient gas flow to avoid rebreathing.

(b) *Inadequate alveolar ventilation secondary to neuromuscular or rib-cage defects*

The $PaCO_2$ rises early at a rate which is inversely proportional to the fall in PaO_2. The hypoxia can be relieved by increasing the inspired oxygen concentration but the $PaCO_2$ can only be corrected by intermittent positive-pressure ventilation or by overcoming the underlying defect.

(c) Inadequate ventilation secondary to upper airway obstruction

These conditions exist in the presence of acute laryngotracheobronchitis (croup). Initially, the child hyperventilates in response to the obstruction but as the resistance to airflow increases the alveolar minute volume falls, resulting in hypercapnia and hypoxia. The hypoxia is again easy to relieve with added oxygen but the CO_2 retention will remain high until the obstruction is by-passed or responds to treatment.

(d) Ventilation perfusion abnormalities

This is the commonest cause of hypoxic respiratory failure and results from a disturbance of the close match between the blood supply and ventilation at alveolar level. It occurs in status asthmaticus, bronchiolitis, wheezy bronchitis and in bronchopneumonia. The child usually

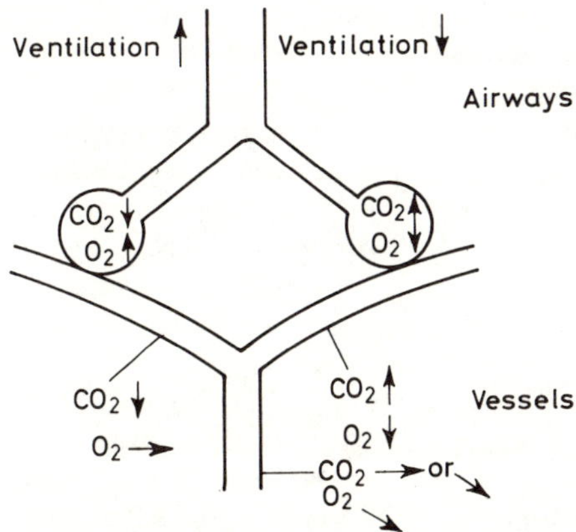

Figure 25.1. Ventilation perfusion mismatch. The blood leaving the hypoventilated alveolae has a high CO_2 and low O_2 content. The blood leaving the hyperventilated unit has a low CO_2 but normal O_2 content so that the mixed blood will be desaturated

hyperventilates in response to the altered lung mechanics so that the $PaCO_2$ is below the normal range of 4.7 to 6.2 kPa (35 to 47 mm Hg) until the obstruction is severe. The blood leaving poorly ventilated units will have a relatively high $PaCO_2$ but this will be more than compensated for by the low $PaCO_2$ in blood leaving over-ventilated units. Unfortunately, this mechanism cannot compensate for the relative desaturation of blood leaving poorly ventilated areas, as blood leaving normally ventilated units is already virtually 100 per cent saturated and little additional oxygen carriage is gained by hyperventilation (*Figure 25.1*).

The hypoxia responds readily to increasing the inspired oxygen concentration. If the underlying mechanical changes are sufficiently severe the child will eventually be unable to maintain his high alveolar ventilation and carbon dioxide retention will occur. This can only be overcome by relief of the mechanical problem or by supportive ventilation.

MANAGEMENT

(a) Hypoxia

Hypoxia can usually be overcome by increasing the inspired oxygen concentration. The young child can be nursed in an oxygen tent or in a Derbyshire chair (Portex Ltd). Alternatively, there are a number of lightweight face masks and nasal cannulae which are tolerated by most older children. The ambient oxygen should either be measured intermittently (every 15 to 30 minutes) using a paramagnetic oxygen analyser, or continuously, using one of the other oxygen-measuring devices available on the market.

As gas from any oxygen source is completely dry the mixture should pass through a humidification system. As long as the upper airways have not been by-passed by an endotracheal tube and there is no other indication for humidification it is not necessary to ensure that 100 per cent saturation has occurred. This will also avoid the problem of soaking the child and obscuring observation with heavy condensation within the tent.

Unlike adults, children rarely lose their carbon dioxide respiratory drive and become dependent on hypoxia, so that there is little danger in giving unlimited oxygen for short periods. There is some evidence to suggest that very high inspired oxygen concentrations (over 70 per cent) may produce lung damage if maintained for more than 48 hours and so it is advisable to restrict the concentration to below that level as soon as the child's clinical condition permits.

(b) Humidification

Humidification is frequently used in acute laryngotracheobronchitis although there is little evidence that standard humidifiers feeding into oxygen tents have any influence on the water content within the larynx or have any effect on the course of the disease. Steam kettles were effective in producing a good mist but these have been abandoned because of the danger of scalding. The ultrasonic nebulizers are the most efficient at producing high water content with relatively small particle size but, even when feeding directly to a face mask, less than 10 per cent of the droplets pass beyond the upper airways. If humidification is to do anything useful the child must be nursed in a dense mist, as the water content of saturated air at room temperature is only half that of the content at body temperature. This makes close observation of the child difficult.

(c) Sedation

Children with obstructed airways, e.g. 'croup', wheezy bronchitis, bronchiolitis and status asthmaticus, are often very restless and, as a result, greatly increase their respiratory efforts. This can be counter-productive as dynamic compression of the airways will occur, making the obstruction worse (*Figures 25.2* and *25.3*). Often, the transfer of the child from the tense home situation to the relatively calm environment of the hospital ward produces a great improvement. It is well worthwhile spending time trying to gain the child's confidence. If the child remains very distressed, sedation can be helpful but respiratory depressants must be avoided. Chloral hydrate* (30 to 50 mg per kg) can be given up to 4-hourly. Promethazine (Phenergan) (1 to 2 mg per kg) is an alternative safe form of sedation. Sedation must only be given when the child can be kept under continuous close observation. Sometimes the child becomes more confused on sedation, resulting in further deterioration.

(d) Intubation (*see also* Appendix 21)

    (i) In an emergency oro-endotracheal intubation is quicker and easier than via the nose. Either a straight or curved laryngoscope blade can be used depending on the operator's preference. A 3.0 to 3.5-mm tube will comfortably fit the larynx of a full-term baby. By one year, a 4.5-mm tube can be passed. Over this age the size is approximately given by the formula:

$$Size\ of\ tube = \frac{Age\ (years)}{4} + 4.5\ mm$$

(Jones and Owen-Thomas, 1971).

---

* Chloral hydrate has a very unpleasant taste; a satisfactory alternative is dichloralphenazone (Welldorm (*Smith and Nephew*)) in the form of an elixir containing 225 mg per 5 ml; the usual dosage is: up to 1 year, 2.5–5.0 ml; 1–5 years, 5.0–10.0 ml; 6–12 years, 10.0–20.0 ml

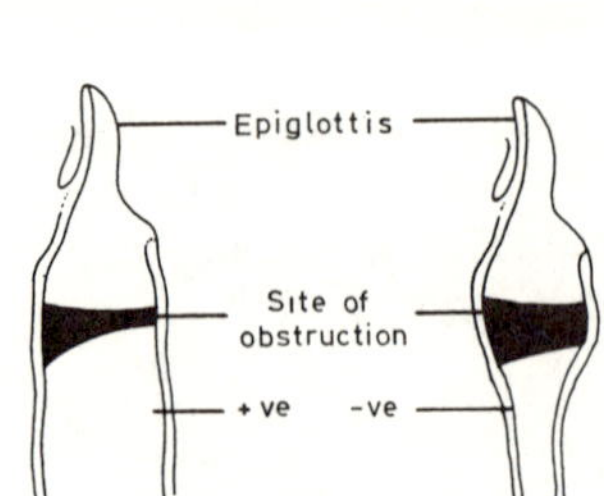

Figure 25.2. Upper-airway obstruction. On inspiration the pressure proximal to the obstruction will drop so that the trachea will tend to collapse on itself, increasing the obstruction. The reverse occurs on expiration

(ii) For resuscitation the dead space should be kept as small as possible. If inflation is achieved by covering the open limb of a T-piece with a finger or thumb it is essential to have a safety blow-off pressure-limiting system in the inspired line since *the pressure delivered by a gas cylinder or wall supply is measured in atmospheres and is very likely to cause a pneumothorax.*

It is rarely necessary to exceed an inflation pressure of 40 cm of water during the resuscitation unless there is severe airways obstruction (status asthmaticus, bronchiolitis) when pressures up to 70 cm of water are sometimes required. It is important to listen over both sides of the chest during inflation to check that the tube has been passed correctly.

(iii) If the tube is to remain in place, adequate humidification is essential because the upper airways are by-passed. Heated nebulizers will provide satisfactory water vapour content provided the temperature at the junction with the endotracheal tube is maintained at 35°C (95°F). Ultrasonic nebulizers are also very efficient and *can provide up to 25 per cent of the child's total fluid requirement.* In addition to using an efficient humidification system it is also necessary to instill $\frac{1}{2}$ to 1.0 ml of normal saline (0.9 per cent NaCl) down the tube at 2- to 4-hour intervals and pass a suction catheter down the lumen to prevent build-up of thick secretions in the airway. Cuffed tubes should not be used in young children because of the risk of subsequent tracheal stenosis.

(e) Tracheostomy

Tracheostomies are now rarely required as an emergency procedure but are still done as an elective measure in children and babies who have been intubated for at least 7 days. Emergency tracheostomy may rarely be required for acute upper-airway obstruction when intubation has failed. Alternatively, tracheostomy may be required when there is no-one sufficiently skilled in intubation immediately available. This procedure will only be carried out if the child is unconscious or anaesthetized. (For technique and maintenance *see* page 341.)

(f) Blood-gas analysis

Blood suitable for analysis can be obtained from the radial, brachial, femoral or even the temporal artery. A 1- or 2-ml syringe can be used. The dead space of the needle and syringe should be filled with heparin (5000 units per ml). Alternatively, blood can be collected in a heparinized capillary tube from a finger or heel prick. To prevent the blood clotting in the capillary tube it is necessary to insert a short metal pin and to run this up and down the lumen of the capillary tube with the aid of a magnet after sealing the tube with plasticine ('Astrup' technique). These capillary samples are satisfactory for hydrogen-ion concentration (pH) and carbon dioxide estimations, but unless the peripheral circulation is very good oxygen-tension results will be unreliable. If the blood is not to be analysed immediately the sample should be stored on ice; at 37°C (98.6°F) the oxygen tension may drop by as much as 0.4 kPa (3 mm Hg) per minute.

(*i*) *Oxygen*   The PaO_2 should, if possible, be maintained above 6.6 kPa (50 mm Hg) since outside the immediate neonatal period this represents 80 per cent saturation at a blood H^+ concentration of 40 nmol per litre (pH 7.40). At a PaO_2 of 4 kPa (30 mm Hg) the blood is only 50 per cent saturated. If the blood H^+ concentration rises by 25 nmol per litre to 65 nmol per litre (pH falls by 0.2 to 7.20) the saturation at oxygen tensions of 6.6 and 4.0 kPa (50 and 30 mm Hg) falls to 70 and 35 per cent respectively, indicating the importance of correcting any metabolic acidosis.

(*ii*) *Carbon dioxide*   When hypoxia is due to a ventilation perfusion abnormality (e.g. status asthmaticus) the $PaCO_2$ will tend to be subnormal secondary to alveolar hyperventilation. A normal or raised $PaCO_2$ indicates that the obstruction is severe and supportive measures may soon be necessary. If the respiratory failure is secondary to an upper-airway obstruction or a neuromuscular problem a moderately raised pCO_2 is less ominous. Many young children can tolerate a $PaCO_2$ of 9 to 10 kPa (70–80 mm Hg) for days and recover without the need for ventilation therapy. Arterial carbon dioxide levels are probably not as good a guide for the need for intervention as an assessment of the clinical state and level of consciousness. The arterial carbon dioxide level does, however, provide a very useful measure of the severity and the course of the condition.

(*iii*) *Acid-base state*   The blood H^+ concentration (pH) alone is of limited value as (for example) an H^+ concentration of 65 nmol per litre (pH 7.20) may indicate a relatively severe metabolic acidosis requiring intravenous bicarbonate or, a normal acid-base balance with a $PaCO_2$ of 10 kPa (75 mm Hg). Under these latter conditions intravenous bicarbonate will only raise the $PaCO_2$ further and may lead to deterioration.

If the $PaCO_2$ and the pH are known the base deficit can be calculated by reference to nomograms. Further adjustments will be necessary if the body temperature or haemoglobin concentration differs widely from the normal range. A base deficit of up to 10 mmol per litre does not require correction providing the condition is otherwise satisfactory. The dose of sodium bicarbonate necessary can be calculated from the standard formula;

$$\text{mmol sodium bicarbonate} = \text{base deficit} \times \text{Wt (kg)} \times 0.3$$

(*See also* page 126).

Conditions associated with respiratory failure

Status asthmaticus

Status asthmaticus is a state of respiratory insufficiency due to severe airways obstruction in which bronchodilator therapy is no longer effective.

The lumen of the medium and small airways is reduced by mucosal oedema, accumulation of sticky secretions, desquamated cells, and to a

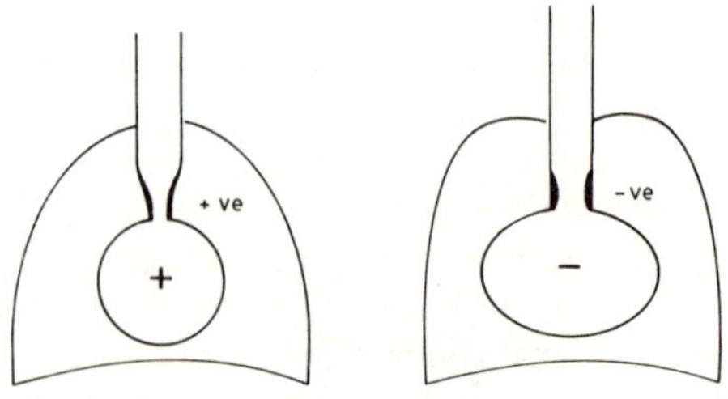

Figure 25.3. Lower airway obstruction on active expiration. The high pleural pressure will compress the airways distal to the obstruction increasing the resistance to breathing

variable extent by muscle spasm. The resistance to airflow is greater on expiration, due to dynamic compression (*Figure 25.3*). This leads to gross over-inflation of the lungs. Some airways become completely obstructed, resulting in areas of atelectasis which are apparent on chest x-ray. Cyanosis occurs early, due to a ventilation perfusion mismatch, but the $PaCO_2$ will initially be low as a result of alveolar hyperventilation. As the obstruction progresses and the child tires the alveolar ventilation will drop and the $PaCO_2$ will rise. There is often an associated metabolic acidosis secondary to hypoxia, poor peripheral perfusion and poor hydration.

RECOGNITION

Most children will have had respiratory symptoms for 24 to 48 hours before admission to hospital although there is the occasional severe asthmatic who can become critically ill within hours. The child is often cyanosed, with rapid pulse rate, expiratory and inspiratory wheeze and laboured respiratory movement. The hyperinflation is apparent clinically and radiologically. The liver is usually displaced downwards by the diaphragm.

Critical signs are:
(a) Rising pulse and respiratory rate.
(b) An apparent reduction in the wheeze not accompanied by an improvement in the child's general condition.
(c) Reduced air entry.
(d) Deterioration in the level of consciousness.

MANAGEMENT

The child should be admitted urgently to hospital, preferably accompanied by a parent.

(a) Bronchodilator therapy

By the time the child reaches hospital and is in established status asthmaticus, he will almost certainly have received significant quantities of sympathomimetic drugs and at least part of his tachycardia may be drug-induced. However, further bronchodilator therapy should be tried. There are several possible alternatives.

(i) 0.5 per cent salbutamol (1 to 2 ml) as a nebulized solution using either a loosely applied face mask or an open-ended mouth tube. This should be diluted to 0.25 per cent for use in children under 7 years of age. The nebulizer can be driven by an electric pump or by air–oxygen from a cylinder or wall supply.

(ii) IV aminophylline (4 mg per kg) is sometimes successful when sympathomimetic bronchodilators are ineffective.

It should be given slowly, over at least 5 minutes, and the pulse rate should be monitored throughout the injection. This drug sometimes produces vomiting in children. Alternatively, salbutamol can be given intravenously in a dose of 4 to 6 μg per kg body weight.

(b) Oxygen therapy

Any child who is cyanosed with asthma will require oxygen using either an oxygen tent, a face mask or nasal cannulae.

(c) Hydration

By the time the child is in need of intensive care he has probably had a severe asthmatic attack for 24 to 48 hours. During this period, respiratory water loss will have been high and oral intake low. Intravenous fluids in the form of 0.18 per cent NaCl in 4 per cent glucose should be given to correct any dehydration and provide maintenance requirements. Normal fluid intake plus 30 per cent is probably adequate. The intravenous line will also provide a route for drug therapy.

(d) Steroids

Any child who still requires oxygen after an adequate dose of bronchodilator drugs should be given steroids. In hospital this should be given as intravenous hydrocortisone to produce as rapid a response as possible (100 to 200 mg 4- to 6-hourly). Hydrocortisone usually takes some hours to be effective (normally 4 hours should be assumed in planning treatment) and can usually be replaced by an oral steroid such as prednisolone after 24 to 48 hours.

(e) Sedation

Reassurance of the child and parents will usually overcome the severe anxiety associated with status asthmaticus and allow the child to breathe in a more relaxed manner. This will avoid excessive dynamic compression on expiration and reduce the respiratory workload. Very occasionally sedation is worth trying using either promethazine (Phenergan) (1 to 2 mg per kg) or chloral hydrate (30 to 50 mg per kg) or dichloralphenazone (Welldorm), (for dosage *see* page 774) but close observation will be needed subsequently.

(f) Physiotherapy

There is little place for physiotherapy in status asthmaticus as this disturbs and tires the child with little relief of the underlying obstruction.

(g) Blood gases

Arterial blood gas analyses are of value in status asthmaticus as they give information about progress. The reduction in audible wheeze is often misinterpreted as an improvement in the child's condition and inappropriate action can be avoided if blood gas data are available. The sampling need not be painful if local anaesthesia is used. Alternatively, a catheter can be inserted transcutaneously in the radial or brachial artery.

(h) Metabolic acidosis

If the blood gases indicate a metabolic acidosis with a base deficit in excess of 10 mmol per litre, sodium bicarbonate should be given intravenously (see page 126). This sometimes produces a striking improvement in the degree of airways obstruction.

(i) Bronchial lavage

The value of bronchial lavage is still in dispute. Sometimes, treatment results in a considerable improvement in the clinical condition, with the removal of large quantities of debris. It involves intubation or bronchoscopy, often under an anaesthetic. Sterile normal (0.9 per cent NaCl) saline (1 to 2 ml per kg) is instilled down the tube. The lungs are overinflated for approximately ten breaths, using an anaesthetic rebreathing bag followed by a sudden release of the inflation pressure and external chest wall compression. This procedure is possibly worth doing once the decision to ventilate has been made.

(j) Supportive ventilation

In some centres the decision to ventilate is based on blood gas data and is carried out when the $PaCO_2$ is greater than 8 kPa (60 mm Hg). Alternatively, the decision can be made on the clinical condition, particularly the *level of consciousness*. This will avoid ventilating some children who recover without IPPV despite a $PaCO_2$ in excess of 8 kPa (60 mm Hg). A light anaesthetic may be necessary to carry out the intubation. Often, high inflation pressures are needed (up to 70 cm H_2O) and as the mechanical characteristics of the lung can change rapidly in the recovery phase a volume-controlled ventilator should be used if this is available. An inspiratory:expiratory ratio of 1:2 is usually adequate. Ventilatory support is rarely required for more than 24 hours.

(k) Later care

Weaning from the ventilator and extubation should be done with great care. Oral steroids and salbutamol should be continued until at least 48 hours after the child has been breathing independently. A chest x-ray should be obtained before removal from the ventilator. The tube, after removal, should be cultured and any clinically evident chest infection should be treated with antibiotics.

Acute pneumonia

Pneumonia is still a common cause of admission to hospital, and death in infancy; but it is relatively rare in the older child.

The majority of pneumonias are caused by viruses, particularly the respiratory syncytial, para-influenza, influenza, and the adenoviruses. Mycoplasma pneumoniae is a relatively common cause between the ages of 5 and 15 years. The pneumococcus is the commonest bacterial pathogen (90 per cent). Staphylococcal pneumonias are rare except in the first year of life. A variety of Gram-negative organisms, e.g. *E. coli, pseudomonas aeruginosa, klebsiella* and *proteus*, are responsible for pneumonia in debilitated infants. Occasionally, the *Streptococcus* and *Haemophilus influenzae* are isolated.

RECOGNITION

There is usually a sudden onset of fever, reluctance to feed and listlessness, with tachypnoea, tachycardia and cough occurring in a child who has had an upper respiratory infection for several days. Apart from the cough and tachypnoea, chest signs are often slight and the diagnosis can only be made with certainty after a chest x-ray; this can be helpful in the identification of the aetiological agent in the acute phase. If consolidation is extensive and some of the lesions are circumscribed, staphylococcal pneumonia is likely. Mycoplasma infections produce patchy, lobar or segmental consolidation. The viral pneumonias rarely produce more than the patchy consolidation.

Other investigations which can help identify the causal agents are:
(a) Full blood picture. A high neutrophil count is suggestive of a bacterial infection.
(b) Throat swab. This should be taken for both bacterial and viral culture.

(c) Blood culture.

(d) Serum for viral antibody titres. Although a single sample can be helpful in the acute phase, a further specimen should be examined in the convalescent stage for confirmation.

(e) Lung tap. This involves inserting a needle into the lung transcutaneously, aspirating with a syringe, and withdrawing the needle. The aspirate can then be cultured. There is a risk of pneumothorax with the procedure and it is not recommended except in immune deficiency states or where there is no clinical evidence of response to adequate antibiotic therapy.

(f) Immunofluorescent identification. Techniques are now available for identifying a number of viruses including the respiratory syncytial virus in respiratory-tract secretions. This can be done within two to three hours of admission.

MANAGEMENT

Although most pneumonias are viral in origin, a number are caused by bacteria and, as this is a potentially fatal condition, antibiotics are almost always indicated. During the first year of life cloxacillin with gentamicin is at present the safest combination. After one year cloxacillin with ampicillin will provide adequate cover for staphylococcal and haemophilus influenzae. Parenteral benzylpenicillin is the recommended treatment for pneumococcal infections unless local strains are penicillin-resistant. Mycoplasma pneumonia responds to tetracycline or erythromycin.

If the child is cyanosed oxygen should be given. Infants with pneumonia are often unable to feed adequately by mouth and will require intravenous or nasogastric feeding.

Aspiration

(a) *Milk*

Aspiration of milk is not rare in childhood. It is particularly common in 'brain-damaged' children with inco-ordination of swallowing. Although recognition is important in the long-term management, the individual episodes should be treated as a lower respiratory-tract infection. Physiotherapy often aids recovery.

(b) *Foreign bodies* (*see* page 206)

(c) *Chemicals*

Children may swallow kerosene-based solutions and require admission to hospital for observation, mainly because of the possibility of inhalation pneumonitis. When inhalation does occur the mucosal inflammation is usually relatively mild and resolves rapidly. Systemic steroids have been given but there is little evidence that they are of value.

Pneumothorax

Spontaneous pneumothorax is rare in children. Pneumothorax does however occur in status asthmaticus and cystic fibrosis, secondary to congenital lung cysts, lung trauma, or in staphylococcal pneumonia, and in a variety of neonatal lung conditions (p. 278).

RECOGNITION

A pneumothorax in an otherwise healthy child produces some breathlessness, often associated with pleuritic pain. A pneumothorax should always be suspected when there is deterioration in status asthmaticus or in a staphylococcal pneumonia. The diagnosis should be suspected if air entry is asymmetrical and there is clinical evidence of mediastinal shift. A chest x-ray will confirm the diagnosis.

MANAGEMENT

Specific treatment is rarely required except for a child who already has a respiratory problem or when a tension pneumothorax occurs. In an emergency a wide-bore needle can be inserted into the third intercostal space in the mid-axillary line. If pus is present the needle should be replaced by a wide-bore catheter. The needle or catheter is connected to an underwater seal or flap valve to prevent a further build-up of the pneumothorax.

Respiratory burns
(*See* page 41).

Acute bronchiolitis

Acute bronchiolitis is a common respiratory emergency in infancy and early childhood. It occurs predominantly in children between the ages of 3 months and 18 months. It is also one of the more frustrating respiratory disorders as so few therapeutic manoeuvres have any effect. This condition is always viral in origin, often the respiratory syncytial virus, although it can also be caused by the influenza, parainfluenza and adenoviruses. The main disturbance is that of acute severe airway obstruction at bronchiolar level due to mucosal oedema, thick secretions and desquamated epithelial cells.

RECOGNITION

There is often a history of nasal discharge, cough and poor feeding for 1 to 3 days before the onset of severe symptoms. The baby has tachypnoea (often over 100 per minute), wheezing and coughing. The chest is clinically and radiologically hyperinflated. As the disease progresses the wheezing becomes less marked, secondary to a fall in alveolar ventilation. Sometimes only râles can be heard throughout the lung fields. Despite the severity of the respiratory problem the babies are often afebrile. The liver is displaced downwards by the hyperinflated lungs and is often easily palpable. This is accompanied by distension of the neck veins giving the appearance of heart failure, but this is rare in acute bronchiolitis. Peripheral hypoperfusion and hypoxia produce a metabolic acidosis. Apnoeic episodes also occur which, if not treated promptly, may progress to cardiorespiratory arrest.

MANAGEMENT

(a) Oxygen therapy

The cyanosis can usually be relieved by oxygen, using either an oxygen tent or a Derbyshire chair.* The inspired oxygen concentration should be monitored but concentrations of up to 60 per cent can be given for short periods without any danger.

(b) Feeding

If there is severe respiratory distress a nasogastric tube should be passed and left *in situ*.

(c) Antibiotics

As this is a viral infection, antibiotics are not indicated. In the acute stage, however, it is often difficult to be sure that the baby does not have a bacterial bronchopneumonia, particularly when seen in the middle of the night. If bronchopneumonia cannot be excluded it is reasonable to give parenteral antibiotics, e.g. cloxacillin and ampicillin or cloxacillin and gentamicin.

(d) Steroids

Treatment with steroids has been used widely but has been shown (Connolly *et al.*, 1969) to be of no value. Nevertheless steroids should be used if there is a possibility of asthma (*see below*).

* Obtainable from Portex Ltd.

(e) Bronchodilator drugs

Clinical trials have shown that bronchodilator drugs are ineffective in the first year of life in this condition. In the older child their place has not been evaluated and it is reasonable to try oral or intravenous salbutamol or intravenous aminophylline *as it is often difficult to distinguish between a severe asthmatic attack and acute bronchiolitis in a young child.*

(f) Cardiac failure

For the reasons already stated heart failure is over-diagnosed in this condition. It does, however, occasionally occur and an increase in cardiac size on serial x-rays is an indication to give digoxin.

(g) Respiratory support

Continuous distending pressure has been suggested for this condition but trials have been conflicting and this form of treatment should probably not be used until further information is available. Intermittent positive-pressure ventilation is hazardous and difficult in affected children and should not be undertaken lightly. Serial blood gas measurements can give useful information on progress but the decision to ventilate should be made on clinical grounds, as many of these babies can tolerate arterial carbon dioxide levels of 8 to 9 kPa (60 to 70 mm Hg) for days or even weeks and then recover without supportive ventilation. The main indication for intermittent positive-pressure ventilation should be a deterioration in the child's level of consciousness, or apnoea not responding to stimulation. The pressures required are likely to be high and often prolonged periods of ventilation are required.

Most babies recover after 7 to 10 days. Occasionally, those with severe bronchiolitis have respiratory symptoms for weeks or even months and are dependent on oxygen for prolonged periods. Even in these babies, steroids are unhelpful and the majority will improve spontaneously.

Acute laryngotracheobronchitis, epiglottitis and 'croup'
(*See* page 217)

Whooping cough in infants and young children

Whooping cough is a dangerous and potentially fatal disease. In industrialized societies the main risk is to infants in the first year of life or before immunization has been completed. In countries in which malnutrition or undernutrition is common there is a particularly high mortality, it being second only to measles in some areas (Morley, 1970). It should be remembered that there is no transplacental immunity to whooping cough from the mother to the newborn infant and therefore an infant can be at risk from birth. Exposure may occur from infected sibs or less commonly from adults including the child's own mother.

RECOGNITION

Infants rarely whoop; common symptoms are:

(a) Paroxysms of coughing with facial congestion, followed by vomiting. These are more frequent at night but the difference between night and day is less marked than in the older child. Paroxysms may be provoked by crying, feeding, change of temperature or any disturbance such as examination of the throat with a spatula.

(b) In severe cases respiratory arrest may follow a paroxysm of coughing, necessitating immediate intubation.

(c) Choking or apnoeic spells may occur without spasms of coughing. Characteristically the lungs are clinically and radiologically clear unless there is a complicating pneumonia or collapse. Periorbital oedema is common in malnourished children. In a proportion of cases there is leucocytosis of between 15 000 and 45 000 with 60 per cent or more lymphocytes; a pernasal swab should be used for bacteriological examination. Symptoms indistinguishable from *B. pertussis* infections may be produced by infection with *B. parapertussis*, *B. bronchoseptica* or the adenoviruses.

MANAGEMENT

Antibiotic therapy has disappointingly little effect on the clinical course of whooping cough unless given in the very early stages. The more important aspect of management is the control of the paroxysms.

(a) Antibiotics

The majority of strains of *B. pertussis* are sensitive to ampicillin and amoxycillin but strains resistant to these drugs are becoming more common; if resistance is thought to be likely (local information) erythromycin should be used. If vomiting is not a major problem amoxycillin can be given orally or parenterally. The use of chloramphenicol does not appear to be justified.

(b) Management of paroxysms

Severe coughing paroxysms can be very frightening and rapidly produce severe anoxia. They are associated with the production of excessive secretions which should be sucked out gently. This is important as the aggressive use of suction catheters will induce further paroxysms. Oxygen given during the paroxysm allows the hypoxia to be relieved more rapidly and may prevent some attacks proceeding to total respiratory arrest.

Facilities for immediate intubation must be available for the severely affected child. Spontaneous respiration usually returns rapidly after intubation so that the child can be extubated within a few minutes.

(c) Prevention of paroxysms

It has been claimed that phenobarbitone (2 mg per kg at night and 1 mg per kg in the morning) or diazepam (1 mg three times daily increasing to 2 mg four times daily for children under 2 years) will reduce the frequency of paroxysms, although there is little objective evidence in favour of either. They are worth trying in a severely affected infant.

Neonatal respiratory emergencies

The maturity and reserve of the respiratory system determine whether a small pre-term baby will survive. The chances of the baby surviving neurologically intact have been greatly improved in the last few years by intensive monitoring and new therapeutic techniques. As these techniques are not without hazards, early and accurate diagnosis has become of great importance in the management. The neonatal respiratory system can respond to pathological disturbances only in a limited number of ways:

(a) tachypnoea (respiratory rate of >60),
(b) sternal and intercostal recession,
(c) expiratory grunting,
(d) cyanosis
(e) apnoea.

If these features are observed in the first 6 hours of life a diagnosis of the idiopathic respiratory distress syndrome (IRDS) is usually made, but many other respiratory, cardiac, neurological and even metabolic conditions may produce an identical picture.

DIFFERENTIAL DIAGNOSIS OF RESPIRATORY DISTRESS SHORTLY AFTER BIRTH

(a) Idiopathic respiratory distress syndrome (IRDS)

The symptoms are always present within the first 6 hours of life and are often detectable from birth. The child tends to get progressively worse for 24 to 48 hours. Chest x-ray shows poorly expanded lungs either with a complete 'white out', ground glass or fine granular appearance with an 'air bronchogram'. The x-ray changes are sometimes asymmetrical.

(b) Pneumothorax

This may mimic IRDS closely but should be suspected if the breath sounds are conducted asymmetrically. A chest x-ray will establish the diagnosis. Pneumothorax may occur after resuscitation, as a complication of IRDS, with meconium aspiration, or in the hypoplastic lung after operation for diaphragmatic hernia. Recently a fibre-optic system has been used to identify large pneumothoraces. The affected side can be transilluminated if a sufficiently bright light source is available (Kuhns *et al.*, 1975).

(c) Pneumomediastinum

This condition is also differentiated from IRDS by chest x-ray.

(d) Meconium aspiration (*see also* page 275)

Meconium aspiration can produce signs which are identical to IRDS but there will have been a history of meconium-staining of the liquor. Chest x-ray shows areas of patchy atelectasis but unlike IRDS the lungs are hyperinflated due to airway obstruction.

(e) Transient tachypnoea

Many babies, particularly those born prematurely, have tachypnoea, sternal recession and sometimes grunting for some hours after birth. In the early stages the symptoms may be indistinguishable from those of IRDS and chest x-ray often shows poorly expanded lungs or central streaking. The main differentiating factor is that the symptoms settle after 6 to 12 hours. Other babies have tachypnoea persisting for several days (transient tachypnoea of the newborn). This is often seen in full-term babies, particularly those born by caesarian section, and is thought to be due to delayed re-absorption of lung fluid.

(f) Cardiac causes of respiratory distress

Cyanotic congenital heart disease, e.g. transposition of the great vessels, is relatively easy to differentiate from IRDS as the air entry is good, the lungs well expanded on chest x-ray, and sometimes a murmur is audible. If cardiac failure is present, either complicating cyanotic congenital heart disease or due to the left-heart syndrome or other obstructive lesions, differentiation can be much more difficult. A rise in PaO_2 of more than 4 kPa (30 mm Hg) when the baby is given a high inspired-oxygen concentration makes cyanotic congenital heart disease extremely unlikely. Similarly, a good response to continuous positive airways pressure (*see below*) is helpful in differentiating the babies with cyanotic congenital heart disease but, of course, an improvement may well be seen if pulmonary oedema is present. An ECG can also be helpful in the differentiation. (*See* Cardiac Emergencies p. 298.)

(g) Shunting

Occasionally the high pulmonary-vascular resistance present during fetal life persists for several days after birth so that the blood continues to shunt from right to left at duct and atrial level. This produces a cyanosis which may be accompanied by tachypnoea but often no other cardiac or respiratory signs. This condition is sometimes fatal. A period of hyperventilation or tolazoline IV (1–2 mg) may reverse this situation.

(h) Neurological causes

 (i) Severe asphyxia and brain trauma may produce a picture very similar to IRDS. These babies always show other neurological disturbances, usually hypotonia and unresponsiveness, and usually become pink if the inspired oxygen is raised.

 (ii) Abnormal breathing patterns are also seen in phrenic nerve palsy. This usually accompanies other brachial plexus injuries (Erb's palsy) but may occur on its own. Elevation of the affected hemidiaphragm will be apparent on the chest x-ray with paradoxical movement.

(i) Surgical conditions

Babies with diaphragmatic herniae often have respiratory symptoms from birth with further deterioration occurring after the first feed. As these are almost always on the left they should be suspected when the heart is clinically shifted to the right (apparent dextrocardia) and when the breath sounds are diminished over the left chest. Tracheo-oesophageal fistulae are unlikely to be confused with IRDS since respiratory symptoms do not arise until after the first feed.

Idiopathic respiratory distress syndrome

The underlying problem in IRDS appears to be a lack of adequate surfactant, preventing satisfactory lung expansion and greatly increasing the respiratory work load. Cyanosis occurs early, due to ventilation mismatch and intrapulmonary shunting. Poor oxygenation and acidosis lead to maintenance of the high pulmonary-vascular resistance present throughout fetal life and a return to right-to-left shunting at duct and probably also at atrial level. As the disease progresses, hypoventilation occurs with hypercapnia, metabolic and respiratory acidosis and, finally, peripheral vascular collapse. The condition is to some extent self-limiting as surfactant production is achieved a few days after birth so that even in severely affected babies, an improvement can be expected at this time.

RECOGNITION

A diagnosis of IRDS is made if two of the following are present within the first 6 hours of life: tachypnoea (respiratory rate >60), sternal and intercostal recession, expiratory grunting—provided the conditions discussed previously have been excluded. The x-ray appearances have already been described; in very severe cases there may be virtually no air remaining in the lungs so that there is no contrast between the heart and the lung shadows.

MANAGEMENT

In severe respiratory distress the physiological reserves of the infant are stretched to their limits so that it is essential to provide the optimal environmental conditions to reduce metabolic demands to a minimum.

(a) Thermal environment

The environmental temperature range over which oxygen requirements of a naked baby in an incubator are at a minimum are narrow and depend on the baby's size and postnatal age. A useful guide to select the appropriate incubator temperature has been provided by Hey (1971). Alternatively, if facilities are available the incubator temperature can be servo-controlled from a skin probe. The temperature usually selected is 36.5°C (98°F) for skin temperature. Despite high environmental temperatures some babies have great difficulty maintaining a normal core temperature; even when the environmental temperature is high the baby may be losing a considerable amount of radiant heat. This heat loss can be reduced by placing a radiant heat shield within the incubator or by covering the baby with a cot blanket.

(b) Feeding

Babies with mild respiratory distress will almost always require naso-gastric tube feeding. If tolerated, feeds can be given appropriate to size and age. If continuous positive airways pressure (CPAP) or intermittent positive-pressure ventilation (IPPV) are required, the baby will almost certainly be too ill to tolerate oral gastric feeds and will then require IV fluids given in two-thirds of the normal oral feed volumes. For the first 24 hours, 5 per cent or 10 per cent glucose can be given but this should be replaced by 0.18 per cent NaCl in 4 per cent glucose at the age of 24 hours, with potassium supplements added after 48 hours.

(c) Oxygen therapy

If the baby has only a tinge of cyanosis then it is usually sufficient to bleed oxygen into the incubator, measuring the inspired oxygen concentration with an oxygen analyser but not repeatedly measuring the blood gases. If more than 30 per cent of oxygen is required a perspex head box (Gairdner Head Box) should be used as this enables nursing care of the infant to be done without disturbing the ambient oxygen concentration. At this level of inspired oxygen it is also essential to measure the blood gases repeatedly to avoid retrolental fibroplasia and unrecognized hypoxia, and to check on the acid-base status. Currently blood-gas analysers require less than 0.3 ml of blood which can be obtained by repeated radial-artery stabs, a technique that requires considerable practice. Alternatively, an umbilical-artery catheter can be inserted with the tip below the origin of the renal arteries (L3,4). Previously it has been standard practice to pass an umbilical-vein catheter at the same time as a route for intravenous fluids. Most centres now use a single catheter in an umbilical artery for both sampling and for fluid requirements.

The aim of oxygen therapy is to maintain the aortic arterial PaO_2 between 6.6 and 12.0 kPa (50 and 90 mm Hg). The upper limit is kept relatively low to allow for right-to-left shunting at duct level as the arterial-oxygen tension in the carotid artery may be 8 to 9 kPa (60 to 70 mm Hg) higher than in the lower part of the aorta. Although radial-artery blood samples do not suffer from this disadvantage, experience with continuous-reading oxygen electrodes has shown that the PaO_2 tends to fall during sampling. Disposable catheters tipped with continuously-recording oxygen sensors are now available commercially. These can be passed up an umbilical artery so that the tip lies within the artery. Their advantage is that the PaO_2 fluctuates considerably minute-by-minute so that even 4-hourly blood-gas estimations may give misleading information. The transcutaneous oxygen electrode is probably unreliable when peripheral perfusion is poor.

(d) Continuous distending pressure

Continuous distending pressure (CDP), whether applied as a positive pressure to the child's upper airway (CPAP), or as a negative pressure applied to the outside of the chest (continuous negative external pressure—CNEP) has generally been accepted as a valuable technique in the management of IRDS. Recent trials suggest that CDP is less effective at reducing the mortality than was initially claimed, particularly in babies weighing less than 1.5 kg (Krouskop, Brown and Sweet, 1975). Nevertheless all agree that in the majority of babies the application of CDP causes a dramatic rise in arterial oxygen, allowing the inspired oxygen concentration to be reduced, and also shortening the course of the disease. The means by which this improvement in oxygenation occurs is not fully understood but probably results from a reduction in the ventilation-perfusion imbalance within the lung.

METHODS FOR CONTINUOUS DISTENDING PRESSURE

(*a*) *The Gregory Box* (Gregory, Kitterman and Phibbs, 1971)

This system consists of a head box with a neck seal achieved either by a soft PVC sleeve attached round the baby's neck by a velcro belt or by a semi-rigid diaphragm and a loose towel of PVC which is wrapped around the baby's neck and acts as a washer. The disadvantages of this system are:

(i) The baby has to be subjected to much handling to obtain an adequate neck seal, and often deteriorates during the procedure.
(ii) A good neck seal is often difficult to achieve without using excessively high pressures and running the risk of hydrocephalus and intracranial haemorrhage. This is usually overcome by increasing the flow of gas and air to the Gregory Box. Sometimes flows as high as 20 to 30 litres per minute are required which have a cooling effect on the baby.

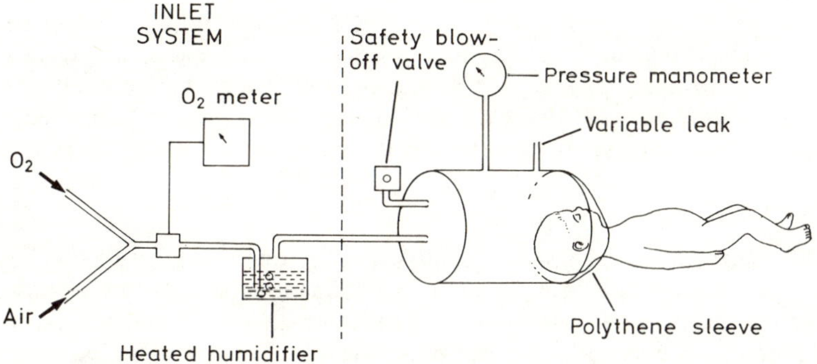

Figure 25.4. Continuous Distending Pressure: Gregory Box. The inlet systems shown are common to apparatus shown in Figures 25.5 and 25.6

   (iii) There is poor access to the head in an emergency.
   (iv) The neck seal may cause skin lesions.
    (v) When the gas flow is high, noise levels of above 80 decibels have
        been recorded, which may well be damaging to the ear.
Polythene bags have been used as a substitute for the Gregory Box and
there is a disposable system costing only a few pounds available on the
market.

(b) Face mask

A soft face mask (e.g. The Bennett mask) can be used to apply the
CPAP. Compliance should be added to the system by inserting an

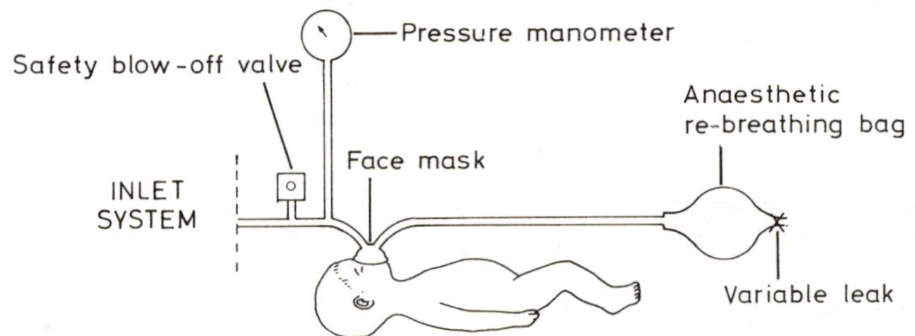

Figure 25.5. Continuous Distending Pressure: Face Mask

anaesthetic re-breathing bag. This will reduce the pressure swings
produced by the baby's tidal breaths. Pressure can be selected by
controlling the leak from the system or by altering the flow. Pressure in
the system can be monitored either with an aneroid device or by a water
column in a thoracotomy bottle. Care must be taken to avoid local
pressure to the occipital region as this has been shown to produce
cerebellar damage. This can be avoided by using either a Netelast
stocking covering the face and face mask or by using a helmet. The face
mask system tends to disfigure the baby temporarily but has proved a
simple system to set up and run in the neonatal nursery.

(c) Nasal cannulae

Soft nasal cannulae are now available commercially mounted either on
a wide bore tube (Portex) or on a small silastic block (Argyle). These
can be set up with minimal disturbance to the child, but are more
difficult to secure than the face mask system. This problem has been
overcome in some units by connecting the ends of the Portex device to
semi-rigid tubes using 90° elbow connectors and strapping these tubes

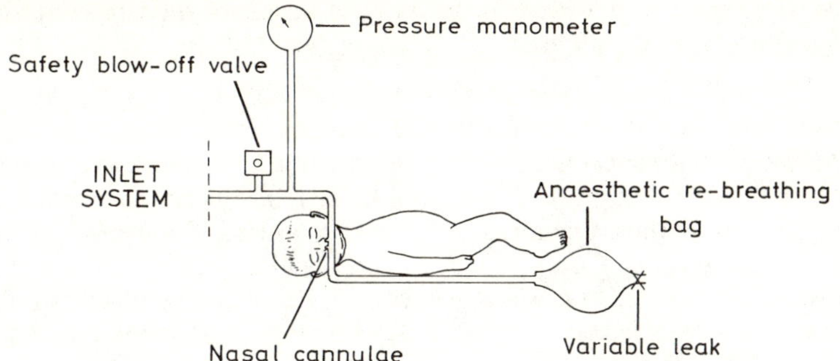

Figure 25.6. Continuous Distending Pressure: Nasal Cannulae

to the sides of the baby's head. The Argyle unit is supplied with angled flanges which allow it to be strapped to the infant's head. It was initially claimed that nasally applied CPAP was less likely to lead to pneumothorax, but recent experience has cast doubt on this. Both units tend to cause ulceration of the nares and have produced areas of necrosis of the septal wall.

Although easier to secure, the Argyle device has a significant dead space which may add to the baby's problems.

These systems also require a compliant reservoir in the system to avoid large pressure swings.

(d) Endotracheal tube

This has been used widely but necessitates intubation. There is little trouble with gastric distension and it is more often possible to continue nasogastric feeding.

(e) Continuous negative external pressure

A commercially available negative chamber is available. This is relatively easy to set up as the neck seal is less difficult than the Gregory

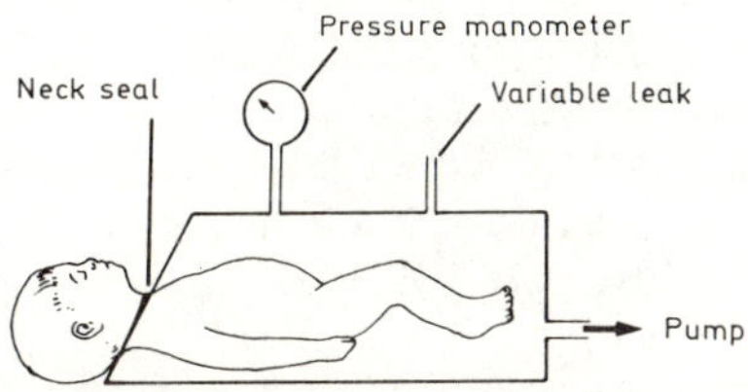

Figure 25.7. Continuous Negative External Pressure Chamber

Box. The main disadvantages are those of access to the baby and the high price of the apparatus.

INDICATION FOR CONTINUOUS DISTENDING PRESSURE

The indications for CDP vary from unit to unit. Most users would now accept that CDP should be started if more than 60 per cent ambient oxygen is required to maintain a PaO_2 of 6.6 kPa (50 mm Hg). Some advocate that CDP should be started early, within the first 2 to 3 hours of birth, but a large number of babies with transient symptoms would have to be subjected to CDP. The distending pressure should be kept below 10 cm H_2O.

INTERMITTENT POSITIVE-PRESSURE VENTILATION (IPPV)

IPPV is indicated if there is deterioration despite attempts to control the acidosis with bicarbonate, and hypoxia with high inspired oxygen concentration and CDP. Most centres would now start IPPV only if the PaO_2 is less than 4.7 kPa (35 mm Hg) with an inspired oxygen concentration of at least 70 per cent with the patient on CDP. A further indication is apnoea not responding to intubation and manual IPPV. Details of ventilation therapy are given elsewhere, but good results in ventilation with IRDS have been obtained by using a high inspiratory:expiratory ratio (2:1 to 3:1) with inflation pressures of 20 to 30 cm of water and a respiration rate of 30 to 50 per minute. Additional improvement is sometimes obtained by adding a positive-end-expiratory-pressure.

The aim should always be to reduce the inflation pressure to below 20 cm water and the inspired oxygen concentration to below 70 per cent as soon as possible, to reduce the risk of further lung damage from exposure to high oxygen concentration and high pressures.

ACID-BASE BALANCE

In addition to the cardiorespiratory effects already mentioned, a severe metabolic acidosis depresses myocardial function. A metabolic acidosis should be treated with intravenous sodium bicarbonate. Ideally this should be given according to the base deficit calculated from nomograms using the arterial H^+ concentration (pH) and $PaCO_2$. The aim should be to make a two-thirds correction assuming that the metabolic acidosis is limited to the extracellular compartment. Alternatively, bicarbonate can be given by rule of thumb on the pH alone.

    55–65 nmol per litre (pH 7.20–7.25): give 1 mmol sodium bicarbonate per kg

    65–70 nmol per litre (pH 7.15–7.20): give 2 mmol per kg

    70–80 nmol per litre (pH 7.10–7.15): give 3 mmol per kg

80–90 nmol per litre (pH 7.05–7.10): give 4 mmol per kg
>90 nmol per litre (pH <7.02): give 5 mmol per kg
These figures do not make any allowance for respiratory acidosis.

Although the sodium bicarbonate often produces a dramatic improvement, the injections should be given over at least 10 minutes and preferably over a 30-minute period as very large changes in osmolality, haemoglobin concentration and circulating blood volume occur during and immediately after the injections which may cause an intraventricular haemorrhage.

DETERIORATION WITH IRDS

(a) *Natural course*

In severe IRDS the baby tends to deteriorate progressively for 24 to 48 hours.

(b) *Pneumothorax*

Pneumothorax is common in IRDS, particularly during CDP (most series have reported rates as high as 25 per cent). A pneumothorax should be suspected if there is a shift in the apex beat and if breath sounds are asymmetrically conducted. A chest x-ray will confirm the diagnosis. If the condition is satisfactory, close observation only is required. With increasing cyanosis peripheral perfusion deteriorates. It may be possible to reverse the situation by aspirating air with a 20-ml syringe and a No. 1 needle. If this is insufficient and there is further deterioration an intercostal drain will be required. A Medicut or similar catheter is inserted through the lateral chest wall and connected to a flutter valve or an underwater seal. Occasionally, particularly when the pneumothorax occurs during CDP, low-pressure suction (10–15 cm water) may be necessary.

(c) *Infection*

Crepitations in the lungs after the first 24 hours of age suggest an infection. A full infection screen should be done and antibiotics should be started.

(d) *Intraventricular haemorrhage*

This now accounts for approximately 70 per cent of the deaths with IRDS. The infant is often unresponsive and hypotonic. Blood pressure falls and the baby has difficulty maintaining a normal core temperature even in an adequately warm environment. Often, fresh blood will be found in the CSF. There is no treatment for this condition but small haemorrhages are compatible with survival.

(e) Severe hypotension

This is sometimes associated with failure of peripheral perfusion. It is probably the result of hypovolaemia, and is most easily detected by repeated measurement of the blood pressure using either a cuff sphygmomanometer and Doppler system or by measuring the blood pressure by a pressure transducer connected to an umbilical-artery catheter.

If the blood pressure is falling and the condition is deteriorating improvement can be obtained by giving the baby small volumes (10–20 ml per kg) of fresh blood or fresh frozen plasma.

Massive pulmonary haemorrhage

This condition is poorly understood. The affected babies have signs of respiratory distress associated with what appears to be fresh or altered blood welling up the trachea. It occurs most frequently in pre-term babies, sometimes as a complication of the respiratory distress syndrome, but is also seen in infants born to diabetic mothers or infants with severe Rhesus haemolytic disease. Chest x-ray shows diffuse reticulation, nodular opacities or opacification of the whole lung field (Avery, 1968).

Occasionally there is evidence of a bleeding abnormality elsewhere. Examination of the fluid has revealed that this is a bloody transudate rather than undiluted blood.

MANAGEMENT

This is generally regarded as a terminal event but recent reports suggest that active intervention with intubation and IPPV will salvage up to 50 per cent of the infants.

Apnoeic attacks

Apnoeic attacks are a frequent cause for concern in the immediate neonatal period and repeated or long apnoeic attacks may cause brain damage.

RECOGNITION

(a) In pre-term babies

Pre-term babies are prone to recurrent apnoeic episodes which appear to be due to a failure or immaturity of the respiratory centre. The attacks usually occur within the first 48 hours of life and usually cease after a few days, but may persist for several weeks. They are at least partially dependent on the ambient temperature and arterial-oxygen concentration. Between the episodes the babies appear to be entirely healthy.

It is essential to identify those babies who are having apnoeic attacks secondary to other disorders if this latter group are to survive.

(b) Infection

Any systemic infection can precipitate apnoea, e.g. urinary-tract infection, pneumonia, septicaemia and meningitis. A full infection screen should be carried out and if there is any doubt antibiotic therapy should be started immediately.

(c) IRDS

Babies with IRDS or other pulmonary problems are likely to have apnoeic attacks, possibly due to the associated hypoxia. Regurgitation of milk into the upper airways is another possible cause and milk is often found on nasopharyngeal suction during apnoeic episodes.

(d) Hypoglycaemia

Hypoglycaemia may present as recurrent apnoea and all babies having apnoeic episodes must have at least a Dextrostix estimation carried out. If a low reading is obtained the blood glucose should be measured and intravenous glucose given (*see* page 449).

(e) Intracranial lesions

Any intracranial lesion, asphyxial, traumatic or haemorrhagic can precipitate apnoeic attacks. Usually, the baby's neurological condition will be grossly abnormal between episodes, with hypotonia or hypertonia, abnormal movements or frank convulsions. It is important to bear in mind the possibility of subdural haemorrhage with expanding head circumference as this is a potentially treatable lesion.

Usually it is not difficult to distinguish the idiopathic from the symptomatic group by the condition of the baby between apnoeic episodes but it is far better to investigate a few pre-term babies unnecessarily than to miss a treatable and potentially fatal underlying condition.

MANAGEMENT

It is essential to monitor the respiration of all pre-term babies and those with a birth weight of less than 2 kg. Several systems are available, e.g. apnoea mattresses, impedance and Doppler systems and mattress transducers. These should be set to give an audible alarm after 15 seconds of apnoea. The sensitivity of the system should be kept down,

K

as it is possible to trigger some of them, particularly the apnoea mattress, with a heartbeat alone.

(a) The apnoeic episode

Many apnoeic episodes end spontaneously with the baby crying. The majority respond to simple superficial stimulation, e.g. flicking the feet, blowing cold air or oxygen over the baby's face. If these fail, mouth suction is often successful, sometimes revealing the presence of regurgitated milk. If this fails, intubation and manual IPPV are necessary. This is almost always followed by a rapid improvement so that the endotracheal tube can be removed within a few minutes. It is bad practice to leave an endotracheal tube in place to avoid the need for repeated intubation, particularly if there is an associated respiratory problem. The tube by-passes the upper airways and the inspired gases will be inadequately humidified; it also prevents the expiratory grunt and so leads to a fall in the arterial-oxygen tension. If the baby fails to improve on manual ventilation, IPPV will be required, often for the next 1 to 2 days. Ventilation is a relatively easy procedure in the majority of these babies as their lungs are normal so that low inflation pressures (15–20 cm water) can be used with a rate of around 30 per minute and an inspiratory:expiratory ratio of 1:2.

(b) Prevention

Several lines of treatment are now available.

(i) *Reduction of environmental temperature*   Reducing the incubator temperature by 1°C (2°F) sometimes reduces the number of attacks. This must obviously only be done when the baby is normothermic.

(ii) *Increasing the inspired oxygen concentration*   Increasing the ambient oxygen to 25 to 30 per cent is also effective in some pre-term infants. This is potentially dangerous as the babies are often very immature and may have normal gas transfer between attacks. *Under these circumstances there is a considerable risk of retrolental fibroplasia if the inspired oxygen is allowed to rise above 30 per cent.* For this reason the inspired oxygen must be monitored continuously.

(iii) *Continuous positive airway pressure*   CPAP reduces the incidence of apnoeic episodes by about 50 per cent and can be very effective. It is important to limit the inspired oxygen to less than 25 per cent unless the baby has associated lung problems and to keep the inflation pressures down to a maximum of 5 cm of water.

(*iv*) *Theophylline*   Rectal aminophylline suppositories have been used, but with uncertain results. Absorption is unreliable and the suppository is often passed unabsorbed. An alternative is to give oral theophylline (3 mg per kg, 6-hourly orally). This has proved to be most successful in the idiopathic group.

(*v*) *Total intravenous alimentation*   There is now evidence that the apnoeic episodes can be stopped by substituting total intravenous feeding for oral feeding and some centres now recommend that if the apnoea is not responding to simple measures oral feeds should be stopped and total intravenous alimentation maintained for at least a week. This is a difficult technique and should only be used in intensive care units experienced in this method.

(*vi*) *Nasojejunal feeding*   When gastric distension causes apnoeic attacks the stomach can be by-passed by feeding direct into the jejunum. Feeds should be isotonic: the modified cow's milk formulae are satisfactory for this purpose.

Meconium aspiration

Meconium-staining of the liquor occurs in approximately 8 per cent of all labours; experience in the United States suggests that about 50 per cent of those with meconium-staining of the skin also have meconium within the trachea (Gregory *et al.*, 1974). In Britain symptoms from meconium aspiration are less common and less than 10 per cent of those with meconium-staining of the liquor have any respiratory distress. Clinical evidence of fetal asphyxia is only found in about 15 per cent of babies with meconium aspiration and it is probable that meconium aspiration is confined to infants who have gasped *in utero* from severe hypoxia.

RECOGNITION

Symptomatically, meconium aspiration closely resembles IRDS as the affected babies have a high respiration rate, recession, grunting, and in severe cases, cyanosis. However, in contrast to IRDS meconium aspiration is rare in pre-term infants. The mechanical problem, however, is very different. There is acute airway obstruction with hyper-inflation of the lungs, often apparent clinically. The x-ray appearance has already been described (p. 263). The gross hyperinflation presents a mechanical problem identical to that of bronchiolitis in the older infant and may be complicated by a pneumothorax.

MANAGEMENT

All babies with marked meconium-staining of the skin, nails and cord should have a laryngoscopy and aspiration of any meconium in the trachea. A wide-bore tube will be needed for this as the meconium tends to be thick and viscous. If meconium aspiration has occurred the baby should be closely observed for the next 3 days as the respiratory signs do not always appear immediately after birth. Cyanosis is usually easily relieved by oxygen but regular blood gas analysis will be required if the inspired oxygen is above 30 per cent. Continuous distending pressure is unlikely to be helpful in this condition; IPPV is occasionally needed, but should only be resorted to reluctantly as high pressures will be required. Prophylactic antibiotics should be given to all these infants as animal experiments have shown that there is an increased incidence of pneumonia after meconium aspiration.

Milk aspiration

The incidence of milk aspiration in the immediate neonatal period is not known, but small aspirations are probably common. Regurgitation of stomach contents into the pre-term infant's mouth is a common finding. Massive aspiration causes respiratory distress, cyanosis or apnoea, with patchy consolidation in the chest x-ray.

MANAGEMENT

If aspiration is suspected the mouth and pharynx should be immediately aspirated using a disposable mouth sucker or low-pressure suction unit (maximum pressure 50 mm Hg). The trachea should be sucked out under direct vision. Antibiotic therapy should be started.

Pneumonia

This is usually associated with septicaemia but may be secondary to aspiration. There is a rising respiratory rate with recession and sometimes cyanosis. In Britain the organisms most commonly implicated are the Gram-negative bacilli, particularly *E. coli*, and the coagulase-positive staphylococci in North America. There have been several outbreaks of streptococcal infections, usually belonging to Lancefield Group B, but also to Group A. These may present as a septicaemia but sometimes produce pneumonia, often accompanied by pleural effusion and empyema. Localizing signs are rarely present, with the exception of crepitations. Diagnosis is confirmed by chest x-ray. Attempts should be made to identify the organism by culture of nose and throat swabs and blood.

MANAGEMENT

The choice of antibiotics for immediate therapy should be based on the sensitivities of the local organisms. An effective antistaphylococcal agent, e.g. cloxacillin, should be combined with a wide-spectrum antibiotic to which the Gram-negative bacilli are rarely resistant, e.g. gentamicin or the recently introduced aminoglycoside, amikacin sulphate. Ampicillin is less effective as there are now many resistant strains of *E. coli.* Cloxacillin should initially be given intravenously to achieve high levels particularly if peripheral perfusion is poor. A 7-day course is usually adequate. For confirmed or suspected group B streptococcal pneumonia large i.m. doses of benzylpenicillin should be used (250 000 units/kg/24 hours; *see also* page 635).

Diaphragmatic hernia

This is due to a failure of closure of the pleuroperitoneal canal. It is almost always left-sided, occurring in about 1 in 2000 deliveries.

RECOGNITION

The presenting symptoms are always respiratory, partly because of the presence of bowel within the chest, preventing lung expansion, but also because there is often associated hypoplasia of one or both lungs. Some infants have respiratory distress from birth while others only develop symptoms when feeding is started.

The diagnosis should be suspected when the apex beat is found to be displaced to the right and there is poor air entry to the left lung. Occasionally bowel sounds may be heard in the left chest. The diagnosis is confirmed on chest x-ray by bowel shadows in the left side of the chest. *If the x-ray is taken immediately after birth the left hemithorax will appear opaque as there will be no air present in the bowel.*

MANAGEMENT

Immediate surgery is required to ensure survival.

If cases require transfer to other units they must be accompanied by someone skilled in intubation and IPPV. If there is any doubt about the baby's respiratory reserve, intubation should be done before transfer. The response to surgery depends to a large extent on the degree of lung hypoplasia and many require supportive ventilation postoperatively.

POSITIVE PRESSURE WITH A FACE MASK MUST NEVER BE USED IN DIAPHRAGMATIC HERNIA.

Tracheo-oesophageal fistula with oesophageal atresia

RECOGNITION
This should be suspected whenever polyhydramnios is present, and a fairly stiff catheter should be passed down the oesophagus to see if an atresia is present. If there is any doubt, the catheter should be left in place and a chest x-ray taken to identify the site of obstruction. No reliance can be placed on attempts to aspirate acid stomach contents. Excessive salivation is often present almost from birth. If the condition is not identified immediately at birth the baby will have a cyanotic attack associated with aspiration at the first feed. An exception is the rare H-type which is not associated with oesophageal atresia. Chest x-ray may show the bowel to be distended with air.

MANAGEMENT
Surgery is required before oral feeding can be started. During transport the infant should be kept in the head-down position and the saliva repeatedly aspirated. If possible, the fistula is closed and an end-to-end anastomosis carried out at the initial operation. If this is impossible the fistula is tied off and a gastrostomy performed to tide the baby over until the definitive repair can be carried out. If aspiration has occurred antibiotics will be indicated.

Phrenic-nerve paralysis

The phrenic nerves arise from the 3rd to 5th cervical nerve roots. One or other may be damaged or even avulsed during difficult deliveries.

RECOGNITION
In approximately half the cases the phrenic-nerve paralysis is accompanied by an Erb's palsy. The resulting paradoxical respiration is often apparent clinically but easier to see on screening. A plain film of the chest shows an elevated diaphragm on the affected side, occasionally with some collapse.

MANAGEMENT
Most babies tolerate this situation but those who have persistent respiratory symptoms should be considered for surgery. This consists of plicating the diaphragm to improve its efficiency.

Congenital lobar emphysema

This is a rare cause of respiratory distress in the neonatal period.

RECOGNITION

Symptoms may not occur for several days. Clinically, there is hyperinflation, usually associated with expiratory wheeze and attacks of cyanosis. Air entry is reduced on the affected side and hyperresonance and mediastinal shift can usually be detected. The diagnosis is made on chest x-ray which shows overdistension of the affected lobe.

Occasionally a simple mechanical cause can be found in the form of a mucus plug within a bronchus or an aberrant artery compressing the bronchial wall from outside. At other times the aetiology is obscure.

MANAGEMENT

If the respiratory symptoms are severe, bronchoscopy should be done without delay, followed by removal of the affected lobe if an obvious bronchial cause is not found.

When symptoms are mild or absent, bronchoscopy is still indicated; but because the hyperinflation tends to resolve spontaneously in some cases, surgical intervention can be delayed. It is, however, important that these babies are kept under close review as deterioration may occur later.

Congenital lung cysts

Congenital lung cysts rarely produce symptoms in the neonatal period. They may be single or multiple. If multiple, they tend to involve several segments of one lobe and rarely occur bilaterally. Occasionally the cysts expand rapidly in the neonatal period, producing dyspnoea, or rupture creating a pneumothorax. In the absence of a pneumothorax the unilocular or multilocular distended area is easily visible but the distinction from lobar emphysema may be difficult.

MANAGEMENT

Surgical treatment is only indicated if there is progressive respiratory distress secondary to air tension within the cyst. Repeated tapping with a syringe and needle has been advocated and can tide the infant over. If surgical intervention is required it is usually possible to limit the resection to a segment of a lobe.

Upper airway obstruction

(*See also under* Neonatal Emergencies and Nasopharyngeal Obstruction)

The Pierre Robin syndrome. In this condition the baby has great difficulty in establishing an airway. The lower jaw is poorly developed and there is often a large palatal defect so that the tongue tends to obstruct the nasopharynx.

MANAGEMENT
Many of the infants can be reared by careful positioning, usually face-down with the head in a cradle so that gravity tends to bring the tongue forward. Occasionally this is insufficient and the baby remains cyanosed and in distress whatever his position. Under these circumstances a stitch can be put into the tip of the tongue and slight traction exerted. The problem may persist for months but gradually improves as the lower jaw grows. Very occasionally a tracheostomy may be necessary.

   This is a simple mechanical problem which all too often results in death. These babies should be closely observed for months before discharge.

Choanal atresia

This is due to a partial or complete obstruction of the posterior nares; the obstruction may consist of bone or soft tissue. Severe symptoms only occur with bilateral atresia; unilaterial atresia causes a purulent nasal discharge. For recognition and management of choanal atresia and other causes of nasopharyngeal obstruction in the newborn (*see* page 650).

Laryngeal bands or stenosis

Inspiratory stridor is a surprisingly rare condition in the neonatal period considering how many babies are intubated. The commonest cause of stridor is a congenital floppy larynx which gradually improves over the next 12 months. A rare cause of inspiratory stridor is a congenital web in the larynx, usually just below the cords; but subglottic stenosis or subglottic haemangioma should also be considered. These may almost completely obstruct the airway producing severe stridor and respiratory distress; in some cases however stridor is absent. The diagnosis is made by direct laryngoscopy.

MANAGEMENT
It may be possible to dilate the airway with endotracheal tubes. This should be done by a highly skilled anaesthetist or operator, as such intervention may produce a rapid deterioration. If dilatation proves inadequate the band can be removed surgically but this is a major undertaking and has to be preceded by a tracheostomy. Fortunately, the majority improve spontaneously.

Laryngeal paralysis
(*See* page 648)

References

Avery, M. E. (1968). *The Lung and its Disorders in the Newborn Infant.* 2nd edn. p. 192. London: W. B. Saunders

Connolly, J. H., Fields, C. M. B., Glasgow, J. F. T., Slattery, C. M. and MacLynn, D. M. (1969). Double blind trial of prednisolone in epidemic bronchiolitis due to respiratory syncytial virus. *Acta Paediat. scand.* **58**, 116

Gregory, G. A., Kitterman, J. A., and Phibbs, R. H. (1971). The treatment of the idiopathic respiratory distress syndrome with continuous positive airway pressure. *New Engl. J. Med.* **284**, 1333

Gregory, G. A., Gooding, C. A., Phibbs, R. H. and Tooley, W. H. (1974). Meconium aspiration in infants—a prospective study. *J. Pediat.* **85**, 848

Hey, E. (1971). The care of babies in incubators. In *Recent Advances in Paediatrics.* 4th edn. Eds. D. Gairdner and D. Hull, p. 171. London: J. and A. Churchill

Jones, R. S., and Owen-Thomas, J. B. (1971). *Care of the Critically Ill Child.* p. 241. London: Edward Arnold

Krouskop, R. W., Brown, E. G., and Sweet, A. Y. (1975). The early use of continuous positive airway pressure in the treatment of idiopathic respiratory distress syndrome. *J. Pediat.* **87**, 262

Kuhns, L. R., Bednarek, F. J., Wyman, M. L., Roloff, D. W., and Borer, R. C. (1975). Diagnosis of pneumothorax or pneumomediastinum in the neonate by transillumination. *Pediatrics* **56**, 355

Morley, D. C. (1970). Whooping cough. In *Diseases of Children in the Subtropics and Tropics.* 2nd edn. p. 222. Ed. D. B. Jelliffe. London: Edward Arnold

FOR BACKGROUND READING

Williams, H. E., and Phelan, P. D. (1975). *Respiratory Illness in Children.* Oxford: Blackwell Scientific Publications

Part VII: Cardiac Emergencies

CHAPTER 26

Cardiac Emergencies

J. L. Wilkinson

Cardiac failure

Causes

The commoner conditions, which may lead to cardiac failure, vary at different ages. The following list contains some of the diseases or abnormalities which are likely to present with heart failure in each age group.

First 2 weeks:	Hypoplastic left-heart syndrome
	Coarctation
	Complex anomalies
2 to 4 weeks:	Coarctation
	Complex anomalies
	Ventricular-septal defect
4 to 12 weeks:	Ventricular-septal defect
	Patent ductus arteriosus
	Coarctation
3 to 12 months:	Onset of failure less common.
	May occur with many defects, often precipitated by superimposed chest infection. May be due to acquired heart disease (*see below*).
After 12 months:	Myocarditis (rheumatic or non-rheumatic). Acute rheumatism and new cases of rheumatic carditis are now relatively uncommon in Western countries.
	Bacterial endocarditis
	Rheumatic carditis
	Terminal feature of complex congenital heart lesions

RECOGNITION

The main symptoms in infants are respiratory, with dyspnoea on feeding or at rest, and tachycardia. Physical signs include tachycardia, tachypnoea, intercostal and subcostal recession, Harrison's sulci and hepatomegaly. Peripheral oedema is unusual in infancy (except terminally) and crepitations in the lung fields are a late manifestation or may be due to superimposed infection. In the first week of life cardiac failure may cause an early increase in weight, the expected initial drop failing to occur. This pattern should always raise suspicion of cardiac disease. Longstanding heart failure is frequently associated with failure to thrive and an abnormal tendency to chest infections. Acute distension of the liver, also due to cardiac failure, may mimic an acute abdominal emergency.

MANAGEMENT

(a) Digitalization

Various dosage regimens are used and there is poor agreement between different units. In general, infants tolerate higher doses weight-for-weight than older children and adults.

TABLE 26.I
Suggested doses

Weight	24-h digitalizing dose		24-h maintenance	
	Oral	i.m.	Oral	i.m.
0–5 kg	0.06mg/kg	0.05 mg/kg	0.015 mg/kg	0.01 mg/kg
5–10 kg	0.3 mg	0.2 mg	0.1 mg	0.06 mg
Above 10 kg	0.04 mg/kg	0.03 mg/kg	0.01 mg/kg	0.005 mg/kg

The digitalizing dose should be given in three equal parts at 8-hourly intervals. In sick infants rapid digitalization by the intramuscular route should be used. In less severe situations oral digitalization may be preferred unless the child is vomiting.

In small premature babies and in newborns, who often tolerate digoxin less well than more mature infants, the doses should be reduced to 2/3 of those recommended above.

Digitalis intoxication   Persistent bradycardia, A-V dissociation or ectopic beats, are indications to stop digoxin for 24 to 48 hours and, if possible, to obtain an estimation of digoxin level. Vomiting should be regarded with suspicion in a child on digoxin and if repeated, or unattributable to other causes, the dose of digoxin should be reduced or checked and a digoxin level performed if possible.

In any child, where digitalis toxicity is suspected, the serum potassium should be checked and, if low, oral potassium supplements should be given.

(b) Diuretics

In severe heart failure in infancy the first-choice diuretic should be frusemide, which may be given initially intramuscularly in a dose of 1 to 1.5 mg per kg (up to 6 mg). The child should have a urine bag on and may be weighed before, and 4 hours after, the dose. If an inadequate diuresis is obtained, further doses may be given, increasing the amount by 1 to 2 mg at each injection. Frusemide may be given intravenously but the initial dose should not exceed 1 mg per kg as a very rapid diuresis may occur. Maintenance oral diuretics should be started as soon as the infant's condition is improving.

In children over a year old initial intramuscular frusemide should be given in a dose of 5 to 10 mg. Even quite large children may have a good diuresis on doses of 5 or 6 mg, so it is safer to start with a relatively small dose and repeat with increasing amounts of drug at 4-hourly intervals if response is poor.

TABLE 26.II
Oral diuretic doses in infancy—to be given once or twice daily

	Initial dose
Chlorothiazide	25 mg/kg
Frusemide	2 mg/kg

Other measures

(*i*) *Oxygen*   Sick infants in heart failure should be nursed in an incubator or a tent in 30 per cent O_2.

(*ii*) *Humidification*   Adequate humidification prevents drying out of respiratory secretions and reduces insensible fluid loss. This is desirable for small infants in incubators and should also be used when a larger child is being nursed in a tent.

(*iii*) *Sedation*   Sedation is necessary if the child is distressed or agitated. Chloral hydrate or dichloralphenazone (Welldorm) may be adequate as an initial measure but if more regular sedation is required phenobarbitone or promethazine are preferable. For doses *see* pages 772, 774. The severely ill child may benefit from a single dose of morphine (*see* section on Pulmonary oedema).

(*iv*) *Position*   The infant is best nursed head-up. This may easily be achieved by tipping the incubator tray. Older infants may be nursed in a chair inside a tent. The infant's temperature should be maintained at or a little below normal, and the ambient temperature should be adjusted if the infant's temperature begins to rise.

(*v*) *Feeding*   Small, frequent feeds are better tolerated than large ones. A total fluid intake of 150 ml per kg should not be exceeded and a lower intake is desirable in the severely ill infant until failure is controlled. If the child is vomiting, diluted feeds or clear fluids may be better tolerated. Low-sodium milk is not necessary with current diuretics.

Pulmonary oedema

Frank pulmonary oedema is a relatively uncommon problem in paediatric practice. It may develop in infants and children with severe untreated heart failure due to many of the previously listed conditions. Characteristically it occurs with lesions associated with severe pulmonary-venous obstruction, such as the hypoplastic left-heart syndrome and some cases of total anomalous pulmonary-venous return. In older children it may occur with severe carditis, either rheumatic or non-rheumatic, and is most often seen after major surgery. Occasionally severe fluid over-load due to excessive transfusion or to large volumes of IV fluids may, in a sick child, produce pulmonary oedema, even in the absence of underlying heart disease. Pulmonary ocdcma may also occur in acute nephritis.

RECOGNITION

Increasing dyspnoea with marked intercostal and subcostal recession and crepitations in the lung fields are the clinical signs of developing pulmonary oedema. Tachycardia, increasing cyanosis and rising pCO_2 are usually present. The diagnosis is confirmed by the chest x-ray appearance of diffuse hazy shadowing with marked perihilar opacification and upper-lobe venous distension. Differentiation from the appearances of diffuse bronchopneumonia may be difficult.

MANAGEMENT

Intramuscular frusemide (1.5 mg per kg—up to 6 mg) should be given on diagnosis and rapid digitalization commenced if the child is not on digoxin already (*see* previous section). The child should be sedated with morphine (0.2 mg per kg) and nursed in 30 per cent oxygen sitting up in a chair or tilted head-up in an incubator. Antibiotics should usually be given, even if no definite evidence of infection exists, as infection is a common precipitating factor. An intravenous infusion should be commenced so that a ready route for administration of drugs is available but the rate of infusion must be carefully controlled to prevent further fluid overload, and should not exceed 80 ml per kg per 24 hours until the situation is under control.

If the condition is deteriorating or the pCO_2 exceeds 12 kPa (90 mm Hg), positive-pressure ventilation should be considered and is the simplest and surest method of controlling severe pulmonary oedema.

Venesection may be tried if the above measures fail, but should not be necessary unless facilities for positive-pressure ventilation are not available. Up to 10 ml per kg of blood may be removed and this may be accomplished by aspirating blood via a tap connected between the IV infusion tubing and the intravenous cannula. Insertion of a central venous line makes removal of blood very much easier.

Cyanosis and cyanotic attacks

The cyanosed infant is prone to develop several complications which may need urgent treatment and which can often be prevented if foreseen in time.

Acidosis

Severe hypoxia with cyanosis frequently leads to the development of a metabolic acidosis. If this results in the blood H^+ concentration rising above 65 nmol per litre (pH falling below 7.20) or the base deficit exceeding 10 mmol per litre this indicates severe hypoxia requiring urgent treatment. Any child with severe cyanosis should have an estimation of blood gases to assess the degree of hypoxia. Capillary blood gives satisfactory values.

Correction of acidosis, is severe cases, is best achieved by intravenous sodium bicarbonate according to the standard formula (p. 126).

In milder degrees of acidosis, bicarbonate (8.4 per cent) may be given orally or by nasogastric tube in a dose of 1 to 2 ml per kg. The dose may be repeated at $\frac{1}{2}$-hourly intervals until adequate correction has been achieved.

Polycythaemia

Polycythaemia is an important cause of vascular thrombosis, especially if dehydration becomes superimposed, as may occur in febrile illnesses of any kind in which fluid loss is increased and intake may be reduced. Maintenance of an adequate fluid intake is therefore of vital importance to the cyanosed child who has a febrile illness. If oral fluids (by mouth or nasogastric tube) are not tolerated intravenous fluids should be given at a rate of 100 ml per kg per 24 hours.

Any cyanosed and polycythaemic child, who is having oral fluids restricted before surgery or dental extractions, should have intravenous fluids to prevent dehydration.

Cyanotic attacks

Severe cyanotic attacks, sometimes leading to loss of consciousness, are characteristic of Fallot's tetralogy, but may occur with other cyanotic lesions.

Attacks are usually precipitated by exertion, feeding or crying, although intercurrent infection and dehydration may play a part. The attacks are distressing to the child who becomes increasingly agitated until consciousness is lost. The continued crying and struggling of the child tend to worsen the attack.

MANAGEMENT

The first-aid treatment of the attack is to quieten the child and stop the crying. This may often be achieved, if attempted early in the episode, by picking the child up, cuddling him and soothing him. Failing this, or if the attack is already well established, morphine 0.2 mg per kg i.m. should be given. Nursing in the knee-chest position may be helpful. (This is equivalent to the squatting position adopted by the older child).

Oxygen (100 per cent) may be given by face mask, but as the benefit achieved by this is slight, there is little to be gained by persisting if the face mask causes further distress to the child, which may in itself prolong the attack.

Severe acidosis may develop during the attack, requiring correction by sodium bicarbonate. In most cases acidosis resolves spontaneously once the attack has been terminated and attempts at intravenous injection (or even blood-gas determination by heel prick) may, by distressing the child further, prolong or worsen the attack.

The use of propranolol or other β-adrenergic blocking drugs in the managment of cyanotic attacks should only be undertaken by specialized cardiac units as they can lead to severe myocardial depression.

The development of cyanotic attacks is an indication for urgent surgical intervention, as they frequently become rapidly more severe and may be fatal. Referral to a specialized unit is therefore a matter of immediate importance.

Arrhythmias

Paroxysmal supraventricular tachycardia

In paroxysmal supraventricular tachycardia a severe tachycardia (rate usually between 180 and 300 per min) develops suddenly. The onset is abrupt and the attack may last from a matter of a minute or two to several days. The paroxysm ends as suddenly as it starts, although there may be a period of sinus tachycardia following its cessation. Attacks may recur frequently (even several in a day) or they may subside for months or years with only very occasional bouts. Between episodes the rhythm is normal. Some patients only ever have one attack.

RECOGNITION

Older children complain of palpitations and sometimes dizziness or faintness. Abdominal pain or chest pain may also occur. In infants pallor, dyspnoea and cardiac failure indicate an attack.

The pulse is very rapid, of small volume and regular. Cough, dyspnoea and hepatomegaly are signs of developing cardiac failure. The ECG shows a regular tachycardia with a rate of 200 to 300 per minute. The complexes are usually relatively normal in configuration but P waves are difficult to see.

MANAGEMENT

Rapid digitalization with intramuscular digoxin will usually end the attack within an hour or two. Should the tachycardia persist for 8 to 12 hours after starting digitalization, intravenous propanolol (0.1 mg/kg) may be given. The injection should be given slowly—over a period of 5 minutes with ECG monitoring and the injection stopped if the rhythm returns to normal. The use of intravenous drugs such as propanolol (or verapamil) may lead to myocardial depression and should only be carried out in consultation with a cardiologist.

An alternative method of stopping an attack is the use of dc. (direct current) shock. This is a quick and sure way of terminating the tachycardia, but involves the use of a synchronized defibrillator which may not be available in many non-cardiac units. General anaesthesia or sedation with intravenous diazepam (0.2 mg per kg) is required. This latter should be given slowly—over 2 to 3 minutes and a further period of 2 to 3 minutes should be allowed to elapse before applying the shock. An initial charge of 25 joules is often sufficient. If this fails 50 joules may be applied. Occasionally 75 or 100 joules may be required. Direct current cardioversion should not be used unless the operator is familiar with the apparatus and with the use of 'synchronization'.

At the end of an attack the child should be maintained on oral digoxin. If bouts are frequent and disabling further anti-arrhythmic drugs may be added, but this should only be considered after referral to a specialist cardiac unit.

Heart block

Heart block, in childhood, may be congenital or acquired. If acquired it is usually due to myocarditis or to surgical damage to the conducting pathways.

Congenital heart block is, in most cases, an isolated abnormality and unassociated with other congenital cardiac anomalies. The rate is faster than that seen in acquired block, Adams–Stokes attacks are rare and most patients are asymptomatic and require no treatment. When congenital heart block is associated with other cardiac defects, these tend to be complex and the prognosis is poor.

RECOGNITION

The slow heart rate, which accelerates poorly in response to exercise, may cause dyspnoea or dizziness on exertion or even at rest. Cardiac failure seldom develops with uncomplicated congenital heart shock unless the rate is below 50 per minute but may occur when other congenital cardiac defects are also present, or in the course of myocarditis. Loss of consciousness or convulsions due to prolonged periods of asystole or other associated arrhythmias (Adams–Stokes attacks) should be viewed very seriously and indicate the need for urgent artificial pacing.

Physical examination shows a slow, but usually regular, pulse with a rate in infants below 100 per minute and in older children of 40 to 60 per minute. The pulse is of large volume. The apex is forceful and may be displaced. Cannon waves are frequently seen in the jugular-venous pulse. An ejection systolic murmur maximal at the base of the heart is common and is due to the large stroke volume. An apical diastolic murmur or third sound is frequently heard and may also be 'functional'.

DIAGNOSIS

The ECG shows heart block, which is usually complete (3rd degree). Occasionally, second-degree block may be seen.

Chest x-ray shows some cardiac enlargement in most cases, even if no other cardiac lesion exists. This results from the large stroke volume.

MANAGEMENT

Treatment is only required if heart failure is present or when Adams–Stokes attacks occur. Rarely, a very slow rate, associated with dizziness or dyspnoea, may merit a trial of oral sympathomimetic drugs.

Cardiac failure should be treated initially with diuretics. Digoxin should be withheld unless failure is severe as it is liable to cause instability of the idioventricular rhythm, resulting in Adams–Stokes attacks. When failure does not respond to diuretics alone however, digitalization may be carried out cautiously.

Adams–Stokes attacks demand immediate consideration of artificial pacing and this will usually involve transfer to a cardiac unit. Intravenous isoprenaline (2 to 10 microgrammes per kg) may be given as an emergency measure to restore the cardiac rhythm if asystole is present, and oral ephedrine (1 mg per kg, 6-hourly) may be started. Long-acting isoprenaline (Saventrine) is useful in older patients but appropriate tablets are not readily available for infants and the tablets should not be split.

Sick sinus syndrome

Persistent sinus bradycardia (rate less than 60 per minute) associated with periodic sinus arrest or sino-atrial block and/or short-lived paroxysms of supraventricular tachycardia are characteristic; it is rare in childhood but is an occasional cause of unexplained syncopal attacks or convulsions.

RECOGNITION

The condition is asymptomatic except for bouts of dizziness or syncope, which may be accompanied by convulsive movements. The attacks occur irregularly with little or no warning. Physical examination during an attack may show marked bradycardia or asystole. Between attacks the pulse is usually slow (50 to 60 per minute) and may be irregular with runs of very slow rhythm interspersed with short runs of tachycardia.

DIAGNOSIS

The diagnosis depends on the characteristic ECG features of sinus bradycardia with runs of tachycardia and periodic severe slowing. In some cases the rhythm may be normal at rest and *the arrhythmia may be evoked by excercise*. The ECG should therefore include a long lead II both at rest and after exercise. Twenty-four-hour tape monitoring may be helpful.

MANAGEMENT

Patients who experience dizziness should be encouraged to lie down or place the head between the knees. Only with recurrent and disabling syncope should insertion of an artificial pacemaker be considered.

Ventricular tachycardia

This serious arrhythmia is occasionally seen in children with myocarditis, or after surgery. It may rarely be due to digitalis intoxication. The rate may vary between 120 and greater than 300 per minute. When the rate is rapid the cardiac output is severely impaired and consciousness may be lost. There is a very high risk of progression to ventricular fibrillation.

ECG   The ECG shows bizarre, wide QRS complexes and the form of the complexes and the rate may vary.

MANAGEMENT

Immediate cardioversion with dc. shock is the treatment of choice. Synchronization is desirable, but not essential. If the arrhythmia recurs lignocaine (1 mg per kg) should be given intravenously and the shock repeated. If tachycardia continues to recur repeatedly or frequent extrasystoles remain after conversion, a continuous infusion of lignocaine at a rate of 1 to 2 mg per kg per hour may be given, while specialist cardiological advice is sought.

Carditis and pericarditis

Acute myocarditis

Acute myocarditis may be rheumatic or non-rheumatic. Rheumatic carditis (now rare) is usually accompanied by other evidence of acute rheumatic fever such as arthritis. Viral myocarditis may be preceded or accompanied by other evidence of viral infection, such as coryzal symptoms, fever or gastrointestinal upset. Non-rheumatic carditis, occurring without clinical or pathological evidence of viral infection, is usually presumed to be viral.

RECOGNITION

Dyspnoea, tachypnoea, tachycardia and signs of cardiac failure in a previously well child with no known heart defect are the major indications of myocarditis. In rheumatic fever murmurs of mitral or aortic incompetence or an apical mid-diastolic (Carey–Coombs murmur) may appear. A pericardial rub is sometimes heard.

Investigations   Chest x-ray; ECG; Hb; WBC; ESR; Blood culture; Viral studies; ASO titre; Throat and nose swabs.

DIAGNOSIS

Chest x-ray usually shows generalized cardiac enlargment with pulmonary-venous congestion and sometimes pulmonary oedema.

ECG will often show T-wave flattening or inversion and reduced voltage of QRS complexes. Conduction defects, such as first degree block (common in rheumatic carditis), bundle-branch block or more severe degrees of block, may occur. Extrasystoles or paroxysm: tachycardia are sometimes seen.

MANAGEMENT

Digitalization and diuretics are the basis of treatment of cardiac failure (*see* Cardiac Failure). The management of arrhythmias may be difficult but digoxin should not be withheld unless it is likely that the rhythm disturbance is digitalis-induced. Patients with myocarditis are, however, unusually sensitive to digitalis and the development of any arrhythmia in a patient who is fully digitalized should give rise to suspicion of digitalis toxicity.

Bed-rest should be enforced in the acute phase of carditis and if necessary the patient may be sedated. In infants this is best achieved with phenobarbitone. In the acutely ill patient, especially if there is evidence of anxiety or pulmonary oedema, morphine (0.2 mg per kg) may be used.

Antibiotics should be given if there is an associated lung infection and in rheumatic carditis penicillin should be given to eliminate any residual streptococcal infection.

Corticosteroids are of little proven value in the treatment of acute carditis except when it is rheumatic in origin (and even then though the effect may appear dramatic at the time they probably do not influence the long-term outcome). If heart block develops a short course of steroids is justified. In infants hydrocortisone 50 mg 6-hourly i.m. or IV should be used. In older children larger doses will be required.

Acute pericarditis and tamponade

Acute pericarditis may be viral, bacterial or, rarely, fungal in origin. It may also occur in association with rheumatic carditis and collagen diseases. It seldom caused a large effusion with risk of tamponade except when of bacterial aetiology and only then is it likely to require urgent treatment.

Cardiac tamponade, which occurs when a large effusion interferes with cardiac function, may also be due to non-infective conditions such as malignant disease, including leukaemia.

RECOGNITION

Retrosternal chest pain made worse by breathing or coughing, and often relieved by sitting up and leaning forward, is characteristic of acute pericarditis. Fever and tachycardia are usually present and a pericardial friction rub may be heard unless a large effusion is present.

With the development of a large effusion dyspnoea, cough and abdominal pain are frequent. Tachycardia, small-volume pulses with pulsus paradoxus and raised jugular-venous pressure are the clinical signs and these, in association with a large, globular heart shadow on x-ray, without other cause should suggest the diagnosis of tamponade. Muffled heart sounds and an increase in the area of cardiac dullness to percussion are additional features but more difficult to detect.

INVESTIGATIONS

Chest x-rays ECG, Hb, WBC, blood culture, viral studies.

The chest x-ray shows a large, globular heart shadow with clearly defined edges. It may be possible to see a denser shadow within it, which is the heart itself.

The ECG may show signs of acute or chronic pericarditis with S-T segment elevation or T-wave flattening or inversion. In a large effusion low-voltage complexes may be seen in all leads.

Differentiation from myocarditis can be difficult and if in doubt a cardiological opinion should be sought. Echocardiography or cardiac catheterization and angiography may be necessary to establish the diagnosis with certainty.

MANAGEMENT

If septic pericarditis is suspected, antibiotic treatment should be started without awaiting results of cultures; a sample of pericardial fluid should be obtained (*see below*) for culture before starting treatment, but this is not always possible. A satisfactory initial antibiotic regime is benzyl-penicillin (50 mg per kg, 6-hourly) and chloramphenicol (50 mg per kg per 24 hours) given IV.

Digoxin is contra-indicated in the presence of tamponade and diuretics should be used with caution. Pericardial aspiration should, ideally, be done only by trained personnel, with electrocardiographic monitoring (i.e. ECG lead attached to the needle) and a defibrillator available.

If transfer to a cardiac unit is not possible and the patient's condition is critical the following technique for pericardiocentesis should be used.

Pericardial aspiration

The patient should be lying supine, propped up with head and shoulders at an angle of 45°. A wide-bore lumbar-puncture needle may be used with a 20-ml syringe and three-way tap. The needle is inserted to the left of the xiphisternum upwards and backwards, at an angle of 45°, behind the sternum. If fluid is not found the procedure should be stopped.

The risks of pericardiocentesis are ventricular fibrillation, or laceration of the heart or a coronary artery resulting in haemopericardium. These can be reduced by connecting the barrel of the aspirating needle via a sterile connector to the V lead of the ECG monitor. Contact between the needle and the ventricular myocardium produces sudden marked elevation of the S-T segment on the ECG thus obtained, and if this is seen the needle should be withdrawn.

An alternative approach is through the fifth intercostal space anteriorly. The needle is inserted lateral to the midclavicular line but internal to the edge of the cardiac dullness. This method carries a greater risk of damage to coronary arteries and can also produce a pneumothorax.

Perinatal cardiac emergencies

First 24 hours

Cyanosis

Cyanosis in the first few hours of life may be due to a variety of conditions. As a general rule non-cardiac causes outnumber cardiac causes at this age. The importance of looking for and, if possible, identifying the cause cannot be overstressed. For non-cardiac causes of cyanosis in the newborn *see* pages 645–646.

'Persistent fetal circulation'

Rarely an infant with no apparent other diseases, respiratory or otherwise may show severe central cyanosis due to persistent right–left shunting via the foramen ovale and the ductus. The condition is indistinguishable from cyanotic heart disease without cardiological investigation, but is entirely benign, resolving spontaneously over a few days. The same disturbance is frequently seen in infants with respiratory or neurological problems and is probably the reason why they may appear to have cyanosis out of proportion to their degree of respiratory distress.

Cardiac failure

Obvious cardiac failure, which is apparent from birth or within the first few hours is rare. The commoner non-cardiac causes include severe haemolytic disease of the newborn or intrapartum fetal haemorrhage. Cardiac causes are discussed under 'First week' (*see below*). Treatment depends upon the cause, which must be identified urgently. Digitalization and diuretics are important. Immediate transfusion or exchange transfusion may be necessary in appropriate cases.

Heart block

Congenital heart block has been discussed under 'Arrhythmias' (p. 292). It is unusual for an infant with isolated congenital heart block to develop severe symptoms in the first few days of life but any infant with evidence of co-existing cardiac defect or developing heart failure should be referred immediately to a cardiac centre.

First week

(a) Cyanosis

Cyanosis persisting beyond 24 hours or appearing after the first day of life, in the absence of other apparent cause (*see above*) is likely to be due to cardiac disease. The commoner conditions which present with cyanosis include:

Transposition of the great arteries.
Tricuspid atresia.
Pulmonary atresia.
Total anomalous pulmonary-venous return.

The assessment of the infant with suspected heart disease is discussed below.

(b) Cardiac failure

Development of cardiac failure at this age is usually due to severe congenital heart disease. An important early sign is failure of the infant to lose weight in the first few days of life—or even weight gain from birth. Cardiac failure may develop in babies with non-cardiac problems such as respiratory distress syndrome or severe infection, particularly septicaemia. Rarely, the only abnormality on full investigation of an infant with severe heart failure is hypocalcaemia and when this is treated the cardiac failure improves (*see* page 141).

The cardiac conditions presenting at this age include:
Hypoplastic left-heart syndrome.
Infantile coarctation syndrome.
Complex anomalies.

(c) Cyanosis with heart failure

The development of both cyanosis and evidence of cardiac failure in the first week of life is almost always due to severe congenital heart disease such as:

Transposition of the great arteries.
Total anomalous pulmonary-venous return.
Complex anomalies.

Emergency assessment

The emergency assessment of infants with suspected congenital heart disease should include the following investigations.

(*a*) *Chest x-ray*   For evidence of cardiac enlargement, abnormal cardiac shape or position, pulmonary plethora or oligaemia.

(*b*) *ECG*   For abnormalities of rate or rhythm, atrial or ventricular hypertrophy.

(*c*) *Electrolytes*. Especially calcium and glucose.

(*d*) *Blood gas analysis*. Estimation of H^+ concentration (pH), pCO_2, standard bicarbonate and base deficit on arterial or capillary blood and estimation of pO_2 in cyanosed patients (*see below*).

(*e*) *Hyperoxia test* (*cyanosed infants*). If significant cyanosis is present this is a useful test and helps to distinguish between cyanosis due to cardiac disease and that due to non-cardiac problems.

An arterial sample, preferably obtained from the right radial artery, as this eliminates desaturation due to persistent right-left ductal shunting, is taken for pO_2 at rest while the infant is breathing air or 30 per cent oxygen. The infant is then nursed in a head box in 100 per cent oxygen (or as close to 100 per cent as can be obtained) for 20 minutes and the arterial sample is repeated. Failure of the pO_2 to rise above 13 kPa (100 mm Hg) in an infant who is ventilating normally strongly suggests cyanotic heart disease.

If the infant is ventilating poorly due to neurological disease or severe respiratory problems the test may be done with the infant intubated and hand-ventilated with 100 per cent oxygen.

A slightly cruder method of doing this test is to observe the infant's colour without taking arterial samples. If the degree of cyanosis improves markedly in high O_2 concentration then it is unlikely that the cyanosis is due to cardiac disease.

When these investigations have been done a decision should be made as to whether the infant should be referred for specialized cardiological assessment. At the same time emergency treatment should be started if indicated.

Emergency treatment may include:

Digitalization if cardiac failure is present.

Diuretics—if there is cardiac failure.

Intravenous fluids, in sick infants, but the volume must be kept low ($\simeq$ 75 ml per kg per 24 hours).

Correction of metabolic acidosis (*see* page 289).

Correction of hypocalcaemia with oral or intravenous calcium gluconate. (*See* page 143 for dangers of IV calcium gluconate)
Correction of hypoglycaemia with intravenous glucose. (*See* page 446)

Indications for referral to a special unit.

(*a*) *Cyanotic infants*

Cyanotic babies require immediate referral for cardiological assessment if there is other evidence of cardiac disease (abnormal x-ray or ECG or presence of loud murmur, etc.) or the hyperoxia test fails to raise the arterial pO_2 above 13 kPa (100 mm Hg) or cyanosis persists.

(b) *Acyanotic infants*

Babies without cyanosis but with evidence of heart disease require immediate referral if cardiac failure appears or if the femoral pulses are reduced or absent, whether or not cardiac failure is present.

If it is decided to transfer a baby to a cardiac unit, the parents must be informed of the reasons for transfer and the gravity of the situation. If one or both parents is not accompanying the child, consent for cardiac catheterization and possible Rashkind septostomy should be obtained at the referring hospital and a signed consent form should accompany the referral letter, notes and x-rays and 5 to 10 ml of the mother's blood, all of which should, if possible, accompany the patient.

Cardiac arrest

Cardiac and respiratory arrest are so closely interrelated—the one following the other rapidly, whatever the cause—that their management must be considered together. The wide variety of circumstances and diseases which may lead to cardiorespiratory arrest need not be considered here except in so far as the immediate management involves, as it always must, an attempt to identify the cause.

Complete cardiorespiratory arrest, shown by apnoea, pallor or cyanosis and absence of the carotid or femoral pulses is usually obvious.

If cardiac arrest or arrhythmia is the initiating factor, *cyanosis and loss of consciousness precede* respiratory arrest which is itself preceded by transient hyperpnoea and then apnoea with occasional gasps before complete respiratory arrest. When respiratory factors are the cause, *the pulse is usually palpable after consciousness is lost* and when respiratory efforts are feeble or absent.

Vomiting may occur, as a late feature, in cardiorespiratory arrest from any cause and aspiration of vomit is likely. While aspiration of vomit is occasionally the primary event in a cardiorespiratory arrest it is more often secondary and, for this reason, it should not be regarded as the initiating factor until other possibilities have been ruled out.

DRILL (*see also* pages 201, 223)

Initiation of treatment for a cardiorespiratory arrest is usually in the hands of the nursing staff. Adequate instruction and training of nurses is therefore vital.

An instruction sheet, as below, should be available in wards, casualty departments, etc., but the drill must be familiar to all staff so that reference to the chart during the emergency should not be necessary.

Cardiac and respiratory arrest procedure

On finding a patient collapsed or unconscious:
(1) Shout for help.
(2) If no pulse is palpable start external cardiac massage. (The femoral or carotid pulse is easier to feel than the radial in a collapsed child).
(3) Clear airway of vomit and mucus by suction or finger, extend neck and elevate chin (to prevent tongue occluding pharynx).
(4) If no spontaneous breathing, ventilate with bag and face mask or start mouth-to-mouth respiration. Ensure adequate chest movement occurs with each ventilation.
(5) As soon as help arrives send someone to summon cardiac arrest team—by pressing emergency bell or telephoning . . . . ..
(6) Send someone to prepare emergency drugs and drip.

POINTS TO REMEMBER.
(1) Child must be on firm surface if cardiac massage is to be effective (use board if necessary).
(2) In infants, place one hand behind infant's chest and massage with fingers of other hand.
(3) Apply firm pressure to centre of chest to compress heart between sternum and spine.
The following points require amplification.

Cardiac massage

The object of external massage is to compress the heart between sternum and spine. Pressure should therefore be exerted over the sternum rather than on the ribcage (which is ineffective in producing an output and tends to result in multiple rib fractures).

In infants, pressure should be applied over the mid- or upper-sternum as depression of the lower third of the sternum can cause rupture of the liver.

An alternative method in infants to that on the drill sheet, is to hold the chest between the hands with the fingers behind and compress with the two thumbs.

A compression rate of 100 per minute is satisfactory for infants and children.

Ventilation

Adequate ventilation can only be achieved by intubation and ventilation with a bag. As an emergency measure, ventilation with a bag and face mask may be performed, but it is essential that the chin is elevated and that an adequate seal is obtained.

Mouth-to-mouth respiration (*see* Acute Respiratory Failures, page 237) is a satisfactory alternative but requires training and some practice to be effective. Whatever method is used it is important that adequate chest movement is occurring and that the airway is kept clear of vomit, mucus, etc.

It is helpful to alternate external cardiac massage with ventilation, giving 5 compressions of the heart between each ventilation of the lungs.

(a) Monitoring

As soon as cardiac massage has been started and ventilation is proceeding satisfactorily the patient should be connected to an ECG monitor. If this shows ventricular fibrillation then defibrillation should be attempted without delay as the likelihood of reversion to a stable rhythm is greater if this is done early.

(b) Intravenous infusion

While the ECG monitor is being obtained or connected, a drip should be commenced for administration of drugs. Either percutaneous cannulation of a peripheral vein or a 'cut-down' may be used, the latter being indicated if peripheral veins are collapsed and cannot be entered percutaneously.

The long saphenous vein at the ankle is the easiest cut-down site, but it can be difficult to cannulate in small infants and occasionally the saphenous vein at the groin or an antecubital vein may be used. The latter techniques carry risks of inadvertent arterial damage and should preferably not be attempted by the inexperienced operator.

The infusion rate should be kept to a minimum until the situation is under control. It is easy to run in large volumes inadvertently if the drip is left unobserved!

Drugs

(a) CORRECTION OF ACIDOSIS

8.4 per cent (molar) sodium bicarbonate may be given by bolus injection over 1 to 2 minutes in a dose of 1 to 2 ml per kg. This will not correct a significant degree of acidosis but if larger doses are to be given the rate of infusion should not exceed 0.5 ml per kg per minute as the solution is extremely hypertonic. If the patient has been hypoxic for a long period further bicarbonate may be given, up to a total of 5 ml per kg. This dose should not be exceeded until blood-gas determination has been performed. Total correction of acidosis may be achieved by using the standard formula (*see* page 126).

(b) CARDIAC STIMULANTS

If the ECG monitor shows bradycardia or asystole, or if no peripheral pulses are palpable despite an apparently satisfactory rhythm and rate, cardiac stimulants should be given.

  (i) Calcium gluconate (10 per cent solution) 0.5 to 2 ml IV ($\simeq$ 0.1 ml per kg)

  (ii) Adrenaline *1:10 000* 1 to 4 ml IV (100–500 μg) or Isoprenaline 10 to 50 μg IV

These drugs may be repeated if no effect is obtained after 2 to 3 minutes.

Direct intracardiac injection is seldom, if ever, worthwhile except as a last resort:

  (iii) *Glucose 50 per cent.* In all infants under a year it is worth giving 2 to 3 ml 50 per cent glucose.

  (iv) *Anti-arrhythmic drugs.* If ventricular fibrillation recurs repeatedly after defibrillation, ensure that adequate acid-base correction has been given; then give lignocaine 1 to 2 mg per kg; if that fails give propanolol 0.1 mg per kg.

If severe bradycardia persists or recurs despite earlier measures: give atropine 0.15 to 0.6 mg.

WHEN TO STOP (*see also* section on stopping ventilator treatment, page 188). The decision to stop is seldom easy. It should always be left to the most senior member of the 'team', who should take into account the following points.

(*a*) *Time elapsed before resuscitation started*

If this is likely to have exceeded 3 minutes then success is very improbable.

(*b*) *Evidence of cerebral activity*

Fully dilated, fixed pupils in the absence of any spontaneous respiratory efforts and which fail to constrict despite adequate external massage for ten minutes, are a strong indication of brain death.

(*c*) *Underlying illness*

If the child's underlying condition is known and is unlikely to be compatible with recovery, or is likely to result in severe, permanent disability, a decision should be sought from the consultant responsible as to whether resuscitation should be abandoned. If a senior person, preferably the consultant, is not available to make this decision, then resuscitation should be continued.

(*d*) *Duration of arrest*

If there is evidence of residual brain activity (respiratory efforts, small pupils) it is reasonable to continue with resuscitative efforts for at least an hour. Successful resuscitation without brain damage can certainly occur after 90 minutes or more of massage. On the other hand, failure to obtain an adequate cardiac output within an hour, despite adequate acid-base correction and cardiac stimulants, strongly suggests an irremediable situation.

Part VIII: Neurological Emergencies

CHAPTER 27

Acute Neurosurgical Emergencies

D. N. Grant

Acute head injuries

Children, particularly babies and infants, are extremely labile in their response to brain trauma; and, though appearing initially to have suffered no harm from a head injury, may rapidly deteriorate while a life-threatening situation may arise. The severity of the damage is not always proportional to the apparent degree of trauma, and significant injury to the brain may result from an incident which might well have left an adult unscathed. It is often difficult to decide whether a child should be admitted to hospital. In case of doubt, one should always err on the side of safety.

CRITERIA FOR ADMISSION TO HOSPITAL
  (a) Any child who has an injury sufficiently severe to cause loss of consciousness, even if only for a period of minutes.
  (b) Any child with a skull fracture.
  (c) Any child who remains or becomes drowsy following the injury.

An exception can sometimes be made in the case of children whose parents are sufficiently intelligent and level-headed to carry out the necessary observations through the night following the injury, with the proviso that there must be no delay in bringing the child back or getting in touch with the hospital at the first suspicion of deterioration.

Children selected for admission can be divided into those about whom there is no present worry, but who may develop complications and those who are clearly seriously injured and in need of urgent attention.

Severe injury

MANAGEMENT

In a severe injury there are a number of essential observations which must be rapidly, but carefully carried out, leading in turn to particular lines of action.

(1) Airway and respiration

In the unconscious patient, particularly if supine, the airway is likely to be obstructed by the tongue; this is reversed in the semi-prone position with the lower jaw pulled forward. If this is inadequate, an oral airway may be effective provided it is of sufficient bore to prevent further obstruction, it is long enough to reach the back of the tongue, and is of rigid material or at least has a rigid portion opposite the incisor teeth to prevent its total obstruction by spasm of the jaw muscles. Accumulated vomitus, blood and mucus must be removed from the mouth and pharynx. If these manoeuvres are ineffective, as they would be for example in profuse haemorrhage into the mouth or nasopharynx, an endotracheal tube must be inserted.

All casualty officers and residents ought to be able to do this without waiting for an anaesthetist. Inadequate respiration demands intubation and ventilation. *It is difficult to over-stress the deleterious effect which airway obstruction, with its resulting accumulation of carbon dioxide in the bloodstream leading to cerebral vasodilation, has on a brain which may already be grossly swollen from traumatic oedema.*

(2) Blood pressure

As soon as the airway is secure, the blood pressure is checked. It is often said that a head injury, unless it has caused catastrophic brain damage, is unlikely itself to cause low blood pressure. While this is true in adults and older children, babies can lose a significant fraction of their blood volume into a scalp haematoma or from a scalp laceration. However, in the absence of such an explanation, the cause of low blood pressure must be sought elsewhere. Bleedings into the thorax, peritoneal cavity, pelvic tissues or around long-bone fractures are the likeliest possibilities. Resuscitation is aimed at restoring the blood pressure according to the cause.

(3) Assessment of vital functions

   (a) The pattern and frequency of respiration previously observed.
   (b) The blood pressure and pulse.
   (c) The conscious level in terms of response to stimuli of increasing intensity such as ordinary conversation appropriate to the age,

shouting, non-painful and, finally, painful stimulation if required. During this stimulation the presence of any obvious limb weakness will be detected.

(d) The size, equality or otherwise, and reaction of the pupils.

These observations form a base-line for later comparisons; *the use of vague terms such as stupor and semi-coma is to be deprecated*. A change from the base-line, will indicate the onset of complications sufficiently early to treat them before irreparable damage is done. Deterioration is usually due to intracranial bleeding and traumatic oedema.

(4) Radiography

Good quality plain radiographs of the skull should be taken, for fractures, sprung sutures, and intracranial air indicative of a compound fracture; but x-ray of the skull is not necessarily an essential emergency investigation.

(5) Warning signs of complications

(a) Progressive deterioration in level of consciousness.
(b) Progressive dilatation and sluggish response to light in a previously normal pupil.
(c) The appearance or worsening of a neurological deficit in the limbs.
(d) All these may be accompanied by bradycardia, rising blood pressure and altered respiratory pattern.

In children there may be a misleading phase of increased activity and irritability with a rising pulse rate during the onset of rising intracranial pressure. However dramatic the onset of signs indicative of complications, there must be time which can profitably be spent in telephoning the nearest neurosurgeon before making the next move.

Extradural haematoma

RECOGNITION

(a) Extradural bleeding may be anticipated even after mild trauma such as a kick on the head while playing football or a fall against the pavement. There may be loss of consciousness for a short period although this is by no means always the case. After this, there is apparent recovery for a few hours, although, during this so-called lucid interval, there is often increasing headache and drowsiness.
(b) By the time of examination in hospital there may be sufficient extravasation of blood outside the skull to result in a boggy

swelling in the scalp. One pupil may already be larger, usually on the side of the haematoma. Plain radiographs of the skull may be helpful in showing a fracture crossing the markings of the middle meningeal vessels or one of the major venous sinuses.

(c) It is possible for extradural bleeding to occur, particularly in children, without the presence of a fracture. The temporoparietal suture may be temporarily separated at the time of injury, rupturing the middle meningeal artery and returning immediately to its normal configuration.

MANAGEMENT

(a) When some or all of the danger signs are present, and particularly when the situation has deteriorated to the extent of one pupil being fixed and dilated, the child's brainstem may be about to undergo irreversible damage and *there may be minutes in which to initiate effective treatment.*

(b) Ideally the haematoma should be evacuated without transfer to a more distant hospital and without more specialized and time-consuming investigation. In a desperate situation shaving the head can be omitted.

(c) Assuming that the situation, although critical, is not desperate, the following sequence should be followed.

(1) An endotracheal tube is inserted, for anaesthesia if necessary, but more importantly, to ensure an adequate airway.

(2) Blood is taken for emergency crossmatching because, although the quantity of blood in the haematoma is unlikely to be significant in relation to total blood volume (except in the very young), profuse haemorrhage which is difficult to control may be encountered when the haematoma is evacuated.

(3) *Preparation* While a theatre and basic instruments are prepared, the head is shaved. If time permits the shave should be complete to allow further burrholes through an uncontaminated field if the first is unproductive.

(4) *In theatre* The patient should be placed on the operating table with a 10-degree head-up tilt to diminish the venous pressure in the head. The relevant side of the head, that on which the pupil first became dilated (or in the absence of that sign, the side with the skull fracture or external evidence of trauma) is turned to face upwards, any tension in the neck being minimized by placing a large sandbag under the shoulder.

(5) *Operative technique (Figure 27.1)* A linear incision about 4 cm ($1\frac{1}{2}$ in) in length is made over the fracture site at the

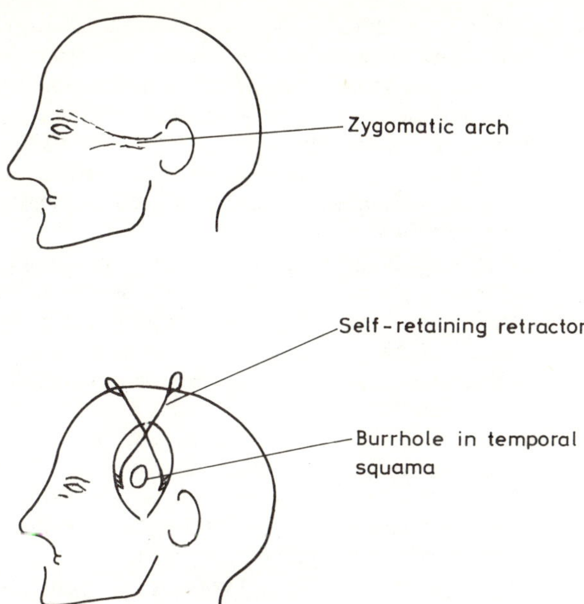

Figure 27.1. Site of skin incision for evacuation of acute extradural haematoma

point of external trauma or, failing these indicators, midway between the external auditory meatus and the posterior limit of the orbital margin. The lower end of this incision must extend down to the zygomatic arch. The incision is carried at one stroke down to the pericranium. A self-retaining retractor, such as a mastoid retractor, is then inserted, both to separate the edges of the incision and to arrest bleeding from the scalp. The pericranium is then incised and scraped aside. A burrhole is made preferably with a brace and bit, but if this is not available, a suitable opening can be made with hammer and gouge or chisel. If the diagnosis is correct, the dura will not be seen at this stage, as it is covered by haematoma which will begin to extrude through the opening. Gentle suction will assist the evacuation of the clot. As soon as a significant quantity of the haematoma has emerged, the pressure upon the brainstem is relieved and the situation is no longer acutely life-threatening. *If expert assistance is expected, it is probably advisable to proceed no further.* If however help is not at hand, the scalp incision should be extended sufficiently widely to allow the burrhole to be enlarged with bone-nibbling instruments into an oval craniectomy some 6 cm ($2-2\frac{1}{2}$ in) in diameter. Through this the remainder of the haematoma can be evacuated, allowing the surface of the dura to be exposed. The ruptured middle meningeal artery may be visible and can be coagulated with diathermy or underrun with a stitch. Occasionally the artery is torn as it emerges from the foramen spinosum. Haemorrhage from this site may be controlled by plugging the hole in the bone with wax, gelatin sponge or muscle. The exposed dura is usually hyperaemic and produces a troublesome amount of blood from multiple sites, which, if not controlled, would result in reaccumulation of the extradural haematoma. This reaccumulation is most readily limited by hitching the dura at a number of points around the edges of the craniectomy to the adjacent pericranium, using sutures which are passed through avascular areas of dura and which ideally penetrate only the outer layer of the dura, thus avoiding puncturing underlying cortical vessels. The wound may then be closed in several layers, including a simple drain if there is doubt about the efficacy of the haemostasis. If the site first selected for the burrhole does not reveal the expected extradural blood two further burrholes should be made, one over the frontal pole and another in the posterior parietal region. If none of the sites show extradural blood and the situation remains critical there is little to be lost in opening the dura, particularly if it appears to be dark blue in colour. Should the lesion in fact be an acute subdural haematoma, sufficient blood may be released to relieve the distortion of the brainstem. It is unfortunately more probable that a thin film of blood will be encountered over a contused cerebral cortex.

Acute subdural haematoma

Acute subdural bleeding usually results from laceration of dural-venous sinuses, from cerebral laceration or from tearing of bridging veins from the surface of the brain to the dural sinuses. Usually the deterioration is less rapid than in extradural bleeding. A rapidly compressing haematoma can arise from a tear in a major venous channel. Whereas in extradural haemorrhage the underlying brain is often intact, in subdural bleeding there is commonly associated damage to the cerebral hemisphere.

RECOGNITION

The clinical picture is less stereotyped and the site of the haematoma less predictable.

MANAGEMENT (*Figure 27.2*)

The patient should, if possible, be transferred to hospital for neuroradiological investigation, ensuring an adequate airway, if need be, by inserting an endotracheal tube. *If the deterioration is rapid and transfer of the patient is not practicable, the haematoma should be sought via multiple burrholes as for extradural bleeding.* The initial exploration

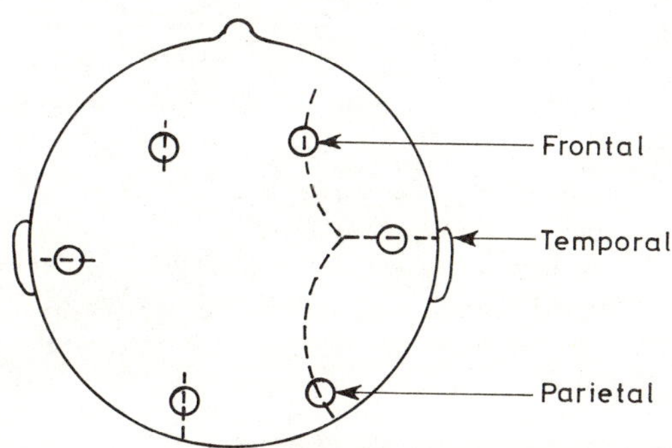

Figure 27.2. Site of burrholes for acute subdural haematomas. The frontal and temporal or temporal and parietal incisions can be connected as shown by the dotted lines in order to turn a formal craniotomy flap with the help of additional burrholes if wider exposure is required

should be at the site of a fracture or external trauma. Three burrholes situated, frontally, temporally, and in the posterior parietal region, are the minimum requirement to cover the surface of one cerebral hemisphere, and it is possible to miss a significant haematoma in spite of such a search. The possibility of a contrecoup injury makes it necessary to explore the surface of the second hemisphere, if the first side is found to be free from haematoma. Posterior-fossa subdural haemorrhage is fortunately rare; this should be considered where a fracture line is seen to pass into the foramen magnum. *Such a patient may deteriorate suddenly with respiratory irregularity or arrest and should preferably be sent for observation to a neurological centre.* Posterior-fossa burrholes are technically more difficult for the inexperienced operator.

Extradural and acute subdural bleeding and the general surgeon

The operations described for the relief of extradural or acute subdural bleeding should be within the capabilities of every general surgeon. If the child's condition is judged to be deteriorating rapidly and transfer time to a neurosurgical unit is measurable in hours rather than minutes, the surgeon on the spot should proceed, encouraged by the fact that prompt evacuation of a haematoma results in a normal child, whereas undue delay all too commonly results in death or severe and irreversible brainstem damage.

Traumatic cerebral oedema

This is much commoner as a cause of deterioration than a surface haematoma. The oedematous area is usually circumscribed and therefore limited in the clinical effect it produces. However the process may be progressive, involving both hemispheres widely, particularly if exacerbated by an inadequate airway. If it is not feasible to transfer the patient for neuroradiological study, the deterioration must be assumed to be due to accumulating haematoma until proved otherwise. Having established that there is no haematoma, cerebral oedema is assumed by exclusion to be the reason for the patient's deterioration and is treated by the measures described in the next section.

Acutely raised intracranial pressure

RECOGNITION
This occurs when a space-occupying lesion, e.g. a neoplasm, abscess or haematoma, reaches such dimensions that compensation by venting of cerebrospinal fluid or venous blood from the intracranial compartment is exhausted.

(a) Cerebral oedema

More diffuse increase in brain bulk by cerebral oedema as in trauma, encephalitis, and lead poisoning, or increase in cerebrospinal-fluid volume in hydrocephalus, has the same ultimate ill-effects. These are impaired respiration and finally cardiovascular activity from interference with brainstem centres either by mechanical distortion, impaired arterial-blood supply or haemorrhagic infarction.

(b) Intracranial tumours

Intracranial tumours in childhood rarely present as life-threatening emergencies without some clue in the history such as alteration in personality, deterioration in school performance, increasing complaint of headache, clumsiness of limbs or gait, or impaired vision.

(c) Cerebral abscess

Intracerebral abscess is found in association with cyanotic heart disease, chronic sepsis in middle-ear or nasal sinuses, following compound skull fracture or associated with dermal cysts or sinuses.

RECOGNITION

When a neoplasm or abscess finally results in an acute rise in intracranial pressure, there is depression of consciousness, eventually leading to unconsciousness. There is likely to be papilloedema, although its absence, particularly when the lesion has evolved rapidly, does not exclude the presence of raised intracranial pressure. The pulse rate is likely to be slow and the blood pressure high. When the brainstem is in danger there is pupillary inequality or gaze palsies and periodic or irregular gasping respiration.

MANAGEMENT
(a) Relief of brainstem compression

It is necessary to relieve brainstem compression without waiting for expert assistance. If in doubt about the efficacy of respiration, immediate intubation and ventilation will diminish the bulk of the vascular compartment and so lower the intracranial pressure by reducing the arterial carbon dioxide tension, but also at the same time this will ensure adequate oxygenation.

(b) Use of osmotic agents

Mannitol 20 to 25 per cent is infused in the dose of 1 to 2 g per kg over the course of 10 minutes. This will reduce brain oedema which is likely to be present in varying degrees under all the circumstances mentioned. The bladder should be catheterized in order to prevent its sudden distention in the unconscious patient. At the same time 10 mg dexamethasone given intravenously will disperse oedema around a tumour or abscess although there appears to be doubt about its efficacy in traumatic oedema. Further management is dependent on neuroradiological investigation and demands early transfer to a neurosurgical department.

(c) Impairment of vision

Papilloedema may be sufficiently severe to result in seriously diminished visual acuity at first evident as transient visual impairment. If permanent damage is to be prevented the intracranial pressure must be reduced by the use of mannitol and dexamethasone.

Under all circumstances of suspected raised intracranial pressure in childhood, valuable confirmatory and sometimes diagnostic evidence may be obtained from good-quality skull radiographs.

Acute hydrocephalus (*See* page 366)

Subdural effusion (*See* page 363)

CHAPTER 28

Convulsions and Status Epilepticus

M. J. Noronha
(*See also* page 687 for Convulsions in the Newborn)

A convulsion or seizure is a symptom: it denotes a sudden, excessive and disorderly discharge of neurones that may be induced by a variety of pathological processes of genetic or acquired origin. The abnormal discharge in the brain may result in a variety of manifestations which include disturbance of movement, sensation, behaviour or consciousness, depending upon the region of the central nervous system involved.

PATHOPHYSIOLOGY

During an epileptic seizure, cerebral metabolism increases by 50 to 100 per cent. In a brief seizure the accompanying increase in cerebral blood flow is sufficient to meet the increased cerebral metabolic needs. However, a prolonged convulsive seizure lasting more than 20 to 30 minutes is usually accompanied by apnoea and in addition an enormous increase in oxygen and energy demand from the contracting skeletal muscles. This results in:

  (a) Hypoxaemia.
  (b) Hypercapnia.
  (c) Lactic acidosis secondary to anaerobic metabolism.
  (d) Arterial hypotension and cardiac irregularities.
  (e) Rise in body temperature secondary to the muscular activity, itself further increasing cerebral metabolic needs.

This chain of events is probably the most important factor in the production of cerebral damage during prolonged convulsive seizures and underlies the importance of their management as acute medical emergencies.

RECOGNITION

A patient is said to be in status epilepticus when seizures occur in succession without intervening periods of recovery. Only the generalized convulsive (tonic-clonic) form presents an immediate threat to life or cerebral damage. Other forms of status epilepticus, such as absence (petit mal or minor seizures), myoclonic, psychomotor and partial-continuous varieties, do not usually require urgent life-saving measures, and there is time for investigation before treatment is commenced.

MANAGEMENT
(a) *The single convulsion*

This is usually self-limiting and, unless prolonged for more than 5 or 10 minutes, does not require immediate anticonvulsant medication, but the patient must have an adequate airway and be protected from self-injury.

(b) *Status epilepticus*

The prolonged convulsion is a true medical emergency and the principles of treatment are:

  (i) An adequate airway must be maintained and oxygen should be given.

 (ii) The patient should be placed in a semi-prone position and protected against self-injury or too zealous therapeutic restraint.

(iii) The seizures should be controlled by drugs (*see below*).

(iv) Fluid and electrolyte balance must be maintained.

 (v) Obvious causes such as infection, tumour, encephalitis, or recent withdrawal of anticonvulsant drugs, should be treated.

(vi) Laboratory investigations should include (but not on an emergency basis) complete blood count and urinalysis, blood glucose, urea and electrolytes, plasma calcium and phosphorus, radiographs of the skull (for intracranial calcification or evidence of raised intracranial pressure (ICP)); lumbar puncture *except when the ICP is raised*.

CONTROLLING THE SEIZURE

(1) Diazepam (Valium), without dilution, should be given by slow intravenous injection over the course of 2 to 3 minutes.

  (a) Recommended dose:

      < 1 year: 0.25 mg per kg.

      1 to 6 years: 2.5 mg.

      7 to 12 years: 5 mg.

      > 12 years: 10 mg.

  (b) Apnoea may occur if the drug is given too quickly.

  (c) The effect is rapid but usually lasts for only 30 to 60 minutes and it may have to be repeated.

(2) A slow intravenous infusion of diazepam can be given instead of repeated bolus injections.

    (a) Diazepam 30 mg in 500 ml of sodium chloride injection (*B.P.*) at a rate of 0.05 to 0.2 mg per minute.

    (b) The total amount of drug given depends on the response, the effect being assessed after each 5 mg is given.

    (c) As soon as the seizures subside the infusion can be stopped, to be started again if they recur.

    (d) A careful watch must be kept for signs of respiratory depression and hypotension: these complications are only likely to occur to a significant degree when other drugs such as barbiturates have been given parenterally.

(3) Alternatively clonazepam (Rivotril, another benzodiazepine derivative) may be given as it is claimed by some to be more effective than diazepam. Clonazepam may be used as a slow intravenous injection of 0.5 mg of active substance freshly mixed with 0.5 ml of diluent (Water for Injection) over a period of a minute, and the injection can be repeated in a few minutes if necessary. Alternatively, clonazepam can be given as a slow intravenous infusion (like diazepam)—3 mg of the drug are dissolved in 250 ml of either sodium chloride injection (*B.P.*) or 5 to 10 per cent glucose, the rate of infusion depending upon the clinical response.

(4) Paraldehyde may be given intramuscularly if there is difficulty in giving an intravenous injection of other drugs. A glass syringe should be used, although an opaque plastic syringe (but not the clear translucent variety) can also be used.

    Dose:

        < 1 year of age: 1.0 to 1.5 ml.

        1 to 5 years: 3 ml.

        6 to 10 years: 8 ml.

        Over 10 years: 10 ml.

(5) The importance of stopping the seizures as quickly as possible, in order to minimize the risk of brain damage, cannot be overemphasized. If this cannot be achieved with the use of the above-mentioned drugs in generous dosage, the aid of an anaesthetist should be sought without delay so that the patient can be anaesthetized with thiopentone sodium. This should only be done in an intensive treatment unit and maintained until seizures no longer recur as the level of anaesthesia is lightened.

CHAPTER 29

Coma

M. J. Noronha

Coma is a state of unconsciousness from which the patient cannot be roused. Consciousness requires intact functioning of the cerebral hemispheres and the reticular activating formation in the upper brainstem.

RECOGNITION

The initial questions are:
  (a) Where does the lesion(s) lie?
  (b) In what direction is the process evolving?
  (c) What is the pathological process and what can be done about it and its effects on the brain?
  (d) Is there a patent airway with sufficient respiratory exchange?
  (e) Is the circulation adequate?
  (f) Is intracranial pressure elevated, and, if so, is the elevation great enough to be life-threatening?
  (g) Is there a focal neurological deficit which might indicate a localized, surgically remediable lesion?
  (h) Is the coma likely to be due to a remediable metabolic disease, e.g. hypoglycaemia?

CLINICAL DIAGNOSIS
  (a) Often a reliable history is unobtainable and the immediate cause obscure, so that great reliance is placed on the clinical examination.
  (b) The major difficulty is to differentiate between primary CNS disease and systemic diseases or poisoning which produce secondary CNS depression.
  (c) Evidence of increased intracranial pressure:
      (i) In infants: full, bulging fontanelle, increased head size, separation of sutures, prominent scalp veins, papilloedema.

(ii) Older children: headache, vomiting and papilloedema.
(d) Serial evaluation of 5 physiological functions (level of coma, pupillary reaction, eye movements, motor functions, respirations) gives important information about the *level* of the brain involved, the nature of the involvement, and the direction the disease process is taking.

Level of coma

Record the actual state of the patient and his response to specific stimuli:

Stage 1 (*stupor*)   The child can be roused for brief periods during which he may be able to make simple verbal and voluntary responses.

Stage 2 (*light coma*)   The child cannot be roused even with painful stimuli but may respond by moans and semi-purposeful avoidance movements.

Stage 3 (*deep coma*)   Painful stimuli fail to produce a response, or they lead to decerebrate posturing.

Stage 4   The patient is flaccid and apnoeic. All brainstem functions are lost although some spinal reflexes may be preserved.

Pupillary reactions

(a) Normally reacting pupils are an encouraging sign.
(b) An unequal, widely dilated and non-reacting pupil usually indicates 3rd nerve damage by tentorial herniation of the brain and is an indication for emergency medical or surgical measures to reduce intracranial pressure.
(c) A dilated pupil may also be due to eye trauma, a transient postconvulsive finding, and is occasionally congenital.
(d) Bilateral fixed dilated pupils often, but not always, imply irreversible brainstem damage when the condition persists for more than 5 minutes.
(e) Pupils may be unreactive in reversible coma from poisoning by sedative or atropine-like drugs, hypothermia, and from previous local instillation of mydriatics.
(f) Pinpoint pupils are seen in poisoning with opiates and with pontine lesions.

Eye movements

   (a) Roving, nonconjugate eye movements suggest a light plane of anaesthesia.

   (b) Conjugate deviation of eyes suggest a destructive process on the same side or an irritative process on the opposite side of the cerebral hemisphere.

   (c) Sixth nerve palsy is usually due to increased intracranial pressure; it does not carry as ominous a prognosis as does 3rd nerve dysfunction.

   (d) 'Doll's eye' phenomenon: with the eyelids open, the head is briskly rotated from side to side. A positive response is a contraversive conjugate eye movement (e.g. turn the head to the right, the eyes move conjugately to the left, then the eyes slowly return to the new head position). Absence of this response in a comatose patient implies disturbance of the brainstem or of the oculomotor nerves.

   (e) 'Caloric stimulation test': this can be done as a less urgent test to investigate brainstem function.

Motor functions

These can be observed by applying painful stimuli and observing the responses.

   (a) Decorticate posturing with arms flexed and legs extended is produced by severe diffuse disturbance of the cerebral cortex and its thalamic connections.

   (b) Decerebrate posturing is characterized by rigid extension and pronation of arms and extension of legs. It indicates mid-brain involvement. When decerebrate posturing is unilateral, it is often caused by tentorial herniation, in which case it may be associated with a contralateral 3rd nerve palsy.

   (c) Flaccid limbs appear when the lower pons and medulla are involved.

Respirations

   (a) Cheyne–Stokes respiration is a pattern of periodic breathing in which hyperpnoea regularly alternates with apnoea. It implies bilateral disturbance of deep cerebral and diencephalic structures.

   (b) Central neurogenic hyperventilation; deep, rapid, regular respirations occur with involvement of mid-brain and pontine structures.

   (c) Ataxic breathing is irregular in rate and depth and indicates involvement of the medulla and the respiratory centre. It is a feature of impending respiratory arrest.

The recognition of the signs of decerebrate rigidity and the accompanying respiratory patterns associated with 'coning' (brain herniation) are most important in any condition in which there is raised intracranial pressure from any cause. This is considered further in the section on lumbar puncture (p. 727) and meningitis (p. 359).

INVESTIGATIONS

Determinations of blood glucose, serum electrolytes, blood gases and H^+ concentration (pH), blood urea, liver function tests and toxicology screening may be required. A lumbar puncture is usually necessary to rule out bacterial meningitis, but this carries the risk of tentorial herniation in the patient with increased intracranial pressure, especially with a focal brain lesion, e.g. cerebral abscess. In any comatose child who has raised intracranial pressure lumbar puncture is therefore contra-indicated. Proper diagnosis of the comatose child with focal neurological signs usually requires cerebral angiography. A computerized axial tomography (CT) brain scan if available may make angiography unnecessary.

DIFFERENTIAL DIAGNOSIS

Information obtained during the examination will usually enable the child to be placed into one of four categories depending on whether intracranial pressure is raised and on whether focal neurological signs are present (Table 29.I).

MANAGEMENT

(1) The airway and oxygenation must be maintained; the child is nursed on the side to minimize the danger of aspiration. Frequent suction of secretions is required. The comatose patient should never be left unattended.

(2) Shock should be treated (p. 90).

(3) An intravenous line should be set up; fluid intake should be carefully monitored as overhydration is common and results in water intoxication (p. 130) because patients often have inappropriate secretion of antidiuretic hormone.

(4) Prompt therapeutic intervention may be life-saving in the comatose child with a marked increase in intracranial pressure (ICP).

    (a) Obstructive hydrocephalus; this is relieved most quickly and effectively by ventricular tap.

    (b) Cerebral oedema; several medical measures may be effective—
IV 20 per cent mannitol (1 to 2 g per kg) administered rapidly

TABLE 29.I
The differential diagnosis of coma

| Without focal signs | | With focal signs | |
Normal pressure	Increased pressure	Normal pressure	Increased pressure
Most metabolic encephalopathies; diabetes, hypoglycaemia, hepatic, uraemia	Some metabolic encephalopathies; water intoxication, Reye's syndrome, severe hypoxia	Vascular disease; (cerebral artery occlusion)	Trauma; subdural, extradural or intracerebral haemorrhage, cerebral contusion
Intoxication	Acute lead poisoning		Brain tumour; usually supratentorial
CNS infection, meningitis, encephalitis	CNS infection; meningitis, encephalitis	CNS infection; encephalitis	CNS infection; brain abscess, subdural empyema, encephalitis especially herpes simplex
Trauma (concussion)	Trauma; subdural haemorrhage in infants, subarachnoid haemorrhage	Trauma; cerebral contusion	
Epilepsy (postconvulsive state)	Brain tumour; mid-line, posterior fossa.	Epilepsy; postconvulsive state with Todd's paralysis	Vascular disease; arteriovenous malformation
	Hypertensive encephalopathy Hydrocephalus		

over 20 to 30 minutes or oral glycerol (1 g per kg) repeated 6-hourly. A urinary catheter should be in place to prevent overdistension of the bladder. The effect of these agents is quick but transient and rarely lasts longer than 6 hours. Dexamethasone 0.2 to 0.4 mg per kg, IV initially, followed by 0.1 to 0.2 mg per kg i.m. every 6 hours is commonly employed but the therapeutic response is not seen for 3 or 4 hours. These measures are non-specific and should not replace or delay definitive therapy of the underlying disease.

(5) Specific treatment is indicated by assessment of the patient, the history, physical examination, laboratory and special investigations.

(6) The child should be repeatedly reassessed with the view to altering treatment or seeking further advice, e.g. focal neurological signs and raised intracranial pressure will usually require neurosurgical assistance.

CHAPTER 30

Acute Paraplegia

Ian A. McKinlay

RECOGNITION
Acute paraplegia is sudden loss of power in the legs.

BASIC PRINCIPLES
  (a) Spinal compression requires urgent investigation and relief.
  (b) Investigation, particularly lumbar puncture, can induce marked
      deterioration if acute paraplegia is due to compression, so it
      should be performed in collaboration with a neurosurgeon.
  (c) Surgical relief of the compression is more important than precise
      preoperative pathological diagnosis.
  (d) Commonly acute paraplegia occurs after acute infection, or as
      post-immunization myelopathy or transverse myelitis. Surgery
      in such cases is potentially harmful.

HISTORY
  (a) A history of recent viràl infection or immunization should be
      sought.
  (b) Evidence of systemic upset suggests continuing viral infection,
      spinal tuberculosis, osteomyelitis or leukaemia.
  (c) Only severe spinal injury causes acute paraplegia. A history of
      minor injury is commonly obtained from patients with spinal
      compression. Sudden movement can disturb the blood supply of
      compressed cord or the compressing lesion.
  (d) There may be a history of recent clumsiness of gait and increased
      tendency to fall as the result of compression.
  (e) Local aching or girdle pain is commonly associated with spinal
      tumours or local infection and helps to localize the lesion.
  (f) Retention of urine is usual in transverse myelitis but a history of
      bowel or bladder-habit change is absent twice as commonly as it

is present in spinal compression. Frequency of micturition and constipation are the commonest symptoms.

(g) A history of sudden, painful and often transient loss of vision in the preceding weeks or months strongly favours a demyelinating disorder (Devic's disease (neuromyelitis optica)).

(h) The more sudden, severe and painless is the onset of weakness the more likely is the cause to be intrinsic inflammation of the cord.

EXAMINATION

(a) The patient may have generalized superficial skin lesions in neurofibromatosis or a local superficial abnormality overlying a congenital lesion.

(b) Scoliosis may be present below a lesion of long standing.

(c) Spinal tenderness elicited by pressure is of great localizing value. It is more marked in the presence of infection.

(d) The legs are weak and usually hypotonic and hyporeflexic in acute paraplegia though, with acute deterioration of unrecognized compression, the legs may be spastic and hyper-reflexic. Plantar reflexes are difficult to elicit or extensor.

(e) Paralysis may ascend progressively (Landry syndrome) with poor prognosis.

(f) It is difficult to delineate sensory loss precisely. The apparent level may be several segments below the lesion. It is to be distinguished from the glove and stocking sensory loss of the Guillain–Barré syndrome when weakness and hyporeflexia in the arms will usually be found.

(g) Spinal angulation (gibbus) is a very late feature of spinal tuberculosis.

DIAGNOSIS

(a) Full blood count, ESR, blood culture, and viral studies on blood, urine and nasopharyngeal secretions should be done.

(b) Plain x-rays of the spine should be taken, including intervertebral foramina (dumb-bell lesions such as neuroblastoma or neurofibroma may widen them). There may be spina bifida occulta or hemivertebrae associated with a congenital lesion. The spinal canal may show widening, sometimes with narrowing of the anteroposterior diameter of a vertebra, or scoliosis in the presence of a slow-growing lesion. The pedicles may be eroded by an infiltrative lesion, disc spaces narrowed by tuberculous infection; a paraspinal soft-tissue mass usually indicates a neuroblastoma though tuberculosis also causes this. Nearly 50 per cent of spinal tumours are in the narrow thoracic canal.

    (c) Lumbar puncture should be performed, preferably by a radiologist, with great caution and using a fine needle. Only a very small volume of CSF should be removed and replaced by contrast medium to delineate any compression. Cisternal myelography may be necessary also to delineate the upper limit of a big lesion. The CSF from a case of compression is often yellow with very high protein content and few cells, though leukaemic cells may be seen in a freshly-prepared specimen. If the fluid is clear there is greater likelihood of myelitis or myelopathy. There may be slight increase in protein, especially the globulin fraction, and lymphocyte count. Heavy blood-staining from an atraumatic tap suggests rupture of an angioma. Very frequent reassessment after lumbar puncture will detect deterioration early.

    (d) Urine collection for vanillylmandelic acid (VMA) and homovanillic acid (HVA) base-line values is often indicated as neuroblastoma is the commonest tumour causing compression. However, surgery may be necessary before the collection is complete.

MANAGEMENT

(1) Nurse in a firm bed, immobilizing as far as is possible and as is consistent with skin care.

(2) Treat pain with analgesics.

(3) Arrange urgent surgical decompression when indicated. Discuss with radiotherapist in addition when appropriate.

(4) Dexamethasone 4 mg i.m. immediately and 2 to 4 mg i.m. 4-hourly is indicated pending surgery when a compressive lesion is present, especially if lumbar puncture is followed by deterioration. Its advantage in acute myelitis or myelopathy is dubious.

(5) Antibiotics (with drainage of a compressing abscess) are indicated in tuberculosis or osteomyelitis.

(6) Attention to bowel and bladder function. Catheterization may be necessary temporarily.

PROGNOSIS

Children recover from spinal compression better than adults so surgery is indicated even when severe disability is present. Recovery is variable after inflammatory disorders but many patients make a good recovery with symptomatic treatment.

CHAPTER 31

Acute Polyneuropathies

M. J. Noronha

The acute polyneuropathies include a group of clinical syndromes of uncertain aetiology characterized by the acute or sub-acute paralysis of the limbs, at times of the trunk, or of muscles innervated by the cranial nerves. A variable degree of sensory disturbance is present with sphincter disturbances and autonomic dysfunction in severe cases.

RECOGNITION

Most of the acute and sub-acute neuropathies do not progress and become life-threatening, but serious respiratory, cardiac and central-nervous-system complications can occur, and deaths have resulted. Although the rate at which symptoms have developed may provide a guide, it is often difficult to predict how rapidly progression will occur.

A thorough general neurological examination should be done to establish a base-line from which the subsequent course may be judged.

  (a) The degree of weakness in the extremities should be assessed; also the presence or absence of the tendon reflexes.

  (b) The degree of bulbar and respiratory muscle involvement:

    (i) Dysphagia, dysphonia and respiratory effort.

    (ii) Ability to cough and the presence of infection in the upper or lower respiratory tract.

    (iii) Optic fundi, blood pressure and respiratory rate should be checked regularly. In older children tidal volume should be measured with Wright's respirometer.

    (iv) Chest x-ray and ECG monitoring are indicated if there is evidence of respiratory or cardiac involvement.

FEATURES OF FAILING RESPIRATORY FUNCTION

  (a) Restlessness and anxiety.

  (b) Increasing pulse rate and respiratory rate.

(c) Cyanosis (if oxygen is not being given).
(d) Signs of CO_2 retention, warm extremities, high pulse pressure, tremor.
(e) If in doubt a blood-gas analysis should be done.
(f) If swallowing mechanisms and/or respiratory function fail (pCO_2 > 6.6 kPa (> 50 mm Hg) or if pO_2 < 9 kPa (< 70 mmHg) provided the patient is not receiving oxygen), expert advice should be sought from the specialist in charge of the intensive treatment unit as the patient may require to be intubated and ventilated (*see* Acute Respiratory Failure, page 233).

CHAPTER 32

Poliomyelitis

B. Heyworth

Since the introduction of immunization, particularly with oral polio vaccine, poliomyelitis has become rare in developed countries, though cases are still imported.

In developing countries poliomyelitis is widespread, mainly in children under five years of age. A common presentation is 'morning paralysis', a flaccid paralysis of a limb in an infant who seems otherwise well, without preceding illness. With improvements in urban sanitation in developing countries, older children may develop respiratory and bulbar paralysis; these are paediatric emergencies.

RECOGNITION

In paralytic poliomyelitis the following respiratory complications may occur:
   (a) Increasing weakness of the respiratory muscles progressing to respiratory failure.
   (b) Upper-airways obstruction from retained secretions, progressing to respiratory failure.
   (c) A combination of the above.
   (d) Superadded pneumonia or atelectasis.
   (e) Coma with bulbar or bulbospinal poliomyelitis.

MANAGEMENT
(1) Ensure an adequate airway by a combination of postural drainage, mechanical suction and perhaps tracheostomy.
(2) Adequate mechanical respiratory assistance and ventilation by intermittent positive pressure via endotracheal intubation or tracheostomy tube, or by a tank respirator.

Tracheostomy

This is indicated when posture and suction fail to relieve airways obstruction.

(a) In comatose or stuporous patients (usually due to polioencephalitis) when restlessness, diminished reflexes, reduced ventilation and increased secretions make drainage and suction impracticable.
(b) In the presence of persistent atelectasis.
(c) In bulbospinal cases where the airway cannot be kept open.
(d) In patients with hypoventilation where a respirator is not available.

Tracheostomy should be done early, before the onset of hypercapnia and hypoxia. Adequate humidification and repeated suction are necessary to avoid repeated changes of the tube. A cuffed tube is used where secretions are retained. It can be removed when swallowing is normal and the patient can cough.

Mechanical ventilation will depend on the type of respiratory paralysis.

Respiratory paralysis

This may occur with or without limb or bulbar paralysis, and may occur suddenly. It can be caused by:

(a) Paralysis of intercostal muscles; asymmetrical, complete or incomplete.
(b) Paralysis of the diaphragm; asymmetrical, complete or incomplete.
(c) Paralysis of the respiratory centre (*see under* Bulbar poliomyelitis *below*).

RECOGNITION

Symptoms of the respiratory insufficiency due to (a) and (b) above are:

(a) Breathlessness.
(b) Restlessness and foreboding of suffocation.
(c) Difficulty in coughing and talking.

Signs of respiratory insufficiency are:

(a) Tachypnoea.
(b) Use of accessory respiratory muscles (alae nasi, sternomastoids, etc.)
(c) Inability to take and hold a deep breath. ⎱ Difficult to
(d) Inability to count 30 after one inspiration. ⎰ determine in
(e) Reduction of the vital capacity.   children

    (f) Reduction of the arterial pO_2 below 11kPa (80 mm Hg) and if
        severe, a reduction of O_2 saturation below 93 per cent, and/or
        respiratory acidosis.

Assessment of the muscles involved must be carried out frequently.

(a) Intercostal muscles

Inspection may reveal paradoxical enlargement of the thorax during
inspiration, with movement of the thorax towards the abdomen. As the
patient tires, or towards the end of the examination, there may be
increasing use of the accessory muscles. Palpation and measurement of
the thorax at several levels and on each side is necessary.

(b) Diaphragm

Unilateral or incomplete involvement may only be revealed by fluoro-
scopic screening. Unless associated with intercostal paralysis it does
not usually cause trouble. Bilateral paralysis results in paradoxical 'see-
saw' movements of the thoraco-abdominal muscles, seen as depression
of the epigastrium during inspiration. Paralysis of the abdominal
muscles will produce abnormal movement of the umbilicus on coughing. They contribute little to the overall respiratory embarrassment,
except indirectly by failing to clear secretions.

    Obstruction of the upper airways by secretions, atelectasis and
pneumonia can all cause respiratory insufficiency in an otherwise mild
case, or increase mortality.

Prognosis   Without ventilation, respiratory failure is said to carry a
90 per cent mortality. Although ventilation can reduce mortality below
50 per cent only half of those surviving return to a normal life.

(c) Bulbar paralysis

Bulbar involvement occurs in 10 to 20 per cent of cases of paralytic
poliomyelitis. 90 per cent of those with bulbar palsy have spinal
paralysis, often of the upper limb girdle and sometimes with diaphragmatic paralysis. Major bulbar poliomyelitis can be very rapid in onset
and progression.

(i) Polioencephalitis   This may involve the medulla or brainstem, and
can only be diagnosed with certainty when hypoxia and hypercapnia
are proved absent. Children seem particularly susceptible, possibly
boys more than girls. Associated upper cranial nerve palsies, especially
of the facial nerve, lethargy, coma and muscular hypotonia simulate
true respiratory paresis. There is often no peripheral paralysis. When

bulbar or medullary centres are also involved, respirations are constantly irregular and the 'circulation centre' may be affected. (*See below*)

(*ii*) *Lower cranial nerves*   Recurrent laryngeal-nerve involvement occurs frequently, causing suffocation before difficulty with swallowing is observed. As it is often associated with dysphagia it is difficult to diagnose. Children may present with coughing and choking especially after eating and drinking. Occasionally, regurgitation of fluids through the nose occurs on swallowing causing refusal to eat or drink, which should be heeded. Respiration is difficult because of obstruction and spilling of fluids into the respiratory tract. Suffocation and salivation, sometimes with frothing, may lead to cyanosis, noisy breathing, and pulmonary atelectasis. But, even when the child has been deeply unconscious, recovery is often complete.

(*iii*) *Respiratory centre*   Involvement is shown by irregular respiration or apnoea for several seconds. Older children may show inability to change the rate and/or depth of respiration. Retention of secretions with increasing cyanosis indicates obstruction and asphyxia. Auscultation may reveal extensive râles and signs of atelectasis.

(*iv*) *Circulation centre*   In the absence of asphyxia, tachycardia is significant. The blood pressure is usually unstable. As in tetanus, hypertensive episodes without hypercapnia are grave, indicating extensive involvement of the brainstem. Just before death, multiple ventricular extrasystoles may appear. Vasomotor and secretory disturbances, with flushing of the face, sweating and excessive salivation may alternate with pallor. Rarely, convulsions, with drowsiness and hallucinations, may occur terminally.

Other cranial nerves can be involved without causing immediate danger.

MANAGEMENT

The management of emergencies in poliomyelitis should start promptly with the major illness, for emergencies can develop with little warning. Pain and paraesthesiae in limbs, trunk or neck are preparalytic symptoms. General management preceding and during an emergency includes:

(a) Rest.
(b) Measurement of the respiratory rate (4-hourly during waking and sleeping); assessment of the ability to cough and clear secretions; and of respiratory effort, especially the use of accessory muscles.
(c) Measurement of temperature and pulse rate, rhythm and volume.

Assessment of colour, speech, eating and drinking, bladder and bowel function, weakness, pain, spasm and tenderness of muscles.

(d) Assessment of motor function of limbs, abdomen and chest.

Bulbar poliomyelitis

Most cases do not need tracheostomy, but a clear airway is essential. Nursing the patient head-down by raising the foot of the bed about 45 cm (18 in) and using a simple shoulder harness to restrict sliding helps in this. If this is not well tolerated, the mattress can be made into an inverted 'V' so that both head and feet are dependent, probably a better position for treatment. A 'baby alarm' system or microphone should be positioned to monitor breathing and possible vomiting.

Respiratory paralysis only

Treatment can be carried out by a tank respirator without the need for tracheostomy. Waiting for severe hypoxia to develop before resorting to artificial respiration is harmful because it increases atelectasis. If a tank respirator is not available, tracheostomy with intermittent positive-pressure respiration can be used. Measurement of tidal flow, full blood gas analysis and clinical and radiological examination for lung pathology should be done periodically.

Other complications

These tend to occur later in the course of the disease and rarely as presenting complications. In decreasing order of frequency these are:

(*a*) *Shock*   In polioencephalitis and bulbar poliomyelitis shock may be due to affected centres and myocardial damage. It is precipitated by hypoxia and hypercapnia. Respirators operating at too high a pressure can impede the venous return and so reduce the cardiac output causing peripheral circulatory failure.

(*b*) *Paralytic ileus and acute gastric dilatation*   These can be due to central damage in bulbar poliomyelitis, but also caused by shock or hypokalaemia. Increased secretions, vomiting and impaired diaphragmatic movement make postural drainage difficult. Aspiration via a nasogastric tube may help to prevent this complication. Continuous suction should be used and a normal fluid and electrolyte balance should be maintained.

(*c*) *Azotaemia*   This is caused by renal failure secondary to shock, and will be associated with a metabolic acidosis; it is also aggravated by increased catabolism.

(*d*) *Hyperpyrexia*   This may occur early in polioencephalitis, or may be the result of secondary infection. Tepid sponging should always be used; β-adrenergic blockers may be tried in polioencephalitis.

(*e*) *Hypertension and cardiac arrhythmias*   These are also seen, like hyperpyrexia, in tetanus, and are usually transient and due to hypercapnia. If they are central in origin β-adrenergic blockade may be successful.

(*f*) *Pulmonary oedema*   This may be secondary to vasomotor centre involvement, hypoxia or ill-judged IV therapy.

One of these complications occurs in 10 to 40 per cent of cases of poliomyelitis with bulbar palsy or respiratory insufficiency. All are associated with a high mortality.

Suggested reading
(Including details of tracheostomy and respirators)

Bower, A. G. (Ed.) (1954). *Poliomyelitis and its Complications*. Baltimore: Williams and Wilkins
Fourth International Polio Conference. (1958). Poliomyelitis. Paper and Discussions. Philadelphia: J. B. Lippincott
World Health Organisation. (1955). Poliomyelitis. *W.H.O. Monogr. Series No. 26.* Geneva: World Health Organisation

CHAPTER 33

Tetanus in Childhood

P. M. Smythe

Tetanus in the child follows a course similar to that in the adult. In only about 50 per cent of cases can the site of injury and invasion of the organism be identified.

Where a recognized injury occurs those with some retained foreign body most predispose to tetanus. Otitis media or a burn can be the site of the infection.

RECOGNITION

The minimum incubation period is 5 days. The longer the period of incubation, and the longer the invasive period between the first signs of trismus and generalized spasms, the milder the disease.

(a) Trismus is the earliest and most constant physical sign.

(b) The risus sardonicus is diagnostic.

(c) Mild forms of the disease show only muscular hypertonicity.

(d) Moderate cases have generalized spasms but these are not prolonged or frequent and do not interfere with respiration or swallowing.

(e) Severe cases have spasms which impair pulmonary ventilation in one or more of the following ways:

   (i) Prolonged or frequent spasms which fix the chest wall and diaphragm.

   (ii) Laryngospasm with complete obstruction of respiration.

   (iii) Pharyngospasm which prevents the swallowing of saliva which lies pooled in the pharynx and is inhaled into the trachea.

Impaired pulmonary ventilation is shown by anxiety, restlessness, a rising pulse and blood pressure, sweating and cyanosis.

Severe forms of tetanus

Very severe forms show signs of impending failure of the vital centres, with circulatory collapse, respiratory failure, hyperpyrexia, ileus and sometimes, terminally, diminished spasms with muscular flaccidity.

(a) Any spasm severe enough to cause apnoea which requires artificial respiration to re-establish breathing is an absolute indication for tracheostomy as a second attack of this type is almost invariably fatal.

(b) Very occasionally, severe forms are associated with only focal spasms of the larynx and pharynx.

(c) Generalized spasms and trismus due to infections of the central nervous system have to be distinguished from tetanus, but in tetanus the state of consciousness is characteristically clear.

(d) Neck stiffness can be confused with meningitis, and abdominal rigidity with peritonitis.

MANAGEMENT

(a) If human antitetanus immunoglobulin is available, 500 units should be given intramuscularly; otherwise 20 000 units of ATS (antitetanus horse serum) (10 000 IV and 10 000 i.m.) after testing for sensitivity.

(b) Wounds are treated solely on their surgical merits; any wound must be examined carefully for the presence of a foreign body.

(c) Procaine-penicillin is given i.m. for 10 days and then stopped.

(d) The sedatives used are diazepam, chlorpromazine or paraldehyde.

TRACHEOSTOMY

(a) All severe cases require tracheostomy. This is best done under general anaesthesia but can be done under local. A high tracheostomy at the level of the third, fourth and fifth rings is essential. If the disease is expected to run a severe course a cuffed tracheostomy tube should be inserted. The tube must lie in alignment with the trachea so that the tip does not cause pressure erosion of the tracheal wall or kink the trachea. The position of the head and neck can determine if pressure effects occur.

(b) The patient should be placed in a humidified atmosphere as soon after the tracheostomy as possible, as blood and mucus can quickly inspissate and lead to obstruction.

(c) Secretions must be kept fluid so that physiotherapy and suctioning are efficient, otherwise bronchial obstruction and infection of the lung are inevitable. A solution of penicillin and colistin (*see under* Neonatal Tetanus, page 342) instilled 4-hourly down the tracheostomy tube is effective in controlling infection.

M

(d) Tracheostomy tubes require to be changed every 4 days as tenacious mucus may adhere to the tube causing obstruction and infection. Auscultation of the chest should be frequent to check on equal air-entry to exclude bronchial obstruction.

(e) Hypersalivation, which seems to be a feature of severe tetanus, requires the mouth and pharynx to be suctioned frequently.

(f) Change of posture from back to side is required every 4 hours to encourage bronchial drainage and prevent pressure sores.

(g) A rising pulse rate, sweating, fever and increased spasms are far more likely to be due to some obstruction of the airway than pulmonary infection or tetanus intoxication. In the older child tracheostomy alone is often enough to break the vicious circle of spasms–asphyxia–increasing spasm.

(h) With sedation and good care of the tracheostomy, recovery can follow. Very severe forms requiring curarization and IPPV are recognized by spasms of such severity as to interfere with respiration and which cannot be controlled by sedation, or which require such heavy sedation as to depress respiration, increasing cardiorespiratory distress with a rising pulse, especially over 160, or hyperpyrexia with a temperature of over 40°C (104°F).

(i) The tracheostomy tube should be removed only after the patient has recovered sufficiently to swallow feeds without difficulty and spasms have ceased to impede respiration. Removal of the trachcostomy tube is made a safer procedure if a smaller tracheostomy tube is inserted, around which the patient can breathe, the stoma of the tube occluded with a bung, and the patient accustomed to breathing through the mouth for 24 hours before the tube is removed.

PREVENTION

(a) When an injury occurs in which tetanus could be a complication, previously fully-immunized individuals need no treatment, providing the last immunizing dose was given not more than a year previously.

(b) If the last immunizing dose was longer than a year ago a booster dose of 0.5 ml of tetanus toxoid should be given intramuscularly.

(c) If the patient was not fully immunized previously, prophylactic human antiglobulin should be given.

(d) If human tetanus antiglobulin is not available, antitetanus horse serum (ATS) should be given; but it is essential that skin tests for hypersensitivity be done, and it is safer if the injection is given starting with a small dosage and increasing the volume every half-hour until the full amount is given.

Horse serum carries a risk of severe, sometimes fatal, hypersensitivity reaction and should it be decided that the risk of the reaction is greater than the likelihood of tetanus following the injury this must be clearly stated to the patient and recorded in the notes, as claims for negligence can follow should tetanus subsequently develop. Although *Clostridium tetani* is sensitive to penicillin, penicillin alone will not prevent tetanus developing.

CHAPTER 34

Neonatal Tetanus: Treatment with IPPV

P. M. Smythe

Neonatal tetanus is due to infection of the umbilical cord by unsterile dressings or ligature.

RECOGNITION

The onset is seldom less than 5 days and never less than 3 days after birth; in general the prognosis is worse the earlier the onset.

(a) Presenting symptoms are: refusal to feed, due to trismus; muscular rigidity or spasms without loss of consciousness.

(b) Other symptoms are:

Risus sardonicus.

Salivation due to pharyngospasm.

Rigidity, especially of the abdominal muscles and spasms causing head retraction or arching of the back.

Respiratory impairment due to spasm of intercostals and diaphragm. Nearly always there is some evidence of umbilical infection.

(c) The differential diagnosis includes:

(i) Intracranial haemorrhage or hypoxia.

(ii) Fits from any cause (such as meningitis).

(iii) Tetany from hypocalcaemia or hypomagnesaemia: in these conditions there is 'jitteriness' or convulsions.

(iv) Kernicterus.

MANAGEMENT

In areas where neonatal tetanus is common, facilities for tracheostomy, muscle relaxants and IPPV are not always available and it is necessary to take account of this lack in presenting any scheme for the management of neonatal tetanus. Conservative treatment has a mortality of over 90 per cent and units without facilities for IPPV but with the possibility of transport of cases to a specialized centre must decide early in the course of the disease which cases require transfer. It is not easy to foresee the course of neonatal tetanus; apnoeic attacks may occur at any time, as may also pulmonary infection. To wait for these complications before transfer to an IPPV unit is to impair seriously the chance of survival.

PROCEDURE
(1) On admission all infants receive 1 to 2 ml of paraldehyde i.m. or 1 to 2 mg of diazepam i.m. Oxygen is given as required.
(2) Antitetanus serum (ATS) 10 000 to 20 000 units is given IV, and 20 000 units i.m. in divided doses at four different sites (there is no fear of sensitivity reaction in this age group) OR human antitetanus globulin 1000 units i.m. (1 ampoule normally contains 250 iu.)
(3) Procaine-penicillin 100 000 units i.m. (or an injection of benethamine, procaine, and benzylpenicillin (Triplopen) in a dose of one vial by deep i.m. injection) with the addition of kanamycin (15 mg per kg per 24 hours) or gentamicin (1 to 4 mg per kg per 24 hours) if thought necessary (e.g. for an umbilical site infected with other organisms).
(4) Indications for tracheostomy and IPPV
   (a) Severe spasms
   (b) A severe cyanotic or apnoeic episode.

MANAGEMENT WITH IPPV (Smythe, Bowie and Voss, 1974).

(a) Tracheostomy

Tracheostomy is necessary; endotracheal intubation cannot be maintained for the necessary length of time without damage to the cords, though obviously intubation could be used as a temporary or emergency expedient.
(1) Give vitamin K_1 (Konakion) 1 mg i.m. before tracheostomy to minimize bleeding.
(2) Tracheostomy should be done under general anaesthesia; a local anaesthetic carries greater risk.
(3) Use a high tracheostomy with vertical incision through 3rd and 4th or 3rd, 4th and 5th rings to avoid pneumothorax. A Pilling–Holinger tube (size 1.5mm diameter) can be used with a T-piece welded on to the side to provide a side attachment to the ventilator and an opening for suction. A cuffed tube is not necessary.
(4) To prevent pressure erosion of the trachea the tapes are not tied too tightly and the tube is kept loose enough to be pulled in and out for 0.5 cm each day to avoid constant pressure on the same area.

(b) Ventilation

A ventilator should be used with which the nursing and medical staff are familiar; an East Radcliff or similar ventilator is recommended, with a warm-water humidifier set so that the gases entering the patient are between 33°C (91.4°F) and 35°C (95°F), using a setting of $\pm$ 60°C (140°F). The ventilator should run at 37 cycles per minute with an initial water pressure of 15 cm water and should be subsequently adjusted to maintain a pCO_2 of 4.2 kPa (32 mm Hg). Air can be used but 30 per cent oxygen is preferable. This concentration should not be exceeded.

(c) Muscle relaxation

Tubocurarine 10 mg i.m. should be used repeating injections whenever muscular twitching occurs but allowing some recovery of muscle activity between injections in order to avoid ileus.

(d) Nursing

The head and the body are inclined upwards at 15° to drain the upper lobes; pressure sores and occipital flattening are avoided by turning the head every half-hour.

(e) Physiotherapy to the chest should be done every 4 hours.

(f) Avoidance of complications

(i) Any deterioration in the infant's condition should suggest airway obstruction; this can be detected by inadequate or unequal air entry on auscultation. Incorrect alignment or inspissation of mucus may obstruct the tracheostomy tube. Aspiration of the trachea and bronchi should be done hourly initially and later at 2-hourly intervals. A sterile No. 3 (English) or No. 8 (French) gauge rubber catheter should be used, with a side and end opening or a tip cut obliquely.

(ii) Saliva should be sucked out of the mouth before applying suction to the trachea and bronchi.

(iii) Airway infection: instil 0.25 ml of a sterile solution of 500 units of penicillin and 500 units of colistin (freshly made up each day) down the tracheostomy tube every 4 hours for the first 2 days. This should be continued or restarted if the secretions become purulent.

(g) Feeds

Routine milk feeds are given using a nasogastric tube, aspirating the stomach before each feed; any residue indicates some degree of ileus. Accumulated faeces (detected by palpation) should be evacuated by a $\frac{1}{4}$ of a bisacodyl (Dulcolax) suppository. Clear fluids are given for the first 48 hours: milk is started when there is no gastric residue.

(h) Weaning from ventilation

After 2 to 4 weeks tetanic twitchings have usually lessened and the interval between tubocurarine injections will be lengthened; spontaneous respiratory movements will start at this time and an attempt should then be made to stop the tubocurarine. Some relaxation can still be maintained by giving phenobarbitone 7.5 mg three times daily down the nasogastric tube. The ventilator should be continued for 4 to 5 days after stopping curare, but with *gradual* reduction of the inspiratory pressure. Extubation should only be done when there is a demonstrable return of sucking movements on a small teat; this can be done by replacing the original tube by a size 00 Pilling–Holinger tube of 3 mm diameter. This tube allows free breathing round the tube and the opening of the tube itself can then be blocked off with a bung. When the tube can be occluded continuously for 24 hours and all feeds can be taken without difficulty the tube itself is removed. Failure to tolerate blocking of the 00 tube indicates granulation tissue above the level of the tube, compression of the tracheal rings above the stoma, or angling or kinking of the trachea with inspiration because of its attachment by fibrous tissue round the stoma to the skin. These complications require expert advice (Smythe, 1964, 1967).

ACTIVE IMMUNIZATION

As soon as the infant is well both mother and baby should be immunized with toxoid. The maternal immunity produced will protect future infants during the neonatal period.

References

Smythe, P. M. (1964). The problem of detubating an infant with a tracheostomy. *J. Pediat.* **65**, 446

Smythe, P. M. (1967). Treatment of tetanus in neonates. *Lancet* **(1)**, 335

Smythe, P. M., Bowie, M. D. and Voss, J. T. V. (1974). Treatment of tetanus neonatorum with muscle relaxants and intermittent positive-pressure ventilation. *Br. med. J.* **1**, 223

CHAPTER 35

Neonatal Tetanus: Treatment without IPPV

Elizabeth Lund

It was felt essential to include a section for the many units in various parts of the world without facilities for IPPV and without any possibility of transferring their cases to an IPPV centre. (Editor)

MANAGEMENT

Note: Antitetanus serum and antibiotics should of course be given as in the previous section on IPPV treatment.

Good nursing and continuous supervision are essential.

(1) On admission: start IV drip with a maintenance electrolyte solution (p. 93) containing 4 to 5 per cent glucose. When spasms have ceased the child can be weighed, and the fluid requirement for the 24 hours can be calculated on the basis of 160 ml per kg plus an additional 50 to 60 ml per kg if dehydration is present. Since all cases are acidotic 20 ml of a 4 per cent solution of sodium bicarbonate (10.0 mmol) should be put in the first bottle of IV fluid, preceded by an initial 'bolus' of 6 ml per kg of the sodium bicarbonate solution (3 mmol per kg) given over 5 to 10 minutes.

(2) As soon as the drip is running satisfactorily, give 2.5 mg diazepam into the rubber bulb at the end of the tubing and run in at least 30 drops of fluid to ensure that the diazepam has entered the circulation; this dose can be repeated at 5- to 10-minute intervals, giving up to 10 doses over a period of 4 hours: occasionally very large amounts up to 120 mg over 4 hours will be required. Respiratory arrest from the diazepam is rare, but facilities for intubation should be at the bedside.

(3) When muscle relaxation and regular breathing have been produced a nasogastric tube should be passed and 12.5 mg of chlorpromazine in the form of a syrup given down the tube, followed by 2 to

3 ml of sterile water to make certain that the whole dose is in the stomach.

(4) Continued treatment:

    (a) Chlorpromazine 12.5 mg every 6 hours through the nasogastric tube; alternating with (b).

    (b) Diazepam syrup 2.5 to 5.0 mg orally every 6 hours (2.5 mg for infants of 2.5 to 3.5 kg and 5.0 mg if over 3.5 kg). Additional doses of chlorpromazine or diazepam can be given IV between the 6-hourly doses if the spasms are severe.

(5) At the end of 24 hours:

    (a) Slow down the drip to give half the maintenance requirement IV and half by nasogastric tube. The IV drip should be kept going for 3 days in case extra doses of IV diazepam are required.

    (b) Give diazepam syrup orally in the previous dose and increasing or decreasing the dose according to the degree of sedation achieved, as assessed by graded stimuli (*see below*). The diazepam should be given at 6-hourly intervals and should be continued for 1 to 2 days after the spasms have ceased.

    Assessment of diazepam dosage by stimulation:

I Lifting the sheet
II Touching the abdomen lightly

(A spasm in response to I or II requires an additional dose or an increased dose, as does a spontaneous spasm)

III Poking the abdomen gently
IV Poking the abdomen harder

(Absence of spontaneous spasms or spasms after III or IV stimulus indicates a satisfactory degree of sedation. Spasms after III or IV require continuation of diazepam in the previous dose)

    (c) Chlorpromazine should be continued for 3 to 5 weeks but the dose can generally be decreased from the 12th day onwards.

CHAPTER 36

Acute Meningitis

J. A. Black

Failure to recognize acute bacterial meningitis and treat it adequately may result in death, or survival with sequelae such as hydrocephalus, spasticity or mental retardation.

The organisms most likely to cause meningitis vary with the age of the child (Table 36.I). When access of bacteria to the brain or meninges

TABLE 36.I
Bacterial meningitis at different ages

| | Neonatal period | Over 1 month and | |
Common	Less common	under 5 years	Over 5 years
Escherichia coli	Streptococcus viridans	Haemophilus influenzae	As for previous column, but H. influenzae is rare
Proteus species	Streptococcus faecalis (enterococcus)	Meningococcus	
Paracolon bacillus	Pneumococcus	Pneumococcus	
Klebsiella species	Staphylococcus	Group A Streptococcus	
Pseudomonas aeruginosa	Meningococcus	Staphylococcus	
Group B strepto-coccus	Salmonella species, Bacillus subtilis	Gram-negative bacilli infections up to age of 6 months	
Listeria monocytogenes	Serratia species Flavobacterium meningosepticum Gonococcus Citrobacter diversus Bacteroides fragilis* Fusobacterium*		

* Anaerobic

is facilitated (e.g. by leaking meningomyelocele, open head injury, communicating dermal sinus), or the resistance of the patient is reduced (e.g. immunosuppression in the treatment of leukaemia or malignancy; congenital or acquired immunological deficiency), infection may occur with organisms which are not normally pathogenic, or are rarely encountered as a cause of meningitis. In post-splenectomy patients or in the older child with sickle-cell anaemia, pneumococcal meningitis is particularly common.

Neonatal meningitis

RECOGNITION

Meningitis should be looked for in any newborn infant with a suspected septicaemia.

Early symptoms and signs, all of which may have other causes

   (a) Sudden lethargy, hypotonia, reluctance to feed, vomiting, abdominal distension.
   (b) Apnoeic spells, tachypnoea.
   (c) Fits, focal or generalized.
   (d) Rapidly developing jaundice.
   (e) Sudden hypothermia or raised temperature.

Late signs, which carry a bad prognosis

   (a) Head retraction or neck stiffness.
   (b) Bulging fontanelle.
   (c) Head circumference increasing at more than 1 mm per day.
   (d) Thickly purulent CSF.

Investigations indicated in suspected cases

   (a) In the infant: blood and urine culture, lumbar puncture, swabs from nose, umbilicus, rectum and from infected sites. Chest x-ray.
   (b) In the mother, if indicated: blood, stool and urine culture; swabs from the genital tract.

LUMBAR PUNCTURE

(a) Difficulty in obtaining CSF

Failure to obtain fluid may be due to thick fluid, very low pressure in a shocked infant, a block higher up, or to incorrect position of the needle.

Gentle aspiration with a syringe may be attempted, or the puncture can be repeated with the infant supported in the sitting position. Occasionally fluid can be obtained by reinserting the needle one space higher up. (*See* page 726 for technique of lumbar puncture in the newborn)

(b) *Interpretation of CSF*

(*i*) *Normal limits for CSF in the newborn*   Cells 20 per mm^3, protein 1.5 g per litre (150 mg%) pre-term infants 2.0 g per litre (200 mg%). Glucose levels as low as 0.5 mmol per litre (10 mg%) are common with an otherwise normal fluid but in such cases hypoglycaemia should be suspected. A raised white-cell count (with a predominance of lymphocytes *or* polymorphs) which cannot be accounted for by the presence of blood, should be considered to be due to meningitis.

(*ii*) *Blood-stained CSF*   Blood-stained fluid may be due to the coexistence of meningitis *and* intracranial haemorrhage (this is not uncommon), intracranial haemorrhage alone, or a traumatic tap. Blood-stained fluid should always be examined fully and even specimens unsuitable for a cell count should be examined by Gram film and put up for culture.

The white-cell count in blood-stained fluid is usually raised; if this is due to a coexistent meningitis the count is likely to be greater than 100 per mm^3, usually with an excess of polymorphs. If blood has been in the subarachnoid space for longer than 24 hours, an increased cell count is likely to be due to the presence of the blood, and counts of 50 to 100 cells per mm^3 may be found. Blood-stained fluid due to a traumatic tap contains the white cells from the original CSF with the addition of white cells from the blood. A normal ratio of red cells to white cells (1 to 500) indicates that they originate from the peripheral blood (a more accurate ratio can be obtained by an actual count on the infant's blood): 0.01 g per litre (1.0 mg%) of protein should be allowed for every 800 red cells per m^3.

(*iii*) *Gram film and culture*   Organisms may be visible on the stained film from fluid with normal cytology and chemistry, and therefore *all* specimens at diagnostic lumbar puncture should be examined by Gram film and should be cultured.

Antibiotics given before the lumbar puncture may alter the staining characteristics and morphology, making identification difficult; or a CSF in which stained organisms have been seen may be sterile on culture.

If the CSF is sterile but no antibiotics had been given before lumbar puncture, and organisms were seen on the film or the cytology is typical

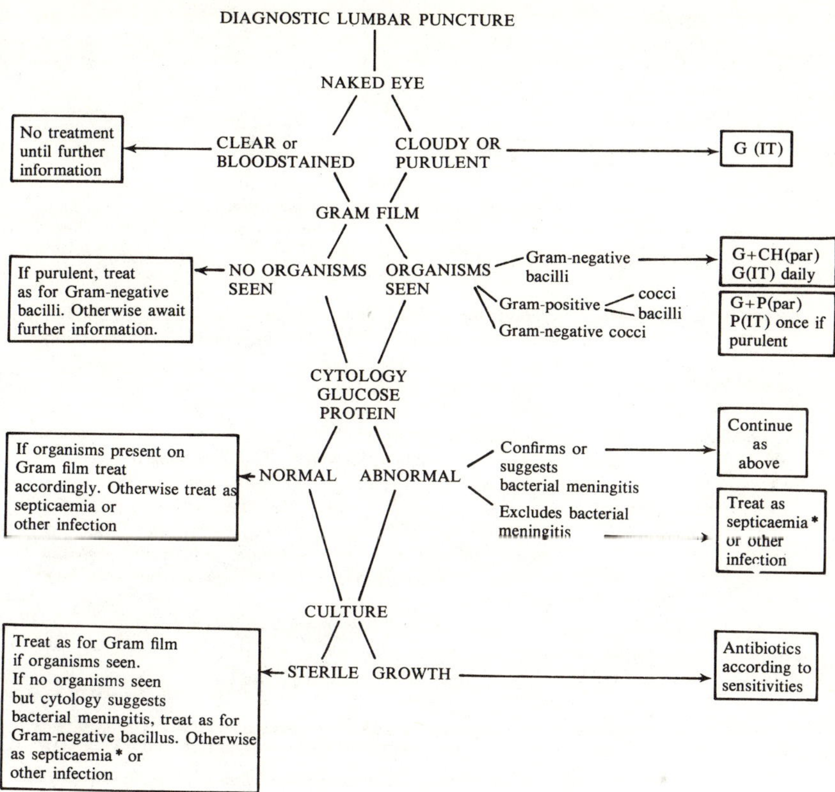

Figure 36.1. Neonatal meningitis: outline of recognition and initial management. CH = *chloramphenicol*, G = *gentamicin*, P = *benzylpenicillin*, IT = *intrathecal*, Par = *parenteral*

* Antibiotics for septicaemic illness with unidentified organism: use G + P parenterally.

of bacterial meningitis, both blood and CSF should be cultured anaerobically.

MANAGEMENT (*See* Table 36.I)

If in doubt, the infant should be treated for meningitis.

NOTE: Diagnostic lumbar puncture must be postponed until after appropriate treatment in severe shock, repeated fits or if there is evidence of brain herniation (p. 359).

(a) Endotoxic shock

This may require IV plasma (pooled plasma is being replaced by Plasma-Protein Fraction (PPF) and hydrocortisone (p. 107).

(*b*) *Anticonvulsants*

Phenobarbitone (7.5 mg i.m. at 12-hourly intervals) should be given to prevent fits. Actual fits may require treatment initially with diazepam i.m. or IV (p. 318).

TABLE 36.II
Treatment of the commoner forms of neonatal meningitis

Infecting organism	Antibiotics: dose per 24 hours	Alternatives[1]
E. coli[2] or no organisms identified	Chloramphenicol IV 50–100 mg per kg[3] + gentamicin i.m. 7.5 mg per kg Gentamicin IT 1–2 mg	Ampicillin IV 200 mg per kg in place of chloramphenicol
Pseudomonas and proteus	Carbenicillin IV 400 mg per kg + gentamicin as above i.m. and IT	Colistin i.m. 2.5–5 mg per kg IT 0.2–0.8 mg in place of gentamicin
Group B Streptococcus[4]	Benzylpenicillin IV 250 000 units per kg	Chloramphenicol in place of benzylpenicillin
Listeria	Benzylpenicillin as above + gentamicin i.m. and IT as above	Ampicillin for benzylpenicillin Gentamicin may be omitted

[1] Alternatives are indicated by the results of bacterial sensitivity or some contra-indication in the infant (penicillin sensitivity is very rare in the newborn).
[2] Similar treatment for other Gram-negative bacilli. except Pseudomonas and Proteus.
[3] For the first week of life in term infants (> 37 weeks) and for the first 4 weeks in pre-term infants the dose of chloramphenicol is 25 mg per kg per 24 hours.
   After the end of the first week of life in term infants and the first 4 weeks in pre-term infants the dose should be 50 mg per kg per 24 hours for all infections except meningitis, in which a dose of 100 mg per kg should be used.
[4] Similar treatment for other streptococci except *S. faecalis* (enterococcus) in which ampicillin should be used.

NOTE: *See* Appendix 9 page 790 for the dosage of parenteral antibiotics singly or in combination, and dosage intervals.

ANTIBIOTICS

Two antibiotics should be used initially and should be continued until the organism and its sensitivities have been identified from CSF or blood culture, and a second CSF has been examined 48 hours after starting treatment. These two antibiotics should consist of one which has adequate penetration into the CSF when given parenterally and one which is suitable for both parenteral and intrathecal (IT) treatment (*see* Table 36.III for IT dosages). McCracken and Mize (1976) have thrown some doubt on the efficacy of IT treatment in infections due to Gram-negative bacilli, but most centres appear to be continuing its use. Currently the most effective *initial* combination consists of chloramphenicol IV with gentamicin i.m. and intrathecally.

(a) Initial intrathecal treatment at diagnostic lumbar puncture
If the fluid is cloudy or purulent, 1.0 to 2.0 mg of gentamicin (intrathecal preparation) should be injected.

(b) Combination of antibiotics based upon Gram film
If the Gram film shows organisms which are likely to be sensitive to benzylpenicillin (Gram-negative or Gram-positive cocci, Gram-positive bacilli) this should be used in combination with parenteral gentamicin, and these two antibiotics should be continued until the results of CSF culture are known. If Gram-negative bacilli are seen, treatment with chloramphenicol and gentamicin should be continued with *daily* gentamicin IT.

(c) Final combination of antibiotics based upon culture and sensitivity

When the actual organism and its sensitivities are known (usually at 24 hours) the best combination of antibiotics can be chosen.

    (i)   If the organism is sensitive to benzylpenicillin further treatment with gentamicin, either parenterally or intrathecally is usually unnccccssary.

TABLE 36.III
Intrathecal preparations of antibiotics currently available

Antibiotic	Birth to 1 year*	Other ages
Ampicillin	5 up to 10 mg	10 up to 40 mg
Carbenicillin	10 mg	Up to 2 years: 10 mg
		2–12 years: 20 mg
		Over 12 years: 40 mg
Cephaloridine	0.5 mg/kg	Adult 50 mg
Chloramphenicol	5–10 mg	10–50 mg
Cloxacillin	as for Ampicillin	
Colistin	0.2 up to 0.8 mg	Adult 2–5 mg
Gentamicin	1–2 mg	Adult 8 mg
Kanamycin	2–3 mg	Adult 10 mg
Benzylpenicillin	1.5 mg (2500 units)	6 mg (10 000 units)
Streptomycin	1.0 mg/kg	Up to 50 mg

* The smaller doses are for newborn infants (up to 4 weeks of age)

    (ii) Penicillin-resistant staphylococcal infections require a change to cloxacillin and one of these should be given IT if the organism is insensitive to gentamicin or the CSF was purulent.

   (iii) Infection due to Gram-negative bacilli requires continued treatment with chloramphenicol and gentamicin unless the sensitivities indicate a change. (For unusual or difficult infections, *see* page 357).

Treatment at 48 hours   (i) In cases not requiring daily IT treatment a second lumbar puncture should be done to assess progress. Failure to sterilize the CSF or an increase in cell count are indications for a review of treatment and a ventricular tap (*see below*). (ii) A persistently positive culture at 48 to 72 hours with daily intrathecal treatment is also an indication for ventricular tap (*see below*)

Penetration into the CSF   Of the commonly used antibiotics, only chloramphenicol, ampicillin and benzylpenicillin achieve effective levels in the CSF when given in high dosage parenterally; but the results with ampicillin have been variable. The advantages of chloramphenicol over ampicillin considerably outweigh the possible dangers of 'Grey syndrome' or marrow depression provided chloramphenicol is used in the correct dosage. Even chloramphenicol however cannot be relied on to prevent ventriculitis.

(*d*) *Duration of treatment*

   (i) Parenteral treatment. For Gram-positive organisms treatment should be continued for two weeks; for Gram-negative bacilli treatment should continue for 3 weeks or for 2 weeks after the CSF has been sterile.

  (ii) Intrathecal treatment. In pneumococcal or staphylococcal infections with purulent CSF daily IT treatment should be continued until the cell count has improved and the fluid is sterile.

      In infection with Gram-negative bacilli daily IT treatment should be continued until the CSF has been sterile on 4 successive days.

Difficult or unusual infections

  (a) No organism identified in spite of clear evidence (clinical picture, cell count) of meningitis. This may be due to treatment with antibiotics before diagnostic lumbar puncture, an anaerobic infection or to a viral infection mimicking bacterial meningitis. Treatment should be given on the basis of an infection with Gram-negative bacilli.

  (b) *Pseudomonas meningitis*. This is particularly difficult to treat because of the limited number of suitable antibiotics, and because those to which the organism is usually sensitive are not those with adequate penetration into the CSF from the blood.

Prolonged intrathecal treatment is therefore always necessary. Antibiotics to which the organism may be sensitive are:
Gentamicin
Colistin
Kanamycin
Tobramycin (contra-indicated since no IT preparation is available)
Carbenicillin
Owing to their chemical similarities, the aminoglycosides (gentamicin, kanamycin, tobramycin) cannot be used in combination without the risk of oto- or nephrotoxicity. Carbenicillin can be used with any of the drugs listed above, but should not be given alone since the organism may become resistant during the course of treatment.

(c) *Anaerobic infections (Bacteroides and Fusobacterium)* An anaerobic infection should be suspected where there is obvious meningitis, but no growth on aerobic culture. Both these organisms are Gram-negative bacilli and may be mistaken for coliforms on the film. They are resistant to benzylpenicillin but sensitive to chloramphenicol and clindamycin, and occasionally to carbenicillin. Clindamycin has poor penetration into the CSF and cannot be injected IT or into the ventricles, therefore chloramphenicol is the drug of choice. In a resistant case with ventriculitis, metronidazole (Flagyl, 30 mg per kg) orally has been successfully used (Feldman, 1976).

(d) *Listeria meningitis.* Initial symptoms are those of a septicaemia, sometimes with dyspnoea or tachypnoea. The organisms are usually sensitive to benzylpenicillin, gentamicin or ampicillin. Intrathecal treatment is not necessary. Treatment should be with benzylpenicillin and gentamicin or with ampicillin alone

Acute complications

(a) Ventriculitis

This is the commonest cause of therapeutic failure (McCracken and Mize, 1976; Yeung, 1976) and should be suspected if:

(i) There is a positive culture after 72 hours of treatment.

(ii) There is no improvement in the general condition after 3 days of treatment, *even if the lumbar CSF is sterile.*

(iii) There is deterioration in the general condition at any time during treatment, with the onset of fits, bulging fontanelle, tonic fits or the head circumference is increasing quicker than 1 mm per day. If any of these indications are present bilateral ventricular taps should be done. Treatment with intraventricular antibiotics, by repeated taps, or an implanted reservoir may require transfer to a more specialized unit.

(*b*) *Increasing intracranial pressure and/or evidence of brain herniation. (See* page 359)

Meningitis after the neonatal period

RECOGNITION
The immediate diagnostic investigation is a lumbar puncture, but blood and nasal swabs should always be cultured at the same time. Necrotic or nodular skin lesions should be cultured, using material aspirated with a syringe and needle.
   Indications for a lumbar puncture.
   (a) Neck stiffness, head retraction, stiff back.
   (b) A convulsion in an ill or febrile child.
   (c) Drowsiness or irritability without obvious cause.
   (d) Petechiae with or without skin haemorrhages in a febrile child.
   (e) Severe shock without obvious cause (usually meningococcal septicaemia).
   (f) Otitis media or upper-respiratory infection in which the child appears more ill than would be expected (usually *Haemophilus influenzae* infection).

INTERPRETATION OF THE CSF (Table 36.IV)
   (a) A turbid or purulent fluid always indicates bacterial meningitis.
   (b) A clear or opalescent fluid (cell count < 1000 per mm^3); treatment should not be started until a Gram film, cell count and chemistry are available. All specimens of CSF should be examined by Gram film and should be cultured, even in the absence of a raised cell count: particularly in very severe meningococcal infection, organisms may be present in the CSF without pleocytosis.
   (c) Meningitis may develop after a lumbar puncture has shown a normal CSF. If this is suspected a second lumbar puncture must be done within 28 to 48 hours (Fischer *et al.*, 1975).

MANAGEMENT
Diagnostic lumbar puncture must be postponed until after the appropriate treatment in cases of severe shock, repeated fits, or if there is evidence of mid-brain or medullary herniation (*See* page 322).
   (a) Suspected endotoxic shock should be treated with IV plasma and high doses of corticosteroids (p. 107).

TABLE 36.IV
Cytology and chemistry in relation to type of infection

Polymorphs in excess		Lymphocytes in excess	
Glucose↓ Protein↑↑	Glucose normal Protein↑	Glucose↓ Protein↑↑	Glucose normal Protein↑ or normal
Bacterial meningitis	Early viral infection	*Tuberculous meningitis*	Viral infection
Mumps meningoencephalitis	Poliomyelitis	Mumps meningoencephalitis	Cerebral abscess
	Cerebral abscess		Septic thrombophlebitis
Tuberculous meningitis rarely			*Tuberculous meningitis*

Rarer causes of increased cell count with low glucose (Kocen, 1972–4) are: lymphocytic choriomeningitis, crytococcal meningitis, herpes simplex encephalitis, meningeal spread of medulloblastoma, leukaemia or other malignancy, and mycoplasma meningoencephalitis (Klimek, Russman and Quintiliani, 1976).

(b) Disseminated intravascular coagulopathy (*see* page 482) should be suspected in severely ill cases (invariably meningococcal) particularly with large necrotic skin lesions, oozing from puncture sites, leucopenia and thrombocytopenia.

(c) Anticonvulsants, either phenobarbitone or phenytoin, should be given prophylactically. Prolonged or repeated fits may require diazepam IV or i.m.

ANTIBIOTICS (*See* Table 36.V for dosage)
(a) Intrathecal treatment.
   (i) *At diagnostic lumbar puncture.* In all severely ill children a syringe containing an intrathecal preparation of benzylpenicillin should be prepared for injection if the CSF is found to be purulent.
   (ii) Repeated intrathecal treatment is rarely required except in infection with an organism which is insensitive to the antibiotics (chloramphenicol, ampicillin, benzylpenicillin) with adequate penetration into the CSF
(b) The initial combination is based upon the results of the Gram film.
   (i) Gram-negative cocci (meningococci): benzylpenicillin IV.
   (ii) Gram-negative bacilli or coccobacilli (probably Haemophilus): chloramphenicol IV or i.m. and benzylpenicillin IV or i.m.
   (iii) Gram-positive cocci (probably streptococci, pneumococci or staphylococci): benzylpenicillin IV. If there is a possibility of staphylococcal infection cloxacillin should be used in addition to benzylpenicillin until the results of culture and

sensitivity are known. Intrathecal cloxacillin should be given if the CSF is purulent and a staphylococcal infection is suspected.

(iv) No organisms seen on the Gram film. This may be the result of antibiotic treatment given before the diagnostic lumbar puncture: if the CSF otherwise suggests a bacterial infection, one should treat as in (ii) above. Rarely, tuberculous meningitis may mimic acute bacterial meningitis (*see* Table 36.IV).

(c) The final combination of antibiotics is based upon results of culture and sensitivities.

(d) At 48 hours a second lumbar puncture should be done to assess progress. A positive culture or no improvement in the cell count requires reassessment of treatment.

(e) If the patient has a history of sensitivity to the penicillin group, chloramphenicol should be used.

Specific infections

(*a*) *Meningococcal meningitis*

Normally, high dosage benzylpenicillin IV for 5 days is adequate treatment. An increasing number of strains are resistant to sulphonamides which are no longer indicated, either alone or in combination.

(*b*) *Haemophilus meningitis*

As in (b) (ii) above. The duration of treatment should be a minimum of 10 days.

(*c*) *Pneumococcal meningitis*

At least one dose of benzylpenicillin should be given IT initially. Cerebral oedema (p. 358) fits, focal signs and brain herniation are common. High-dosage benzylpenicillin IV should be given for a minimum of 10 days. Penicillin-resistant strains of pneumococci have been recently identified in South Africa and may become more common; if penicillin resistance is likely chloramphenicol should be used IV and, in severe cases, IT also.

(*d*) *Tuberculous meningitis*

Usually the onset is less acute than in other forms of bacterial meningitis, but occasionally the history is short and the CSF findings may mimic an acute bacterial or viral infection (Table 36.IV). If there is any possibility of tuberculous meningitis, tubercle bacilli should be looked

TABLE 36.V

Treatment of the commoner forms of meningitis after the neonatal period

Infecting organism	Antibiotics: dose /24 hours*	Alternatives†
No organism identified	Chloramphenicol 100 mg/kg IV or i.m. Benzylpenicillin 300 000 units/kg IV or i.m.	Ampicillin 400 mg/kg IV or i.m.
H. influenzae	As above	As above
Meningococcus	Benzylpenicillin 300 000 units/kg IV or i.m.	Chloramphenicol 100/kg IV or i.m. for benzylpenicillin
Pneumococcus	As above	Chloramphenicol as above
Staphylococcus	Benzylpenicillin in twice above dose + cloxacillin 100–200 mg/kg IV until sensitivity is known	Chloramphenicol as above

* *See* Appendix 9 for methods of giving parenteral antibiotics singly or in combination, and intervals of dosage.

† Alternatives are indicated either by the results of bacterial sensitivities or a history of penicillin sensitivity in the patient. For patients sensitive to the penicillin group, chloramphenicol is the best alternative antibiotic in meningitis.

for in the deposit of from 10 to 20 ml of centrifuged fluid. Additional evidence of tuberculous meningitis:

(i) Choroidal tubercles.

(ii) Enlarged spleen.

(iii) Miliary appearance on a chest x-ray or unilateral hilar enlargement with or without lobar or segmental consolidation.

(iv) A strongly positive tuberculin test (if B.C.G. has not been given previously) is not conclusive evidence; nor is a negative or weakly-positive test evidence against tuberculous meningitis.

Treatment should consist of 5 days of streptomycin i.m. (40 mg per kg at 12-hourly intervals; maximum dose 1 g) and IT (10 to 50 mg according to age), combined with continued treatment with oral rifampicin* (25 mg per kg; maximum dose 600 mg) and isoniazid (20 mg per kg; maximum dose 500 mg) with pyridoxine 10 mg daily.

Mid-brain compression due to cerebral oedema or obstructive hydrocephalus requires the same treatment as an acute bacterial meningitis (*see below*).

Unusual forms of meningitis

(a) Cryptococcal meningitis (torulosis): flucytosine is now recommended in place of amphotericin (Watkins *et al.*, 1969; McDonald, Greenberg and Kramer, 1970).

* Produces harmless but alarming red urine, tears and sweat

(b) Amoebic (Naegleria) meningoencephalitis: amphotericin should be used (Apley *et al.*, 1970).

(c) Mycoplasma meningoencephalitis (Klimek, Russman and Quintiliani, 1976); in lung infections erythromycin or tetracycline are effective and may be equally so in infections of the CNS.

(d) Plague meningitis (pasteurella pestis); chloramphenicol appears to be the most useful in this form or complication of plague (Tuan Phan Dinh, 1975).

Acute complications in the older child

(*a*) *Subdural effusion*

This is particularly common in *Haemophilus influenzae* meningitis, but may occur in other types of infection. This complication should be suspected in the following circumstances:

(i) There is sudden or progressive increase in head circumference.

(ii) There is a sudden increase in tension or bulging of the fontanelle which persists after the first 48 hours of treatment.

(iii) The development of papilloedema which was not present at the onset of meningitis.

(iv) The child remains unwell or febrile in spite of improvement in the lumbar fluid.

The diagnosis is confirmed by a subdural tap through the anterior fontanelle or a burrhole: if no fluid is obtained a ventricular tap should be attempted. Initially both sides should be explored.

(*b*) *Acute cerebral oedema or obstructive hydrocephalus in bacterial meningitis*

(i) Acute cerebral oedema is particularly common in pneumococcal meningitis, and the child may have signs of brain herniation (decerebrate rigidity etc., *see* page 321) when first seen, or the herniation may be precipitated by a lumbar puncture.

(ii) Similar complications may occur with obstructive hydrocephalus in late-diagnosed cases, particularly in *Haemophilus influenzae* infections.

(iii) *Brain herniation whether related to lumbar puncture or not is probably the commonest cause of death in acute bacterial meningitis.*

RECOGNITION

(a) Acute cerebral oedema is difficult to recognize and papilloedema is often absent.

(b) The symptoms and signs of brain herniation are more fully described on pages 321–322 but Williams, Swanson and Chapman (1964) have described the progression of events in acute bacterial meningitis with brain herniation.

(1) Hemiplegic signs with bilateral extensor plantar reflexes.
(2) Unilateral clonic convulsions.
(3) Cheyne–Stokes respiration progressing to hyperventilation.
(4) Decerebrate attacks (tonic spasms) progressing to decerebrate rigidity (*see* pages 322, 728).
(5) Pupils may become fixed in mid-position, later becoming fixed and dilated.

MANAGEMENT (for essential information on management *see* pages 323, 728)

(a) *Evidence of brain herniation is an emergency and an absolute contra-indication to lumbar puncture.*
(b) *Development of neurological evidence of brain herniation during or after a lumbar puncture is an emergency.*
(c) If bacterial meningitis is suspected in the presence of papilloedema, probable cerebral oedema or evidence of brain herniation, A LUMBAR PUNCTURE MUST BE DELAYED UNTIL AFTER TREATMENT OF THE RAISED PRESSURE AND SHOULD BE DONE ONLY WHEN EVIDENCE OF BRAIN HERNIATION HAS DISAPPEARED.
(d) CSF obtained from the subarachnoid space or lateral ventricle may be helpful in diagnosis.
(e) Parenteral antibiotics should be started *before* a lumbar puncture even if this reduces the possibility of culturing an organism from the lumbar CSF later.

References

Apley, J., Clarke, S. K. R., Roome, A. P. C. H., Sandry, S. A., Saygi, G., Silk, B. and Warhurst, D. G. (1970). Primary amoebic meningoencephalitis in Britain. *Br. med. J.* **(i)**, 596

Feldman, W. E., (1976). Bacteroides fragilis ventriculitis and meningitis. *Am. J. Dis. Child.* **130**, 880

Fischer, G. W., Brenz, R. W., Alden, E. R. and Beckwith, J. B. (1975). Lumbar punctures and meningitis. *Am. J. Dis. Child.* **129**, 590

Klimek, J. J., Russman, B. S. and Quintiliani, R. (1976). Mycoplasma pneumoniae meningoencephalitis and transverse myelitis in association with low cerebrospinal fluid glucose. *Pediatrics,* **58**, 133

Kocen, R. S. (1972–74). Infective and inflammatory disorders. In *Diseases of the Nervous System* (4). *Medicine* **No. 34**, 1989

McCracken, G. H. and Mize, S. G. (1976). A controlled study of intrathecal antibiotic therapy in Gram-negative enteric meningitis of infancy. *J. Pediat.* **89**, 66

McDonald, R., Greenberg, E. N. and Kramer, R. (1970). Cryptococcal meningitis. *Archs Dis. Childh.* **45**, 417

Tuan, Phan Dinh (1975). In *Pediatric Therapy,* 5th edn. Ed. H. C. Shirkey. pp. 451–452. St Louis: C. V. Mosby

Watkins, J. S., Campbell, M. J., Gardner-Medwin, D., Ingham, H. R. and Murray, I. G. (1969). Two cases of cryptococcal meningitis, one treated with 5-fluorocytosine. *Br. med. J.* **(iii)**, 29

Williams, C. P. S., Swanson, A. G. and Chapman, J. T. (1964). Brain swelling with acute purulent meningitis. *Pediatrics* **34**, 220

Yeung, C. Y. (1976). Intrathecal antibiotic therapy for neonatal meningitis. *Archs Dis. Childh.* **51**, 686

CRITICAL REVIEW OF ANTIBIOTICS IN ACUTE INFECTIONS

McCracken, G. H. and Eichenwald, H. F. (1974). Antimicrobial therapy: therapeutic recommendations and a review of newer drugs. *J. Pediat.* **85**, Part I, p. 297; Part II, p. 451

CHAPTER 37

Expanding Lesions in the Head

Ian A. McKinlay

Most expanding lesions in the head do not require emergency treatment at the time of diagnosis. Exceptions are those in patients with signs of raised intracranial pressure, status epilepticus, cerebral abscess or empyema, subdural or large intracerebral haematomas and those with bulbar palsy.

RECOGNITION

Signs of raised intracranial pressure

> (a) Rising pulse rate, respiratory rate and blood pressure.
> (b) Deteriorating conscious-level—initially loss of highest mental functions.
> (c) Stiffness of the neck, stridor and dysphagia.
> (d) Tense fontanelle or intracranial bruit.
> (e) Papilloedema (only found in 50 per cent cases).
> (f) Dilatation or constriction and sluggish reaction of pupils.
> (g) Bradycardia and Cheyne–Stokes respiration.

MANAGEMENT

Hazards of lumbar puncture in raised intracranial pressure (see also page 727)

Lumbar puncture is not an appropriate means of routine investigation of intracranial tumours (or subdural haematomas) or even abscesses except in special circumstances, e.g. for air-encephalography or if meningitis is thought to coexist with an abscess. The CSF is usually normal in patients with gliomas and is often unhelpful in patients with cerebral abscess, when it may be normal or show a slight lymphocytosis if the abscess is near the meninges. CT, electroencephalography and angiography are much safer and more reliable investigations in most cases. If not available, transfer of the patient should be arranged. If, after discussion with a neurosurgeon, a lumbar puncture is performed a fine needle should be used and the pressure directly measured (rate of drip of fluid is unreliable). Queckenstedt's test should never be attempted and the patient should be frequently monitored for evidence of deterioration for 24 hours as 'coning' can occur many hours after the lumbar puncture. As little CSF as possible should be withdrawn. (*See also* page 728).

Cerebral abscess

RECOGNITION

This should be suspected in the following circumstances:
  (a) Unexplained raised intracranial pressure with a short history.
  (b) Patients whose conscious level or neurological state does not seem consistent with an obvious infection, e.g. meningitis, sinusitis, acute or chronic otitis media (abscess is now more common in acute than chronic otitis media). 40 per cent cases have fits. The site of the known infection may give a clue to the site of the abscess.
  (c) After compound head injury with neurological deterioration.
  (d) In vague illness with malaise, vomiting, failure to thrive, fits and often drowsiness or irritability. There may be focal neurological signs. 30 per cent cases have no fever, leucocytosis or raised ESR. Toddlers and older children with cyanotic congenital heart disease are especially susceptible.

INVESTIGATIONS
  (a) Skull x-ray (sutures, sinuses, mastoids, fractures, osteomyelitis).
  (b) EEG—focal slow-wave activity is helpful evidence.
  (c) Cerebral scan; isotope or computerized axial tomography if available.
  (d) Blood culture.
  (e) Full blood count and ESR.
  (f) Angiography (blush round avascular area and associated oedema; multiple abscesses may be demonstrated. Often not suitable in polycythaemic patients.

MANAGEMENT
  (a) Empirical antibiotics (e.g. intravenous cloxacillin and ampicillin or gentamicin) are often indicated before drainage which, if performed prematurely, may be unsuccessful and even harmful.
  (b) Drainage by a neurosurgeon is indicated if the patient is deteriorating or when the situation is more stable.

Subdural empyema

Presentation and primary source of infection are similar to cerebral abscess. It is commoner in later childhood and in boys more than girls. Early neurosurgical drainage by burrhole is indicated; bilateral collections are common.

Subdural effusion or haematoma (*See* section on Neurosurgery, page 312, for *Acute* Subdural Haematoma)

The commonest causes are trauma (often non-accidental) and meningitis.

RECOGNITION
  (a) More than half the patients show vomiting, tense anterior fontanelle and/or suture separation, fits, retinal haemorrhages and irritability. About 40 per cent are anaemic, 30 per cent have big heads and 10 per cent have skull fractures. If no explanation is forthcoming a full social history should be obtained, skeletal-survey x-rays requested and the child carefully inspected for bruises, state of hygiene and nutrition.
  (b) The only certain diagnostic test is a subdural tap performed by an experienced person. A size-19 subdural needle is introduced at the lateral angle of the anterior fontanelle at least 1 cm from the mid-line. The tip of the needle is advanced a few mm under the frontal and parietal bones at right-angles to the bones. The fluid may be viscous and slow to drip. Very gentle suction by syringe is sometimes necessary initially for the diagnostic tap but not for subsequent taps (performed on account of clinical state, not just because fluid is known to be present). Not more than 15 ml should be removed from each side at any one time. Air (5 to 10 ml) should be introduced slowly after dripping has ceased in the diagnostic tap to demonstrate the extent of the collection (lateral brow-up and brow-down x-rays). The lesions are commonly bilateral.
  (c) Cerebral scan and angiography are commonly positive but often unnecessary. Echo-encephalogram can be misleading with bilateral collections (i.e. no shift) and the electroencephalogram is usually normal unless there is coexisting brain injury.

Intracerebral haematoma

Sudden bleeding from a vascular malformation may cause raised intracranial pressure with an intracerebral haematoma. Urgent neurosurgical opinion is required as to the advisability of removing the clot.

Gliomas

Gliomas may cause raised intracranial pressure (*see above and below*), convulsions (*see* chapter on epilepsy), or bulbar palsy (usually brain-stem lesions). The latter may produce acute problems by causing aspiration or respiratory failure. Tube feeding or intravenous fluid, and sometimes assisted ventilation may be needed pending full investigation. Ataxia, hemiplegia or squint are usually present.

Other causes of raised intracranial pressure and differential diagnosis

Sudden, often painful, visual failure with a central scotoma, especially for red objects, occurs with optic neuritis (*compare* peripheral-field loss in papilloedema). Though the optic-nerve head is oedematous there are no haemorrhages and usually no other neurological sign unless a myelitis coexists. Optic nerve 'Drusen', a congenital malformation, can be mistaken for papilloedema in patients presenting with headache. Sagittal sinus thrombosis can be diagnosed by angiography. Benign intracranial hypertension is diagnosed after investigation, e.g. air-encephalogram. Hypertensive encephalopathy, acute encephalitis and toxic encephalopathy need to be considered. Occasionally migraine with focal signs may cause difficulty in diagnosis, especially from cerebral haemorrhage.

MANAGEMENT OF RAISED INTRACRANIAL PRESSURE
See section on Coma, page 323.

CHAPTER 38

Spina Bifida and Hydrocephalus

Ian A. McKinlay

Spina bifida: examination of newborn

(1) Inspect the lesion and record the extent.
(2) Cover with a non-adherent dressing, e.g. a *single* layer of tulle or mellolin + swabs. It may be useful to mark the lesion, e.g. with a sterile pipe-cleaner for x-ray purposes.
(3) Lie the patient prone or on one side to avoid pressure on the lesion.
(4) Examine the patient for generalized abnormalities or other congenital lesion (lesions may be multiple).
(5) Examine the head for evidence of obvious hydrocephalus or encephalocele. Record the occipitofrontal circumference (OFC) with paper tape and plot on a standard chart.
(6) Assess voluntary movement below the lesion by observation and by stimulation above the site of the lesion.
(7) Assess the state of sphincters and bladder function.

INVESTIGATIONS

(a) X-ray the skull, whole spine, chest and hips for evidence of splayed sutures, lacunar skull, hemivertebrae, other occult spina-bifida lesions, rib anomalies, cardiac abnormality, sacral abnormalities and hip dislocation.
(b) Air ventriculography may be indicated if there is doubt as to degree of hydrocephalus. Lacunar skull or silver-beaten appearance on x-ray need not mean severe hydrocephalus. A cortical thickness of less than 22 mm is unlikely to be associated with normal intelligence when present in the newborn.
(c) Assess the family situation and parental attitudes to the baby's problem. Most will rely on the informed opinion of the doctor with regard to the prognosis.

Early operation is less important than careful assessment and, in selected patients, repair by an experienced surgeon. Factors often considered to make repair inadvisable, unless parents wish it to be done, include marked hydrocephalus, hemivertebrae, congenital scoliosis, lack of voluntary leg movement other than hip flexion, and other major congenital abnormalities.

The patient not selected should be kept comfortable with attention to warmth, feeding on request, adequate relief of pain and regular sedation. This may need to be discussed with parents and colleagues.

Acute hydrocephalus

Ninety per cent of patients with spina bifida have an associated Arnold–Chiari malformation, though only 10 per cent have frank clinical hydrocephalus at birth. The clinical features of acute hydrocephalus are irritability, drowsiness, vomiting, stridor, raised blood pressure, tachycardia or bradycardia, tachypnoea or Cheyne–Stokes ventilation, tense fontanelle, distended scalp veins, pupillary abnormalities, ophthalmoplegia, papilloedema, 'setting sun' sign (not diagnostic of raised pressure, however) and neck stiffness. Apart from risks to vital functions the main hazard is rapid visual failure.

Acute hydrocephalus can occur at any time in infancy and childhood, though it is commonest in the first few weeks after birth. The OFC should be measured daily in the newborn period and regularly thereafter with a paper tape and charted to gain early evidence of unduly rapid head growth, which is more important than large head size but normal growth rate. Compensated or arrested hydrocephalus may deteriorate acutely often in the course of an infection (usually upper-respiratory tract infection) or after a head injury. Ventricular tapping of CSF through the anterior fontanelle or a burrhole may be life-saving.

The skin is shaved and cleaned with iodine-containing surgical scrub. If the anterior fontanelle is patent a lumbar puncture needle is introduced at the lateral angle and aimed for a line between the glabellum and the occiput. Ventricular CSF is obtained at about 4.5 cm in the normal neonate, and 6 cm at 1 year of age. CSF is usually obtained earlier if hydrocephalus is present. The pressure is reduced by allowing the fluid to drain spontaneously down to a pressure of not less than 80 to 90 mm of CSF. Either a reservoir for repeated tapping of fluid or an indwelling catheter with continuous external drainage will usually be instituted before later insertion of a valve. If a burrhole is necessary the best site is frontal on the hairline in the sagittal plane of the pupil. If CSF is not obtained, repeated attempts should not be made as intraventricular haemorrhage or post-traumatic porencephalic cysts can be caused. It is better to try the other side or seek expert help.

Valve problems

Every opportunity should be taken to assess the feel of valves in different circumstances. Many children with apparently blocked valves are asymptomatic and require no treatment unless there is acute deterioration. In an emergency with a distal catheter block CSF can be obtained by direct puncture of the shunt chamber.

INFECTION OF THE VALVE

Bacteraemic spread of *Staphylococcus albus* or coliforms leads to ventriculitis (and septicaemia with ventriculo-atrial shunts). This is a very rapidly destructive condition and removal of the shunt is urgently required as well as intravenous and intraventricular antibiotic treatment. After valve removal regular removal of CSF and ventricular instillation of antibiotics may be achieved either by ventricular punctures or through a reservoir inserted half an hour after removal of the contaminated shunt and an intravenous high dose of antibiotics (e.g. gentamicin and cloxacillin). The intrathecal dose of gentamicin in the presence of hydrocephalus is 2 to 3 mg and the intravenous dose 6 mg per kg. The intrathecal dose of cloxacillin is 5 mg.

CATHETER DISCONNECTION

This can occur proximally or distally. The radio-opaque markers can be found by x-ray if not palpable or visible. There may be swelling due to accumulation of CSF at the site of distal disconnection. The disconnected part usually has to be replaced, but seldom as an urgency.

OVERACTIVITY OF THE VALVE

This can cause an alarming state of 'upward coning' with shock, very depressed fontanelle, abnormal pulse rate, blood pressure, respiratory pattern, ophthalmoplegia and disturbed conscious-level, or some of these. This is commonest following insertion of the valve and also can lead to an acute subdural haematoma. The patient should be nursed head-down with liberal oral or intravenous fluids. It is commonly transient but if persistent a valve draining at higher pressure may need to replace the existing valve.

Septicaemia

This is relatively common in children with spina bifida and blood cultures should be taken in any significant infective illness. Urinary-tract infection, related to disturbed bladder function and sometimes associated hydronephrosis, or infected valves are common sources. A chronically-infected valve is sometimes associated with splenomegaly, anaemia, haematuria, cor pulmonale or nephrotic syndrome.

Fractures

These are quite common in the legs of paraplegic patients and are usually painless. The presentation is an audible crack or crepitus, swelling and bruising of the limb or abnormal mobility. Immobilization in a functional position should be achieved in the least cumbersome way and only until the callus is stable.

Abandonment of treatment

It is as well to take stock of the general state of the child if this is known, before launching into vigorous resuscitative measures for their own sake.

CHAPTER 39

Acute Lead Poisoning

Ian Shellshear

Two factors are present in most children who present with lead poisoning.

Exposure to lead based paints

This is possible in most housing built before 1950, as it was not until then that titanium began to replace lead extensively as a paint base.

Pica

This behavioural disturbance, often associated with anaemia, is so common as to be regarded as normal from 1 to 2 years of age, but usually regresses after the age of 2 years. The age of children most affected, 1 to 5 years, is closely related to mobility and exploration of the environment. Inadequate supervision and poor social circumstances are also important.

The onset of symptoms in summer, and especially in association with upper-respiratory infections, may be related to lead mobilization within the body.

RECOGNITION

Lead poisoning may present as:
  (a) Acute encephalopathy: this is usually preceded by anorexia, lethargy, irritability, loss of co-ordination and occasional vomiting. It is followed by gross ataxia associated with forceful vomiting, stupor, convulsions and finally coma. Papilloedema is usually present. Lead toxicity should always be suspected in any unexplained 'encephalitis'.

N

(b) Vague symptoms such as anorexia, constipation and colicky abdominal pains. Peripheral neuropathy as seen in adults rarely occurs in children.

(c) In the course of a screening programme or during the investigation of an iron-deficiency anaemia. Treatment with iron may mobilize lead and precipitate encephalopathy.

Increased lead intake may also be suspected when a plain abdominal x-ray shows radio-opaque flakes in the gut and especially if the x-ray is being taken because of abdominal pain. X-rays of the long bones may show radio-opaque metaphyseal lead lines. These are best recognized at the knee, wrist or costochondral junction. Less frequently lead poisoning may be found on investigation of unexplained glycosuria or aminoaciduria. Any of the following investigations may be used for rapid confirmation of a diagnosis of lead poisoning.

CONFIRMATION OF THE DIAGNOSIS

(a) The U.S Public Health Service regards a blood-lead level of greater than 80 μg per 100 ml as unequivocal evidence of lead poisoning and recommends that such a case be treated as a medical emergency.

(b) Children with a blood-lead level between 40 and 80 μg per 100 ml should be tested by a calcium disodium versenate (calcium EDTA) mobilization test. If more than 0.5 mg of lead are excreted in 24 hours after an i.m. test dose of 25 mg per kg of calcium EDTA, the child has a potentially dangerous lead burden and treatment should be started.

(c) The definitive test is to measure the blood lead, preferably by the dithizone method. For this method 10 ml of heparinized blood are required. The atomic absorption micromethod is less reliable unless the laboratory is routinely carrying out lead estimations; 1 to 5 ml of whole blood (lithium heparin) are required.

In any unexplained encephalopathy the urine should be tested for coproporphyrin and x-rays of the abdomen and long bones should be taken.

MANAGEMENT

Acute encephalopathy

Lumbar puncture carries a high risk of death by 'coning' (*see* page 727) if lead encephalopathy is present and is contra-indicated. If CSF was obtained before the disease was considered, it is usually found to have a raised protein level.

Treatment is aimed at:
(a) Reduction of cerebral oedema (*see* page 323).
(b) Control of convulsions (*see* page 317).
(c) Reduction of the blood-lead level; initially dimercaprol (BAL) should be used in a dose of 4 mg per kg i.m. 4-hourly on the first day reducing to 2.5 mg per kg by the fourth day and then stopping. Four hours after starting BAL, calcium disodium versenate (CaEDTA) is started in a dose of 50 mg per kg per day IV as divided 'push' doses, or i.m. 4-hourly, for 5 to 7 days. The gut is emptied with an enema to remove the remaining ingested lead.

Acute poisoning without encephalopathy

(a) Chelation therapy as above (BAL, CaEDTA).
(b) The gut should be emptied as above but using oral laxatives.
(c) The home environment must be checked for a source of lead which should include:
> Chewed window sills or cot sides.
> Putty containing red lead.
> Lead soldiers, crayons, coloured newsprint.
> Batteries burned for heat, soft water in lead pipes.
> Stoneware storage of drinking fluids (especially if slightly acid, as lemon juice or cider).
> Housedust, soil around the house.
> Proximity to motorways and lead-processing industries.
> The father's occupation both past and present should be investigated.
(d) Whatever the presentation, the affected child MUST NOT be returned to an environment where there is still a source of lead. Prevention may involve stripping paint from walls and removing the paint chips, or covering walls with board.
(e) It may be necessary to move the family to other accommodation.
(f) A long-term plan should be considered which might involve cyclical chelation therapy as described, every 3 to 4 weeks, while the blood lead remains grossly elevated. The use of oral d-penicillamine 40 mg per kg per day, once the blood lead is reduced below the dangerous level, would then be appropriate. *D-penicillamine should not be used if there is any possibility of continuing exposure, as it will increase the absorption of ingested lead.* Treatment of the anaemia with iron therapy should be delayed until the blood lead is reduced to safe levels since iron can mobilize lead from red cells.

(g) The management of associated social difficulties and the education of parents should be considered.

(h) Siblings with a history of pica should have their blood lead checked and anaemia (if present) treated.

References

Betts, P. R., Astley, R. and Raine D. N. (1973). Lead intoxication in children in Birmingham. *Br. Med. J.* **(1)**, 402

Chisholm, J. J. (1968). The use of chelating agents in the treatment of acute and chronic lead intoxication in childhood. *J. Pediat.* **73**, 1

Chisholm, J. J. (1973). Screening for lead poisoning in children. *Pediatrics* **51**, 280

Committee on Environment Hazards. (1971). Lead content of paint applied to surfaces accessible to young children. *Pediatrics* **49**, 918

Hardy, H. L., Chamberlin, R. I., Maloof, C. C., Boylen, G. W. and Howell, M. C. (1971). Lead as an environment poison. *Clin. Pharmacol. Therapeut.* **12**, 982

Part IX: Gastrointestinal Tract Emergencies

CHAPTER 40

Acute Abdominal Emergencies

Lewis Spitz

Examination of the infant and child with acute abdominal pain

HISTORY

An accurate and detailed history is an essential initial step in arriving at the correct diagnosis. In most cases the history will be obtained from the parents, but, when feasible, the child should be consulted on the finer details.

Pain

(a) Onset

The sudden onset of acute abdominal pain in a previously well child usually signifies a surgical condition unless there is a clear history of dietary indiscretion such as eating unripe fruit.

(b) Situation

Localization is characteristically inaccurate in the young child, who, irrespective of the site of the disease, invariably points to the umbilical region. Vague periumbilical pain in the older child, except in early appendicitis, is usually of little significance, whereas pain localized to one or other abdominal quadrant is suggestive of local organic disease.

(c) Nature

It is often difficult for a child to describe pain, though he may do so by analogy (e.g. 'It pricks'; 'It feels like squeezing'). The pain may be intermittent and colicky in intestinal obstruction; continuous, intense and sharply defined as in acute appendicitis with peritonitis; or a vague dull ache.

(*d*) *Persistence*

Persistence of the pain means persistence of the cause. An attack of abdominal pain lasting more than 3 hours should be regarded as an abdominal emergency until proved otherwise. It is helpful to ascertain whether the pain is persisting, subsiding or getting worse.

(*e*) *Radiation*

Periumbilical pain which radiates and localizes in the right iliac fossa is practically diagnostic of acute appendicitis, but such a history is rarely obtainable from a child.

Vomiting

(*a*) *Relation to the onset of pain*   In surgical conditions vomiting usually occurs after the onset of abdominal pain.

(*b*) *Type*   The presence of bile in the vomitus is indicative of intestinal obstruction unless proved otherwise.

(*c*) *Frequency*   In acute appendicitis vomiting may occur on only two or three occasions. It may then cease and not reappear until peritonitis supervenes. In intestinal obstruction the vomiting lasts as long as the obstruction and is usually frequent and copious.

Bowel function

Constipation occurs in the majority of abdominal emergencies. It is important to appreciate that some parents will have given a laxative to the child before the medical consultation, and that diarrhoea from this cause should not be misinterpreted.

Micturition

Dysuria, frequency and haematuria may suggest a urinary tract infection.

PREVIOUS HISTORY
A history of previous similar attacks of abdominal pain which resolves spontaneously, especially if vague and periumbilical in location, suggests a functional rather than an organic cause (*see below*, page 388).

EXAMINATION
While obtaining the history, it is essential to gain the confidence of the

child. The position and comfort of the child are more important than that of the doctor. The most suitable position for the child may be the mother's lap or curled up in an armchair.

In the older child the examination can be done in the conventional manner, whereas in the tense or unco-operative patient subtle variations are of great value. It is wise to palpate the abdomen before inspecting it. Gentle palpation with the warm hand under the bedclothes may provide more valuable information than baring the abdomen and upsetting the child. Palpation should start well away from the suspected site of disease while the child's facial expression is observed for signs of pain, such as wincing. Having obtained the maximum information from palpation, the rest of the examination can be conducted, reserving rectal examination and inspection of the ears and throat until the end. Rebound tenderness is a sign with limited clinical value in children, is acutely distressing to the child with peritoneal irritation, and attempts to elicit it should not be made.

The acute abdomen

The spectrum of disease which may cause abdominal symptoms in the child is so wide and diverse that a complete discussion of all the conditions is beyond the scope of this chapter.

It is intended to present a practical diagnostic approach to some of the more common conditions involved in the differential diagnosis of the acute surgical abdomen encountered in the child, and to outline briefly the principles of management.

Intestinal obstruction in the neonate and infant

RECOGNITION

The classical presenting features of neonatal intestinal obstruction are: (a) Vomiting; (b) Delay in the passage of meconium; (c) Abdominal distension.

A practical diagnostic approach to vomiting in the infant is given in *Figure 40.1*.

(a) Vomiting is the only absolute sign of intestinal obstruction and when the vomitus contains bile-stained material its significance should be obvious. Unless a non-surgical cause for the bile-stained vomiting has been confirmed, a mechanical cause for the intestinal obstruction should be assumed.

(b) It is important to recognize that small amounts of meconium may be passed rectally even in the presence of a complete intestinal atresia. Failure to pass meconium within the first 24

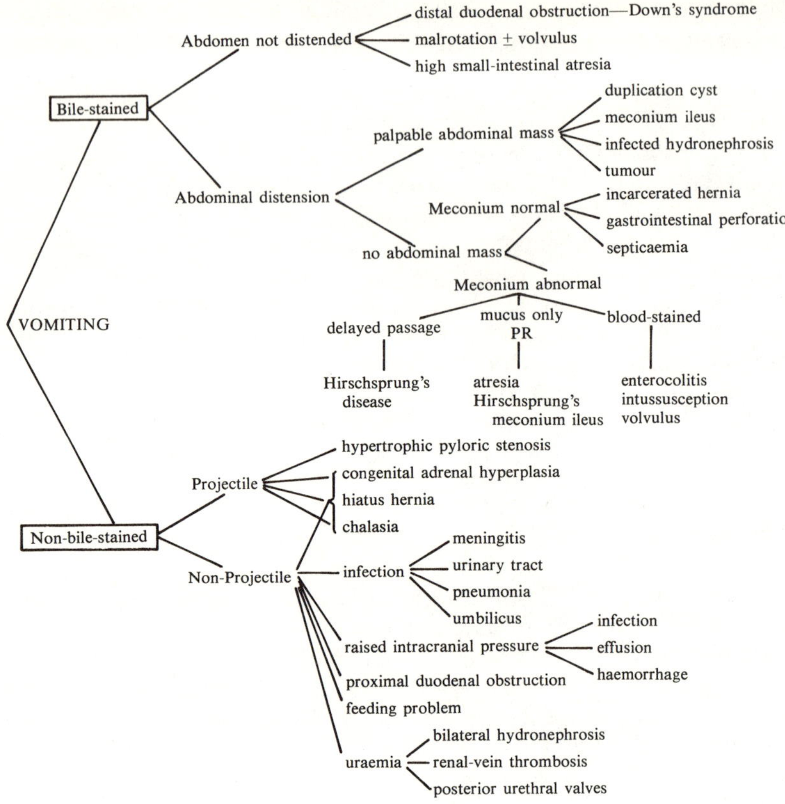

Figure 40.1. Diagnostic approach to vomiting in the newborn

hours of life is abnormal. If, in addition to this delay in the
passage of meconium, other symptoms of intestinal obstruction
are present, which are relieved by the evacuation of a large plug
of meconium following either digital examination or a saline
rectal wash-out, a presumptive diagnosis of Hirschsprung's
disease should be made, and only excluded after negative radiological, histopathological, or manometric examination.

(c) The degree of abdominal distension is related to the level of the
intestinal obstruction. In duodenal obstructions there may be
only minimal upper-abdominal fullness, whereas in low-colonic
lesions massive distension with elevation of the diaphragms,
sufficient to produce respiratory embarrassment, may be
present.

The presence of periumbilical erythema and/or oedema of the anterior abdominal wall, in addition to the above signs, signifies an intraperitoneal complication such as peritonitis or intestinal gangrene.

RADIOGRAPHY

Radiography of the abdomen is the most useful special investigation. The initial examination should consist of straight erect and supine views of the abdomen, as air is a safe and effective contrast at this age. Barium enema is reserved for cases in which the diagnosis is uncertain, and only if doubt still exists after a barium enema should a barium meal and follow-through examination be performed.

The main causes of intestinal obstruction are listed below:

Mechanical

(a) Intraluminal.
    (i) Meconium ileus.
    (ii) Meconium plug syndrome.
    (iii) 'Inspissated milk' syndrome.
(b) Intramural.
    (i) Intestinal atresia and stenosis.
    (ii) Hirschsprung's disease
(c) Extraluminal.
    (i) Malrotation with or without associated volvulus, including anorectal anomalies.
    (ii) Duplication cysts.
    (iii) Obstructed hernia.
    (iv) Intussusception.
    (v) Adhesions from previous surgery.

Paralytic (Ileus)

(a) Gastrointestinal perforation.
(b) Necrotizing enterocolitis.
(c) Septicaemia, usually with one of the following:
    (i) Pyelonephritis.
    (ii) Meningitis.
    (iii) Pneumonia.
    (iv) Umbilical sepsis.
(d) Hypothyroidism; a rare cause of ileus in the newborn.

Septicaemia and intestinal obstruction

The onset of septicaemia is usually acute, with instability of temperature, jaundice, moderate hepatosplenomegaly and thrombocytopenia, in addition to the usual signs of intestinal obstruction. The poor general condition of the infant with septicaemia, the presence of jaundice, and the diagnostic importance of the thrombocytopenia (jaundice and thrombocytopenia are not invariably present) should alert one to the possibility of septicaemia. The diagnosis is confirmed by positive blood cultures but a full 'infection-screen' should be done including lumbar puncture, examination of the urine, x-ray of the chest and swabs from nose, umbilicus, axillae, rectum and any septic skin lesions. In addition to the basic conservative measures for intestinal obstruction, i.e. naso-gastric decompression and intravenous infusion, broad-spectrum anti-biotic therapy with parenteral gentamicin, and benzylpenicillin or ampicillin should be started immediately. *Inadvertent operative intervention should, if possible, be avoided. See also* page 632 for further discussion on septicaemia in the newborn.

MANAGEMENT OF INTESTINAL OBSTRUCTION

Gross fluid and electrolyte imbalances should be corrected by intra-venous infusion before the infant is transferred to a hospital equipped to deal with neonatal surgical problems. A large-calibre nasogastric tube should be passed and the stomach evacuated of its contents before the infant leaves the base hospital and at regular intervals during transpor-tation, to prevent vomiting and aspiration. The ideal method of trans-portation for the newborn infant is in a portable incubator, accom-panied by an experienced medical attendant. In all circumstances great care should be paid to maintenance of normal body temperature. It is also important to send a valid consent form for surgery, and a specimen of maternal blood for crossmatching purposes. For a detailed descrip-tion of the surgical management of the specific lesions, the reader is referred to the standard paediatric surgical texts.

Necrotizing enterocolitis

RECOGNITION

Reluctance to feed, abdominal distension and bile-stained vomiting with the passage of blood and mucus rectally, are the first symptoms of necrotizing enterocolitis. It is more commonly seen in low birth-weight infants, and occurs especially in infants who have undergone some perinatal stress such as hypoxia, hypothermia, hypotension, or have required an exchange transfusion or infusions through the umbilical vein. The diagnosis is confirmed radiologically by the presence of gas within the wall of the intestine (pneumatosis intestinalis). Pneumoperi-toneum signifies the presence of an intestinal perforation (Plate I).

MANAGEMENT
Early intensive medical therapy, including nasogastric decompression, parenteral nutrition and parenteral broad-spectrum antibiotics (gentamicin and ampicillin) facilitate complete resolution of the pathological process in the majority of cases. It is important to continue with the total parenteral nutrition and systemic antibiotics for at least 14 to 21 days. Oral feeds may then be commenced with extreme caution. Surgical intervention is indicated in the presence of an intestinal perforation, as shown by pneumoperitoneum or signs of local peritonitis, mechanical intestinal obstruction due to stricture formation, or profuse gastrointestinal haemorrhage, and in those cases failing to respond within a reasonable period to vigorous medical therapy. The surgical procedure consists of the resection of obviously gangrenous intestine and the establishment of a proximal and distal enterostomy. Restoration of bowel continuity by primary end-to-end anastomosis in the acute stage of the disease is hazardous and contra-indicated because the intestine immediately adjacent to the necrotic segment has also suffered relative ischaemic damage. The anastomosis between the proximal and distal enterostomies should be carried out when the infant has completely recovered from the acute episode, and is thriving.

Intussusception

Intussusception is the most common cause of intestinal obstruction in infants between the ages of 3 months and 2 years. The peak incidence is from 6 to 9 months of age. The ileocaecal region is the site most commonly involved, although any part of the intestine may be affected.

RECOGNITION
Clinical presentation:
  (a) Colicky abdominal pain.
  (b) Vomiting.
  (c) Presence of a 'sausage-shaped' abdominal mass.
  (d) Passage of blood and mucus *per rectum*.
The onset of an intussusception is usually acute, with the development of the classical paroxysms of screaming and drawing up of the knees, accompanied by pallor but in 10 per cent there is no obvious colic. Attacks usually last between 1 and 2 minutes and the interval between the attacks varies from 15 to 30 minutes. Vomiting is usual, but not invariable, and is initially confined to gastric contents only, but in the neglected case with longstanding intussusception the vomiting becomes faecal. The presence of the 'sausage-shaped' abdominal mass is often difficult or impossible to detect, as it may lie beneath the edge of the liver. The mass may be easier to find in a sleeping relaxed child

(sedation may be helpful). The passage of blood and mucus *per rectum* may be delayed for a number of hours (and in some cases is not seen); its appearance on the examining finger after a rectal examining may lead to a diagnosis, but to wait for its occurrence is not good practice. Early diagnosis is important, for after 24 hours the complications rise significantly.

CONFIRMATION OF THE DIAGNOSIS

The diagnosis of intussusception is usually based on the clinical features. A plain film of the abdomen may show air outlining the head of the intussusception which appears as a soft-tissue mass. It may show evidence of intestinal obstruction or an absence of gas in the right iliac fossa. The barium enema for purely diagnostic purposes is reserved for cases in which the clinical diagnosis is inconclusive.

MANAGEMENT

Nasogastric decompression and correction of fluid and electrolyte imbalance are essential before definitive treatment.

Hydrostatic reduction by barium enema is the treatment of choice for the early uncomplicated case. It is contra-indicated in the presence of intestinal obstruction and in the ill, toxic infant who may need resuscitation. Surgical management is the preferred method in cases with prolonged symptoms (over 24 hours), in infants under the age of 3 months, and in the older child where a primary cause for the intussusception, for example polyp, diverticulum or duplication, is more likely to be present. The intussusception may recur after hydrostatic reduction by barium or after operative reduction but is rare after resection.

Appendicitis

Acute appendicitis is the condition which most frequently requires emergency abdominal surgery in childhood. It is rare below the age of 2 years, but becomes progressively more common thereafter. *However, this condition must be considered in the differential diagnosis of almost every acute abdominal emergency in children of all ages.*

RECOGNITION

(*a*) *The older child*

The clinical features are:
> (i) Abdominal pain which may follow the classic pattern of initial vague colicky periumbilical discomfort, and subsequently radiates to and localizes in the right iliac fossa, where it becomes continuous and more intense. But the pain is often

felt to commence over the appendix itself. It is important to recognize that the pain of acute appendicitis may be atypical in presentation, especially in cases with prolonged delay in diagnosis.

(ii) Vomiting is such a constant feature that in its absence the diagnosis of appendicitis should remain suspect. The vomitus is rarely profuse. and usually contains only stomach contents.

(iii) Low grade pyrexia ($\pm$ 38°C (100°F)); a higher fever in the absence of frank perforation or localized abscess is against the diagnosis of acute appendicitis and is more in favour of mesenteric adenitis of viral origin.

(iv) Bowel habits are generally normal. Mild constipation is common but diarrhoea may occur in the presence of a pelvic abscess.

(v) Frequency and pain on micturition are not uncommon and may indicate an inflamed appendix lying in contact with the bladder.

(vi) Loss of appetite is characteristic.

(vii) On examination the child usually lies still and in one fixed position, as movement of the abdomen is painful. It is often obvious that respiratory movement of the lower abdomen is restricted. Localized abdominal tenderness and guarding in the right iliac fossa are the physical signs of an unruptured appendicitis. Rebound tenderness is of no diagnostic value in the child. Involuntary muscle spasm (rigidity) in the right iliac fossa generally indicates a perforated appendicitis with localized peritonitis. A rectal examination, which should be performed as gently as possible, may reveal tenderness or a mass projecting into the anterior wall of the rectum.

(b) The child under 2 years of age

Appendicitis in infancy is usually characterized by a prolonged delay in diagnosis due to the absence of recognizable abdominal signs, a high incidence of perforation (over 80 per cent) and significant mortality (10 per cent) and morbidity (50 per cent) rates. The young infant usually presents with non-specific symptoms such as lethargy, irritability, vomiting and pyrexia. Abdominal distension and tenderness are late signs and usually consequent upon rupture and peritonitis. *Diarrhoea is more common than constipation.*

DIAGNOSIS

Appendicitis is generally a clinical diagnosis based on objective signs, but investigations may be helpful. A polymorphonuclear leucocytosis of 12 000 to 18 000 per mm³ is commonly but not invariably present. The plain abdominal x-rays may reveal localized ileus in the right iliac fossa. The presence of a calcified faecolith should be regarded as pathognomonic of appendicitis. In early acute pyelonephritis pus cells may not be found in the urine but pain is likely to be felt in the costovertebral angle, i.e. even higher than with a retrocaecal appendicitis. The final diagnosis should be based on objective abdominal findings: *when these are absent or inconclusive the child should be kept under observation in hospital and the physical signs reviewed at regular intervals.*

MANAGEMENT

The acutely ill child with a longstanding perforated appendicitis and peritonitis may present with dehydration and shock. In such cases surgery should be delayed while intensive preoperative resuscitation is carried out. This should include nasogastric decompression, intravenous fluid therapy commencing with 20 ml per kg of plasma (or plasma-protein fraction) delivered within the first hour followed by half-normal saline (0.45 per cent NaCl with 2.5 per cent glucose) solution. Preoperative parenteral antibiotics (gentamicin 6.0 mg per kg per day and lincomycin 10 to 20 mg per kg per day) should be started immediately. This choice of antibiotic cover will provide protection against Gram-positive and negative organisms, as well as the anaerobic bacteroides. The surgical treatment is removal of the inflamed appendix whenever possible. In the case of localized perforated appendicitis with abscess formation where the appendix is difficult to isolate, drainage of the abscess cavity should be performed and the child submitted to appendicectomy 6 to 8 weeks later.

Trauma

Accidental injuries of various types are responsible for over half the deaths in boys between 5 and 14 years of age and for nearly 40 per cent of the total in girls of the same age group. Over 90 per cent of abdominal injuries in childhood are caused by blunt trauma. In order of frequency, the spleen, genito-urinary tract, liver, gastrointestinal tract and pancreas are the organs most commonly involved. A complete physical examination is essential to exclude injuries to other parts of the body, e.g. head injury. Injuries to the abdomen may also result from a blow from the hand (*see* Non-Accidental Injury, page 515).

RECOGNITION

Persistent abdominal tenderness is the most consistent physical sign of an abdominal visceral injury. When this is accompanied by the overt

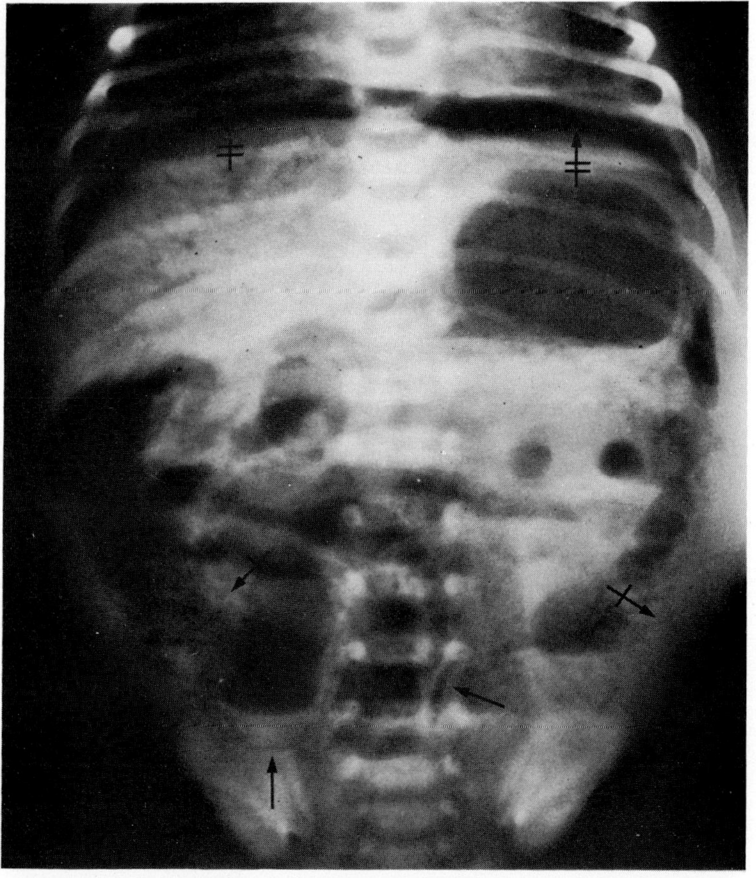

Plate I. *Radiological appearances which may be seen in necrotizing enterocolitis. In addition to gas in the portal venous system in the liver, the following can be seen: Intramural gas producing a halo effect (arrows); Small gas bubbles in the bowel wall producing an appearance similar to that of faecal contents, which is not a normal finding in this age group (single-barred arrows); Free air under the diaphragm (pneumoperitoneum) (double-barred arrows)*

signs of hypovolaemic shock the diagnosis of a ruptured liver, spleen, or kidney is readily apparent. Splenic injury may present less dramatically, with a persistent tachycardia or unexplained pallor. The presence of haematuria, whether macro-or microscopic, demands urgent investigation with intravenous pyelography. Routine erect and supine x-rays of the abdomen and haematological investigations including haematocrit, leucocyte count and serum amylase should be carried out in all cases with suspected visceral injury.

MANAGEMENT

Laparotomy should be performed only after adequate resuscitation and when sufficient quantities of compatible blood are available for transfusion. *In cases with severe liver trauma continuing rapid loss of blood may preclude attempts at resuscitation and urgent exploration may be life-saving.*

Gastrointestinal bleeding (blood in the stool)

(*See* page 396 for further discussion including haematemesis)

The main causes of gastrointestinal haemorrhage in infancy and childhood can be conveniently divided into conditions occurring in the first year of life and those occurring in the older child (Table 40.1).

TABLE 40.I

< 1 year of age	> 1 year of age
Acute peptic ulceration	Oesophageal varices
Volvulus and gangrene of the intestine	Peptic ulceration
Necrotizing enterocolitis (neonatal period)	
Meckel's diverticulum	Meckel's diverticulum
Intussusception	Intussusception
Duplications	Crohn's disease
Anal fissure	Ulcerative colitis
	Polyps
	Anal fissure

Infectious diarrhoea (especially due to Salmonella and Shigella) at any age often produces blood and mucus in the stool. *See Figure 40.2* for diagnostic scheme for gastrointestinal haemorrhage.

INVESTIGATION OF GASTROINTESTINAL HAEMORRHAGE

    (a) Particular attention is given to the age of the child, the quantity and colour of the blood passed, the general physical condition of the patient and the presence or absence of associated signs of intestinal obstruction. The anus should be carefully inspected for the presence of a fissure before digital rectal examination.

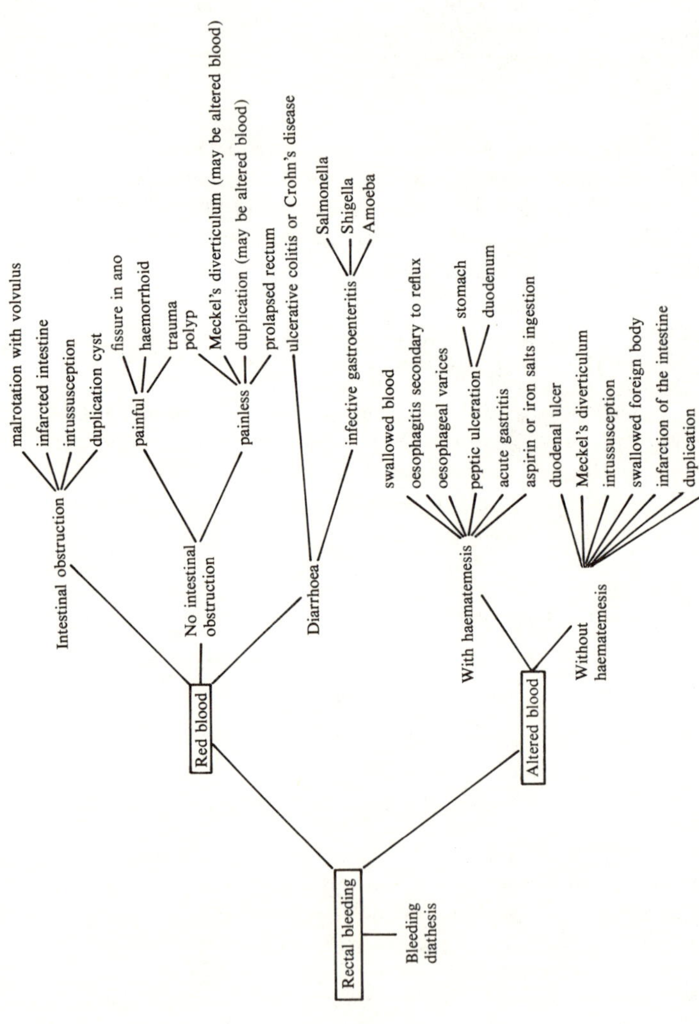

Figure 40.2. Diagnostic approach to rectal bleeding

(b) Ancillary investigations include full blood count, platelet count and screening tests for coagulation disorders (p. 482), sigmoidoscopy, barium enema and/or meal and follow-through. Technetium scan of the abdomen may reveal the presence of ectopic gastric mucosa (Meckel's diverticulum, duplication).

Rectal bleeding associated with bile-stained vomiting and shock in the neonate or in early infancy is indicative of an intestinal volvulus and requires urgent surgical intervention. Where intestinal obstruction coexists with rectal haemorrhage, surgery is indicated on the assumption that the haemorrhage and the obstruction are due to the same pathological process. In the majority of cases with minor rectal bleeding, no cause is found even after exhaustive investigation. In cases where the rectal bleeding is severe enough to warrant admission to hospital, or where repeated minor episodes occur, 50 per cent are found to have a localized gastrointestinal lesion, 10 to 20 per cent have a systemic disturbance (e.g. septicaemia, haemorrhagic diathesis) while in approximately one-third of cases no cause can be identified.

Abdominal masses

The finding of an abdominal mass in a child constitutes a surgical emergency requiring urgent and precise elucidation. Hepatomegaly and splenomegaly, which together account for approximately 50 per cent of all abdominal masses, require further investigation but rarely constitute an emergency. Of the masses which are clearly not due to enlargement of the liver or spleen, half are due to cystic lesions of the kidneys, and the rest must be considered malignant until proved otherwise. It is impossible to distinguish with any certainty intra-abdominal from retroperitoneal masses in infancy and childhood. An excretory urogram (IVP) is an essential initial investigation. Skeletal survey and x-ray of the chest are necessary to detect distant metastases. Routine haematological investigations and urinalysis including catecholamine estimation are useful ancillary tests. Arteriography may be helpful when the true nature of the lesion remains in doubt, but surgical excision and histopathological examination are the only unequivocal methods of diagnosis. The common malignant conditions encountered in infancy and childhood are neuroblastoma, nephroblastoma (Wilms' tumour), teratoma, and the various soft-tissue retroperitoneal sarcomata. The best results in the treatment of childhood malignant tumours are achieved by the combined approach of a paediatric surgeon, a radiotherapist, chemotherapist, oncologist, and radiologist working together as a single unit and adhering strictly to recognized treatment protocols.

Scrotal pain and swelling
(*See also* page 424 for other causes of acute scrotal swelling)

The two conditions which mimic an acute abdomen are irreducible inguinal hernia and testicular torsion.

(a) Irreducible inguinal hernia

The incidence of irreducibility in inguinal hernia is greatest in the first three months of life. For this reason herniotomy is recommended on diagnosis without 'delaying until the child is older'. The early signs and symptoms of incarceration are crying, irritability and vomiting, associated with a swelling in the groin extending for a variable distance into the scrotum. Only later do the features of frank intestinal obstruction and strangulation supervene. Reduction of the hernia by gentle manual pressure may be successful in the early stages. Operation can then be done within 24 to 48 hours. In the presence of intestinal obstruction or overt signs of intestinal strangulation, emergency exploration and herniotomy are indicated.

(b) Testicular torsion

The acute onset of pain and swelling of the testis is an absolute indication for surgical exploration on the provisional diagnosis of testicular torsion. The affected testis should be untwisted and anchored to the scrotum. The testis should always be retained even in the presence of apparent total gangrene. The other testis should likewise be anchored to the scrotum at the same time to prevent a similar episode occurring in the future on the opposite side.

Recurrent abdominal pain and the acute abdomen

A difficult diagnostic problem is the child who has previously been classified as suffering from recurrent abdominal pain, which implies at least three episodes of pain, severe enough to restrict activity and extending over a period in excess of three months. Such a child may at any time develop a true abdominal emergency such as acute appendicitis. Familiarity with the benign course of the previous attacks may delay the realization on the part of the parents or the doctor that the present attack is different from its predecessors, and the actual diagnosis may be greatly delayed. This situation may arise in one of two ways.

   (a) The previous attacks were caused by an organic condition and were NOT of psychosomatic origin, e.g. malrotation with episodes of incomplete mid-gut volvulus; or hydronephrosis.

(b) The previous attacks were genuinely those of recurrent abdominal pain of psychosomatic origin, but the current attack is due to an acute abdominal emergency.

It is important to emphasize the manner in which the clinical presentation of an acute abdominal emergency differs from attacks of psychogenic recurrent abdominal pain.

(i) The attack is 'different' from previous attacks.

(ii) An additional feature not experienced in previous attacks is present, e.g. pyrexia, vomiting (especially if bile-stained), abdominal distension, pain which is sharply localized (especially if lateralized).

(iii) The attack may last longer than usual.

The child with abdominal pain of organic origin will not sleep, nor will anyone else in the household.

References

GENERAL

Dennison, W. M. (1974) *Surgery in Infancy and Childhood*. Edinburgh and London: Churchill Livingstone

Hendren, W. H. (1973). Pediatric Surgery (Medical Progress). *New Engl. J. Med.* **289**, 456, 507, 562

Jones, P. G. (1976). *Clinical Paediatric Surgery*. 2nd edn. Oxford: Blackwell Scientific Publications

Nixon, H. H., and O'Donnell, B. (1976). *The Essentials of Paediatric Surgery*. 3rd edn. London: Heinemann

Raffensperger, J. G., Seeler, R. A., and Moncade, R. (1970). *The Acute Abdomen in Infancy and Childhood*. Philadelphia: J. B. Lippincott

NEONATAL SURGICAL EMERGENCIES

Haller, J. A., and Talbert, J. L. (1972) *Surgical Emergencies in the Newborn*. Philadelphia: Lea and Febiger

Rickham, P. P. and Johnstone, J. H. (1969). *Neonatal Surgery*. London: Butterworths

CHAPTER 41

Medical Conditions which may Mimic an Acute Abdominal Emergency

J. A. Black

The newborn and young infant

TABLE 41.I

Conditions mimicking acute intestinal obstruction in the newborn and young infant

Medical condition	Clues to diagnosis	Diagnostic tests	Remarks
Septicaemia with or without meningitis.	Sudden onset of lethargy, pallor, reluctance to feed, abdominal distension, jaundice, bile-stained vomiting.	Lumbar puncture Blood culture Platelet count Full blood count.	*See* page 354.
Hypothyroidism (cretinism) with ileus.	'Physiological' jaundice prolonged beyond 14 days.	Skeletal age at the knee will be delayed in term infants. P.B.I., T_3 or T_4 low. T.S.H. raised.	Occasionally occurs in older infants (*see* page 462).
Cardiac failure with acute hepatic enlargement causing abdominal distension and discomfort.	Large tender liver and tachypnoea; paroxysmal tachycardia the commonest cause in previously healthy infant, with apex beat > 250 per minute during paroxysms.	ECG may be abnormal X-ray of chest may show cardiac enlargement.	*See* page 286.

Older children

TABLE 41.II

Conditions mimicking acute appendicitis in older children

Medical condition	Clues to diagnosis	Diagnostic tests	Remarks
Diabetic ketoacidosis.	(a) Known diabetic (b) Previously undetected diabetic; history of thirst and polyuria.	Urine shows + + of sugar and acetone. Plasma glucose or Dextrostix > 25 mmol per litre (> 450 mg%).	Diabetics can also develop acute appendicitis, pyelonephritis, pneumonia, etc. (*see* page 432).
Acute pyelonephritis.	Frequency and pain on micturition; high fever and loin tenderness: sometimes previous attacks.	Urine microscopy shows white cells and organisms.	Pelvic appendicitis may cause similar urinary symptoms and slight pyuria but no organisms on microscopy (*see* page 383).
Right basal (lobar) pneumonia.	Sudden onset with tachypnoea, and high fever.	X-ray of chest shows lobar consolidation.	Pneumonia and acute appendicitis may co-exist.
Acute mesenteric adenitis.	High fever, abdominal pain and vomiting, sometimes with constipation or diarrhoea. Acute tonsillitis is commonly present.	If the pain and tenderness are localized in the right iliac fossa, acute appendicitis may only be excluded at laparotomy. White cell counts are generally unhelpful.	*See* page 383.
Acute mesenteric adenitis due to infection with *Yersinia enterocolitica*.	Continuous fever of 38.5–40°C (101–104°F) with abdominal pain; stools may contain mucus and occasionally blood.	Leucocytosis is not common. The organism can be grown from mesenteric glands but is easily confused with Proteus sp.	Infection from contaminated food (*See* page 408)
Acute toxic staphylococcal food poisoning.	Acute onset of severe epigastric pain followed by vomiting and diarrhoea. Others in family, school or other close group often simultaneously affected.	Staphylococci may not be isolated from stool, or from suspect food if this was cooked after the formation of the heat-stable toxin.	*See* page 407
Pre-icteric hepatitis. Commonly infective hepatitis A, in children.	Vomiting and abdominal pain with mild fever and anorexia.	Serum transaminases are raised before clinical jaundice. Bilirubin usually	

TABLE 41.II (*continued*)

Medical condition	Clues to diagnosis	Diagnostic tests	Remarks
	Liver enlarged and tender. Spleen may be palpable in young children.	present in urine in immediate pre-icteric phase; increased urobilin less constant.	
Sickle-cell crisis (very rarely in children with sickle-cell trait who are not usually anaemic but have positive screening test).	Commonly but not exclusively in children of African race. Anaemia and hepatomegaly; jaundice and splenomegaly are common in young children.	Sickle cells usually visible on direct blood film in sickle-cell disease, but in trait only when cells are mixed with reducing agent.	'Sicklers' are as liable as others to develop acute appendicitis, etc. Pneumococcal infections, particularly meningitis and peritonitis are common.
Faecal impaction in cystic fibrosis (*see below*).			

TABLE 41.III
Conditions mimicking acute intussusception in older children

Medical condition	Clues to diagnosis	Diagnostic tests	Remarks
Acute bacillary dysentery (commonly *Shigella sonnei* in United Kingdom). Similar symptoms may be due to Salmonella infections.	Sudden onset with high fever, severe colicky pain and blood and mucus in stool.	Microscopy of stool showing white cells, may help.	Misdiagnosis may cause admission of a dysentery case to a surgical ward or intussusception to an infectious unit, both undesirable (*see* pages 381, 406).
Henoch–Schoenlein (anaphylactoid) purpura.	Severe abdominal pain may precede or accompany one or some of the following: rash, joint-swelling, haematuria (often on microscopy only), fresh blood or melaena in the stool.	Careful clinical examination: rash if present, is usually typical; platelet count is *always* normal; ESR and ASO titre are sometimes raised but rarely helpful.	Ileus or intussusception may occur.
Meningococcal septicaemia (with or without meningitis) and attacks of screaming. Ascaris obstruction (*see below*).	Petechiae or skin haemorrhages. Meningitis may be obvious.	Lumbar puncture. Blood culture. Evidence of DIC (*see* page 482).	

TABLE 41.IV
Other conditions causing ill-defined acute abdominal pain in older children

Medical condition	Clues to diagnosis	Diagnostic tests	Remarks
Severe constipation.	History of chronic constipation; hard faecal masses in lower abdomen, rectum, and anal canal.	Relief after enema.	Acute retention of urine may also occur causing severe lower-abdominal pain.
Faecal impaction in cystic fibrosis.	The diagnosis is generally already known. Obstruction usually occurs in older children. It may mimic acute appendicitis, and intussusception may be a complication.	Sweat test. Sodium level > 70 mmol per litre.	
Mumps pancreatitis with or without salivary gland swelling: upper-epigastric pain and vomiting.	Usually other evidence of mumps. Close contact with a known case may help.	Serum amylase is raised in mumps but this may be due to involvement of the salivary glands.	
Ascaris (roundworm) obstruction.	Affects children born or living in a highly infected environment who have heavy infestation. Occasionally a mass of worms may mimic intussusception.	Microscopy of stool for ova. Ill-defined mass may be palpable. Plain film of abdomen may show worms or barium meal may outline them.	Ascariasis is almost universal in some communities, therefore the presence of ova in the stool is difficult to evaluate.
Tuberculous adenitis or peritonitis.	Masses of glands in omentum, ± ascites.	Tuberculin test usually positive. Calcified glands sometimes visible in chest x-ray. Diagnostic laparotomy is sometimes necessary.	
Acute lead poisoning with colicky abdominal pain.	History of pica sometimes obtained but often denied.	Opaque flecks in plain film of abdomen; dense lines at the metaphyses. Raised blood level of > 50 μg per 100 ml. Punctate basophilia and blue gums quite unreliable.	*See* page 369.

TABLE 41.IV (*continued*)

Medical condition	Clues to diagnosis	Diagnostic tests	Remarks
Haemophilia with haemorrhage into rectus sheath or retroperitoneal tissues.	Diagnosis usually known.	Prolonged partial thromboplastin time (PTT). Whole blood coagulation time too insensitive and *may be normal* in haemophilia. Lowered factor VIII (or X in Christmas disease).	Genuine acute appendicitis may cause diagnostic difficulty. (*See* page 479).
Malignant tertian (falciparum) malaria, with acute abdominal pain, with or without diarrhoea or blood in the stool.	Liver may be palpable and tender: splenomegaly variable.	Blood film examination *repeatedly*	*See* page 558.
Iliac adenitis	Inguinal glands may also be enlarged. Restriction of movement at the hip sometimes present.	Primary infection on leg or perineum.	
Osteomyelitis of the pelvis (iliac bone).	Onset more acute, with higher fever than in appendicitis. Abdominal rigidity and tenderness on rectal examination may be present. Occasionally fixed flexion of the hip or limitation of medial rotation.	Polymorph leucocytosis, positive blood culture. X-ray only shows changes in late cases (over 10 days).	

TABLE 41.V
Less common conditions causing acute abdominal pain in older children.

Medical condition	Clues to diagnosis	Diagnostic tests	Remarks
Primary peritonitis (pneumococcal or streptococcal)	May complicate nephrotic syndrome. Abdominal distension, with rigidity later unless ascites is present.	Needle aspiration of the peritoneal cavity.	

TABLE 41.V (*continued*)

Medical condition	Clues to diagnosis	Diagnostic tests	Remarks
Polyarteritis nodosa.	Skin rashes, joint pains, proteinuria, haematuria are common.	Skin or muscle biopsy may be diagnostic.	
Familial Mediterranean fever.	History of recurrent pain in joints, chest (pleuritic) or abdomen (peritoneal irritation).	Rectal or renal biopsy may show amyloid.	Inherited as a dominant. Mainly in Sephardic (N. African, Mediterranean) Jews. Occasionally in Armenians, Arabs, or Turks.
Hyperlipidaemia, type I.	Hepatosplenomegaly, xanthomata.	Marked lipaemia of serum.	Inherited as a recessive.
Acute intermittent porphyria.	Attacks of abdominal pain and constipation. Usually with barbiturates or other precipitating drugs. Urine may be dark, but is not a useful diagnostic point.	Elevated urinary porphobilinogens.	This type of porphyria is inherited as a dominant.
Hereditary angio-oedema.	Previous attacks of localized oedema after trauma, or laryngeal oedema. Abdominal pain due to oedema of intestinal wall.	Low level of complement C 1-esterase inhibitor, or more rarely, normal levels of an inactive molecule.	Inherited as a dominant. History of recurrent abdominal pains or sudden death from laryngeal oedema in parent or close relative (*see also* page 494).

CHAPTER 42

Gastrointestinal Bleeding (including Haematemesis)

J. A. Black

This may show itself as the vomiting of blood (haematemesis) which may be fresh or altered ('coffee-grounds'), or by the presence of fresh or altered blood (melaena) in the stool. Occasionally symptoms of shock, pallor, or hypotension may precede the appearance of blood (fresh or melaena) in the stool. Small amounts of fresh blood if not intimately mixed with the stool are easily visible, but much larger quantities have to be present to produce obvious malaena.

Haematemesis

(*a*) *Vomiting due to the presence of blood in the stomach*

Large amounts of blood in the stomach, whether swallowed or originally in the oesophagus or stomach, cause vomiting of the blood which is usually unaltered.

Common causes in the newborn:

    (i) Maternal blood swallowed during labour or delivery in an accidental (partly concealed, usually) haemorrhage. Less commonly, small amounts of maternal blood are swallowed due to bleeding from a cracked nipple, mastitis, papilloma, or carcinoma of the breast.

    (ii) Swallowed blood: epistaxis, dental extraction, a cut in mouth or nose, post-tonsillectomy.

    (iii) Oesophageal or gastric varices: this may cause a massive haematemesis. The primary cause is usually known, i.e. portal hypertension from cirrhosis or portal-vein thrombosis.

    (iv) Gastric bleeding from aspirin ingestion, either from single or repeated ingestion. This is not uncommon in previously normal individuals (Bergman, Philippidis and Naiman, 1976), but children with coagulation defects, thrombocytopenia, or defective platelet function are particularly at risk (p. 478).

(b) Vomiting of small amounts of blood

This may be due to repeated vomiting from any cause, or the blood may be vomited as part of a disease causing both bleeding and vomiting. Small amounts of blood which have been in contact with the gastric juice are usually altered, but in oesophageal disease the blood may be either fresh or altered.

Common causes are:
  (i) In oesophageal atresia, duodenal atresia or stenosis, the vomits may contain small amounts of blood.
  (ii) Hiatus hernia: this commonly presents in early infancy with repeated vomits containing fresh or altered blood.
  (iii) Haemorrhagic disease of the newborn (*see* page 663).
  (iv) Pyloric stenosis: massive haematemesis may occur in neglected cases.
  (v) Duodenal ulcer is a rare cause of haematemesis; usually in children over 8 years of age.
  (vi) Stress ulcers may cause a massive haematemesis in severe infection or trauma, and especially in severe burns. (p. 47).
  (vii) Henoch–Schoenlein purpura: a rare cause of haematemesis.

MANAGEMENT

Any large haematemesis requires immediate assessment for shock, per cent haemoglobin, blood for grouping and crossmatching; if the immediate site and cause of the bleeding are not known, platelet count and screening tests for coagulation defects should be done (p. 482). In the presence of shock, a transfusion with normal saline or other suitable fluid (p. 92) should be started and changed to blood as soon as it is available. It should be recognized that in many cases the amount of blood vomited may represent only a fraction of that which has been lost and has been retained in the intestinal tract.

In most cases the treatment is that of the blood loss and of the primary condition, but specific treatment to arrest or prevent further haemorrhage is necessary in:
  (a) Haemorrhagic disease of the newborn (p. 663).
  (b) Bleeding oesophageal or gastric varices. Initially vasopressin (Pitressin) 0.3 units per kg in 5 per cent glucose should be given IV over 10 minutes. Failure with this method may require the use of a Blakemore–Sengstaken tube.

(c) Thrombocytopenia or coagulation disorders (p. 482).

(d) Continued bleeding from epistaxis (p. 212), dental extractions (p. 169), and after tonsillectomy (p. 214).

The diagnosis of swallowed maternal blood in the newborn is usually obvious from the obstetric history, or by examination of the breasts or milk in the breast-fed infant. If in doubt, do Apt's test on the vomited material (p. 399): however, this test can only be used on unaltered blood.

Blood in the stool

RECOGNITION

(*a*) *Small amounts of fresh blood*

This rarely produces anaemia in infancy or childhood, since most of the causes are self-limiting and the loss of blood is quite small.

Common causes:

(*i*) *In the newborn*   Small streaks of fresh blood on or in the stool are quite common in the first 2 weeks of life, particularly in pre-term infants. The cause is uncertain but may be small superficial ulcerations of the lower rectum or anal canal; there appears to be no connexion between these small, usually single, bleeds and haemorrhagic disease of the newborn. An important cause of blood in the stool is necrotizing enterocolitis in which the passage of loose motions containing blood may be an early sign; but there is usually abdominal distension and vomiting (*see* page 380).

Other conditions to be considered in the newborn are acute intestinal infections with enteropathogenic *E. coli* and *Salmonella typhimurium* or related organisms (p. 406).

(*ii*) *In the older infant*   Anal fissure is common in bottle-fed infants.

(*iii*) *Between 3 months and 2 years*   Intussusception (*see* page 381) is an important cause of the passage of blood mixed with mucus (redcurrant jelly stool), with spasms of severe colic and pallor. Intussusception may occur in newborn infants and older children.

(*iv*) *At any age*   Acute intestinal infections (bacillary dysentry, *S. typhimurium*, polyp, adenoma, haemangioma, amoebic dysentery; schistosomiasis in children who could have been exposed to this infection (*Schistosoma mansoni* in Africa, Arabian States, Brazil; *Sch. japonicum* in the Far East).

(b) *Large amounts of fresh blood*

This may originate in the small intestine from a Meckel's diverticulum.
   Less common causes are:
   (i) Volvulus (under 1 year).
   (ii) Duplication of the bowel (under 1 year).
   (iii) Ulcerative colitis (over 1 year).
   (iv) Crohn's disease (over 1 year).
   (v) Henoch–Schoenlein purpura (over 1 year).
   (vi) Typhoid or paratyphoid fever.
   (vii) Acute tuberculous ulceration of the intestine (rare).
   (viii) Intestinal amoebiasis (p. 571).
   (ix) Haemorrhagic fever (Dengue) (p. 575).

(c) *Altered blood* (*melaena*) *in the stool*

For melaena to be obvious a large amount of blood must be in contact
with the intestinal contents for long enough to break down some of the
blood. In the newborn infant the passage of the blood may be so rapid
that, even if the blood has been swallowed, it may traverse the whole of
the intestinal tract and be passed in a partly changed form, with a dark
beetroot or maroon colour.
   Conditions mimicking melaena are:
   (i) Taking iron-containing preparations.
   (ii) Taking bismuth-containing preparations.
   (iii) Pica: eating earth or coal.
All will give a negative reaction for the usual tests for blood.
   Common causes of melaena:
   (i) In the newborn, swallowed maternal blood; an accidental (usu-
      ally partly concealed) haemorrhage; haemorrhagic disease of
      the newborn; Meckel's diverticulum. In all these conditions the
      blood is usually partly altered.
         To distinguish between maternal (swallowed) and fetal blood
      in the stool, use Apt's test:
      Soak the blood-stained napkin or other material in water or mix
      some of the stool, until a pink solution is obtained. Filter or
      centrifuge to obtain a clear solution. Add one part of 10 per cent
      sodium hydroxide (NaOH) and wait for 1 to 2 minutes. An
      unchanged pink colour indicates fetal blood and a yellow-brown
      colour indicates maternal blood. If in doubt, do control tests
      using blood of known origin.
   (ii) In other age groups: blood swallowed from epistaxis, or after
      dental extraction or tonsillectomy; bleeding oesophageal or
      gastric varices in portal hypertension, acute gastric haemor-
      rhage from aspirin ingestion, stress ulcer (*see* page 47), peptic

ulcer, Henoch–Schoenlein purpura, Crohn's disease, Meckel's diverticulum.

MANAGEMENT

(*a*) *Small amounts of fresh blood*

No specific treatment for the bleeding itself is required; but the treatment is that of the primary conditions.

(*b*) *Large amounts of fresh blood*

If there is shock, treatment and investigation are as for haematemesis (p. 397). The primary condition should be treated if a Meckel's diverticulum is suspected. The only method of diagnosis apart from a laparotomy (which may be required in persistent or severe bleeding) is a technetium scan in which the ectopic gastric mucosa may be demonstrated when it takes up the technetium.

(*c*) *Melaena*

Treatment and investigation is as for haematemesis. Haemorrhagic disease of the newborn requires specific treatment (p. 663), as do thrombocytopenia, and coagulation defects.

Reference

Bergman G. E., Philippidis P. and Naiman J. L. (1976). Severe gastrointestinal haemorrhage and anaemia after therapeutic doses of aspirin in normal children. *J. Pediat.* **88** 501

CHAPTER 43

Acute Gastrointestinal Infections

J. A. Black

A wide variety of organisms can cause acute gastrointestinal infections, depending upon the age and condition of the child and the climatic and hygienic conditions. The more important diseases are considered in this chapter.

General points in the management of acute gastrointestinal infections

DRUGS IN THE TREATMENT OF ACUTE DIARRHOEA
> (i) Oral antibiotics are in general ineffective but may be indicated in outbreaks of exceptionally severe *E. coli* gastroenteritis (p. 640). Neomycin and streptomycin should not be used. Ampicillin or amoxycillin may be required in bacillary dysentery (shigellosis) or salmonellosis, but in septicaemic salmonella infections parenteral treatment may be required (*see below*).
> (ii) Purgatives (such as the traditional dosing with magnesium sulphate) increase the diarrhoea and dehydration.
> (iii) Opiates such as tincture of opium and paregoric, and related drugs such as diphenoxylate (Lomotil) and loperamide (Imodium), are potentially dangerous and should NOT be given to children with acute diarrhoea.
> (iv) Charcoal, kaolin, pectin and bismuth are of no value.

ORAL REPLACEMENT OF FLUIDS IN ACUTE DIARRHOEA (for use in outpatient clinics)
(*See* Appendix 7 for details of other oral repair solutions)
Very mild cases need no treatment but should be kept under observation by the parents, and brought back if they do not get better.

O

TABLE 43.I

Organism	Age	Disease	Importance
Enteropathogenic *E. coli*	Mainly < 6 months	Gastroenteritis	Deaths from dehydration; cerebral damage from hypertonic dehydration.
Viruses (numerous).	As above	Gastroenteritis	As above but usually less severe illness.
Shigella sp.	Usually > 6 months	Bacillary dysentery (shigellosis)	Dehydration, fits, toxaemia.
Salmonella sp. (mainly typhimurium and related organisms); excluding typhoid and paratyphoid	Any age	Salmonellosis	Septicaemia, meningitis, or osteitis in newborn; septicaemia occasionally in older children.
Staphylococcus aureus (coagulase positive).	Usually > 6 months	(a) Staphylococcal toxin gastro-enteritis.	Vomiting, acute diarrhoea and abdominal pain of short duration.
		(b) Acute staphylococcal enterocolitis.	Very severe diarrhoea.
Yersinia enterocolitica.	Usually under 2 years.	Gastroenteritis	May mimic acute appendicitis.
Campylobacter enteritis.	Any age, but mainly young children.	Enteritis.	May cause severe illness with diarrhoea, occasionally with very severe pain suggestive of peritonitis.

Other infections which
  may cause acute
  diarrhoea are:
  Amoebiasis (p. 569).
  M.T. (falciparum)
    Malaria, (p. 558)
  Cholera (p. 560);
  Measles (in
    malnourished
    children).

Oral replacement of water and electrolytes may be attempted in infants with mild dehydration (up to but not exceeding 5 per cent dehydration; *see* page 88) who are able to retain fluids whether given by bottle, cup, teaspoon, or nasogastric tube, and providing the diarrhoea is not very profuse.

(a) Infants who can drink and retain fluids

If breast-fed, this should be continued and a glucose-electrolyte solution (*see below*) should be given until the infant will accept no more. This replacement should be given over a period of 4 to 6 hours and the total amount given is recorded by measuring the volume of each feed or by subtraction from the volume initially prepared. A total volume of up to 100 ml per kg over 4 to 6 hours should be adequate if breast-feeding is continuing, and up to 120 ml per kg if not.

(b) Infants who cannot drink but can retain oral fluids.

A nasogastric tube should be used, with the same glucose-electrolyte solution as in *(a)*. A volume of up to 100 to 120 ml per kg should be given over a 6-hour period. The fluid can be given initially with a 20- or 50-ml syringe and subsequently by a drip set. Intermittent giving of fluids is less likely to cause vomiting due to the gastric dilatation than is a constant slow drip.

(c) The volume to be given for maintenance and replacement over the first 24 hours

Matthews (1970) has published a simple method of calculating the fluid requirement for various degrees of dehydration (*see also* page 97), based upon a maintenance requirement of 150 ml per kg per 24 hours and 50 ml per kg for replacement of mild (5 per cent) dehydration. This chart can safely be used for mild dehydration using the oral route, but for more severe dehydration plasma electrolyte estimations should be used as a guide to treatment (p. 94) (unless an emergency arises where laboratory control is not available) and admission to hospital should be arranged if possible.

Example   Rapid replacement by the oral route over 6 hours.
   Infant of 5.0 kg with 5 per cent dehydration.
   $\therefore$ deficit $= 50$ ml per kg $= 250$ ml
   Maintenance requirement $= 5$ (kg) $\times 150 = 750$ ml per 24 hours
   $\therefore$ Maintenance over 6 hours $\dfrac{750}{4} = \sim 190$ ml

   Total volume over 6 hours: maintenance and replacement $= 190 + 250 = 440$ ml.
   This amount can be given in 3 feeds of 140 to 150 ml ($4\frac{1}{2}$–5 oz) over 6 hours.

(d) Continued oral replacement

If there is persistent diarrhoea but acceptance and retention of oral fluids, oral replacement can be continued in 'blocks' of 6-hour periods provided that the clinical signs of dehydration are decreasing and the weight is increasing. With very profuse diarrhoea the stools should be

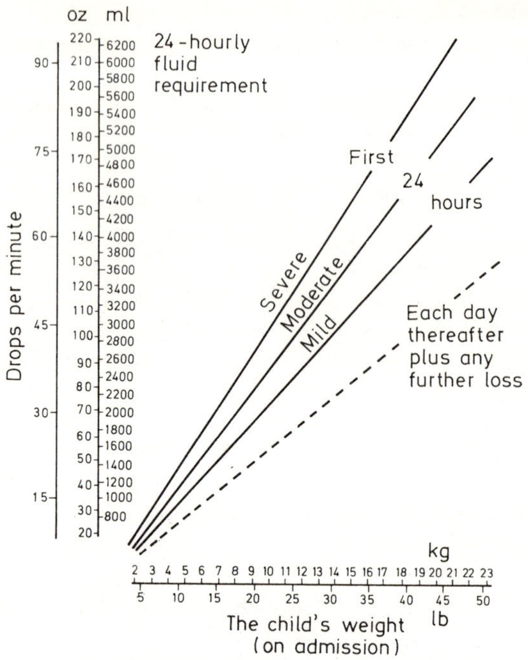

Figure 43.1. Dehydration fluid replacement chart for mild *dehydration.* (Reproduced by kind permission from Matthews (1970))

collected and the volume passed over a timed period should be used as a guide to replacement (*see also under* Cholera, p. 560).

(e) Choice of oral fluids

This is controversial: the correct replacement fluid depends upon the circumstances. In well-nourished infants fed on one of the modifications of cow's milk, isotonic or hypertonic dehyration is usual, whereas in infants in whom breast-feeding (human milk has a sodium content of 7 mmol per litre) has been continued during the diarrhoeal illness, or who are malnourished, or both, are more likely to develop hyponatraemic dehydration. Also, in cholera and other diarrhoeas of cholera-like severity the sodium content of the stools increases with the rate at which fluid is lost through the bowel (Nalin and Cash, 1976), and therefore a relatively high concentration of sodium is required in the replacement fluid. If isotonic or hypertonic dehydration is expected, one of the numerous standard glucose-electrolyte solutions should be used; e.g. GE-SOL. (*U.S.P.*), which is convenient for general purposes and has an electrolyte content in mmol per litre of sodium 81, potassium 18, chloride 71, bicarbonate 28, with glucose 7.7 per cent. This solution can be made up, roughly but sufficiently accurately, as follows:

Sodium chloride—$\frac{1}{2}$ teaspoon
Sodium bicarbonate—$\frac{1}{2}$ teaspoon in 1 litre of
Potassium chloride—$\frac{1}{4}$ teaspoon   water
Glucose—2 tablespoons

This is very similar in composition to that recommended in the W.H.O. (1976) booklet. Alternatively Darrow's solution can be diluted with equal parts of 5 per cent glucose (Matthews, 1970), giving a solution containing, in mmol per litre, sodium 61, potassium 18, chloride 52, lactate 26, with glucose 2.5 per cent. The formula in the British National Formulary (1976–8) with a sodium content of 35 mmol per litre is probably too low in sodium content for general purposes now that low-sodium modifications of cow's milk are in common use.

In conditions likely to be associated with hypotonic dehydration or very high sodium losses in the stool a replacement fluid with a higher sodium content should be used, e.g. that suggested by Nalin and Cash (1971, 1976) with the following composition in mmol per litre, sodium 120, potassium 25, chloride 98, bicarbonate 48, with glucose 6 per cent.

(*f*) *Preparation and dispensing of oral replacement fluids*

Hirschhorn and Denny (1975) make the following recommendations for non-medical personnel.

The constituent chemicals should be prepared and packaged so as to be stable in tropical conditions for some months. The packets should carry simple pictorial instructions and each packet should be sufficient to make up 0.25 to 2.0 litres of the solution. If an area has a common-use container (e.g. quart beer bottles) the contents of the packet should be adapted to this volume. The solution must be prepared daily, preferably with boiled water. Cultural preferences for colour, taste and packaging should also be considered. The addition of glucose to these solutions appears to facilitate the absorption of sodium across the intestinal wall in cholera, but it is uncertain whether this is true in other infections. Sucrose (beet or cane sugar) is NOT a safe substitute for glucose. *These solutions should not be boiled or autoclaved.*

Acute gastroenteritis

This condition has its most serious effects in the newborn, especially in pre-term infants, and in malnourished infants.

RECOGNITION (*See* page 638 as for newborn.)

MANAGEMENT
    (a) Newborn and older infants: including administrative aspects of gastroenteritis in a special care unit (p. 64).
    (b) Dehydration requiring IV fluids (p. 94).
    (c) Treatment of dehydration with oral fluids (*see above*).

Bacillary dysentery (Shigellosis)

In temperate climates this is a relatively mild disease due usually to *Sh. sonnei* or *flexneri;* in the subtropics and tropics infections with other strains may be more severe (*Sh. boydi* or *dysenteriae*).

RECOGNITION
    (a) Newborn: the infection may be acquired from the mother (p. 632).
    (b) Other age groups.
        (i) Typically this is an acute condition with high fever, colicky abdominal pain and vomiting, which precede the sudden onset of tenesmus and diarrhoea with blood and mucus. Occasionally the colicky pain may be so severe as to suggest intussusception, particularly in the age group most affected by intussusception (6 months to 1 year).
        (ii) Very severe infections may resemble cholera, with rapidly developing dehydration.
        (iii) In the so-called 'toxic' forms, there may be a very high temperature, with convulsions and sometimes head retraction, suggesting meningitis.
    (c) Identification of the infecting organism is by culture of a stool or rectal swab. The organism cannot usually be cultured from the blood except in infections due to *Sh. boydi* and *dysenteriae*. Microscopy of the stool, particularly portions with blood or mucus, shows large numbers of leucocytes and red cells.

MANAGEMENT
    (a) Dehydration should be treated, as in gastroenteritis.
    (b) Antibiotics: in the acutely ill child ampicillin or preferably amoxycillin should be given orally, or parenterally if very ill and septicaemia is suspected.

Salmonellosis (infection with *S. typhimurium* and related organisms)

This is a very variable infection which may produce mild symptoms but can cause septicaemia.

RECOGNITION
    (a) Newborn: the infection may be acquired from the mother (p. 632), or from infected feeds. Symptoms may be mild with slight diarrhoea and with occasional flecks of mucus, or a septicaemic illness complicated by meningitis or osteitis.
    (b) Other age groups.
       (i) Acute gastrointestinal symptoms may occur with fever, headache, vomiting, abdominal pain and watery stools.
      (ii) A typhoid-like condition may develop, with a high remittent fever.
     (iii) A septicaemia may resemble tuberculous meningitis, with lethargy, stiff neck (without meningitis) and splenomegaly.
     (iv) Osteitis is a common complication in Africa in children with sickle-cell anaemia.
    (c) Identification of the infecting organism is by culture of the blood (or CSF in meningitis) and stools or rectal swab.

MANAGEMENT
    (a) Dehydration should be treated, as in gastroenteritis.
    (b) Antibiotics: ampicillin or amoxycillin should be given orally in acutely ill children, but ampicillin or amoxycillin should be given parenterally in a septicaemic illness, or chloramphenicol in meningitis (p. 357). In mildly affected children there is no indication for antibiotics since they do not appear to hasten the disappearance of the organism from the intestine, nor do they reduce the incidence of the carrier state.

Staphylococcal infections

(a) Staphylococcal toxin enteritis

This is really a form of 'food poisoning' in which the toxin has been already formed in infected food, but there is no *bacterial* infection. Vomiting and diarrhoea develop suddenly, often with acute abdominal pain which initially may suggest acute appendicitis. *This is a self-limiting condition, usually of a few hours duration.*

(b) Staphylococcal enterocolitis

This is an acute staphylococcal infection of the gastrointestinal tract, usually resulting from the elimination of the normal flora by a wide-spectrum antibiotic, typically one of the tetracyclines, clindamycin, or lincomycin. Dehydration may be severe and require urgent IV correction. Antibiotics parenterally, and possibly orally also, should be given with any of the antibiotics with a high degree of activity against the staphylococcus (e.g. one of the cephalosporins). Acute pseudo-membranous colitis may result from treatment with clindamycin or lincomycin.

Yersinia infections

This is usually acquired from infected food and appears to be commoner (or more commonly recognized) in Scandinavia and North America. It may cause a moderately severe acute gastroenteritis but may also mimic acute appendicitis. The organism is usually sensitive to gentamicin, kanamycin and the sulphonamides but is not sensitive to ampicillin. Most of the cases have occurred in children under 2 years of age.

Campylobacter infections (Skirrow, 1977)

RECOGNITION
Acute febrile illness with colicky abdominal pain and watery diarrhoea, occasionally with blood in the stool. The source is usually infected food (usually chicken) or from an adult to a child. *Campylobacter jejuni* or *coli* can be cultured from the blood and from the stools using appropriate conditions (43°C and 5 per cent oxygen, 10 per cent carbon dioxide and 85 per cent hydrogen; Skirrow, 1977).

MANAGEMENT
Erythromycin stearate appears to be the most suitable antibiotic, using the usual dosage.

References

Hirschhorn, N. and Denny, K.M. (1975). Oral glucose-electrolyte therapy for diarrhoea: a means to maintain or improve nutrition? *Am. J. Clin. Nutr.* **28**, 189

Matthews, T.S. (1970). The nursing and general medical care of sick children. In *Diseases of Children in the Subtropics and Tropic*. Ed. D.B. Jelliffe. 2nd edn. p. 951. London: Edward Arnold

Nalin, D.R. and Cash, R.A. (1971). Oral or nasogastric maintenance therapy in pediatric chlolera patients. *J. Pediat.* **78**, 355

Nalin, D.R. and Cash, R.A. (1976). Sodium content in oral therapy for diarrhoea. *Lancet* **(ii)**, 957

Skirrow, M.B. (1977). Campylobacter enteritis; a "new" disease. *Br. Med. J.* **2**, 9

Wolman, Irving J. (Ed) (1976–77). Rehydration treatment of acute diarrhoea with inexpensive oral fluids. *Clinical Pediatrics Handbook II*. p. 237–243. Interleaved in *Clin. Pediat. (1977)*. **15** and **16**

World Health Organisation (1976). *Treatment and Prevention of Dehydration in Diarrhoeal Disease*. Geneva: W.H.O.

Part X: Genito-Urinary Tract

CHAPTER 44

Acute Renal Failure

S. R. Meadow

Acute renal failure is characterized by the sudden impairment of glomerular and tubular function. There are many consequences, the most important of which are failure to eliminate waste products and disturbance of acid-base, electrolyte and water balance. In general the blood urea and creatinine levels are raised and there is diminished urine output.

'Acute on chronic' renal failure refers to the sudden accelerated deterioration in renal function in someone whose kidney function is already impaired.

Causes

Although acute renal failure is often the result of a combination of different causes, it is useful to classify it into three main groups: (a) Prerenal; (b) Renal; and (c) Postrenal.

Prerenal

Poor perfusion of the kidneys does not allow the previously healthy kidney to work efficiently. The infant is more liable to prerenal failure than is the older child.

Important causes are:

Dehydration.
Severe haemorrhage.
Severe trauma or burns.
Major surgery, e.g. open-heart surgery.

Renal (intrinsic renal failure)

Despite normal kidney perfusion the kidneys do not work satisfactorily because of intrinsic disease. Important causes are:

Acute glomerulonephritis.
Acute tubular necrosis—following hypovolaemia or toxins.
Disseminated intravascular coagulation (including the haemolytic-
    uraemic syndrome).
Renal venous thromboses.
Pyelonephritis, particularly in neonates.

Postrenal

Acute obstruction of the urinary tract is uncommon in childhood.
Congenital obstructions may, however, be partial and then present as
'acute on chronic' renal failure at the time of an infection or sodium
depletion.

RECOGNITION

A careful history usually reveals the cause of the renal failure. The
possibility of 'acute on chronic' renal failure should be considered.
Previous failure to thrive, short stature, anaemia, abnormal thirst,
disturbances of micturition (e.g. poor urine stream or wetting) may
indicate longstanding renal impairment.

On physical examination the state of hydration *should be assessed*
(*see* page 95) and particular emphasis placed on careful palpation of the
kidneys and bladder. Large renal masses may be polycystic kidneys or
obstructed hydronephrotic kidneys. A large bladder may mean urethral
obstruction. A raised blood pressure is likely to mean intrinsic renal
failure, and longstanding hypertension may be associated with hypertensive retinopathy.

OBSERVATIONS

The child should be weighed every 12 hours. The weight chart will
provide the most useful guide to the fluid-balance.

Temperature, pulse and respiration should be charted at least every 4
hours and, in most renal-failure situations, much more frequently.
Blood pressure should be recorded every 4 hours using the same cuff
(whose diameter should be recorded on the chart).

Fluid input and output measurement are recorded. In most acute
renal-failure situations the bladder should be catheterized using a Foley
or other in-dwelling catheter which is left in position during the critical
first few days. This serves several purposes; the initial catheterization
ensures against urethral obstruction and allows urine to be examined
immediately. Subsequently, the catheter allows accurate measurement
of urine output and ease of access for further urine tests.

INVESTIGATIONS
Urine

(a) Ward tests.
  (i) Dipstix tests: Haematuria and significant albuminuria (Albustix ++ or more) may be associated with urine infection and obstructive lesions, but are much more likely to indicate intrinsic renal disease. Glycosuria may occur with acute intrinsic renal disorders and also be associated with longstanding renal disorders such as congenital dysplasia or cystinosis.
  (ii) Specific gravity: The most reliable method is with a refractometer, which requires only one or two drops of urine. A cheap and reliable instrument is available. * The approximate correlation between specific gravity and osmolality is:

Specific gravity		Osmolality (mosm/kg)
1010	$\hat{=}$	300
1020	$\hat{=}$	700
1030	$\hat{=}$	1000

If the urine contains ++ or more protein (by Albustix), or sugar, the specific gravity is misleadingly high. A specific gravity above 1020 indicates 'good quality' urine and suggests prerenal failure.
  (iii) Microscopy: Initially the sediment in prerenal failure may be normal. Intrinsic renal disease is likely to yield urine containing abundant red cells, white cells, and red cell or granular casts. Postrenal obstructive lesions are often associated with infected urine—bacteriuria with or without excess white cells.
(b) Laboratory tests.
  (i) Urea, sodium and osmolality: These critical measurements which can be done on 5 ml of urine, or less, usually allow differentiation between prerenal and intrinsic renal failure. Prerenal failure is associated with good quality urine of high osmolality (> 400), high urea concentration and low sodium content. Intrinsic renal disease produces poor quality urine of low osmolality (< 320), low urea concentration, and a high sodium content. The test is even more useful if combined with plasma electrolyte and osmolality measurement:

* Uricon Refractometer: ChemLab Instruments Ltd. 16 Seven Kings Road, Ilford, Essex

TABLE 44.I

	Prerenal	Renal
Urine urea: Plasma urea ratio	> 5	< 4
Urine osmolality: Plasma osmolality ratio	> 1.2	< 1.1
Urine Na (mmol/l)	< 20	> 30

(ii) Colony count culture.

Blood

Urea, electrolyte and creatinine levels are measured initially and repeated regularly. Routine haemoglobin and white cell counts are done.
If there is any likelihood of haemolytic-uraemic syndrome or disseminated intravascular coagulation, the haematologist should be asked to
look for red cell fragmentation and consumption of coagulation factors
(low fibrinogen titre, low platelet count); fibrin degradation products
are likely to be raised in these conditions (*see* page 482).

Blood culture is essential: up to one-third of children presenting with
acute renal failure have an associated septicaemia. Blood should be
taken for measurement of plasma proteins, ASO titre, C_3 complement,
and uric acid, as these results may allow more accurate diagnosis in the
long term. Serum calcium, phosphate and alkaline phosphatase are
similarly useful and in infants should be done at once together with
serum magnesium (which is sometimes significantly low).

Radiology

(i) X-ray of abdomen for renal size and symmetry and for
opacities.
(ii) Chest x-ray for evidence of cardiac failure or infection.
(iii) X-ray of lateral spine and a wrist and hand for renal osteodystrophy (suggesting longstanding renal disease).
(iv) At the time of bladder catheterization it may be useful to inject
30 to 50 ml of contrast. Even though full micturition cystography may not be possible, a film of the bladder may be helpful, for
example, in revealing ureteroceles.
(v) Early intravenous urography using tomography is invaluable as
soon as the patient is out of shock and not dehydrated. The
possibility of this investigation will depend upon local facilities
as well as the experience of the radiologist.

ECG

For evidence of electrolyte abnormalities or cardiac arrhythmias.

MANAGEMENT
The child will require a good intravenous line.

Correction of the cause

Prompt correction of the cause of the renal failure is sometimes possible.

(i) Prerenal failure requires measures which increase renal perfusion, e.g. by fluid or blood replacement. If there is any possibility of hypovolaemia it is reasonable to try the effect of 20 per cent mannitol. A test dose of 0.2 g per kg (1 ml per kg) is given intravenously in 3 to 5 minutes. If this produces an appreciable increase of urine output, then 1 g per kg mannitol solution is given by intravenous infusion.

(ii) Intrinsic renal failure is less often reversed quickly. However, large doses of frusemide early in the course of the renal failure are sometimes effective. Intravenous frusemide 2 mg per kg should be given and if the oliguria persists 5 ml per kg can be tried.

(iii) Postrenal failure requires removal of the obstruction by catheterization or by surgery.

Correction of the consequences

Children with acute renal failure are likely to have several of the following problems, each of which may require treatment in its own right.

(i) Shock and dehydration

Blood, plasma or fluid replacement need to be given with care, since if kidney function does not improve, there is an increased risk of cardiac failure. Control by means of central venous pressure measurement is helpful. Alternatively the pulse rate, respiratory rate and liver size are checked frequently for signs of heart failure.

(ii) Electrolyte and fluid overload

Hypertension, cardiac failure, peripheral and pulmonary oedema, are the features. Frusemide (*see above*) should be given. Sodium is restricted and avoided as far as possible in any intravenous infusions. Resistant fluid and sodium overload will require dialysis.

Severe hypertension and hypertensive encephalopathy require prompt drug therapy. Diazoxide 5 mg per kg is given rapidly as a single bolus intravenously. It should act within 10 minutes and be effective for up to 5 hours. If the first dose is ineffective, a second injection can be given after 15 minutes using 10 mg per kg. In less acute situations hydrallazine (Apresoline) should be given by slow intravenous injection in a dose of 0.4 to 1.0 mg per kg. It acts in 20 minutes and is effective for about 4 hours. It is important to remember that fits, encephalopathy and other serious consequences of hypertension can occur at relatively low diastolic blood pressures, for instance, a diastolic pressure of 105 mm may be most dangerous in an infant used to a pressure of 50 mm Hg, particularly if the rise has been sudden.

(*iii*) *Acidosis*

Severe acidosis requires correction with 8.4 per cent sodium bicarbonate in a dose of 2 mmol per kg. It is sometimes dangerous to give the usual full corrective dose of bicarbonate (*see* Chapter 13) in acute renal failure because of the sodium load, and because sudden correction of the acidosis may induce tetany from hypocalcaemia. General measures to relieve acidosis include adequate calorie intake and correction of factors contributing to a hypercatabolic state, e.g. sepsis or hypoxia.

(*iv*) *Hyperkalaemia* (*See also* Chapter 13, page 136)

Children withstand hyperkalaemia better than adults. Nevertheless, the serum potassium in infants should not be allowed to exceed 7 mmol per litre in infants or 8 mmol per litre in children over the age of one year.

Emergency treatment of hyperkalaemia is:
- (a) 10 per cent calcium gluconate 1.5 ml per kg by slow intravenous injection.
- (b) Insulin 0.1 units per kg subcutaneously together with 10 per cent glucose intravenously (2.5 g of glucose being given for each 1 unit of insulin).
- (c) An exchange resin (sodium polystyrene) 1 g per kg per day rectally or orally.
- (d) Correction of metabolic acidosis (*see* (*iii*) *above*).
  Careful control with an ECG or cardiac monitor is necessary during these procedures.

(*v*) *Fits*

Fits may result from hypertension, uraemia, hyper- or hypo-osmolar states, hypocalcaemia and hypomagnesaemia. Each requires specific correction; in addition anticonvulsant therapy with diazepam 0.2 mg per kg can be given intravenously. Phenytoin is also a safe drug in renal failure; barbiturates are best avoided.

(*vi*) *Infection*

Infection is common in renal failure, contributes to the catabolic state, and is a frequent cause of death. Prompt identification and antibiotic treatment is important. Care must be taken in the choice of drugs (*see below*).

(*vii*) *Anaemia*

Severe anaemia may require transfusion. This must be done with care for the fluid load can be lethal to a child whose kidneys are not working. Packed cells should be given slowly in a small amount, e.g. 10 ml per kg, and a careful watch kept for evidence of cardiac failure. Less severe anaemia is best left uncorrected.

(*viii*) *General measures*

Food and fluid   Apart from aiming to correct any initial deficiency or excess of fluid, plans are made to give fluid on the basis of insensible loss (500 ml per m^2 per day); adding an extra 75 ml per m^2 per day for each 1°C or 2°F of fever plus urine or other daily fluid output. In practice a common problem is that the solutions required for treatment of acidosis, hyperkalaemia, etc. may take up nearly all this allowance.

A satisfactory calorie intake reduces catabolism, uraemia and acidosis. In the long term a high-calorie low-protein diet may be required, but in the initial acute situation, any food which the child will either take or not vomit is acceptable.

Drugs   All drugs are dangerous, and in renal failure may lead to death. No drug should be given unless it is essential, and no drug should be prescribed without first finding out if it can safely be given in renal failure, and the appropriate dose.

Drugs metabolized in the liver are preferable to those excreted by the kidneys.

If a drug has to be given which is excreted by the kidneys it is usually safe to give the standard initial therapeutic dose, but to increase the time interval between doses by a factor of 2 to 6 depending upon the drug and the severity of renal failure.

The following drugs can be given in full doses regardless of the severity of the renal failure:

Cloxacillin	Phenytoin
Erythromycin	Diazepam
Oxacillin	Paraldehyde
Chloramphenicol	Pethidine
Methicillin	Nitrazepam
Fusidic acid	Chloral hydrate
Nalidixic acid	

The papers listed in the References give details of the modifications necessary in drug dosage for almost all drugs that may be needed in an ill child with renal failure. *See also* Appendix 10 for lists of relevant drugs.

Indications for dialysis

In the acute situation peritoneal dialysis is the method of choice. It is highly effective in children. Although peritoneal dialysis appears to be both convenient and simple, it should not be undertaken in a unit unfamiliar with its use in children. The child with acute renal failure has a multiplicity of problems which makes peritoneal dialysis a hazardous procedure. Moreover, the child is likely to need a series of further investigations that only a specialized unit can provide. A good outcome is more likely if the child is transferred to a paediatric renal unit.

Selecting the ideal moment to transfer a patient for dialysis is difficult. There is no single absolute determining factor. It is better to transfer too early than too late. It is likely to be a combination of findings and a trend in the events which points the way towards transfer for dialysis. Relative indications are: hypertensive heart failure in the presence of continued oliguria, a progressively rising serum-potassium level, severe anaemia (as in haemolytic-uraemic syndrome) associated with oliguria. Any child with a hypercatabolic state in which the blood urea is rising by as much as 10 mmol per litre (60 mg%) per day is more likely to need dialysis than one in whom the urea is rising at a rate of 2.5 mmol per litre per day (12–30 mg%). The probable course of the renal failure has to be considered also. If the kidneys seem to be recovering function, or seem about to do so, transfer for dialysis may be delayed.

Once the decision to transfer for dialysis has been taken, every effort must be made to continue the optimal treatment outlined above during the period of transfer. All the observations and recordings should be maintained. The notes, charts, x-rays and investigation results should go with the child together with any urine or blood specimen that may be available.

Prognosis

The outcome will depend upon the cause of the renal failure. Nevertheless, acute renal failure is a rewarding condition to treat in childhood; a large proportion have reversible lesions.

References

DRUG DOSAGE IN RENAL FAILURE
Bennett, W. M. and Coggins, C. H. (1970). A practical guide to drug using in adult patients with impaired renal function. *J. Am. med. Ass.* **214**, 1468

Kunin, C. M. (1967). A guide to the use of antibiotics in patients with renal disease. *Ann. Internal Med.* **67**, 151
Sharpstone, P. (1977). Prescribing for patients with renal failure. *Br. med. J.* **2**, 36

FURTHER READING

Barratt, T. M. (1974). Acute renal failure, In *Urology of Childhood.* Ed. D. I. Williams. *Encyclopedia of Urology, XV Suppl.* Berlin/New York: Springer Verlag
Kaplan, B. S. and Drummond, K. N. (1975). Acute renal failure. In *Pediatric Nephrology.* Ed. M. I. Rubin. Baltimore: Williams and Wilkins
Meadow, S. R., Cameron, J. S., Ogg, L. S. and Saxton, H. M. (1971). Children referred for acute dialysis. *Archs. Dis. Childh.* **46**, 221

CHAPTER 45

Genito-Urinary Emergencies

J. A. Black

Acute retention of urine

This is defined as the sudden inability to pass urine.

RECOGNITION

It is necessary to distinguish between:

(a) Anuria.

(b) Extravasation of urine from rupture of the bladder or urethra.

(c) Acute retention.

If anuria is suspected a catheter should be passed and left *in situ* long enough to determine whether urine is being formed or not. In rupture of the urethra or bladder there is a history of trauma. Drops of blood are usually visible at the tip of the penis or coming from the vagina; in urethral rupture there is extravasation of urine into the perineal region, and in rupture of the bladder there is pain and rigidity of the lower abdomen.

Acute retention occurring in a previously normal child causes severe discomfort. The tender bladder may be palpable (and is dull to percussion) above the symphysis pubis. In older children the bladder may not be palpable, due to rigidity of the rectus muscles, but suprapubic tenderness is still present.

In infants and young children who are unable to explain what they feel, the discomfort from the bladder may be mistaken for pain in an abdominal organ or even an 'acute abdomen'.

In the unconscious or semiconscious patient acute retention is common even in the absence of paralysis, and a distended bladder should always be considered as a cause of unexplained restlessness in such patients.

If pain and tenderness are absent it is necessary to consider the possibility of acute retention (possibly due to an acute infection of the urine) supervening on longstanding bladder-neck obstruction, or a slowly-developing neurogenic bladder. In such cases there is usually a previous history of an inadequate stream or dribbling of urine.

Acute retention due to a sudden paraplegia is also painless but other evidence of paraplegia is obvious.

CAUSES OF PAINFUL ACUTE RETENTION

    (a) Spasm of the detrusor due to 'holding on' so long that the spasm occurs. This may occur in a child (usually a boy) who is too embarrassed to ask about the nearest lavatory.

    (b) Meatal ulcer in a recently circumcized child. The meatus becomes blocked by a scab forming on an ulcer. The diagnosis is obvious on inspection of the meatus.

    (c) Chronic constipation. Very large masses of faeces are palpable in the descending colon.

    (d) Pelvic tumour. The mechanism of retention is the same as in constipation. The tumour may not have been recognized previously.

    (e) An acutely inflamed pelvic appendix. (*See* page 383)

    (f) Other causes include clot retention with massive haematuria from trauma, or occasionally in Henoch–Schoenlein purpura. Impaction in the urethra of a stone, foreign body or pedunculated vesical polyp may also occur. A large ureterocele may cause acute retention.

MANAGEMENT

(a) Spasm of detrusor

Reassurance and avoidance of panic are important. The child may be able to pass urine if left in peace in a lavatory without any adults standing over him. If this is ineffective a warm bath and a sedative are usually successful.

(b) Meatal ulcer

The scab should be softened with warm water and then removed. Further scab formation can be prevented by a gauze pad smeared with Vaseline sewn into the front of the trousers, or inserted between the napkin and the penis.

(c) Chronic constipation

An enema is all that is necessary; catheterization should not be required.

(d) *Pelvic tumour*

Catheterization may be necessary as an emergency measure. Further investigation will be required to discover the nature of the tumour.

(e) *Pelvic appendicitis*

Operation for the appendicitis is required; however if there is much pain, catheterization should be done before the operation.

(f) *Clot retention*

This can be relieved by catheterization; wash-outs may be necessary to remove the clot.

(g) *Impaction in the urethra*

The method of removal depends upon the site and type of obstruction. If there is likely to be difficulty the opinion of a urologist should be obtained.

Haematuria

Haematuria itself rarely constitutes an emergency, except when clot retention occurs, but it may draw attention to a previously unrecognized renal disease. It is sometimes possible clinically to get a clue to the origin of the blood. Renal colic clearly indicates the passage of a blood clot or stone down the ureter, and the diameter of a blood clot may reveal the size of the tube in which it formed.

Haematuria may have to be distinguished from other causes of red or pink urine: haemoglobinuria or myoglobinuria may occur under special circumstances and are easily distinguished after centrifuging the urine and by the absence of red cells on microscopy; spectroscopy will distinguish between haemoglobin and myoglobin in the urine. There are numerous drugs which cause red urine, also benign beeturia may occur in otherwise normal people after eating beetroot. A detailed history of drug treatment, food or sweet ingestion will usually provide the answer; and a negative test for blood excludes both haematuria and haemoglobinuria. A positive chemical test for blood may be found in genuine haematuria when subsequent microscopy fails to confirm the presence of red cells; this occurs when the red cells have lysed, and is likely to occur in an early morning specimen, or if the urine has stood for some hours before microscopy.

RECOGNITION
(a) *In the newborn infant*

Haematuria in the newborn is rare, though the pink urate crystals seen on the napkin during the first 2 to 3 days after birth are often mistaken for blood. The distinction is easy, either by microscopy of the deposit, or by testing the suspended crystals for blood. True haematuria usually indicates renal-vein thrombosis which can be unilateral or bilateral (*see* page 455). Rarely, a Wilms' tumour causes haematuria in the neonatal period; an even rarer cause is hereditary tyrosinosis. The vaginal 'withdrawal' bleeding which sometimes occurs towards the end of the first week of life may be mistaken for haematuria, but the cause is usually obvious after examination of the vaginal opening.

(b) *After the neonatal period*

(i) Meatal ulcer (*see* page 421).

(ii) Between the ages of 2 to 5 years painless haematuria without other symptoms (a tumour may not be palpable) should raise the suspicion of Wilms' tumour; this tumour also occurs in the older child, but less commonly.

(iii) Henoch–Schoenlein purpura is a common cause of haematuria in the 2 to 5 years period but may occur at any age. Haematuria may be the first symptom but is usually followed after an interval of a few hours or days by the characteristic rash, joint pains, abdominal pain, with or without gastrointestinal bleeding.

(iv) Trauma, as a cause of haematuria, is commoner in older children, and may be due to bleeding from a hydronephrotic kidney or from a previously normal one. Trauma to the bladder or urethra also causes haematuria (*see above*).

(v) Other causes of haematuria usually with pain and frequency are renal stone, acute pyelonephritis, acute urethritis, foreign body in the bladder, haemangioma in the ureter or bladder, and vesical papilloma. Bilharzia (*Schistosoma haematobium*) should also be considered in children who could have been exposed to infection (Iran, Iraq, Egypt, Africa, Near East, Western part of India).

(vi) Acute nephritis is becoming a rare cause of haematuria in Western European communities, but continues to be common in some other parts of the world where streptococcal (particularly skin) infections are frequent.

(vii) Other forms of nephritis, such as Alport's syndrome, and focal nephritis, also cause haematuria, which is usually recurrent.

(viii) Sickle-cell anaemia (homozygous sickle-cell disease) should be considered in any child of African descent with painless haematuria.

(ix) Coagulation disorders and thrombocytopenia. Haematuria occurs, usually without obvious trauma in haemophilia, also in Christmas Disease (factor IX deficiency) and, rarely, in von Willebrand's disease.

(x) Drug-induced haematuria. Cyclophosphamide is the most important drug likely to cause haematuria, which is due to a haemorrhagic cystitis. A high urine flow must be maintained while the drug is being given.

(xi) Vaginal bleeding in the prepubertal girl may present as apparent haematuria.

MANAGEMENT

(*a*) *In the newborn*

Investigation and treatment depend upon the cause; an intravenous pyelogram should be done if renal-vein thrombosis or Wilms' tumour are suspected.

(*b*) *After the neonatal period*

(i) Apart from severe haematuria due to trauma an IVP is not usually required as an emergency but if Wilms' tumour is a possibility an urgent IVP should be arranged. In suspected rupture of the kidney, pyelography will confirm the presence (or absence) of a normally functioning kidney on the unaffected side, and will indicate whether the bleeding is coming from the renal substance itself.

(ii) In haemophilia, haematuria is often difficult to control even with adequate treatment with factor VIII concentrates, but usually subsides with rest.

(iii) In vaginal bleeding an endocrine cause should be considered if no local cause for the bleeding is apparent.

Acute swellings in the genital region

It is always necessary, and sometimes difficult, to determine whether the swelling is due to an acutely swollen testis, a rapidly developing hydrocele or haematocele, or a tense inguinal hernia.

(*a*) *In the newborn infant*

(i) After a breech delivery, one or both testes may be swollen, with a hydrocele or haematocele. Though partial testicular atrophy has been recorded after breech delivery, this rare sequel cannot be prevented except by avoiding breech delivery itself.

(ii) A tense or obstructed inguinal hernia is common in the newborn infant, particularly in low birth-weight infants. A careful examination will show that the swelling does not involve the testis (*see* page 388).

(*b*) *After the neonatal period*

The commoner causes of an acutely swollen testis, in order of frequency (Jones, 1976) are the following:

(i) Torsion of the testis.

(ii) Torsion of one of the testicular appendages.

(iii) Epididymo-orchitis and orchitis.

(iv) Idiopathic scrotal oedema.

Less common causes (Jeffs, 1975) include:

(i) Direct trauma (kicks).

(ii) Lymphangitis of the perineal region.

(iii) Extravasation of urine due to urethral rupture from a straddle injury.

(iv) Funicular swelling due to a Richter's hernia.

(v) Passage of blood or pus into a communicating hydrocele from peritoneal bleeding or peritonitis.

(vi) Scrotal staining with blood from retroperitoneal bleeding.

(vii) Testicular involvement in Henoch–Schoenlein purpura.

RECOGNITION

(a) In the infant born after a breech delivery the cause of the testicular swelling is obvious.

(b) After the neonatal period:

(i) Torsion of the testis is the most important condition to consider in the absence of any other obvious cause for the swelling. Even a history of trauma does not necessarily exclude torsion. Typically there is a sudden pain in the testis or *in the abdomen;* fluid quickly collects causing a hydrocele. Occasionally the testis may be drawn up into the superficial ring where it may mimic an obstructed inguinal hernia.

Rarely there is a more gradual onset of symptoms which may make the diagnosis less obvious. In both types of presentation there is often a previous history of brief episodes of pain, due to incomplete or spontaneously resolving torsion.

(ii) Torsion of an appendage of the testis. The symptoms are similar to but less severe than in torsion of the testis. Localized tenderness or, rarely, a tender lump may be identified at the upper pole of the testis.

(iii) Orchitis due to mumps is commoner over the age of 12 years and is usually unilateral. Other evidence of mumps usually makes the diagnosis obvious. Acute epididymo-orchitis is occasionally secondary to an infection of the urinary tract and may be a complication of an in-dwelling catheter. Acute tuberculous epididymo-orchitis is rare and is associated with obvious tuberculous lesions elsewhere.

(iv) In idiopathic scrotal oedema the scrotal skin is swollen and reddened but the testis is normal. The oedema may spread across to the other side.

(v) The less common causes of scrotal swelling can usually be distinguished by careful examination and by evidence of disease elsewhere.

MANAGEMENT
Torsion of the testis

If there is any possibility that the swollen testis has undergone torsion, immediate exploration is necessary. If torsion is found, it should be untwisted and 'fixed'. There is no indication for removal of the testis even if it appears to be necrotic. At the same operation the other testis should also be explored and 'fixed' to prevent torsion at a later date.

Torsion of an appendage

Exploration is required.

Direct trauma

A closed testicular injury will resolve with rest. Exploration is required if there is a possibility of torsion, or if rupture of the testis or continued bleeding are likely.

Paraphimosis

This occurs when the prepuce has been retracted beyond the base of the glans, and cannot be returned because of pain and swelling.

Reduction can often be done by pressing the fluid out of the oedematous foreskin and bringing the foreskin slowly back over the glans. If this is unsuccessful a dorsal slit or circumcision will be required.

Penis-tourniquet syndrome

This is due to a hair becoming wound tightly round the shaft of the penis, causing swelling and oedema distal to the constriction. It is commoner in the infant or pre-school child but occasionally occurs in older children, perhaps as a result of experimentation.

RECOGNITION

The appearance is similar to that of paraphimosis, but the constriction is usually obvious on careful examination.

MANAGEMENT

A general anaesthetic is usually required in order that the encircling hair can be identified and cut.

Zip-fastener injuries (Watson, 1971)

The foreskin may be trapped in the zip during the fastening or unfastening of the zip. This accident is common in boys who arc not wearing underpants. The condition is both embarrassing and painful and distress may be increased by inability to pass urine.

With care it may be possible to free the zip by gentle manipulation of each tooth of the zip separately, but if this is not possible the trapped foreskin should be freed under general anaesthesia.

References

Jeffs, R. D. (1975). Urologic injuries. In *Care for the Injured Child*. The Surgical Staff, the Hospital for Sick Children, Toronto. p. 165. Baltimore: Williams and Wilkins
Jones, P. G. (1976). *Clinical Paediatric Surgery*. 2nd edn. pp. 271–276. Oxford: Blackwell
Watson, C. C. M. (1971). Zipper injuries. *Clin. Pediat.* **10**, 188

Part XI: Metabolic and Endocrine Emergencies

CHAPTER 46

Diabetes Mellitus

J. D. Baum

In this section an outline is given of the emergency management of: Diabetic ketoacidosis; A surgical operation in a diabetic child; Hypoglycaemia; Neonatal hyperglycaemia.

Diabetic ketoacidosis

RECOGNITION

This somewhat imprecise title covers conditions ranging from relatively asymptomatic hyperglycaemia with ketosis, to dehydration in association with ketoacidosis, hyperglycaemia and coma.

The presenting symptoms of ketoacidosis in diabetes of recent onset are:

(a) Vomiting, abdominal pain, headache, thirst, polyuria, and constipation.

(b) Hyperventilation.

(c) Occasionally 'sore throat' (dry mouth from dehydration and hyperventilation).

(d) Drowsiness or coma.

Preceding symptoms, for days or weeks, in addition to the above, are frequency of micturition, the recent onset of bed-wetting, loss of weight, and lethargy. An acute infection may precipitate symptoms of ketoacidosis.

In ketoacidosis in an established diabetic the symptoms are of shorter duration, due to earlier recognition, and may be preceded by a period of unsatisfactory control or precipitated by an acute infection.

In prepubertal girls episodes of ketoacidosis may occur at 4-weekly intervals or less regularly, while after puberty, ketoacidosis may appear regularly during the 2 to 3 days before the actual menstrual period.

In the severely ill child there is evidence of loss of weight and dehydration, and occasionally of shock, but oliguria or anuria is extremely rare. The main differential diagnosis is between:

(a) Acute respiratory disease, particularly lobar pneumonia. The deep pauseless hyperpnoea (Kussmaul) respiration of metabolic acidosis is quite different from the rather jerky respiration of pneumonia. *However, diabetes and pneumonia may occur together.*

(b) Acute salicylate poisoning, particularly in the pre-school child. Many features of severe salicylate poisoning mimic diabetes; there is a severe metabolic acidosis, with hyperglycaemia, glycosuria, and ketonuria. Plasma glucose in salicylate poisoning is usually <14 mmol per litre (<250 mg%) and >22 mmol per litre (>400 mg%) in diabetic ketoacidosis. A positive test for salicylate in the urine is of little diagnostic value since a diabetic may have taken a few aspirin tablets, but in severe salicylate poisoning the plasma-salicylate level is usually >40 mg% (in small children acute symptoms may occur with levels as low as 20 mg%).

(c) Acute abdominal conditions. The 'diabetic abdomen' with abdominal pain and rigidity may present diagnostic difficulties even when diabetic ketoacidosis is recognized, since *a genuine acute abdominal condition may also be present.* A surgical opinion should be obtained.

MANAGEMENT

Initial resuscitation and rehydration

(a) The child should be weighed whenever possible. If this is not possible the weight should be assessed from published growth charts: as an approximation a 1-year-old weighs 10 kg: a 6-year-old, 20 kg: and a 10-year-old, 30 kg.

(b) If there is impending circulatory collapse or 'shock' oxygen is given by face mask.

(c) If the child is in coma the duty anaesthetist should be called.

(d) An intravenous infusion must be set up.

(e) If there are signs of gastric dilation, especially if there is a history of persistent vomiting, a stomach tube (narrow gauge) is passed. Empty the stomach and allow free drainage of stomach contents. The volume of the aspirate is measured.

(f) Routine urethral catheterization is not recommended. After rehydration has commenced it is necessary to check for a full bladder if the child is not passing urine. Catheterization at this later stage may become necessary.

Clinical observations

A half-hourly record of heart rate and respiratory rate is established and an hourly record of blood pressure and axillary (or rectal) temperature. An ECG monitor should be set up for continuous assessment of heart rate and wave form.

Assessment of the degree of dehydration

(a) This involves the assessment and recording of: skin turgor, sunken eyes, dry mouth (*this may be misleading if there has been mouth breathing*), anterior fontanelle tension in infants, heart rate, blood pressure and peripheral skin temperature—ideally this should be measured and compared with rectal temperature Aynsley-Green and Pickering, 1974; *see also* section on Shock and Dehydration, p. 95). Children with Kussmaul respiration are usually severely dehydrated.

(b) As an aid to calculating fluid replacement for a child the degree of dehydration should be classified as:
>Minimal dehydration—5 per cent dehydrated.
>Moderate dehydration—10 per cent dehydrated.
>Severe dehydration—15 per cent dehydrated.

These percentages refer roughly to the percentage of total body weight lost as water and represent the deficit to be made up during the period of rehydration.

Laboratory measurements

(a) Blood is taken as soon as possible for base-line values of: glucose, urea, Na, K, Cl, HCO_3, osmolality, haematocrit and blood culture.

(b) An arterial blood sample is taken (or failing this a venous sample) for measurement of H^+ concentration (pH).

(c) Cultures for bacteriology from nose, throat and urine should be taken and a portable chest x-ray arranged as soon as possible.

Intravenous fluids

The first 6 hours.

(a) The pattern of rehydration is indicated in *Figure 46.1*. Give 20 per cent (1/5) of the calculated fluid deficit as 0.9 per cent NaCl (without glucose) in the first hour; 10 per cent (1/10) as 0.9 per cent NaCl in the second hour; and 10 per cent (1/10) as 0.9 per cent NaCl in the third hour.

Example   A 10-year-old child weighing approximately 30 kg and

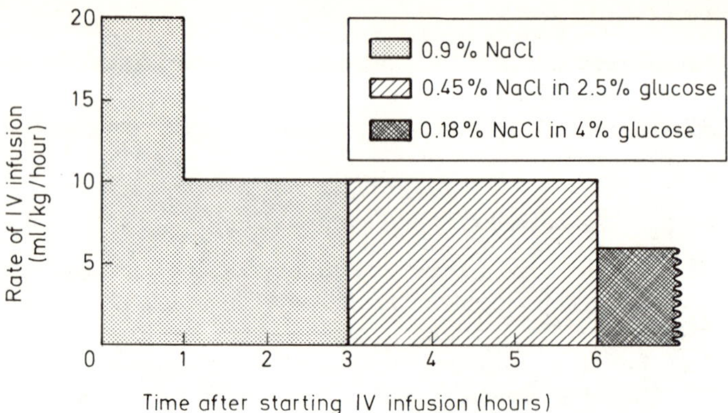

Figure 46.1. A graphic representation of rehydration appropriate for a 10-year-old child estimated to be 10 per cent dehydrated. This should not be taken as a rigid rule for rehydration but represents the sequential change of rate of infusion and change from normal saline to half-normal saline to glucose saline

assessed as 10 per cent dehydrated would have a calculated deficit of approximately 3 litres and would receive: 600 ml of 0.9 per cent NaCl in the first hour (20 per cent of the 3-litre deficit corresponding to a rate of 20 ml per kg per hour); 300 ml of 0.9 per cent NaCl in the second hour (10 per cent of the 3-litre deficit corresponding to a rate of 10 ml per kg per hour); and similarly 300 ml of 0.9 per cent NaCl in the third hour.

(b) This would be followed over the next 3 hours by 0.45 per cent NaCl with or without 2.5 per cent glucose given at a rate of 10 ml per kg body weight per hour. (0.45 per cent saline without glucose is not available in every hospital and the more commonly used 0.45 per cent NaCl in 2.5 per cent glucose would normally be quite appropriate, unless blood-glucose levels are still very high.)

(c) Over these first 6 hours while hydration is improving the blood-glucose level is falling. It is a matter of measurement and judgement when to change from a glucose-free solution to a glucose-containing solution. The fluid therapy should be reviewed after 6 hours in the light of the clinical and biochemical condition of the patient: frequently the blood glucose falls below 11 mmol per litre (200 mg%) within 6 hours and a change from half-normal saline to 0.18 per cent NaCl in 4 per cent glucose is indicated.

Peripheral circulatory failure (shock)

RECOGNITION

Peripheral circulatory failure is indicated by hypotension, tachycardia, vasoconstricted cold white peripheries, and is almost invariably associated with loss of consciousness and Kussmaul respiration. In such a case plasma (or plasma-protein fraction) should be given at a rate of 25 ml per kg over the first hour. Thus for a 30-kg child (a 10-year-old) in a state of 'shock' 750 ml of plasma should be run in during the first hour.

While the blood-glucose concentration is above the renal threshold there is a continuing osmotic diuresis. If the child is not catheterized there is a danger that the fluid balance sums will be seriously misleading unless account is taken of the intermittent passage of large volumes of urine. Whether or not the child is catheterized, a careful input-output chart is essential since once the blood glucose falls below the renal threshold there may be an abrupt change in fluid requirements.

After the first 6 hours

After the first 6 hours if there has been no further vomiting and if the patient has clinically and biochemically responded to intravenous fluids, the rate of infusion should be slowed down to correspond with the maintenance requirements for a child of the appropriate age; approximately 6 ml per kg per hour.

Potassium supplements
(*See also* page 133)

(a) There is invariably a total body deficit of potassium in patients presenting with ketoacidosis (Soler *et al.*, 1972).

   The child with newly developed diabetes will frequently have been in a potassium-losing state for many weeks, with polyuria and glycosuria. He is likely to be more severely potassium-depleted than the established diabetic with a more acute onset of ketoacidosis.

(b) There is no simple guide to the state of total body-potassium depletion but it is important to remember that potassium supplements may be required after the initial resuscitation and rehydration.

   Initially 13 mmol of potassium (1 g KCl) should be added to each 500 ml of fluid (26 mmol per litre). It is important that the child should receive the first dose of insulin before potassium is added to the infusion since it is the insulin which drives the potassium out of the vascular compartment into the cells.

(c) It is unnecessary to wait for urine to be passed before adding potassium *unless* there is peripheral circulatory failure when ischaemic renal damage may have occurred. In such a situation potassium should not be added until the second set of biochemical data has been obtained and urine has been passed.

(d) If a concentration of 26 mmol of potassium per litre of fluid is maintained throughout the period of rehydration hypokalaemia will usually be avoided. Nevertheless it is advisable to follow the T-wave pattern on the ECG monitor (*see* page 137).

Insulin

The priorities in the initial management of diabetic ketoacidosis are: first to set up a drip and start intravenous fluids; and secondly to give insulin.

(a) INSULIN SHOULD NOT BE GIVEN SUBCUTANEOUSLY SINCE ITS ABSORPTION WILL BE POOR AND IRREGULAR IN A DEHYDRATED CHILD.

(b) It is important to avoid the use of large depots of insulin since the insulin may be absorbed irregularly, with the danger of delayed and uncontrolled hypoglycaemia.

Single strength (20 units per ml) soluble insulin (if this is available) should be used.

(c) Insulin may be given either as repeated small doses intramuscularly or by continuous intravenous infusion using a completely reliable pump.

Repeated intramuscular insulin (Baum, Jenkins and Aynsley-Green, 1975)

Initially 0.5 units of insulin per kg should be given up to a maximum dose of 10 units; subsequent doses of 0.1 units of insulin per kg are given at 2-hourly intervals.

These subsequent doses of insulin may need to be modified as follows:

(i) If the blood glucose at 2 hours is higher than the initial base-line value the second dose of insulin should be 0.5 units per kg.

(ii) If the blood glucose falls below 11 mmol per litre (200 mg%) at any time the dose of insulin should be omitted and the child reassessed after two hours.

Intravenous infusion of insulin (Malleson, 1976)

20 units of insulin are added to 100 ml of 0.9 per cent NaCl in a given set. It is not necessary to add albumin. Using an infusion pump the

initial rate should be 0.1 units per kg per hour over the first hour, up to a maximum of 10 units (equals 50 ml of the infusion). Subsequently the rate of the infusion is modified according to blood-glucose levels.

The insulin in 0.9 per cent NaCl infusion is separate from the main rehydration fluid line but joins it by a Y connection.

Insulin resistance

Occasional cases of ketoacidosis which are 'resistant' to insulin have been reported; these require much higher doses of insulin in the initial phase of therapy. Measurement of the blood glucose after starting insulin will ensure that such cases are recognized and treated with appropriately larger doses of insulin.

Bicarbonate therapy

If there is hyperventilation (Kussmaul respiration) or the initial plasma bicarbonate is less than 12 mmol per litre or an arterial H^+ concentration is >65 nmol per litre (pH <7.20), bicarbonate should be added to the infusion. A guide to the approximate dose is as follows: mmol of bicarbonate = the base excess $\times$ the body weight in kilogrammes $\times$ 0.1. This dose is calculated to partially correct the acidosis since the concurrent rehydration will improve tissue perfusion and reduce further lactic acid production and the insulin will suppress further lipolysis and ketoacid production (Zimmet *et al.*, 1970). If bicarbonate has been given the H^+ concentration (pH) must be checked after two hours. For each mmol of bicarbonate, give an extra 1 mmol of potassium in the subsequent intravenous fluids but not exceeding a potassium concentration of 26 mmol in each 500 ml (this is a concentration of 52 mmol per litre which should not be given without careful monitoring of serum potassium and ECG (p. 137)).

Subsequent management

(i) Once the initial resuscitation therapy has been started a flow chart is started to record clinical and biochemical data.

(ii) A second blood sample is taken two hours after the initial baseline biochemical measurements. At the very least, the measurements of blood glucose and potassium, and bicarbonate or H^+ concentration (pH) should be repeated if the child was initially acidotic.

(iii) Additional samples should be sent to the laboratory at least for the measurement of blood glucose and potassium during the period of clinical recovery, initially at 2-hourly intervals. THE

MAIN DANGERS ONCE TREATMENT HAS STARTED ARE HYPOGLYCAEMIA AND HYPOKALAEMIA.

(iv) Blood-glucose levels may be followed at the bedside by the use of Dextrostix* and the Ames Reflectometer*, and the potassium level by observation of the T-waves on the ECG monitor.

(v) *Clinical evidence of recovery*

Rehydration should have been achieved and glucose homeostasis restored. Vomiting should have stopped; the peripheral circulation should have been restored; consciousness regained (allowing for an exhausted child being sleepy!); acidosis corrected; and the blood glucose should be at around 11 mmol per litre (200 mg%). The excretion of ketones in the urine may continue for a day or two: this need not delay subsequent management.

From the onset of resuscitation to the stage of stabilization usually takes from 6 to 24 hours.

(vi) IF THE CHILD FAILS TO RESPOND TO TREATMENT IN THIS PREDICTABLE WAY HIS CLINICAL CONDITION SHOULD BE REVIEWED PARTICULARLY FOR EVIDENCE OF PREVIOUSLY UNDETECTED INFECTION, SILENT URINE INFECTION OR UNDETECTED PNEUMONIA.

(vii) *At 12 to 24 hours after resuscitation*

During the early stage of recovery, small sips of fluids are offered. Once oral fluids are tolerated insulin is given less frequently. For children treated with intramuscular insulin the intervals between injections are extended to 4-hourly and then to three times a day before the main meals. For children treated with an intravenous infusion of insulin the transition is made to deep subcutaneous injections of insulin 4-hourly and finally insulin is given before meals. The doses of insulin used are gauged against the urine tests using the sliding scale supplemented by blood-glucose measurement, especially when the urine-glucose concentration is 6 or 5 per cent.

Sliding scale

This provides a reasonable guide to insulin dosage in this transitional period between resuscitation and stabilization.

A range from 0 to 5 per cent glycosuria can be used for the sliding scale using the 'two-drop Clinitest method' (Belmonte, Sarkozy and

* Ames Company Ltd (Division of Miles Laboratories), Stoke Poges, Slough, UK. (The Ames Eyetone Meter now replaces the Reflectometer.)

Harpur, 1967; Griffin *et al.*, 1979): two drops of urine plus ten drops of water give a colour scale accurately measuring for 0 to 5 per cent glycosuria. The colour chart for this scale may be obtained from Ames.

The maximum dose of insulin given during the period of 4-hourly insulin should be 10 units, corresponding to 5 per cent glycosuria. An indication of the other points on the sliding scale are shown in Table 46.I.

At this stage in the treatment ketonuria is universal and is not an indication for additional insulin dosage.

TABLE 46.I
Sliding scale for insulin dosage

Urine sugar (g/100 ml)	Insulin dose (units)
5	10
2–3	8
1	6
0.5	4
0–Trace	2

An example of a sliding scale of insulin dose according to urine testing using the 2-drop Clinitest method. This is suitable for most 4-hourly insulin regimes, but would require alteration depending on the individual child's response.

Prevention of ketoacidosis

In established diabetics episodes of ketoacidosis indicate a failure in the system of education of the parents and family, and of communication between the family and the hospital. Ketoacidosis should be avoidable in the majority of cases if the early signs of loss of control are recognized and acted upon. Reasons for the failure of early identification and communication should be sought after the child has recovered so that repeat episodes may be prevented.

There will be the occasional established diabetic child who develops an acute intercurrent infection which precipitates ketoacidosis of rapid onset. There are also occasional 'brittle' diabetic children, especially teenage girls before the onset of the menarche, who abruptly start vomiting and become ketoacidotic without previous warning. For example, one girl had six such episodes beginning in the early hours of the morning in as many months before she had had any periods.

In new cases of diabetes, ketoacidosis can only be prevented by awareness of the condition by the general practitioner, with early diagnosis and referral to hospital.

Surgery on the diabetic child

Elective surgery

Even minor surgical procedures in diabetic children such as teeth extraction requiring a general anaesthetic, should be performed in hospital. The child should be admitted to hospital the afternoon before the operation and put first on the operation list for the next morning.

On the day of the operation the usual dose of insulin is omitted, also breakfast. At 0800 hours an IV drip of 0.9 per cent NaCl in 5 per cent glucose is started at a normal maintenance rate and 1/6th of the normal 24-hour dose of insulin is given by deep subcutaneous injection using 20 units per ml soluble insulin.

During the period of the operation the blood glucose is monitored using Dextrostix and the Ames reflectance meter. Postoperatively with the intravenous infusion running insulin is given 4-hourly according to the sliding scale described previously.

Elective operations can alternatively be managed using a continuous infusion of insulin with frequent monitoring of blood glucose as described above.

Difficulties in controlling postoperative hyperglycaemia or the occurrence of refractory ketosis are pointers to complications of the operation or anaesthetic, such as wound sepsis or atelectasis.

Emergency surgery or major surgery

The principles of management are the same as those for the management of diabetic ketoacidosis. The emphasis will vary with the nature of the surgical procedure: thus for an emergency laparotomy the emphasis may be on adequate hydration and the treatment of acidosis: for elective prolonged reconstructive surgery the emphasis may be on the prevention of hypoglycaemia.

Hypoglycaemia

For diabetic children hypoglycaemia represents a condition of relative insulin excess.

RECOGNITION

It is important that a diabetic child and his parents recognize the symptoms of hypoglycaemia, which tend to be consistent for each individual child. For most new diabetic children it is reasonable to allow them to experience mild hypoglycaemia while in hospital, by delaying breakfast following their morning dose of insulin.

The causes of hypoglycaemia
(*See also* page 445)

(a) An alteration in the child's insulin requirements: this may happen in the weeks following the initiation of treatment in new diabetic children (so-called 'honeymoon period').

(b) The change from a regular insulin such as Lente to one of the purified insulins such as the Monocomponent insulin when the dose of insulin required may fall over a matter of weeks by as much as 50 per cent (Griffin, Smith and Baum, 1979).

(c) It may follow any occasion when the insulin has been temporarily increased to deal, for example, with an intercurrent infection.

(d) A mistake in the strength of insulin used, for example confusion arising when changing from 40 strength to 80 strength insulin.

(e) An overdose of insulin, accidental or intentional.

(f) When meals are delayed or missed or as a result of vomiting. Some children are also prone to hypoglycaemia in early summer partly as a result of increased exercise, but possibly as a result of decreased insulin requirements. In susceptible children increased exercise one day may result in hypoglycaemia in the early hours of the following morning.

NOCTURNAL HYPOGLYCAEMIA

In some children this is a particularly difficult and recurrent problem. It may present as nightmares, night cramps, morning headaches, or more obviously night-time hunger, disorientation or convulsions.

MANAGEMENT OF HYPOGLYCAEMIA

Prevention

This depends on the successful education of the child and his parents about the interrelationships between insulin, diet and exercise together with an adequate system of home urine testing. It is also essential that the child recognizes his symptoms as hypoglycaemia.

MANAGEMENT

The diabetic child presenting in coma should have a blood glucose measured immediately by Dextrostix. If it is low, <2.5 mmol per litre (<45 mg%) and there is doubt about the level, it is safer to give IV glucose while awaiting laboratory confirmation of the glucose level (which should always be determined). Clinically there is really little similarity between the child in hypoglycaemic coma and the child in coma with ketoacidosis and dehydration.

(*a*) *Early hypoglycaemia*

The child should eat sugar lumps or glucose tablets or drink glucose or sucrose-sweetened drinks. The proper use of emergency glucose in this way depends upon the adequate instruction of the family and school about carrying glucose tablets, having glucose available at school, taking extra portions of carbohydrates before periods of exercise, etc. Where possible, if a child has had to take glucose for symptoms of hypoglycaemia he should advance the time of his next meal.

(*b*) *Severe hypoglycaemia*

In this situation the child has become unconscious and is unable to take drinks of sugar by mouth. The treatment of choice is intravenous glucose. The parents should be instructed to contact their family doctor at once or take the child to the nearest Casualty department. The dose of intravenous glucose given is somewhat arbitrary and depends upon observing the child's response to treatment.

THE MANAGEMENT OF THE HYPOGLYCAEMIC EPISODE IS NOT COMPLETE UNTIL THE CAUSE OF THE HYPOGLY-CAEMIC ATTACK HAS BEEN IDENTIFIED.

Thus a mistake in the dose of insulin (particularly the long-acting insulins) may require continued intravenous glucose if recurrent hypoglycaemia is not to follow. Hypoglycaemia in the morning following exercise the previous afternoon needs to be recognized, and the parents instructed to give extra carbohydrate portions at bedtime on sports days.

(*c*) *Recurrent hypoglycaemia in 'brittle' diabetic children*

Some children are prone to recurrent hypoglycaemia especially in the early hours of the morning. They require detailed attention to the distribution of food in their diet and to the dosage and type of insulin. In some cases the family should be given glucagon for use at home. Glucagon may be stored in the ordinary compartment of a refrigerator and in an emergency a whole vial (a 1-ml ampoule contains 1 mg) is given as an intramuscular injection. This is usually adequate for the child to regain consciousness and take sugar by mouth.

(*d*) *Hypoglycaemic convulsions*

Episodes of hypoglycaemia may result in convulsions. The management of such children requires detailed attention to the prevention of hypoglycaemia, the treatment of hypoglycaemia in the attack, and in some children the addition of an anticonvulsant, e.g., intravenous diazepam. Children prone to recurrent hypoglycaemic convulsions may require long-term anticonvulsant therapy.

Hyperglycaemia in the newborn

Hyperglycaemia may occur in the newborn in the following situations.
  (a) The pre-term low birth weight infant on intravenous glucose: this is the commonest form of neonatal hyperglycaemia which remits when the concentration or rate of the glucose infusion is reduced.
  (b) The very ill very low birth weight pre-term infant: this is not an uncommon event and is part of the biochemical derangements of terminal illness. It is frequently associated with an intraventricular haemorrhage and perhaps represents a hypothalamic disturbance.
  (c) Transient diabetes in the newborn: this is an uncommon but characteristic condition which is discussed below.
  (d) Permanent diabetes mellitus with the onset in the newborn period: this is very rare and the initial management is the same as that for the transient form of neonatal diabetes.

Transient diabetes in the newborn (Ferguson and Milner, 1970)

RECOGNITION

This condition occurs characteristically in the low birth weight infant, especially the small-for-dates infant. More than one such case may present in an individual family. The onset is usually within the first week or two after birth, but may be in the first 24 hours. The infant develops polyuria, loses weight, appears emaciated and dehydrated: however it is exceptional for the infant to become comatose and frequently an appearance of 'wide-eyed alertness' is noticed.

The blood glucose is raised, frequently to levels up to 56 mmol per litre (1000 mg%); blood urea is elevated as is the potassium, and the plasma sodium is low. There is frequently a metabolic acidosis but characteristically no frank ketosis. This condition may be confused with adrenal insufficiency unless glycosuria and hyperglycaemia are looked for.

MANAGEMENT

Once recognized the treatment consists of rehydration and the continuous infusion of insulin in a dose of between 1 to 3 units per kg per 24 hours by an infusion pump. The dose of insulin delivered is modified according to the blood-glucose response which must be measured frequently, at least by Dextrostix.

As in the older child, potassium supplements are important in addition to rehydration and insulin therapy and an ECG monitor should be employed to view the T-wave pattern.

After initiating treatment the subsequent management is variable according to the individual case. In some infants the condition lasts only a matter of days while at the other extreme it may last months and blend into the condition of permanent diabetes with onset in the newborn period. At the outset it is not possible to be certain with which condition one is dealing.

Depending on other aspects of the case it may be simpler to continue with the continuous infusion of insulin daily or, if the child is otherwise well, to give small (quarter to half a unit of soluble insulin) intermittent subcutaneous doses of insulin 3-hourly with feeds or perhaps twice a day.

PATHOGENESIS

The pathogenesis of transient diabetes in the newborn is incompletely understood. It is presumably related to immaturity of the controlling mechanisms in the β-cells of the pancreas responsible for insulin secretion and release.

References

Aynsley-Green, A., and Pickering, D. (1974). Use of central and peripheral tempera-ture measurements in care of the critically ill child. *Archs Dis. Childh.* **49**, 477

Baum, J. D. and Smith, M. A. (1976). The diabetic child. *Update*, **12**, 1235

Baum, J. D., Jenkins, P., and Aynsley-Green, A. (1975). Immediate metabolic response to a low dose of insulin in children presenting with diabetes. *Archs Dis. Childh.* **50**, 373

Belmonte, M. M., Sarkozy, E. and Harpur, E. R. (1967). Urine-sugar estimation using the 2-drop Clinitest method. *Diabetes* **16**, 557

Ferguson, A. W. and Milner, R. D. G. (1970). Transient neonatal diabetes mellitus in sibs. *Archs Dis. Childh.* **45**, 80

Griffin, N., Smith, M. A. and Baum, J. D. (1979). Reduction of insulin dose on changing diabetic children from standard to monocomponent insulins. *Archs. Dis. Childh.* (In press)

Griffin, N. K., Smith, M. A., Jenkins, P. A., Whether, G. and Baum, J. D. (1979). The relationship between urinary and blood glucose in diabetic children. *Archs. Dis. Childh,* (In press)

Malleson, P. N. (1976). Diabetic ketosis in children treated by adding low-dose insulin to rehydrating fluid. *Archs Dis. Childh.* **51**, 373

Soler, N. G., Bennet, M. A., Dixon, K., Fitzgerald, M. G. and Malins, J. M. (1972). Potassium balance during treatment of diabetic ketoacidosis. *Lancet* **2**, 665

Zimmet, P. Z., Taft, P., Ennis, G. C. and Sheath, J. (1970). Acid production in diabetic acidosis: a more rational approach to alkali replacement. *Br. Med. J.* **3**, 610

Hypoglycaemia

J. A. Black

The newborn

Hypoglycaemia is common in the newborn infant and if untreated, whether symptomatic or not, is likely to cause brain damage. Neonatal hypoglycaemia can be classified as follows:

(*a*) *Transient*

This implies a temporary cause: it may be symptomatic, asymptomatic, or associated (i.e. hypoglycaemia occurring in an infant acutely ill from some other cause; the hypoglycaemia may or may not be contributing to the clinical picture).

Symptomatic or asymptomatic transient hypoglycaemia may be due to:
- (i) Hyperinsulinaemia in the infant of the diabetic mother (IDM; *see* page 691).
- (ii) Glycogen depletion and inadequate intake in small-for-dates (SFD) infants and the smaller of twins.

Associated transient hypoglycaemia may occur in:
- (i) Acute hypoxic states.
- (ii) Respiratory distress syndrome.
- (iii) Acute infections.
- (iv) Intracranial haemorrhage.
- (v) Acute cardiac failure.
- (vi) Cold injury (severe hypothermia).
- (vii) Severe Rhesus isoimmunization.

(*b*) *Persistent or recurrent hypoglycaemia*

This may be symptomatic or asymptomatic and may be due to:

  (i) Galactosaemia.

  (ii) Fructose intolerance.

  (iii) Glycogen storage disease (usually type I in the neonatal period).

  (iv) Adrenocortical insufficiency (*see* page 454).

  (v) Hyperinsulinaemia due to β-cell hyperplasia, β-cell adenoma or β-cell nesidioblastosis (Cornblath and Schwartz, 1976a).

  (vi) Leucine sensitivity.

  (vii) Beckwith's syndrome (macroglossia and visceromegaly).

Symptomatic hypoglycaemia

RECOGNITION

The symptoms are extremely diverse; hypoglycaemia should be considered in all infants with:

  (a) Jitteriness (jerking of the limbs, usually when disturbed).

  (b) Fits: focal, unilateral or generalized.

  (c) Unexplained cyanosis, cyanotic or apnoeic attacks.

  (d) Lethargy, unresponsiveness or coma.

Confirmation of hypoglycaemia should be in the first instance by Dextrostix <1.4 mmol per litre (25 mg%) and confirmed by a plasma-glucose estimation. Levels of <1.7 mmol per litre (<30 mg%) of true glucose require treatment ('blood-sugar' methods give a result 0.5 to 0.8 mmol per litre (10–15 mg%) higher and with these the critical level is 2.2 mmol per litre (40 mg%)).

MANAGEMENT

Intravenous glucose should be given to relieve symptoms when hypoglycaemia has been confirmed, or, in an emergency, to relieve symptoms without chemical confirmation, though a specimen of blood for later analysis should be taken *before* injecting the glucose.

Confirmation that hypoglycaemia is responsible for the symptoms is suggested (though not proven) by the prompt return of the infant to normality. An exception to this is the infant who has been hypoglycaemic for many hours, in whom recovery of cerebral function may be slow or incomplete. Failure of the symptoms to respond to an adequate dose of IV glucose, accompanied by a rise in plasma glucose to normal levels, shows that the symptoms were not due to hypoglycaemia; other possible causes of the symptoms should then be investigated. It is possible that a transient improvement in cerebral symptoms of any sort might on occasion be due to the osmotic effect of hypertonic glucose.

  (a) As an initial diagnostic test 20 ml of 10 per cent glucose (6 ml per kg) are given into a peripheral vein (the umbilical vein should only be used as a last resort) over 10 minutes.

(b) If symptomatic hypoglycaemia is confirmed, the IV infusion of 10 per cent glucose should be continued at a rate of 2 to 3 ml per kg per hour (50–75 ml per kg per day) repeating the Dextrostix or plasma-glucose estimations at 4-hourly intervals and aiming to keep the level between 1.7 and 6.6 mmol per litre (30 mg% and 120 mg%). Failure to maintain a level >1.7 mmol per litre (>30 mg%) requires:

(i) A change to 20 per cent glucose at the *same rate*, rather than increasing the rate of the 10 per cent solution.

or (ii) Hydrocortisone 5 mg i.m. given at 12-hourly intervals or more frequently as indicated by the plasma-glucose levels.

or (iii) Glucagon 0.3 mg (300 μg) per kg i.m. or IV as a single dose or at 6-hourly intervals if necessary: a single dose should not exceed 1.0 mg (Cornblath and Schwartz, 1976b).

NOTE

(1) Glucagon is unlikely to be effective if the liver glycogen is depleted (SFD infants, or the smaller of twins), or when glucose release from glycogen is impaired (glycogen storage disease, untreated galactosaemia or fructose intolerance). It also acts as a stimulant to insulin production and should not be given repeatedly in states of hyperinsulinaemia.

(2) Fructose (laevulose, invert sugar) should NEVER be used for the treatment of neonatal hypoglycaemia since it will produce severe, possibly fatal hypoglycaemia in unrecognized cases of fructose intolerance, and is liable to produce a metabolic acidosis in the normal neonate.

(c) Subsequent management.

(i) In transient hypoglycaemia the IV glucose should be slowly reduced, overlapping with an increasing oral intake of milk. Oral glucose or other hypertonic sugar solution should not be used; oral glucose is a potent stimulus to insulin production.

The IV glucose should not be stopped suddenly, and should be run at a slow rate until it is clear that oral feeds are adequate to maintain normal plasma-glucose levels.

(ii) In persistent or recurrent hypoglycaemia treatment depends upon the cause. An attempt should be made to stop IV glucose and to maintain normal glucose levels on oral feeds as described above. In hyperinsulinaemic states this may require 2-hourly feeds (to prevent fasting hypoglycaemia) and occasionally the addition of diazoxide in a dose of 5 mg per kg per 24 hours divided into 3 doses or oral steroids. In the metabolic disorders the hypoglycaemia will respond to appropriate treatment of the primary condition.

Asymptomatic hypoglycaemia

The management is similar to that of symptomatic hypoglycaemia except that a diagnostic rapid infusion of glucose is not required. Specific treatment is again required where a metabolic disorder has been recognized.

Associated hypoglycaemia

It is often impossible to assess whether hypoglycaemia is contributing to the clinical picture, but it is essential that a normal plasma glucose is maintained, usually by a continuous IV drip of 10 per cent glucose.

Hypoglycaemia after the neonatal period (*See also* Diabetes mellitus, page 440)

Prolonged or repeated attacks of hypoglycaemia may cause irreversible brain damage, with intellectual impairment or the development of epileptic fits, so that a child starting off with hypoglycaemic fits may become an established epileptic with fits unrelated to the level of plasma glucose. For practical purposes hypoglycaemia in the child is usually symptomatic, though unrecognized asymptomatic hypoglycaemia may be detected during the investigation of various endocrine disorders, particularly hypopituitarism or adrenocortical insufficiency.

The causes of hypoglycaemia in children can be classified as follows:
(a) Continued symptoms in unrecognized or inadequately treated conditions with an onset in the neonatal period or early infancy:
    (i) β-cell hyperplasia, β-cell adenoma, β-cell nesidioblastosis.
    (ii) Leucine sensitivity.
    (iii) Fructose intolerance.
(b) Metabolic or endocrine disorders with the onset of symptoms in childhood:
    (i) Glycogen storage disease, Types I, III, IV, VI (Farquhar, 1978).
    (ii) Ketotic hypoglycaemia.
    (iii) Addison's disease or adrenocortical insufficiency (*see* page 454).
    (iv) Hypopituitary states.
    (v) Pre-diabetic states.
    (vi) Protein-energy malnutrition (PEM, p. 589).

(c) Drug effects, intoxications:
  (i) Overdosage with insulin (*see* page 440).
  (ii) Accidental ingestion and overdosage with salicylates (p. 77), alcohol, oral hypoglycaemic agents.
  (iii) Acute toxic hypoglycaemia in Jamaica (Ackee poisoning, p. 594).

RECOGNITION
  (a) It is difficult to give an absolute figure for a glucose level which is diagnostic of symptomatic hypoglycaemia, since the development of symptoms depends partly on the rate of fall of the plasma-glucose level and partly on the level of plasma glucose to which the brain has become adapted. *Therefore a rapid fall from hyperglycaemia may cause symptoms at a plasma glucose of around 2.8 mmol per litre (50 mg%)* whereas levels of <2.2 mmol per litre (<40 mg%) are normally regarded as necessary for the production of symptoms. Conversely children who are persistently hypoglycaemic may be asymptomatic at levels at which symptoms would normally be expected.
  (b) Rate of recovery from hypoglycaemic coma: the longer the duration of hypoglycaemia and the lower the plasma-glucose level the longer the time taken to regain consciousness. This has three important aspects:
  (i) Failure to respond rapidly and completely to IV glucose after prolonged or severe coma (proved to be hypoglycaemic) does not mean that the diagnosis of hypoglycaemia was wrong, though obviously it is necessary to look carefully for an additional cause for the coma.
  (ii) A normal plasma-glucose level, taken just *after* a fit does not exclude the possibility of hypoglycaemia.
  (iii) A CSF glucose level of <1.7 mmol per litre (30 mg%) in an otherwise normal fluid should suggest the possibility of hypoglycaemia, particularly in a lumbar puncture done after a convulsion. The CSF glucose level returns to normal more slowly than does the plasma glucose.
  (c) Symptoms of hypoglycaemia: these are extremely diverse and may be:
  (i) Fits, often in the fasting state, during the night, or before breakfast.
  (ii) Episodes of hunger, anxiety, tremulousness, visual disturbances, pallor, sweating, tachycardia, abnormal behaviour, ataxia, slurred speech.
  (iii) Episodes of coma, usually with pallor and sweating.
  (iv) Repeated nightmares, followed by early-morning headache.

(d) Confirmation of the diagnosis. With the reservations discussed previously, the diagnosis of symptomatic hypoglycaemia requires:
   (i) A plasma-glucose level of <2.2 mmol per litre (40 mg%) or initially a Dextrostix level of <2.5 mmol per litre (45 mg%).
   (ii) A prompt (within 10 or 15 minutes) return to normality, or marked improvement after an adequate amount of IV glucose.

MANAGEMENT
   (a) 50 per cent glucose should be given IV, in a dose of 0.5 g (1 ml) per kg up to a maximum dose of 25 g (50 ml). If the injection is made over 5 to 10 minutes it is often obvious that recovery is occurring and further injection is therefore unnecessary. As in the newborn, fructose (laevulose, invert sugar) should not be used where the diagnosis is not certain.
   (b) Unless the cause is known to be self-limiting and of short duration it should be assumed that the hypoglycaemia may recur; this is particularly likely with an overdose of one of the long-acting insulins or in Ackee poisoning. Therefore an IV drip of 10 per cent glucose (or if necessary a stronger solution) should be set up, at a rate not to exceed the normal fluid requirements. Plasma-glucose levels should be measured at regular (4-hourly initially) intervals and the level should be maintained above 2.2 mmol per litre (40 mg%).
   (c) For insulin overdosage glucagon may be useful (*see* page 442).
   (d) Failure to respond clinically but with an adequate rise in plasma glucose: severe cerebral damage or an additional cause should be considered (*see above*).

References

Cornblath, M. and Schwartz, R. (1976a,b). *Disorders of Metabolism in Infancy*. 2nd edn. (a) pp. 183, 184. (b) p. 370. London: W. B. Saunders

Farquhar, J. W. (1978). Hypoglycaemia. In *Textbook of Paediatrics*. 2nd Edn. Eds. J. O. Forfar and G. C. Arneil. p. 1026. Edinburgh and London: Churchill Livingstone

CHAPTER 48

Adrenocortical Insufficiency and Ambiguous Genitalia in the Newborn

J. A. Black

The newborn

Salt losing conditions

A salt-losing crisis is the most important sign of adrenal disease in the newborn. This possibility should always be considered when an infant with ambiguous external genitalia is born, whether the appearance suggests a partly masculinized female or an incompletely masculinized male (Table 48.I). *However salt-losing crises can occur in infants of either sex with normal external genitalia.* The various conditions in

TABLE 48.I
Causes of ambiguous external genitalia

Genetic males (chromatin-negative)	Genetic females (chromatin-positive)
Incompletely masculinized males*	Masculinized females, variable degree
(i) 20,22-desmolase deficiency: lipoid hyperplasia (CAH)**	(i) 21-hydroxylase deficiency (CAH)
(ii) 3β-hydroxysteroid dehydrogenase deficiency (CAH)	(ii) 11β-hydroxylase deficiency (CAH)
(iii) Intersexes of various types (sex-chromosome aberrations).	(iii) 3β-hydroxysteroid dehydrogenase deficiency (CAH)
(iv) Total or partial testicular feminization	(iv) Some cases of gonadal dysgenesis (Turner's syndrome) with enlarged clitoris
(v) Some patients with autosomal chromosomal disorders (Smith, Lemli and Opitz, 1964)	(v) Androgenic drugs during pregnancy, or masculinized mother
	(vi) Intersexes of various types (sex-chromosome aberrations)

* A genetically male fetus exposed to reduced or absent androgenic influence will retain a female or partially female external genitalia; such cases are not therefore actively feminized
** Congenital adrenal hyperplasia

which salt-losing crises occur are given in Table 48.II. The rarer conditions are included to emphasize that salt-losing states are not confined to the 'classic' type (21-hydroxylase deficiency) of congenital adrenal hyperplasia (CAH).

INVESTIGATION OF INFANTS WITH AMBIGUOUS EXTERNAL GENITALIA
Investigation is a matter of considerable urgency, for two reasons: first, because a proportion of such infants may develop an acute salt-losing crisis; and second, to allay parental anxiety about the correct sex of the infant: the latter does not however constitute an acute emergency and is not considered here.

(a) Buccal smear

This can be done rapidly and indicates whether the genetic sex is the same as that suggested by the external genitalia. When an adrenal cause has been excluded further investigation of the anatomy and of the chromosome pattern is indicated.

(b) Urine steroid pattern

(i) In the commonest form of CAH (21-hydroxylase deficiency) there is a diagnostic combination of raised 17-oxosteroids (17-ketosteroids) and raised pregnanetriol which does not occur in the other forms of CAH. As indicated in Table 48.II, in the other types of salt-losing states the 17-oxosteroids may be increased or decreased.

(ii) Though it is desirable to obtain a full 24-hour specimen in all cases before starting treatment, the collection may be interrupted by a salt-losing crisis, or urine may have to be collected with difficulty in a desperately ill child (*see below*); in such cases appropriate treatment should always be started and an adequate 24-hour collection is made while initial treatment is being given. There is no evidence that the activity of the adrenal in CAH is significantly suppressed after 24 to 48 hours on treatment with hydrocortisone or similar preparations.

(iii) Levels of up to 2.5 mg per 24 hours of 17-oxosteroids may occur in the normal infant up to the age of 3 weeks (Zurbrügg, 1969) and in doubtful cases serial estimations should be made. If there is difficulty in obtaining a complete 24-hour collection the '11-oxy' index (ratio of 11-oxy:11-deoxy compounds) may be done on as little as 5 ml of urine, but results need later confirmation by estimation of the steroid pattern in a complete 24-hour urine.

(iv) Pregnanetriol is either absent, or present in a trace in the urine of

TABLE 48.II

Salt-losing conditions in infancy

Name	External genitalia		Urinary 17-oxosteroids *(17-ketosteroids)*	Response to mineralocorticoids
	Genetic male (chromatin-negative)	*Genetic female (chromatin-positive)*		
21-hydroxylase deficiency (classic type of CAH)*	Normal (N) or enlarged penis	Masculinized (various degrees)	Raised (pregnanetriol raised)	+
20,22-desmolase deficiency (lipoid hyperplasia)* (Rare)	Small penis, hypospadias, scrotolabial folds, cryptorchidism	N	Lowered	+
3β-hydroxysteroid dehydrogenase deficiency* (Rare)	As above	Enlarged clitoris, single perineal opening, fused labia	Raised	+
18-hydroxylation, 18-oxidation deficiency (hypoaldosteronism)* (Rare)	N	N	N	+
Congenital adrenal hyperplasia* (Rare)	N	N	Lowered	+
Adrenal haemorrhage	N	N	Lowered	+
Adrenal suppression due to corticosteroid treatment during pregnancy	N	N	Lowered	+
Tubular insensitivity to mineralocorticoids (Rare)	N	N	N	0
Renal salt-losing states (Rare)	N	N	N	0
Neonatal diabetes† (Rare)	N	N	N	0

Data from Hamilton (1978a) and Visser (1969)

* Inherited as an autosomal recessive (there are incomplete data for the rarer forms but a recessive mode should be assumed)

† Polyuria with glycosuria: (may show hyponatraemia with hyperkalaemia). (*See* page 443)

the normal newborn. Levels greater than 0.5 mg in 24 hours are diagnostic of 21-hydroxylase deficiency.

(v) Normal or low values for 17-oxosteroids and pregnanetriol do not exclude an adrenal disorder and in difficult cases the urine (or the infant) should be sent to a centre where more specialized investigation can be done.

(vi) It should be noted that there are two types of CAH without a salt-losing tendency, of which the 11β-hydroxylase deficiency is the only one likely to be recognized in infancy since the females are masculinized and the males may have an enlarged penis; in this condition the 17-oxosteroid output is raised but not the pregnanetriol.

Infants with normal external genitalia requiring investigation

(a) The most important group are those with a family history of:
    (i) Unexplained neonatal death in sib or sibs.
    (ii) Sibs with precocious puberty who were abnormally tall in childhood and dwarfed as adults.
(b) Infants developing a salt-losing crisis (*see below*).

Salt-losing crisis

Symptoms usually develop within the first 2 to 3 weeks of life but occasionally later.

RECOGNITION

Some or all of the following symptoms develop, usually rapidly:
(a) Failure to gain weight.
(b) Intermittent fever.
(c) Vomiting, sometimes projectile (*may be mistaken for pyloric stenosis*).
(d) Watery stools.
(e) Shock and dehydration.
(f) Hypoglycaemia (uncommon).

Confirmation of a salt-losing state is shown by:
(a) Low plasma sodium (<130 mmol per litre, commonly <120).
(b) Raised plasma potassium; this may precede the hyponatraemia.
(c) In the presence of definite hyponatraemia, a high content of sodium in the urine. In the ward Fantus' test* is useful and in a salt-loser with hyponatraemia shows a sodium chloride content of >3 g per litre (Hamilton 1978b); this would be equivalent to >50 mmol of sodium per litre.

* Fantus' test: *see* Appendix 15.

MANAGEMENT

(a) A complete 24-hour specimen of urine should be collected (*see above*) but survival must not be jeopardized by withholding effective treatment.

(b) An IV drip of 0.9 per cent NaCl in 5 per cent glucose should be started at the rate of 100 to 120 ml per kg per 24 hours, given at an initial rate of 20 ml per kg per hour for the first 1 or 2 hours, until shock is relieved or improved.

(c) In severely shocked infants, plasma (or plasma-protein fraction) should be substituted for the glucose saline, at 20 ml per kg per hour for 1 hour.

(d) Aldosterone (Aldocorten (*Ciba*)) IV 500 μg (0.5 mg) should be given at 4- to 6-hourly intervals during the first 24 hours and reduced to nil over the next 48 hours (Hamilton, 1978c).

(e) Hydrocortisone should be given IV in an initial dose of 100 mg followed by a dose of 2 mg per kg i.m. or IV at 4 to 6-hourly intervals.

(f) Doca is started in a dose of 1 mg i.m. daily. If Doca is unobtainable, the injections of aldosterone should be continued until oral fludrocortisone can be given.

(g) When vomiting has ceased and shock has been relieved, oral feeding should be started:

   (i) Additional oral sodium chloride at 15 to 30 mmol of sodium per day initially; additional salt should not be necessary once the plasma sodium has been stabilized and fludrocortisone has been given for 2 days. *Additional salt and fludrocortisone together may produce hypertension.*

   (ii) Fludrocortisone is given orally in a dose of 0.1 to 0.2 mg daily.

   (iii) Oral cortisone acetate should be given daily, at 6 to 8-hourly intervals in a dose of 10 to 30 mg daily.

Acute adrenal haemorrhage in the newborn

This condition may occur without warning or as part of a septicaemia. One or both adrenals may be affected and a mass may be palpable in the flank. Adrenal haemorrhage must be distinguished from renal-vein thrombosis, the differential diagnosis being discussed on page 656.

RECOGNITION

The sudden onset of shock and pallor, with or without jaundice, in the newborn should raise the possibility of adrenal haemorrhage. Symptoms are due to a combination of blood loss into the adrenal gland or glands, and acute adrenal failure. An IVP should be done if the infant is well enough; in adrenal haemorrhage the kidney on the affected side excretes normally but is displaced downwards and the upper calyces are flattened.

MANAGEMENT

    (a) Initial investigation should include haemoglobin, blood grouping and crossmatching, blood and urine culture, plasma urea, sodium and potassium, urine microscopy for red cells (marked haematuria occurs in renal-vein thrombosis and on the left side it is possible that thrombosis of the renal vein may affect both adrenal and kidney).

    (b) IVP as above.

    (c) Blood should be given as soon as available (p. 654) preceded if necessary by plasma (or PPF*) or 0.9 per cent NaCl in 5 per cent glucose, if necessary.

    (d) If the diagnosis is suspected or confirmed additional treatment should be as for salt-losing crisis in the newborn (*see above*).

    (e) Antibiotics should be given as for a suspected septicaemia: normally benzylpenicillin and gentamicin should be used.

    (f) There is no place for surgical removal of the enlarged adrenal.

Adrenocortical insufficiency after the neonatal period

Acute adrenocortical insufficiency presenting for the first time after the neonatal period is uncommon but may occur in the following situation.

Addison's disease

This is rare in childhood, but may occur as a familial (autosomal-recessive) condition, or as a late result of partial destruction by haemorrhage of the adrenal glands in the neonatal period.

RECOGNITION

An acute crisis is usually preceded by a history of weakness and anorexia, and sometimes hypoglycaemic attacks. Symptoms of the crisis are nausea, vomiting and diarrhoea, dehydration and shock. Pigmentation of the skin, areolae and oral mucosa may be present.

Confirmation of the hyponatraemia and hyperkalaemia are as for the newborn (*see above*). A plain film may show calcification of the adrenals, indicating haemorrhage in the neonatal period.

Waterhouse–Friderichsen syndrome

Bilateral adrenal haemorrhage develops as a complication of a severe septicaemia, usually, but not exclusively, due to the meningococcus.

* Plasma-protein fraction

Confirmation of the diagnosis can only be provided at postmortem, unless (very rarely) the enlarged adrenals are palpable.

RECOGNITION

The diagnosis is a clinical one and should not be dependent upon the presence of hyponatraemia or hyperkalaemia. This condition should be suspected and treated in any child with severe septicaemia, especially with skin haemorrhages, who is moribund or in whom the usual resuscitative measures have failed to produce improvement.

Suppression of the adrenal cortex by exogenous corticosteroids

RECOGNITION

This may occur within two years of stopping corticosteroid treatment and is likely to develop as a result of an acute infection, trauma or an operation. There is no preceding history of weakness or other symptoms of adrenocortical hypofunction, nor is there any abnormal pigmentation. Since the symptomatology appears to be due mainly to an acute deficiency of cortisol production in response to stress rather than a salt-losing crisis, the diagnosis depends upon acute shock with hypotension, while plasma sodium and potassium may remain normal.

MANAGEMENT

(*a*) *Acute crisis*

Treatment is similar to that described for the newborn using appropriately large doses.

(1) IV hydrocortisone should be given in an initial dose of 100 mg. Subsequent dosage: 150 to 250 mg per 24 hours by continuous IV drip.

(2) IV 0.9 per cent NaCl in 5 per cent glucose at 100 ml per kg per 24 hours, with plasma (or PPF) initially if necessary at 5 ml per kg over 1 hour.

(3) Aldosterone IV 500 to 1000 μg (0.5–1 mg) IV as for the newborn.

(4) If there is severe hypotension, adrenaline (1:1000) can be given in a dose of 0.1 to 0.2 mg (0.1–0.2 ml) by deep subcutaneous injection, or noradrenaline (Levophed) or metaraminol (Aramine) can be given by slow IV drip (*see* page 116 for dosage).

(5) Doca 2 to 3 mg i.m. daily.

(*b*) *Steroid cover in children with presumed adrenal suppression*

This regime (i.e. corticosteroids given for longer than 1 week at any time during the previous 2 years) should be used to cover:

(i) Planned or emergency operations.

(ii) Accidental trauma of sufficient severity to require admission to hospital.

(iii) Any acute infection or other stress such as diabetic coma, acute haemorrhage.

A commonly used method of steroid cover (Wood, 1977) is:

12 hours before operation:	100 mg cortisone i.m.
1 hour before operation:	100 mg cortisone i.m.
First 24 hours postoperatively:	50 mg cortisone orally every 6 hours or 100 mg i.m. at 12-hourly intervals.
Second 24 hours postoperatively:	50 mg cortisone orally every 8 hours or 75 mg i.m. at 12-hourly intervals.
Third 24 hours postoperatively:	50 mg cortisone 12-hourly orally or i.m.
Fourth 24 hours postoperatively:	25 mg cortisone, as above.

During operation and for 24 hours afterwards hydrocortisone for IV use must be *immediately* available in the theatre or at the bedside. An emergency dose should not be less than 100 mg.

If the daily dose up till operation has been more than 100 mg of cortisone or its equivalent the preoperative and postoperative doses should be doubled, returning to the previous dose by the 4th day.

(c) Steroid cover of potential salt-losers

Many children with ambiguous genitalia require surgical correction. In addition to the above scheme, Doca 1 to 2 mg i.m. should be given preoperatively and IV fluids should cover the total previous sodium intake (i.e. maintenance and previous daily supplements). If Doca is not available, aldosterone should be given IV at 4 to 6-hourly, as described above.

References

Hamilton, W. (1973a,b,c). Disorders of the endocrine glands: *Textbook of Paediatrics*. 2nd Edn. Ed. J. O. Forfar and G. C. Arneil. (a) pp. 971–974; (b) p. 972; (c) p. 976. Edinburgh and London: Churchill Livingstone

Smith, D. W., Lemli, L. and Opitz, J. M. (1964). A newly recognized syndrome of multiple congenital anomalies. *J. Pediat.* **64**, 210

Visser, H. K. (1969). Hypoadrenocorticism. In *Endocrine and Genetic Disorders of Childhood*. Ed. L. I. Gardner, pp. 452–53. London: W. B. Saunders

Wood, B. (1977). *A Paediatric Vade-Mecum*. 9th edn., p. 1971. London: Lloyd-Luke

Zurbrügg, R. P. (1969). Congenital adrenal hyperplasia. In *Endocrine and Genetic Disorders of Childhood*. Ed. L. I. Gardner, p. 417. London: W. B. Saunders

CHAPTER 49

Disorders of the Thyroid Gland

J. A. Black

The newborn

Goitre in the newborn

The immediate importance of goitre in the newborn infant lies in the danger of asphyxial death from tracheal compression. *The actual size of the goitre can easily be underestimated since the gland may almost completely encircle the trachea and part of it may be retrosternal.*

RECOGNITION

Any condition likely to be associated with neonatal goitre requires a careful examination of the infant immediately after delivery.

(*a*) *Maternal disease*

    (i) Overtreatment of maternal thyrotoxicosis with antithyroid drugs during the last trimester. This can also cause clinically obvious hypothyroidism (*see below*).

    (ii) Maternal thyrotoxicosis, usually when previously treated by partial thyroidectomy, may cause thyrotoxicosis in the fetus and newborn infant (*see below*).

    (iii) Endemic iodine deficiency; the mother is likely to have a large goitre and the infant may have an enlarged thyroid with or without clinical evidence of hypothyroidism.

(*b*) *Obstetric conditions*

A goitre should be suspected in all infants born after a face or brow presentation unless there is some obvious cause for the malpresentation, such as cord round the neck.

(c) Familial (genetically determined) goitrous cretinism

There are a number of recessively determined conditions in which the synthesis of the thyroid hormone is defective. The condition should be suspected if a previous infant was affected. Affected infants appear normal at delivery, apart from a moderately enlarged thyroid. The gland is rarely large enough to cause tracheal compression. One variety of goitrous cretinism (Pendred's syndrome) is associated with deafness.

(d) Long continued ingestion of iodides

This is usually the result of self-medication with iodide-containing cough mixtures for asthma or chronic bronchitis, which is not usually noted in the obstetric history. The mother may have an enlarged thyroid and is sometimes slightly hypothyroid. Other goitrogens are occasionally responsible. They may produce a very large goitre, but the infant is not clinically hypothyroid at birth.

Evidence of tracheal compression

   (a) An early sign of compression is that the infant lies with the head extended.
   (b) Stridor is sometimes, but not usually, a marked feature and may be completely absent.
   (c) Evidence of severe compression is likely to be shown by a rising respiration and pulse rate, cyanosis, and in-drawing of the sternum or lower ribs. A thyrotoxic infant may however also show tachypnoea and tachycardia from cardiac failure.

MANAGEMENT
   (a) All infants with an enlarged thyroid gland should be carefully observed for at least a week for evidence of compression, or in appropriate cases for the development of thyrotoxicosis (*see below*).
   (b) A lateral radiograph of the neck should be done in all cases to show narrowing of the airway.
   (c) Severe compression requires emergency surgery, preferably by partial thyroidectomy which is easier than tracheostomy. Temporary relief may be produced by intubation.
   (d) For less severe compression, the infant should be nursed with the head extended on a sandbag or folded towel.
   (e) The cause of the thyroid enlargement should be treated (*see below*).

Hypothyroidism present at birth

RECOGNITION

Severe hypothyroidism present at birth may be due to maternal over-treatment with antithyroid drugs or to endemic cretinism.

Clinically the infant shows the usual signs of cretinism. Apart from the possibility of tracheal compression the main dangers are:
  (a) Respiratory obstruction (which may occur only intermittently) from the large floppy tongue.
  (b) Feeding difficulty due to (a) and to the hypothyroid state.
  (c) Hyperbilirubinaemia which results from a combination of inadequate fluid intake and the effect of hypothyroidism on bilirubin metabolism.

MANAGEMENT
  (a) If there is evidence of obstruction from the tongue the infant should be nursed in the semiprone or prone position, or in extreme cases with an oropharyngeal airway.
  (b) Fluid intake should be maintained at normal levels by tube feeding.
  (c) Hyperbilirubinaemia should be treated according to the usual indications (p. 666) but exchange transfusion should be avoided unless absolutely essential.
  (d) Thyroxine should be started at once, using an initial dose of 0.0125 mg daily increasing to 0.025 mg daily after 1 week and finally to 0.05 mg daily. Subsequent treatment should be indicated by clinical response and serum PBI or T_4 levels. A too rapid increase in the dose of thyroxine may cause sudden death, possibly from arrhythmia.

Hypothyroidism developing after birth

RECOGNITION

(a) *Before clinical hypothyroidism is obvious*

  (i) Jaundice, of a non-obstructive, non-haemolytic type, persisting for longer than 2 weeks may be due to hypothyroidism. Confirmation of the diagnosis is by a low PBI or T_4 level or raised TSH level and sometimes by a markedly retarded skeletal age (e.g. skeletal age of <36 weeks in a term infant).
  (ii) Acute ileus.
     This is a rare but important manifestation of hypothyroidism which may be accompanied by persistent jaundice. Obstructive

symptoms rarely develop before the age of 1 week. The diagnosis is as in (i) above, having excluded other causes of ileus.

(*b*) *Complications in the clinically hypothyroid infant*

   (i) Respiratory obstruction (may be intermittent or occasional) from the large tongue. Management as above.
   (ii) Carotinaemia, which may be mistaken for jaundice, may develop in hypothyroid infants when on mixed feeding. No treatment of the carotinaemia itself is required.

MANAGEMENT

   (a) Persistent jaundice: this will respond rapidly to treatment with thyroxine. Treatment for hyperbilirubinaemia is as indicated on page 671.
   (b) Acute ileus: gastric suction should be started and IV fluids given as required. Treatment with thyroxine 0.0125 mg daily should be started as soon as the ileus has been relieved mechanically and oral feeding is possible.
   (c) Clinical hypothyroidism alone: treatment as in (d) above.

Thyrotoxicosis in the newborn

This is due to the passage across the placenta of long-acting thyroid-stimulating globulins (LATS) from a mother who has high circulating levels. This situation may occur in:

   (a) Thyrotoxicosis previously treated surgically, rendering the mother euthyroid but without reducing the levels of LATS. Women with persistent or marked eye signs and pretibial myxoedema appear most likely to produce an affected infant.
   (b) Medically treated thyrotoxicosis when the effects of maternal medication on the infant thyroid have worn off, generally after 7 to 10 days.
   (c) Untreated, inadequately treated or unrecognized thyrotoxicosis during pregnancy.

RECOGNITION

   (a) Fetal thyrotoxicosis. This should be suspected if the fetal heart rate is constantly >140 per minute and if the mother's LATS level is very high.
   (b) Evidence of thyrotoxicosis in the newborn:
       (i) A moderately enlarged thyroid.
       (ii) Persistent tachycardia >140 per minute, often up to 200 per minute.

  (iii) Restlessness, sweating, persistent crying, poor feeding, tremulousness, exophthalmos and/or lid retraction.

  (iv) Plethoric appearance.

   (v) Failure to gain weight on a conventionally adequate intake.

 (vii) Cardiac failure may develop very suddenly.

(c) Confirmation of the diagnosis is afforded by a raised serum PBI or T_4, and occasionally an advanced skeletal age.

MANAGEMENT

(a) Antenatal treatment

If there is evidence of fetal thyrotoxicosis or the mother has a high LATS level, antithyroid drugs should be given to the mother, even if she appears clinically euthyroid. Carbimazole appears to be the most satisfactory. The dose should be adjusted to maintain the fetal heart rate below 140 per minute. Treatment should be started as soon as the fetal heart is constantly over 140 per minute. High-risk mothers are those with eye signs and/or pretibial mixoedema *and those who have had a previously affected infant.*

(b) Postnatal treatment

  (i) If treatment has been given to the mother for her own thyrotoxicosis there is no certain way of knowing whether the infant will develop symptoms when the effects of the transplacental antithyroid treatment has worn off. Such infants should be observed closely for 7 to 14 days.

 (ii) If treatment has been given to the mother for treatment of fetal thyrotoxicosis, the same drug (normally carbimazole; for dosage *see below*) should be given to the infant starting immediately.

(iii) Symptomatic thyrotoxicosis may require treatment with the following drugs:

     Carbimazole, 1 mg per kg divided into 3 doses given 8-hourly.

     Propanolol to control tachycardia, 1 mg per kg in 3 doses at 8-hourly intervals.

     Digoxin for cardiac failure at 8-hourly intervals (dosage: *see* page 286).

    There appears to be no indication for iodides or Lugol's iodine, with the risk of causing enlargement of the gland.

 (iv) Carbimazole and other antithyroid drugs are excreted in breast milk, and breast-feeding is therefore contra-indicated if the mother continues on treatment after delivery, since the infant would receive an unpredictable amount of antithyroid drug.

(v) Duration of treatment.

The half-life of LATS is difficult to predict on present evidence since some infants appear to require treatment for longer than would be expected from the normal decay of a globulin (LATS) foreign to the infant. Treatment with carbimazole should be continued for not less than 30 days and if necessary for 3 months. Treatment with propanolol may be stopped when other signs of thyrotoxicosis have been controlled and digoxin is only required until the tachycardia and cardiac failure have been controlled.

Thyroid disease after the neonatal period

There are no emergencies specifically related to thyroid disease in childhood, apart from the possibility of acute thyrotoxicosis, for which appropriate textbooks on adult medicine or endocrinology should be consulted. The effective dose of carbimazole for controlling acute symptoms of thyrotoxicosis in a child of 8 to 12 years is 10 mg three times daily.

Part XII: Haematological Emergencies

CHAPTER 50

Haematological Emergencies

Judith M. Chessells

Sudden anaemia in childhood
(*See* pages 652, 658 for anaemia in the newborn infant)

RECOGNITION

The symptoms depend on the rate of development of the anaemia. If this happens rapidly as a result of blood loss or sudden haemolysis the child may become acutely ill with pallor, tachycardia and shock. A slower onset over days or weeks may result in pallor, lethargy and anorexia progressing in extreme instances to congestive cardiac failure. Recognition and assessment of anaemia are notoriously difficult without haemoglobin estimation and not infrequently the diagnosis of chronic anaemia is made only when a child presents with incidental symptoms, e.g. respiratory infection.

Other symptoms such as bruising or limb pains are referable to the cause of the anaemia, e.g. marrow infiltration.

THE CAUSES OF SUDDEN ANAEMIA

(*a*) *Acute blood loss*

    (i) Obvious: gastrointestinal (p. 396).
    (ii) Not obvious: internal haemorrhage (p. 21).

(*b*) *Failure of red cell production*

Anaemia usually becomes apparent over days rather than hours. An aplastic crisis may be the presenting feature of *hereditary spherocytosis* and may complicate most haemolytic anaemias due to enzyme deficiencies. There is a resultant drop in the haemoglobin and reticulocytes;

white cells and platelets are not usually affected. Examination of the child shows only pallor and sometimes splenomegaly.

An aplastic crisis may occur in sickle-cell disease, and in young children sequestration of cells in the reticuloendothelial system may cause sudden anaemia (page 472). The *unstable haemoglobins* are a rare group of disorders inherited as an autosomal dominant and characterized by congenital non-spherocytic anaemia of variable severity, often associated with splenomegaly. They may be complicated by episodes of red-cell aplasia or drug-induced haemolysis. Sudden anaemia is uncommon in the *thalassaemias* except for Hb H disease. Most children with homozygous β-thalassaemia present with chronic anaemia, hepatosplenomegaly, and growth failure after the first few months of life; occasionally the diagnosis is not made until heart failure from anaemia supervenes. Children with severe iron deficiency occasionally present as an emergency, usually with incidental infection.

Occasionally a previously normal child may present with anaemia due to *transient* red-cell aplasia. This must be distinguished from the true Diamond–Blackfan anaemia (both present with anaemia with reticulocytopenia, the diagnosis being confirmed on bone marrow examination).

Acute leukaemia may present as anaemia alone; there may be no symptoms suggestive of thrombocytopenia or infection but usually some other clinical clue is present, e.g. limb pains. Children with *aplastic* anaemia invariably have bruising or symptoms referable to neutropenia.

(c) Acute haemolysis

This, especially when intravascular, can be very rapid in onset and cause a shock-like picture resembling haemorrhage or septicaemia.

Common causes include:

G-6PD deficiency (*see below*).

Oxidant drugs (*see* Table 50.II) may also cause an exacerbation of haemolysis in patients with Hb H disease and unstable haemoglobins.

Auto-immune haemolytic anaemia in children often follows an acute infection and may cause intravascular haemolysis and haemoglobinuria.

Sudden pallor is often a symptom of the *haemolytic uraemic syndrome*; the diagnosis should be suggested by the previous history and the finding of fragmentation and thrombocytopenia on the blood film.

The possibility of malaria should be considered in patients who have been abroad; thick and thin films should be examined.

MANAGEMENT

(1) Blood should be taken for Hb, PCV, film, WBC and differential platelets, reticulocyte count, direct antiglobulin (Coombs) test, blood grouping and crossmatching, urea and electrolytes. The results of Hb or PCV and blood film should be available within 30 minutes and may give a clue as to the cause of the anaemia and the further investigations indicated (*see* Table 50.I). If a transfusion is indicated and no diagnosis has been made, blood should be taken into EDTA tubes and a sample of serum saved to facilitate subsequent investigation.

(2) Urine must be saved to examine for haemoglobinuria and stools for evidence of blood loss.

(3) Transfusion of blood should be given as necessary. Crossmatching of blood should present no problems but in auto-immune haemolytic anaemia transfusion may be necessary as a life-saving measure despite apparent incompatibility of all crossmatched blood. *If possible seek advice from the regional centre before transfusing* in these circumstances.

TABLE 50.I

Sudden anaemia in childhood—clues to the cause

Blood film	*Possible causes*	*Further investigations*
1. Microspherocytes	Congenital spherocytosis	Family studies. Osmotic fragility
	Auto-immune haemolytic anaemia	Direct antiglobulin test. Red cells (in ACD) and serum for investigation
2. Thalassaemic film	Hb H disease. Other thalassaemias unlikely to cause *acute* anaemia	Reticulocyte preparation (Hb H). Electrophoresis, F and A_2. Family studies
3. Fragmentation—reduced platelets	Haemolytic uraemic syndrome	Clotting studies, fibrin degradation products. Urea, creatinine, electrolytes
4. Shrunken cells (not invariable)	G-6PD deficiency	Enzyme assay
5. Sickled forms. Target cells	Sickle-cell disease	Electrophoresis, F and A_2
6. Reduced platelets, neutropenia ± blast cells	Leukaemia. Aplastic anaemia	Bone marrow
7. No diagnostic features WBC and platelets normal. Low reticulocytes	Congenital haemolytic anaemia in aplastic crisis. Pure red-cell aplasia	Assay enzymes, e.g. pyruvate kinase; test for unstable Hb. Bone marrow
8. Severe hypochromia	Iron deficiency ± thalassaemia trait	Serum iron and total iron-binding capacity. Serum ferritin. Electrophoresis, F and A_2

(4) Further management depends on the cause of the anaemia.
  (a) A bone marrow examination is indicated if there is suspicion of
      pure red-cell aplasia, leukaemia or aplastic anaemia.
  (b) A list of drugs to be avoided should be given to the parents and
      family doctor of patients with G-6PD deficiency, unstable Hb
      and Hb H disease.
  (c) Folic acid supplementation is desirable in all chronic haemolytic
      anaemias.
  (d) In auto-immune haemolytic anaemia arrangements should be
      made to identify the antibody. In many children haemolysis is
      complement-mediated and no antibody can be detected; such
      cases recover very rapidly and no specific therapy may be
      indicated. In most patients treatment with prednisolone (2 mg
      per kg per day) is indicated.

Glucose-6-phosphate dehydrogenase deficiency (G-6PD)

This is the commonest red-cell enzyme deficiency, affecting many
millions of people and present in all ethnic groups, particularly in West
Africa, the Mediterranean, the Middle East, Thailand and parts of
China (p. 670). There are many different isoenzymes of G-6PD which
vary in electrophoretic mobility. The gene is carried on the X chromosome, and carrier females have intermediate levels of G-6PD activity;
deficiency in females is not uncommon. Patients with G-6PD deficiency have normal Hb values and slightly reduced red-cell survival
but, following oxidant stress to the red cell, may become acutely
anaemic and jaundiced. The usual source of oxidant stress is a drug (*see*
Table 50.II) but haemolysis may be precipitated by infection. The
African (A) G-6PD in deficient (A−) individuals is associated with
enzyme levels of 10 to 20 per cent. Much lower levels (0 to 7 per cent)
are found in Mediterranean patients with deficiency.

RECOGNITION

(a) Neonatal jaundice (see page 666)

Neonatal jaundice occurring usually after the first few days of life is
uncommon in Negro (A−) deficiency except in pre-term babies, but
common in the Mediterranean and Far East.

(b) Acute haemolytic anaemia

This usually occurs 3 to 36 hours after drugs and may cause collapse
and haemoglobinuria.

(*c*) *Favism*

Rapid intravascular haemolysis may be triggered in Mediterranean deficiency after eating the broad bean (*vicia fava*) or inhaling its pollen. The offending agent has not been identified.

(*d*) *Chronic haemolytic anaemia*

This may occur in rare Caucasian variants.

DIAGNOSIS
Deficiency of G-6PD should be considered among the causes of acute anaemia in a previously well child. The blood count shows anaemia with normal platelets and possibly a raised white-cell count. The film may show irregular cells in which the haemoglobin appears shrunk away from the cell membrane (diagnostic of a crisis due to G-6PD deficiency). Heinz bodies may be seen in the recovery phase.

Drug-induced haemolysis may also occur in Hb H disease and in patients with unstable haemoglobins.

The diagnosis is confirmed by enzyme assay; screening tests may give false negative results, particularly when there is a reticulocytosis in the recovery phase. Blood taken into EDTA will keep at 4°C for several days.

MANAGEMENT
   (a) Acute haemolysis may necessitate urgent blood transfusion, particularly in Mediterranean deficiency.
   (b) The patients should be given a list of drugs and chemicals to be avoided (Table 50.II).

TABLE 50.II
Agents commonly associated with haemolysis in G-6PD deficiency, Hb H disease and unstable haemoglobins

Anti-malarials: chloroquine, primaquine, pamaquine, and quinacrine.
Analgesics: aspirin, phenacetin, acetanilide.
Sulphonamides and sulphones.
Antibacterial compounds: nitrofurantoin, chloramphenicol.
Others: vitamin-K analogues, methylene blue,
   benzene and naphthalene (moth repellant)
   broad beans (*vicia fava*) in Mediterranean variant
   acute infections
   diabetic ketoacidosis.

Sickle-cell disease

A chronic haemolytic anaemia punctuated by episodes of crisis. This includes sickle-cell anaemia, Hb S/β-thalassaemia and Hb S/C disease. Possession of the sickle-cell trait does *not* cause problems except in conditions of severe hypoxia. The diagnosis of sickle-cell disease must be confirmed by haemoglobin electrophoresis and family studies. A blood count and sickling test will not distinguish between sickle-cell trait and conditions with a near normal Hb (e.g. S/C disease).

NOTE
The sickle-cell gene occurs in Greece, parts of India and the Middle East as well as Africa.

Infarctive crises

Intravascular sickling can cause a multiplicity of symptoms. In this type of crisis there is usually *no drop* in the Hb level (6–10 g per 100 ml).

RECOGNITION
In infants, pallor, infection or painful swelling of the dorsum of the hands and feet are common. Older children may have pain in the limbs, chest, back or abdomen often with prostration and fever. The pains may be diffuse and generalized or localized and must be distinguished from osteomyelitis. Prolonged pulmonary episodes resemble pneumonia. Less common problems are priapism, headache, meningismus cerebro-vascular symptoms, haematuria, haemoptysis.

MANAGEMENT
(1) Identify and treat any precipitating cause, e.g. infection.
(2) Warmth, rest and analgesics (remembering the risk of addiction).
(3) Adequate hydration with IV 5 per cent glucose if necessary.
(4) There are no specific measures of proven benefit but in a very severe crisis partial exchange transfusion may be indicated.
NOTE
Patients with sickle-cell disease are unable to concentrate their urine, and may unexpectedly become dehydrated during an acute illness.

Aplastic crisis

RECOGNITION
Sudden increase in pallor may occur in more than one member of a family. A blood count shows a fall in Hb and reticulocyte count.

MANAGEMENT
Transfusion with packed cells.

Sequestration crisis

RECOGNITION

A catastrophic fall in the Hb results from pooling of blood in the reticuloendothelial system. This is particularly common in young children and may be precipitated by pneumococcal infection. Patients may present *in extremis* with enlarged liver and spleen.

MANAGEMENT

Urgent transfusion of packed cells is required. Treatment should be the same as for pneumococcal septicaemia (*see below*).

Haemolytic crisis

True haemolytic crises are uncommon and must be distinguished from hepatitis, gallstones and coexistent G-6PD deficiency.

Infections in sickle-cell disease

Infection with the pneumococcus is particularly common in young children with sickle-cell disease who may die rapidly from meningitis or septicaemia. Any acute febrile illness should be promptly treated with benzylpenicillin. The patients are also particularly susceptible to salmonella osteomyelitis which must be distinguished from a painful crisis. Prophylactic penicillin or pneumococcal vaccine should be considered in these patients.

Prevention of crises

It is important to maintain good general health by adequate housing and nutrition, avoidance of chilling and regular folic acid supplementation. There are no more specific measures available at present.

Acute leukaemia

RECOGNITION

Common presentations of acute leukaemia include sudden or gradual anaemia, limb pains, bruising, acute infection. On examination there is usually enlargement of lymph nodes, liver and spleen; signs of complications may or may not be present. An uncommon presentation in older children (usually boys) is with a mediastinal mass, sometimes with obstruction and pleural effusion.

DIFFERENTIAL DIAGNOSIS

(a) Other haematological disorders, e.g. idiopathic thrombocytopenia (ITP), aplastic anaemia.
(b) Disseminated malignancy, e.g. neuroblastoma.
(c) Musculoskeletal disorders, e.g. Still's disease (juvenile rheumatoid arthritis), osteomyelitis.

INVESTIGATION

Except in children with a high white-cell count ($> 50\ 000$ per mm^3) who are at risk from intracranial haemorrhage, or those with mediastinal obstruction, treatment of leukaemia itself is *not* an emergency, but *prevention and treatment of complications should start at once.*

Blood should be taken for Hb, WBC and differential count, film, platelet count, and blood group. Serum is saved for crossmatching. Blood should also be saved for uric acid estimation. A chest x-ray postero-anterior and lateral should be taken.

Within the next 24 to 48 hours a bone marrow specimen should be examined *before* starting antileukaemic drugs. If necessary, films can be made and left unfixed and unstained for 2 to 3 days. Occasionally it is impossible to aspirate marrow, and a trephine biopsy of bone is needed.

Before starting antileukaemic drugs, blood is also taken for urea and electrolytes, plasma proteins and liver-function tests. Cell-typing (classification of blast cells) if at all possible should be arranged.

MANAGEMENT

The management of infection and bleeding is discussed below. Packed cells are given as necessary for anaemia. Allopurinol 50 to 100 mg should be given orally three times daily, and adequate hydration must be ensured to prevent uric acid nephropathy; this is especially important in children with a large leukaemic cell mass. If there is doubt about the type of leukaemia, treat at first as for lymphoblastic leukaemia.

Initial treatment of lymphoblastic leukaemia

Prednisolone 40 to 60 mg per m^2 per day orally in 2 to 3 doses.
Vincristine 1.5 mg per m^2 intravenously (to be repeated at weekly intervals for 4 to 5 doses).
A laxative is given to avoid the constipating effects of vincristine.

Initial treatment of myeloblastic leukaemia

Children with myeloblastic leukaemia should be referred to a special centre for remission induction. If this is impossible the TRAP regime is recommended:

Thioguanine 100 mg per m^2 per day by mouth for 5 days.

DaunoRubicin 40 mg per m^2 intravenously on day 1.

Cystosine Arabinoside 100 mg per m^2 IV or subcutaneously, for 5 days.

Prednisolone 30 mg per m^2 per day by mouth, days 1 to 5.

This combination is repeated approximately every two weeks.

IT IS EMPHASIZED THAT MORE PROBLEMS ARISE FROM PARTIAL TREATMENT OF PATIENTS IN WHOM PROPER DIAGNOSIS AND ASSESSMENT HAVE NOT BEEN MADE, THAN FROM DELAYING ANTILEUKAEMIC TREATMENT FOR A FEW DAYS TO SEEK A SPECIALIST OPINION ABOUT DIAGNOSIS AND MANAGEMENT.

Complications during remission induction

(a) Haemorrhage

This is usually due to thrombocytopenia. Platelet concentrates are effective in a dose of 5 units per m^2. Bleeding may also be due to DIC (*see below*) in which case it usually responds to antileukaemic drugs, treatment of any infection, and liberal use of platelet concentrates.

(b) Bacterial infection

This is particularly serious when children are neutropenic ($<$ 500 neutrophils/mm^3); this is usually at presentation or in relapse. The classic signs of infection are often absent and prompt investigation and treatment are essential. Common organisms include: staphylococci, *E. coli, Pseudomonas aeruginosa*. The neutropenic child with sustained pyrexia should have cultures of blood, nose, throat, urine, rectum, any skin lesions and a chest x-ray, also lumbar puncture if clinically indicated. Empirical antibiotic therapy should be started, and as no oral combination is effective against the organisms likely to be responsible for infection, *intravenous* antibiotics should be used. Initially a combination of gentamicin 6 to 8 mg per kg per day with carbenicillin 400 mg per kg per day if pseudomonas is suspected, is a suitable regime. These antibiotics should be given separately at 6-hourly intervals. The treatment is reviewed as soon as results of cultures become available at 24 and 48 hours. The gentamicin levels at 24 hours should be measured to ensure adequate dosage. Blood urea and electrolytes should also be estimated if continued long-term antibiotic treatment is necessary.

(c) Metabolic problems

Patients with a large cell mass are at risk of early metabolic problems (hyperkalaemia, hypocalcaemia and late urate nephropathy. Ensure adequate urine output with IV glucose saline and attempt to alkalinize urine with IV $NaHCO_3$ (1–2 mmol per kg per day) in divided doses. Monitor for hyperkalaemia. Consider leucophoresis in children with very high counts ($>100\,000/mm^3$).

Problems during remission

Minor infections should be treated in the usual way with antibiotics if indicated; it is not usually necessary to stop antileukaemic drugs.

Live virus vaccines should not be given. Toxoids or killed vaccines may be given if necessary. Patients should avoid contact with chicken-pox and measles. Zoster-immune globulin (dose 1 g per m^2) should be given as soon as possible after chickenpox contact. Children who have been in contact with measles should receive immune globulin (dose 0.25 ml per kg).

Pneumonia in remission may be due to non-bacterial infections, e.g. with measles virus or *Pneumocystis carinii*. Antileukaemic drugs must be stopped and samples sent for virological and bacteriological investigations. Cough, tachypnoea, silent chest with bilateral x-ray infiltration is suggestive of *Pneumocystis carinii* pneumonia. The diagnosis is confirmed by identification of the organism on aspirate or lung biopsy. If this cannot be arranged within 12 to 24 hours treatment should be started pending biopsy with trimethoprim–sulfamethoxazole (co-trimoxazole, Septrin) 20 mg trimethoprim, 100 mg sulfamethoxazole per kg per day in two 12-hourly doses by mouth.

The CNS in leukaemia

(a) Leukaemic infiltration

This occurs in about 5 per cent *despite* routine prophylaxis. Clinical features include: headache, vomiting, giddiness, papilloedema and undue weight gain. These findings warrant lumbar puncture with measurement of CSF pressure. The CSF specimen is saved for cytology, and methotrexate (intrathecal preparation) is given in dose of 10 mg per m^2 (maximum dose 12 mg) intrathecally. This can be repeated at weekly intervals until the CSF is clear. The diagnosis must

TABLE 50.III
Drugs used in acute leukaemia

Drug	Trade name	Route(s) of administration	Toxicity					
			Bone marrow	Nausea/ Vomiting	Gastrointestinal	CNS	Alopecia	Other
Vincristine	Oncovin	IV*	±	—	Constipation Ileus	Neuropathy Convulsions	+	—
6-Mercaptopurine (6-MP)	Puri-Nethol	Oral	++**	+	Jaundice	—	—	—
Thioguanine	Lanvis	Oral	++	+	Jaundice	—	—	—
Methotrexate	Methotrexate	Oral i.m., IV, IT	+	+	Mouth ulcers Diarrhoea Hepatitis	Arachnoiditis (IT) Encephalopathy	—	Photosensitivity Pneumonitis Osteoporosis
Cyclophosphamide	Endoxana	Oral IV	++	++	—	—	+	Cystitis
Daunorubicin	Cerubidin	IV*	+++	++	—	—	+	Cardiotoxic
Doxorubicin	Adriamycin	IV*	+++	++	Mucositis	—	+	Cardiotoxic
Cytosine arabinoside (Cytarabine)	Cytosar	Oral s.c., i.m., IV, IT	+++	+++	—	—	—	—
Colaspase (L-Asparaginase)	Crasnitin	IV, s.c.	+	+	Hepatitis Pancreatitis	Confusion	—	Hypofibrinogenaemia Anaphylaxis

* These drugs are sclerosant if they leak outside the vein.
** 6-MP dose should be quartered if given with allopurinol.
± Infrequent.
+++ Marked.

be confirmed by the presence of *blast cells* in the CSF; if they are not found other causes of CNS disease must be considered or excluded.

(*b*) *Convulsions*

These are an uncommon symptom of CNS infiltration. Other causes include haemorrhage (in relapsed patients), vincristine and methotrexate toxicity, and encephalitis. Dystonic reactions from extrapyramidal symptoms due to phenothiazines must be distinguished from a convulsion. Fits should be controlled with anticonvulsants; a lumbar puncture should be done and the CSF specimen saved for cytology.

(*c*) *Progressive neurological deterioration*

This may be due to drug encephalopathy, postinfective encephalomyelitis (measles, mumps, herpes simplex), progressive multifocal leucoencephalopathy. Advice should be sought about further investigation rather than assuming that the symptoms are due to CNS infiltration.

Haematological relapse

RECOGNITION
This may be diagnosed on routine marrow examination or suspected from symptoms like those at presentation, e.g. limb pain.

A fall in the blood count (especially platelets) may be due *either* to relapse or drug toxicity.

MANAGEMENT
If the only feature is a fall in the blood count it is reasonable to do without antileukaemic drugs for a few days and to repeat the count. Other features warrant marrow aspiration as soon as convenient. Complications are treated as at presentation but remembering that the chances of long-term remission are slender in children who relapse on modern combination chemotherapy.

Acute thrombocytopenia

For thrombocytopenia in the newborn infant *see* page 663.

RECOGNITION
A sudden onset of bruising in a previously well child who has not been traumatized is usually due to idiopathic thrombocytopenic purpura (ITP) (*see* Table 50.IV for differential diagnosis). Inquiry should be made about recent viral infections and drug ingestion. Bruising in ITP

TABLE 50.IV
Thrombocytopenia in childhood

Mechanism	Bone marrow	Examples
Decreased platelet production	Megakaryocytes, decreased or absent	Aplastic anaemia* Leukaemia* Disseminated malignancy
Excessive destruction of platelets	Megakaryocytes, normal or increased	Postinfective, e.g. rubella, varicella, infectious mononucleosis Idiopathic* Drug-induced* Systemic lupus erythematosus
Utilization of platelets	Megakaryocytes, normal or increased	Disseminated or localized intravascular coagulation*
Splenic pooling of platelets	Megakaryocytes, normal	Portal hypertension Thalassaemia Gaucher's disease

* Acute onset common

may be widespread and accompanied by palatal petechiae and mucous-membrane haemorrhage. Other signs are uncommon. The absence of anaemia, limb pains, lymphadenopathy and hepatosplenomegaly distinguish ITP from leukaemia. Acute aplastic anaemia usually causes anaemia and infection. The child with DIC is ill from the underlying cause (usually infection). The distribution and type of rash distinguish ITP from anaphylactoid (Henoch–Schoenlein) purpura.

INVESTIGATIONS
The diagnosis of ITP is confirmed by:

(a) Full blood count and film

The results should be made available within the hour. In ITP the only abnormal result usually is a low platelet count (unless substantial blood loss has occurred). Abnormal mononuclear cells may be seen in postviral thrombocytopenia, e.g. infectious mononucleosis.

(b) Bone-marrow aspiration

This should be arranged within the next 24 to 48 hours because although leukaemia and marrow failure are unlikely in the presence of a normal Hb and film they cannot be excluded with certainty. If steroids are to be given, a marrow examination *must* be done first.

MANAGEMENT
ITP in children is a benign condition. If bruising has been sudden in

onset, or is severe, admission to hospital for observation and restriction of activity is warranted. A short (2 to 3 weeks) course of steroids (2 mg prednisolone per kg per day) may be indicated in children with extensive mucous-membrane bleeding but prolonged steroid therapy should be avoided. Occasionally blood transfusion is needed for epistaxis or gastrointestinal bleeding. Platelet concentrates are ineffective since infused platelets are rapidly destroyed.

Haemophilia and related disorders

Previously undiagnosed patients

RECOGNITION

Haemophilia (factor VIII deficiency) and Christmas disease (factor IX deficiency) are clinically indistinguishable and one-third of patients have no family history of bleeding. Presenting features of both depend on the levels of factor VIII or IX. Severely affected boys present late in the first year with bleeding from tongue or mouth, lumpy bruises and muscle bleeds. Haemarthroses are common after age 2 to 3 years. Mild cases bleed after trauma, surgery or dental extraction. Neonatal bleeding is uncommon unless after circumcision or trauma.

Von Willebrand's disease is inherited as an autosomal dominant; the usual symptoms are epistaxes and mucous membrane bleeding.

INVESTIGATIONS

An atraumatic venepuncture with citrated blood sample filling the bottle is needed. DO NOT puncture femoral or jugular veins or cut down on veins in children with suspected bleeding diathesis. *See* Table 50.V for results of emergency screening tests which should be available within the hour. Plasma which is saved must be deep frozen for further investigations. The PTTK is prolonged in all save mild deficiency of factors VIII and IX but does *not* distinguish between them. For this *assays* are essential. If these cannot be obtained, mixing tests will distinguish between haemophilia and Christmas disease; fresh frozen plasma is the only therapeutic material containing both factor VIII and factor IX.

Management of bleeding episodes

RECOGNITION

Haemarthroses are commonest in the knee, elbow and ankle joints; acute bleeds are very painful. Muscle bleeds can occur in limbs (especially the forearm), or abdomen (mimicking appendicitis). Older boys may complain of pain or discomfort in a joint which should be treated as a bleed even in the absence of signs. Haematuria is common in older boys.

MANAGEMENT

Treatment is urgent because delay can result in permanent joint damage or injury to nerves and blood vessels.

IF IN DOUBT TREAT AS A BLEED

Adequate levels of the missing clotting factor must be achieved by prompt intravenous infusion (preferably via 'butterfly' needle) of an adequate amount of the appropriate replacement material. Everything else is of secondary importance.

Haemophilia
(*See* Table 50.VI for treatment)

Example of dose calculation   A 30-kg boy has a severe haemarthrosis. To raise his factor VIII level to 40 per cent requires $30 \times 20 = 600$ units of factor VIII. This will have to be given as concentrate *or* cryoprecipitate. One bag of *cryoprecipitate* contains on average about 60 units of factor VIII, so the estimated dose is 10 bags.

Christmas disease

Early bleeds can be treated with fresh frozen plasma 10 to 15 ml per kg infused as rapidly as possible *or* factor IX concentrate 10 to 15 units per kg. More severe bleeds require a dose of 40 to 50 units per kg which must be given as concentrate.

Von Willebrand's disease

Treatment with fresh frozen plasma or cryoprecipitate results in a prolonged rise in factor VIII level.

These instructions for the treatment of haemophilia, Christmas disease and von Willebrand's disease are based on estimations of dose and in any complicated bleed treatment *must* be monitored by factor VIII/IX assay (*see* further advice).

The early complications of treatment

Circulatory overload limits the use of fresh frozen plasma. Allergic reactions to plasma and cryoprecipitate can result in pyrexia, urticarial rash, abdominal pain and headache. Bronchospasm can occur in severe reactions. These complications should be treated with intravenous antihistamines (e.g. chlorpheniramine 5 to 10 mg); in severe reactions intravenous hydrocortisone and subcutaneous adrenalin may be necessary. In children who react to cryoprecipitate, the injection should be 'covered' by giving antihistamines beforehand orally or intravenously with the plasma.

(*a*) *Pain*   This is relieved by prompt treatment. Severe bleeds may necessitate analgesics but aspirin must be avoided and the risk of addiction kept in mind. DO NOT give intramuscular injections.

(*b*) *Admission to hospital*   This is not usually needed for early bleeds. Some indications on admission include: established haemarthrosis of knee or ankle, risk to nerve or blood supply (e.g. a large forearm bleed), head and mouth injuries, suspected intra-abdominal bleeding, wounds requiring suturing.

(*c*) *Rest*   Initially the limb must be rested. The arm should be elevated in a forearm bleed.

(*d*) *Further replacement therapy*   This is given according to the type and severity of the bleed. One infusion is often enough for early haemarthroses or minor bleeds. The half-life of factor VIII is 12 hours, so treatment twice daily is needed to achieve high enough levels for surgery or following head injury. The half-life of transfused factor IX is about 18 hours so that daily treatment is usually adequate.

(*e*) *When to seek help*   In any complicated case treatment should be monitored by assay of clotting factors. Advice is available from designated haemophilia centres at all times. Surgical procedures even in the mild haemophiliac should *only* be carried out at such centres.

TABLE 50.V
Screening tests of haemostasis

Condition	Platelet count	PT	Screening test PTTK	TT	BT++
Haemophilia	N	N	ABN	N	N
Christmas disease	N	N	ABN	N	N
Von Willebrand's disease	N	N	ABN	N	ABN
Fibrinogen deficiency	N	ABN	ABN	ABN	ABN
ITP	ABN	N	N	N	++
DIC	ABN	ABN	ABN	ABN	+++

+++ *See* text for additional tests; N = Normal result; ABN = Result usually abnormal; PT = Prothrombin time; PTTK = Partial thromboplastin time with kaolin; TT = Thrombin time; BT = Bleeding time; ++ = Test not usually indicated in thrombocytopenic patients

TABLE 50.VI
Treatment of haemophilia (factor VIII deficiency)

Type of bleed	Desirable level after treatment (% normal)	Level 24 hours later (% normal)	Dose of factor VIII (units/kg body weight)*
Spontaneous bleed Early haemarthrosis	20	5	10–15
Major haemarthrosis	40	10	15–30
Serious accident (Major surgery)	100	25	55–70

* 1 unit of factor VIII = amount of factor VIII present in 1 ml fresh normal citrated plasma. For treatment of Christmas disease *see* text.

Disseminated intravascular coagulation

RECOGNITION

Disseminated intravascular coagulation (DIC) occurs as a complication of disease and is not a disease in itself. It should be suspected when bruising, bleeding from venepuncture sites, or, less commonly, thrombosis, occurs in an ill child. The usual underlying cause is septicaemia (e.g. meningococcal infection) but DIC may also occur in acute leukaemia and after cardiopulmonary bypass.

PATHOPHYSIOLOGY

Pathological activation of coagulation results in increased utilization of platelets (causing thrombocytopenia) and clotting factors (particularly V and fibrinogen). Secondary fibrinolysis results in formation of fibrin degradation products (FDP) which are in themselves anticoagulant. Fibrin deposition may be generalized or confined to one site or organ (e.g. the kidney in haemolytic-uraemic syndrome or in a cavernous haemangioma). Fragmentation of red cells (micro-angiopathic haemolytic anaemia) can occur as a result of fibrin damage induced in small blood vessels and is more common in localized fibrin deposition.

Tests of haemostasis (*see* Table 50.V), will give variably abnormal results depending on the timing of blood samples, the rate of regeneration of platelets and clotting factors, and whether the stimulus to coagulation is a continuing one.

MANAGEMENT

(*a*) *Recognition and treatment of the underlying cause*

The causes and differential diagnosis of DIC in the newborn are discussed elsewhere (*see* page 664 and Table 50.V). In older children the diagnosis of DIC is usually apparent clinically and urgent steps to investigate and treat the underlying cause (usually septicaemia) are indicated. All other considerations are of secondary importance.

(b) Assessment of DIC

Blood should be taken for Hb, PCV, film, platelet count and screening tests of haemostasis (results available within 1 to 2 hours). Estimation of FDP may be available and a sample can be saved for assay of clotting factors. Fragmentation of red cells is an inconstant finding but is always marked in haemolytic-uraemic syndrome; thrombocytopenia is usual and FDPs are present but other clotting tests may be normal in this disorder.

(c) Treatment of DIC

Treatment of DIC itself is often unnecessary since the coagulation status improves as the underlying cause of DIC is removed. In children with serious bleeding or overt thrombotic complications heparin is indicated. Heparin should be given intravenously at a dose of 25 units per kg body weight per hour as a continuous infusion or 100 units per kg every 4 to 6 hours as a push dose. Response to therapy is judged by clinical improvement; normalization of clotting tests and platelet count is often delayed for some days and the results are masked by heparin but the prothrombin time may shorten if previously prolonged. Laboratory control of heparin dosage is also difficult in these circumstances but the thrombin time should be checked at 12 to 24 hours; if this is markedly prolonged it indicates a heparin effect and protamine neutralization may be used to estimate heparin levels.

Use and availability of blood products

Whole blood

Whole blood should be used only when the patient needs both plasma and red cells as in severe haemorrhage. It is *not* a useful source of platelets and clotting factors. Blood taken into acid citrate dextrose (ACD) or citrate phosphate dextrose (CPD) can be used for up to 21 days. Blood taken into heparin (e.g. for the neonate) should be used within 24 hours.

Packed cells

Packed cells are preferable to whole blood in treatment of anaemia.

The volume in ml of packed cells needed = desired rise in grams Hb × 2 × wt in kg. For example to raise Hb from 4 g to 8 g/100 ml in a 20-kg child, requires $4 \times 20 \times 2 = 160$ ml packed cells.

Red cells are now usually packed by the transfusion service in a system of plastic bags; if prepared by aspiration of plasma from bottled blood they should be used at once. For patients needing repeated transfusions, washed or frozen cells are available from some centres.

Platelet concentrates

Platelet transfusions are of use in treatment of thrombocytopenia due to marrow failure (e.g. leukaemia) but of little value in ITP. They are prepared by transfusion centres as concentrates (usually from 2 to 5 donors) and should be given within 24 to 48 hours of preparation (where possible give 5 units per m^2). They have a short life after transfusion (half-life: 1 to 2 days). Where a cell separator is available sufficient platelets to achieve haemostasis can be obtained from one donor.

Granulocytes

Granulocytes for treatment of proven infection in neutropenic patients can be obtained in sufficient numbers from normal donors only by use of a cell separator. Cells from patients with chronic granulocytic leukaemia are available in some areas.

Fresh frozen plasma

Plasma stored at or below $-20°C$ contains all clotting factors. It can be used for minor bleeds in factor VIII and IX deficiency or in bleeding due to liver disease. The dose is up to 15 to 20 ml per kg as quickly as possible. Do NOT confuse with freeze-dried plasma stored at room temperature which is used only as a volume expander. Do NOT confuse with the plasma left after removal of cryoprecipitate which no longer contains factor VIII or fibrinogen.

Cryoprecipitate

Cryoprecipitate contains factor VIII and fibrinogen and is available from most transfusion centres. It is used in the treatment of haemophilia (*see* page 481). It must be stored at or below $-20°C$ ($-4°F$): bags must be aspirated with care to avoid leaving much of the factor VIII activity behind. The content of factor VIII is extremely variable and should be monitored regularly.

Human AHG concentrate

Factor VIII concentrate is used in treatment of haemophilia, is freeze-
dried and of guaranteed potency. Supplies of the NHS concentrate are
very limited. Concentrate is available commercially and despite the
expense is now used to treat many haemophiliacs. Concentrate is the
most suitable preparation for home therapy.

Factor IX concentrate

Concentrates rich in factor IX (which also contain II, X, and sometimes VII) are made by the plasma fractionation centres at Oxford and
Edinburgh and are available to designated haemophilia centres for
treatment of Christmas disease.

Purified protein fraction

This contains mainly albumin and is used as a volume expander or to
replace protein loss. It is of no use in clotting disorders.

Part XIII: Acute Skin Conditions

CHAPTER 51

Acute Skin Conditions

A. E. Walker

Toxic epidermal necrolysis
(Lyell's disease, Ritter's disease, Scalded Child syndrome)

The commonest cause in children is a staphylococcal infection with a phage type 71 organism. Drug eruptions, particularly sulphonamides, barbiturates and butazones may present an identical picture. In some cases no causative factor can be established.

RECOGNITION

The child is fretful and frequently febrile with ill-defined patchy red areas of skin, most commonly on the face and trunk. Within hours these areas are denuded of the superficial epidermis leaving raw, red areas resembling scalds. The stripped epidermis hangs in shreds or folds around the raw areas. The reddened areas are tender to touch. Shallow erosions may be visible on the mucous membranes.

The condition must be distinguished from:
(a) Bullous erythema multiforme; this is usually less acute in onset. Lesions of the skin are more regular in appearance, and the erosions deeper. The two conditions may appear simultaneously.

(b) Bullous impetigo. The child is not in discomfort and the blisters appear on normal skin.

MANAGEMENT

(*a*) *Nursing*   Admission is necessary if the lesions are extensive, with isolation and barrier nursing because of the danger of cross-infection. The child should be nursed as a burns patient, i.e. unclothed and with the raw areas exposed.

(*b*) *Investigations*   Swabs from the skin should be taken for culture and phage-typing. A blood culture should also be taken.

(*c*) *Local treatment*   Gentle swabbing of the skin will remove necrotic and loose skin, and topical antibiotic ointment should be applied to the raw areas.

(*d*) *Fluids*   Attention must be paid to fluid and electrolyte balance if the condition is extensive or the oral mucosa affected.

(*e*) *Drug treatment*   Cloxacillin orally should be given if the condition is staphylococcal in origin.

(*f*) *Corticosteroids*   Systemic steroid treatment may be required where the condition is drug induced.

   Spontaneous recovery without scarring usually occurs within 7 to 10 days.

Erythema multiforme (Stevens–Johnson syndrome)

A specific pattern of skin response to multiple factors including herpes simplex, smallpox vaccination and drugs. In 50 per cent of cases the cause remains unknown. The condition may be recurrent.

RECOGNITION

Typical target lesions are present, the maculopapular central area is purplish or purpuric with a surrounding ring of erythema.

   Emergency treatment is required when the lesions become bullous and/or extensive erosions of the mucous membranes are present. The lips quickly develop haemorrhagic crusting. Purulent conjunctivitis is common. The condition must be distinguished from toxic epidermal necrolysis.

MANAGEMENT

(*a*) *Nursing*   Isolation and barrier nursing are necessary.

(*b*) *Drug treatment*   Systemic steroids will be required if the condition is extensive, also a broad-spectrum antibiotic (N.B. a careful drug history is vital; an antibiotic might be the cause of the eruption).

(*c*) *Fluids*   The body temperature should be monitored and fluid and electrolyte balance carefully checked.

(*d*) *Local treatment*   Crusts should be removed with warm vegetable oil. Tetracycline paint (250 mg in 10 ml sterile water) is applied 4-hourly to give symptomatic relief where mucosal erosions are present. Antibiotic ointment is applied to the lips or vulva. Large intact skin blisters should be punctured with a sterile needle (but not de-roofed), then covered with a non-adherent dressing.

Conjuctivitis should be treated with antibiotic eye drops, and the lids bathed frequently to prevent adhesions.

Erythroderma with exfoliation

In children this is usually due to secondary infection in atopic eczema, and occasionally due to psoriasis or drugs (penicillin, barbiturates and gold). The history will usually indicate the underlying aetiology.

RECOGNITION
There is widespread redness and shedding of skin.

MANAGEMENT

(*a*) *Nursing*   Isolation with barrier nursing is required.

(*b*) *Drug treatment*   Broad-spectrum antibiotics should be given, and systemic steroids in severe cases.

(*c*) *Fluid and body temperature*   The body temperature should be measured frequently with a low-reading thermometer because of the danger of hypothermia. Fluid and electrolyte balance should be carefully observed. All may be grossly disturbed in severe exfoliation.

(*d*) *Investigation*   The plasma proteins and blood folic-acid should be estimated since depletion may occur in severe exfoliation.

(*e*) *Local treatment*   A bland emolient should be used as a local application.

Kaposi's varicelliform eruption
(Eczema vaccinatum and Eczema herpeticum)

In children with atopic eczema, even if this is relatively mild, following vaccination against smallpox or contact with herpes simplex, a widespread eruption may occur. (Nursing staff recently vaccinated or suffering from herpes simplex should not nurse children with atopic eczema.)

RECOGNITION

Within 10 days of vaccination or contact with herpes simplex a widespread vesicular eruption develops. The lesions appear in crops, are umbilicated and rapidly become pustular. The vesicles may be confined to areas of eczema or may be generalized. Differentiation between the vaccinial and herpetiform eruptions may be impossible clinically but the history may be helpful. Cytological smears may give a rapid differentiation but in most centres virus culture and antibody estimation must be awaited.

MANAGEMENT

(*a*) *Nursing*   The child must be isolated, particularly from susceptible children and nursing staff who suffer from atopic eczema.

(*b*) *Drug treatment*   Antibiotics should be given for the control of secondary infection. Systemic and local steroids are contra-indicated but must NOT be discontinued in children already receiving them. Long-acting antihistamines can be given systemically for the relief of itching.

(*c*) *Local treatment*   An antibiotic ointment will give symptomatic relief and prevent the adherence of dressings.

(*d*) *Gamma globulin*   A hyperimmune vaccinial gamma globulin is indicated in the vaccinial type (*See* Appendix 9, Table A9.XII for dose).

(*e*) *Complications*   Encephalitis occurs in the herpetic more than in other forms and may require treatment with idoxuridine. Corneal ulcers should be treated with topical idoxuridine.

The condition must be distinguished from smallpox (variola); this may be very difficult though in smallpox the rash is centrifugal. If in doubt, the condition should be treated as smallpox (*see also* page 578).

Wiskott–Aldrich syndrome

A hereditary syndrome with atopic eczema, thrombocytopenia and increased susceptibility to infection. This is due to a sex-linked recessive gene, only boys being affected.

RECOGNITION

This condition should be considered with severe eczema in a male child in association with any of the following.

(a) Recurrent infections.
(b) Purpura.
(c) Bleeding tendency.
(d) Bloody diarrhoea.
(e) Hepatosplenomegaly.

MANAGEMENT
Antibiotics should be given according to the current infection. After full investigation transfer factor may help the immune deficiency state.

Sunburn

In the mild form erythema develops a few hours after exposure and no treatment is needed. In more severe cases local applications of steroid creams reduce inflammation and relieve symptoms. In severe cases there is marked erythema with blisters. Children should be nursed as for thermal burns. Systemic steroids may be indicated.

Erysipelas

An acute infection of the skin and subcutaneous tissues with a virulent strain of *Streptococcus pyogenes*.

RECOGNITION
This is an acute febrile illness associated with a tender browny-red change of the affected skin. The overlying epidermis may blister. Commonly affected areas in infants are the abdominal wall, and in older children the limbs or face. Recurrent attacks are frequently associated with impaired lymphatic drainage.

MANAGEMENT
(a) Benzylpenicillin should be given for 7 days. If the patient is penicillin sensitive erythromycin or a cephaloridin should be used.
(b) A careful search should be made for a possible source of entry of the infection such as fissures around the ears, anus or athlete's foot. If the condition is recurrent a maintenance dose of oral penicillin may be necessary.

Anhidrosis or hypohidrosis

Absence or malfunction of sweat glands gives rise to hyperpyrexia and heat exhaustion in warm climatic conditions or during exertion. Symptoms include lethargy, headache, nausea and vomiting. The temperature may be 39°C (102°F) or higher, with tachycardia and tachypnoea (*see also* page 335). Absence of sweat glands occurs in anhidrotic ectodermal dysplasia, which is a genetically determined syndrome, usually sex-linked and affecting male children. In icthyosis there may be diminished numbers of sweat glands or hypofunction because of plugging of the sweat ducts. Similarly in extensive psoriasis, eczema and bullous eruptions of the skin, sweating may be greatly impaired.

MANAGEMENT
The child is nursed in a cool environment with tepid sponging. In hyperpyrexia associated with extensive skin disorders, ointments and creams in the form of topical applications must be avoided as they may block sweat ducts. Shake lotions should be used.

Angio-oedema
(*See also under* Venomous Bites and Stings, page 542; Ear, Nose and Throat section, page 209; and page 111)

Urticaria as such does not usually present as an emergency, but when associated with angio-oedema in which the subcutaneous tissues are involved urgent treatment may be required. If the lips, tongue or larynx are swollen and with the danger of obstruction of the airway, subcutaneous adrenaline should be given combined with antihistamines.

Hereditary angio-oedema

This is a rare disorder, inherited as an autosomal dominant. It presents with severe swelling of the mucous membrane, often in the mouth following dental treatment. Recurrent abdominal pain is not uncommon. Usually a family history is known and will warn of the possible dangers.

MANAGEMENT
Systemic steroids and antihistamines do not help, but in an emergency with airway obstruction, one unit of fresh frozen plasma will relieve the swelling. Epsilon-amino-caproic acid (Epsikapron) an inhibitor of fibrinolysis, can be given on a long-term basis and in acute attacks. (For dosage *see* Appendix 9.)

INVESTIGATION
Estimation of the C1 esterase inhibitor should be performed; this is low or absent. In rare cases the inhibitor is present but is inactive.

Neonatal emergencies

CONDITIONS ASSOCIATED WITH BLISTERS

Epidermolysis bullosa

A group of hereditary disorders characterized by blisters provoked by minimal trauma. Both the dominant letalis type and the recessive dystrophic type present at birth. The child is born with bullae or extensive raw areas. Lesions are present in the mouth and larynx. Mild trauma leads to new lesions. The mortality rate is high.

MANAGEMENT

Unnecessary trauma should be avoided and the incubator or cot should be padded. If the infant is in an incubator the erosions can be left uncovered, but otherwise non-adherent dressings and topical antibiotic ointment should be used. If oral lesions are present, special feeding with a soft teat may be required.

Systemic steroids are indicated if there are extensive bullae and/or oesophageal lesions. This can often be given in a relatively high dose for a short period. Supplementary iron is indicated because of the loss through the denuded areas of skin. Systemic antibiotics should be given for secondary infection. At an early stage it is important to try to establish the type of disorder in order that advice can be given about future children.

DIFFERENTIAL DIAGNOSIS

This group of conditions must be distinguished from epidermal necrolysis (Ritter's disease) in which the lesions are not present at birth, the nails not involved, and the erosions much more superficial. However, the differentiation may be exceedingly difficult.

Herpes simplex (*Herpesvirus hominis*)
(*See also under* Acute Infections of the newborn, page 630)

Neonatal herpes simplex is usually secondary to a type II herpes infection of the maternal genital tract.

RECOGNITION

The main clinical features are:
  (a) Solitary or grouped vesicles present at birth.
  (b) Development of an erosion with vesicles at the periphery.
  (c) Evidence of CNS involvement.

Confirmation of the diagnosis can be obtained by culture of the vesicular fluid and swab from the genital tract of the mother.

MANAGEMENT
The infant should be nursed in isolation. No specific treatment is of proven value. There is a high mortality rate and in the survivors a high incidence of CNS damage.

Haemangioma with thrombocytopenia (Kasbach–Merritt syndrome)

This complication usually presents within the first few weeks of life. Characteristically it presents with a rapidly enlarging angioma with surrounding ecchymoses, but bleeding can occur anywhere including the gut. Platelets are sequestered in the angioma but multiple coagulation defects may be present.

MANAGEMENT
Transfusion with fresh blood is required. Systemic steroids should also be given and irradiation of the angioma if the bleeding is not controlled by steroid therapy.

DISORDERS OF KERATINIZATION

Icthyosis

This is a disorder of keratinization of the skin. There are four common inherited types.

Clinical syndrome	*Mode of inheritance*
Icthyosis vulgaris	Dominant
Icthyosis vulgaris	Sex-linked recessive (male children)
Icthyosiform erythroderma	Autosomal recessive
Bullous icthyosiform hyperkeratosis	Dominant

The first two conditions do not present until infancy and do not present acute problems in management.

Icthyosiform erythroderma

The essential features are erythroderma and hyperkeratosis.
    The severe form presents at birth as a collodion fetus. The baby is

encased in a thick yellowish-brown horny layer with fissures revealing erythematous skin in the cracks.

It is associated with ectropion, ear deformities and clawing of the hands and feet. The rigidity of the skin may restrict respiratory movements, sucking and swallowing, and be incompatible with life. In less severely affected babies the horny layer is quickly shed leaving a variable degree and distribution of erythema. In others hyperkeratosis persists throughout life.

MANAGEMENT

In the collodion fetus treatment is largely supportive, with intravenous feeding and antibiotics if the skin is fissured, bathing of the eyes, and emulsifying lotions for cleaning the shed scales from the skin.

Bullous icthyosiform hyperkeratosis

In this condition there is disordered keratinization, but also impaired cohesion between the cells of the upper epidermis leading to the formation of bullae.

The condition may present at birth or within the first few days of life with large crops of bullae, redness and peeling of the skin (and may be difficult to distinguish from epidermolysis bullosa, urticaria pigmentosa and incontinentia pigmenti (girls only)).

MANAGEMENT

This is symptomatic only. The tendency to blister decreases with age although the hyperkeratosis may become more marked.

CONGENITAL SYPHILIS

The treponema is transmitted through the placenta from the fourth month of pregnancy onwards.

RECOGNITION

This will of course be suspected if the mother is known to have syphilis. Skin lesions; maculopapular eruption, brownish-red in colour on the palms, soles, anogenital region and around the mouth. Haemorrhagic bullae occur, particularly of the palms and soles. Paronychia and anal condylomata may also be present. There may be a nasal discharge which is often blood-stained. Mucous patches may be seen on the lips, tongue or palate.

Other, non-cutaneous signs.

(a) Prematurity or low birth weight.

R

(b) Hepatomegaly, splenomegaly, lymphadenopathy.
(c) Meningitis. Convulsions may occur; the CSF has a raised protein with an increased cell count up to 100 lymphocytes per mm^3.
(d) Haemolytic anaemia, thrombocytopenia.
(e) Osteochondritis, dactylitis.

Any of the above signs may be present at birth but most frequently appear between the second and sixth week of life.

The diagnosis can be confirmed by dark-field examination of smear from skin lesion or nasal discharge and serology of infant and mother. A higher titre in the infant than the mother is diagnostic. This may have to be repeated at weekly intervals.

MANAGEMENT

The infant should be isolated until treatment has been completed. Intramuscular benzylpenicillin (150 000 units divided into 3 doses) is given daily for 15 days, or procaine penicillin 150 000 units (150 mg) i.m. daily for the same period.

General References

Paediatric dermatology (1971). *Pediat. Clins N. Am.* **18**, (3)
Soloman, L. M. and Esterley, H. B. *Neonatal Dermatology*. London: W. B. Saunders

Part XIV: Psychiatric Emergencies

CHAPTER 52

Acute Psychiatric Conditions

F. G. Thorpe

Psychiatric emergencies are not common in paediatric practice and apart from anorexia nervosa, non-accidental injury, and some adolescent suicidal attempts, they are seldom life-or-death situations. Nevertheless prompt action is necessary to prevent further suffering to the child and family, and, in the case of the young pre-adolescent, to interrupt behaviour patterns which are adversely affecting personality development. A careful history will usually reveal that the crisis is the culmination of increasingly maladaptive behaviour which has been manifest for some time. Children presenting with phobic anxiety states will have shown similar reactions before, such as the school-phobic child who experienced separation anxiety on starting school, or returning to school after every holiday, until finally attendance became impossible. The aetiology of psychiatric disorder in childhood is multifactorial. The initial contact with the parents is of vital importance and many parents may require psychiatric treatment in their own right; those who rationalize their own failure by blaming the school, other children in the neighbourhood, or accept the child's escape into somatic illness as a means of avoiding stress. The real urgency of the problem may sometimes be related to the parents' guilt or shame rather than to the true nature of the problem.

Suicidal attempts

RECOGNITION

Children and adolescents who make suicidal threats or attempts require urgent help. The clinician is sometimes uncertain whether or not to request a psychiatric opinion, particularly as there may well be a tendency to cover up suicidal attempts because of the social stigma and the desire by the parents to regard such events as being due to 'irresponsible hysterical behaviour'. This is more common in girls than boys, but boys are often more seriously disturbed. The frequency increases with age and reaches its peak in adolescence. Serious mental illness in the form of schizophrenia or depressive psychosis is rarely the cause of the suicidal attempt; the majority are reactively depressed, being faced with an unbearable situation from which they want to escape. In many cases the attempt is staged without the real goal of death, and the clinician must remember that the younger child does not comprehend the finality of death, and imagines himself being able to witness the impact of his act upon his parents and others causing his unhappiness. The younger generation see their parents taking tablets, or hear them expressing suicidal thoughts or making actual attempts, so it is not surprising that they do the same. The commonest method used is the ingestion of tablets, usually the property of their parents, many of whom are themselves depressed or have personality disorders.

The attempt may be caused by anger internalized as guilt and depression, is an attempt to manipulate another person to gain love and affection, or is designed to punish another person. It is a signal of distress and warrants immediate psychiatric help because of the tendency, in both the parent and the child, to suppress information concerning motives and underlying family tensions. When the act is a desire to join a dead relative, usually combined with the withdrawal of love by the remaining depressed parent, the motive is usually obvious.

MANAGEMENT
The paediatrician's role

Direct authoritative approaches which go straight into the details of the attempt and its motives are invariably met with denial. It is better to adopt a more gentle, non-demanding, unhurried approach and this usually requires the skills of someone with child-psychiatric training. A minimum of questioning by casualty officers and paediatric housemen is indicated, and they should restrict their activities to the management of the immediate medical problem and the child's admission to a place of safety where psychiatric assessment can take place.

The psychiatrist's role

Most of the affected children will reveal severe family and environmental stresses which require urgent attention, and many of their mothers will be suffering from depressive illness. Paternal rejection, desertion, or even death are common. Although the majority settle in hospital some remain depressed and need to be transferred to an appropriate psychiatric in-patient unit where they can be treated with antidepressants and given psychotherapy over a prolonged period. The treatment of acute depression is considered below. The resolution of family tensions requires all the skills of a psychiatric team, and casework for the parents, and possibly other members of the household, by a skilled psychiatric social worker is essential.

Anorexia nervosa

Although anorexia nervosa is typically a condition of adolescent girls, it is seen sometimes in pre-adolescent children and also in boys. These young people present in a state of extreme emaciation and a resolute determination not to eat food. Their parents are extremely concerned about their welfare but may have become rejecting and hostile after long periods of tempting with tasty morsels, bribing, leading finally to unsuccessful attempts at force-feeding.

RECOGNITION

The following criteria are essential in making the diagnosis.

(a) Attitude to food

The patient has a characteristic attitude towards food and will avoid carbohydrates, which are regarded as fattening. The subsequent loss of weight is marked and, depending upon parental concern, may well have fallen below the 3rd centile. In addition, other methods may be used to lose weight and get rid of nutrients, such as purging, self-induced vomiting, excessive indulgence in exercise and the hiding away of food which is claimed to have been eaten.

(b) Amenorrhoea

In pubertal girls there is amenorrhoea, or in younger children, if the condition persists, delayed onset of menstruation when all secondary sexual characteristics are fully developed. The output of pituitary gonadotrophin is reduced but pituitary function is otherwise normal and the long held view that it resembles Simmonds' disease is now recognized as incorrect.

(c) Fear of obesity

There is a distinctive psychopathology in all cases centred around a morbid fear of becoming obese and an aspiration to an ideal weight far below the mean. Anorexic patients may have a perceptual distortion of body image which accounts for this. Depression superimposed upon an obsessive-compulsive personality is a common feature and may precede the onset of food refusal. Self-mutilation is sometimes observed, and characteristically these patients remain very active and apparently full of energy until the terminal stages of the illness, which can be fatal.

(d) Past history

Often the child has had an above-average birth weight, with infant-feeding problems, obesity in infancy and an early menarche.

Anorexia nervosa may be seen psychologically as a subconscious reluctance to reach sexual maturity, and most of these girls have sexual problems which require psychotherapeutic help and which sometimes persist into adulthood. There is invariably conflict with the mother and problems of identification.

(e) Clinical features

These are secondary to the nutritional deficiency, and include bradycardia, hypotension, acrocyanosis, growth of lanugo hair, dry skin, reduced basal metabolic rate and avitaminosis.

MANAGEMENT

(a) General approach

Treatment is a matter of extreme urgency as the condition can be fatal, and admission to hospital is required. All cases of anorexia nervosa encountered in paediatric practice require the involvement of a child psychiatrist at the earliest opportunity, and, in addition to the treatment of the patient, the parents will require help to sort out their own attitudes towards their child. Unless the patient is extremely debilitated, requiring intravenous feeding and specialized medical care, treatment is better carried out in a psychiatric unit, as the patients are extremely manipulative and unreliable. They can become very depressed and possibly suicidal as they begin to gain weight, and sometimes develop an insatiable appetite. A kind but firm, well-structured approach is required and will test to the limit the nursing skills of the staff. The younger patient will probably be amenable to psychotherapy but the ability to respond diminishes with age, so that it may be almost impossible to establish a rapport with the older adolescent.

(b) Diet

In the early stages an 8400-joule (2000-calorie) liquid diet containing glucose and protein hydrolysate may be necessary but with skilful nursing the patient can soon commence a 12 600-joule (3000-calorie) solid diet. The unpleasant taste of the liquid diet appeals to the self-punitive aspects of the anorexic personality, and it is generally taken well.

(c) Drugs

Chlorpromazine is the drug of choice and high doses such as 75 mg to 100 mg three times daily may be required in older adolescents. Vitamin deficiencies require treatment and when food intake is reasonable the use of anabolic steroids such as nandrolone decanoate (Deca-Durabolin *Organon*) i.m. 12.5 to 25 mg every three weeks may increase food uptake.

School phobia

RECOGNITION

Background

Certain children display abnormal reactions to school of such intensity that they are now commonly termed school phobia, or, more appropriately, neurotic school refusal. They must be regarded as emergencies, firstly because of the nature of the impact they make upon the parents, teachers and various educational officers responsible for school attendance; and, secondly, because the condition may become chronic in the absence of therapeutic intervention. Neurotic school refusal can sometimes be overlooked when the child expresses anxiety predominantly through somatic pathways (e.g. complaints of pain) and the unwary clinician becomes preoccupied with excessive, unnecessary physical investigations. The symptoms may occur either during a child's initial school experience, at the beginning of each new school term, but most commonly reach crisis level on commencing secondary education at the age of eleven or twelve years, often following absence for a minor illness. A phobia is an irrational fear and the reaction is one of intense anxiety, amounting in many cases to panic about the school from which the child protects himself by withdrawal. The psychopathology is usually one of separation anxiety, the child and mother having developed a neurotic bond so that neither can function adequately alone. It is not uncommon to find a mother with agoraphobia, but in every case the attitude towards the child will be one of anxious overprotection, and fathers tend to be passive or sometimes absent. The children function well academically, are frequently of above-average intelligence, and overachieve because they fear the teacher's reprimand, or escape into work to avoid social contact with other children. They will rationalize their absence from school by finding fault with their teacher or peer group and the mother is only too willing to accept this.

Physical symptoms

Children who escape into physical illness display less overt anxiety but present with nausea, vomiting, abdominal pain, headache or limb pains, and both they and their parents lose sight of the true nature of the neurotic conflict. Enquiry will usually reveal that the child wants to go to school if only he could understand his problems, in contrast to the truant who wilfully avoids school as part of a delinquent syndrome, and whose parents are unaware of his absence and not particularly interested. Symptoms are at their worst first thing on school mornings, and minimal at weekends and during school holidays. The child's immaturity may also be shown in aggressive ways leading to ambivalent feelings about parents, which in older children may find actual verbal expression.

MANAGEMENT

(a) General approach

All cases of school phobia require urgent referral to the Child Psychiatric Services as their treatment is complex, time-consuming and aimed at breaking down the neurotic bond between the child and parent. This will involve psychotherapeutic treatment for both and in severe cases separation may only be achieved by admitting the child to a psychiatric unit. The child should be returned to school at the earliest opportunity and in order to do this it will be necessary to get the close co-operation of the Educational Services. Behaviour-modification techniques using progressive desensitization are useful methods of treatment for these cases.

(b) Drug treatment

Medication alone will never resolve the problem but may diminish anxiety while the above procedures are carried out. Diazepam 2 to 5 mg three times daily or medazepam 5 to 10 mg three times daily, according to the age of the child, may be used. The mother herself may well need psychiatric treatment for neurotic depression when she finally releases her child.

(c) Psychometric assessment

This should always be done by an educational psychologist to exclude the rare case with a specific learning difficulty, inappropriate school placement, or any other real stress in school.

(d) Resistant cases

These sometimes occur in adolescence, the personality remaining too immature to cope with the complexities of comprehensive education.

Such cases are best transferred to day schools for maladjusted children, with a more supportive regime.

Acute depression

RECOGNITION

(a) Background

Depressive states are not as common in children as in adults. They are neurotic depressions in which anxiety is partly or completely replaced by depressive mood. They are sometimes masked, taking the form of behaviour disorders of various types, often with a self-punitive content, or even habit disorders such as encopresis. These conditions are not acute and should be dealt with in the usual way.

(b) Common presenting symptoms

The child who presents with a history of increasing weepiness, loss of interest in his surroundings, anorexia, despondency, withdrawal and morbid ideas about death or related subjects, requires urgent help. The possibility of a suicidal attempt must always be considered, especially in adolescence, and the management of this has already been described. The child with acute depression is usually facing overwhelming environmental stress within the family, such as sudden rejection or the death of a parent, or he has been exposed to the loss of one or two favoured grandparents to whom he was very attached. Boys sometimes become very depressed when a father has deserted the family, without any previous hint of marital disharmony, and makes no attempt to maintain contact. The child coping with a chronic handicap may also develop severe depressive reactions.

(c) Possible endogenous depression

The depression becomes of psychotic intensity only when there is loss of contact with reality, and this is very rare in the pre-adolescent child. However, depressions do sometimes develop in a secure, stable environment and respond dramatically to appropriate antidepressant medication and so appear to have been endogenous in type. The parents of such children may themselves exhibit a cyclothymic temperament, with alternating depression and exuberance.

MANAGEMENT

(a) General approach

All the patients require urgent psychiatric help and, if the depression seems profound, admission to a paediatric ward pending psychiatric consultation should be considered, particularly if there have been suicidal threats. The only firm contra-indication to such an admission is the child still in mourning after bereavement. Reactive depressions in young people respond well to psychotherapeutic help once the nature of the stress has been identified and dealt with. The resolution of conflicts in very disturbed families can be a long-term problem; social work skills have to be used and inpatient care may be appropriate.

(b) Drug treatment

Tricyclic antidepressant drugs or monoamine oxidase inhibitors may be life-saving in the adolescent case, but should be prescribed only on the recommendation of a psychiatrist and the normal dietary precautions* taken with the latter. Adolescents will require between 50 and 150 mg daily of imipramine, the dose being gradually increased over a period of two to three weeks, or phenelzine 30 to 60 mg daily, in divided doses. It is rarely necessary to give ECT to young people with acute depression.

Hysteria

RECOGNITION

Background

It is important not to confuse hysteria with the somatic symptoms produced by anxiety, such as recurrent abdominal pain, headaches, nausea, vomiting, frequency of micturition and diarrhoea. In hysteria the somatic symptoms are based upon the patient's inability to cope with reality and his attempt to resolve his conflict by 'dissociation', in which the anxiety about his basic conflict is 'converted' into an hysterical symptom. This symptom usually has secondary gain, commonly avoidance of the original situation, and may also have a symbolic meaning or be imitative of a near relative with a similar symptom due to organic causes. Thus a child may develop a disorder of gait because for some reason he is unable to leave his mother; he may also be immature and literally 'unable to stand on his own two feet'. Because the anxiety has been converted into a somatic symptom, patients with hysteria sometimes show a singular lack of concern for their disability,

---

* Avoidance of Bovril, Oxo, broad beans, Marmite and other yeast extracts, wines, beers or other alcohols, yoghurt, pickled herrings, flavoured textured vegetable proteins (*Monthly Index of Medical Specialties*, 1976); applies to monoamine oxidase inhibitors.

a state known as 'belle indifférence'. Although at one time this was an essential criterion for the diagnosis of hysteria, it is less common in hysterical patients today.

Hysteria is rare in childhood and increases only slightly in frequency during adolescence. The diagnosis must be made with extreme caution as nearly half the cases will eventually be found to have organic illness, especially those with disorders of vision. Although obvious emotional causes for the condition can sometimes be found this is not always so. In pure hysteria there is often a rapid onset of symptoms and a family history of hysterical symptoms. In pre-adolescence it is equally common in both sexes but in adolescence and adulthood females predominate. Epidemic hysteria is also seen in groups of adolescent girls.

Clinical features

Hysteria may present in any of the following ways.
- (a) Disorders of mobility, including abnormalities of gait, psychogenic paralyses, aphonia.
- (b) Disorders of perception, including loss of vision, deafness, insensitivity to pain, and other disorders of sensation.
- (c) Disorders of consciousness, including fits and fugues which are more common in adolescence.

Signs not compatible with known organic disease are demonstrable in many cases as the condition portrayed is the creation of the patient's own mind. A few cases however will be extremely difficult to diagnose with any degree of certainty and prolonged observation will be necessary.

MANAGEMENT

A high proportion of young people with hysterical symptoms find themselves admitted to paediatric wards for further assessment. Whether or not this is the case, early psychiatric involvement and a full neurological investigation is a matter of urgency as early intervention improves the prognosis. These cases require the closest co-operation between paediatricians and child psychiatrists, and in some cases prolonged treatment is necessary. A full psychosocial investigation is required to try to uncover the source of stress, either exogenous or endogenous, which if successful will give psychotherapeutic directives to be used to enable the patient to 'reconvert' to normal function. Although environmental manipulation is seldom successful with adults, some success may be achieved with children. Opportunities should be given for the patient to give up symptoms without 'losing face'. Strong suggestion can be used but hypnosis has its dangers and should be attempted only by a psychiatrist with special skills. Drugs have little to offer in treatment unless abreactive techniques are used, which is unlikely in young patients.

Drug abuse and dependence

RECOGNITION

Background

The possibility of drug abuse must always be considered in patients with toxic confusional states or psychotic-like reactions. At one time this problem was uncommon but in recent years adolescent drug-taking has increased in Western countries, and experimentation with drugs may also occur in young teenage children. It usually starts at parties or group meetings in an attempt to produce uninhibited relaxation or excitement, and, although sometimes a substitute for the alcoholic habits of previous generations, the two can be mixed for extra 'kicks' with dangerous results. Therefore, many young people presenting for emergency treatment may not be drug addicts, but nevertheless nearly every case warrants further investigation.

Toxic substances

(*a*) *Glue sniffing*   Glue sniffing or the inhalation of solvents is a form of addiction that may be encountered in the younger child and can produce symptoms very much like alcoholic intoxication, progressing to stupor. The characteristic odour is usually evident. It is important that the habit should be broken before the patient develops liver and kidney damage.

(*b*) *Soft drugs*   The clinician is more likely to meet patients in early adolescence on 'soft drugs' which cause the minimum of physical dependence but considerable psychological dependence because of the enjoyment obtained. If a drug provides a personality need, dependence is more likely to occur and there may be progression to 'hard drugs', but this is by no means the rule. The 'soft drugs' include stimulants, like caffeine, amphetamine (including Drinamyl) and cocaine, and hallucinogens such as cannabis (marihuana, 'pot') or lysergic acid diethylamide (LSD). Since the medical profession has virtually ceased to prescribe amphetamines and the chemists do not need to carry stocks which may be stolen, amphetamine dependence is probably not on the increase. It does however sometimes produce a psychotic state with delusions and hallucinations not unlike an acute attack of schizophrenia. Methedrine is often self-administered by intravenous injection.

Euphoria, flight of ideas and vivid hallucinatory experiences dominate the picture with LSD and less so with cannabis. The former can produce states very similar to schizophrenic excitability and may precipitate latent psychosis in vulnerable subjects. It is usually taken on blotting paper or a sugar lump and cannot be reliably detected in the urine.

(*c*) *Sedatives*   Barbiturates and compound drugs such as glutethimide, methaqualone with diphenhydramine (Mandrax) are also used by adolescents and may present varying clinical pictures. They are more readily available on the drug market and are frequently taken with alcohol. When dependence develops, withdrawal should only ·be attempted in hospital as it can be complicated by convulsions and hyperpyrexia.

(*d*) *Hard drugs*   It is very unlikely that the paediatrician will encounter patients on 'hard drugs' like narcotics (opiates, pethidine, methadone and others). Should this occur specialist psychiatric services will be urgently required.

(*e*) *Drunkenness in adolescence*   Fashions in adolescent cultures are constantly changing and there are indications that teenagers are becoming increasingly attracted to alcohol. The pub is becoming the social club and one recent study showed that 15 per cent of 14-year-old girls frequent pubs regularly. Alcohol is more readily available in family homes and parents permit their children a drink on social occasions. Alcoholism is not seen in young children; but among adolescents, in addition to those sufferring from acute alcoholic poisoning it is not uncommon to find those whose drinking causes social rather than medical problems. Such patients may eventually become psychologically dependent upon alcohol. The association between drinking alcohol and antisocial behaviour is well known and the resulting violence may bring young intoxicated patients to casualty departments with a variety of physical injuries. Frequent attenders require further investigation by a social worker, and those individuals who need alcohol to cope with life as a form of psychological crutch should be referred for psychiatric opinion as a matter of urgency.

MANAGEMENT

The clinician must use his knowledge of toxicology in dealing with the immediate medical emergency and identifying the overdose syndrome. Urine and blood samples should be taken where appropriate. When psychotic-like states are encountered psychiatric opinion may be needed to exclude acute schizophrenia. All cases of suspected drug abuse ultimately require thorough medical, psychological and sociological investigation, particularly to determine the source of the offending drugs and warn the appropriate authorities. When drug dependence is present skilled psychiatric treatment is a matter of urgency and referral to a drug addiction unit may be necessary.

References

Connell, P. H. (1965). Suicidal attempts in childhood and adolescence. In *Modern Perspectives in Child Psychiatry*. Ed. J. G. Howells. p. 403. Edinburgh: Oliver and Boyd

Crisp, A. H. (1967). Anorexia nervosa. *Br. J. Hosp. Med.* **1**, 713

Hersov, L. (1976). Hysteria. In *Child Psychiatry. Modern Approaches*. Ed. M. Rutter and L. Hersov. p. 437. Oxford: Blackwell

Kahn, J. H. and Nursten, J. P. (1968). *Unwillingly to School*. Oxford: Pergamon Press

Part XV: Medico-Social and Medico-Legal Conditions

CHAPTER 53

Injury: Non-Accidental (Child Abuse)

(Non-Accidental injury, Battered Baby syndrome, Concealed parental violence, Silverman's syndrome).

J. A. Black

It should be remembered that actual physical injury is only one aspect of child abuse and that others include nutritional deprivation, 'imprisonment' within the home, emotional deprivation or abuse, sexual abuse, the giving of harmful drugs and withholding of essential medical care.

The first attempts to modify the law in relation to baby battering were made in the U.S.A.

The legal procedures described here apply only to England and Wales.

RECOGNITION

Ideally, the child at risk for non-accidental injury should be recognized before any physical injury has occurred. Common early warnings are:
- (a) Feeding difficulties in infancy: persistent crying or vomiting, failure to gain weight.
- (b) Severe chronic napkin eruptions with ulceration or scarring.
- (c) Frequent attendances at Casualty Departments, or hospital admissions for vomiting and diarrhoea or other complaints which are not observed during admission.
- (d) In the pre-school child, accidental ingestion of household remedies or drugs.
- (e) In the school child, poor school attendance, persistent lateness for school, unkempt or neglected appearance, apathetic or withdrawn behaviour. Loss of weight or failure to gain weight. Sudden and apparently unexplained scholastic failure.
- (f) Any of the above occuring in a sib.
- (g) A cot death in a sib.

'At risk' parents and families should be recognized. Specific factors which predispose to non-accidental injury are one or more of the following:

The unsupported unmarried mother.

Very young parents.

Maternal depression (often unrecognized).

Deprivation during the childhood of one or both parents.

Parental (usually paternal) criminal record.

Alcholism or drug usage.

Overcrowding $\pm$ poor economic circumstances.

A physically malformed (rejected) child.

A child who returns home having remained in hospital for weeks or months from the moment of birth (inadequate opportunity for the development of the normal bonding between mother and child).

When injury has occurred the explanation may not fit the type or severity of the injury, or the sequence of events appears improbably complex or contrived. The interval between the time of injury and attendance at hospital may be inexplicably long or does not agree with the clinical appearances. The attitude of the parents is often one of unconcern or, less commonly, extreme overconcern, in either case a degree of anxiety inappropriate to the injury. Occasionally it is suggested by them that the child has a tendency to self-injury.

TYPES OF INJURY

    (a) Bruises: these are often of different ages; commonly on the face, round the eyes or at the elbow. A pattern of finger impressions may be visible.

    (b) Swelling of the joints, usually the elbow joint.

    (c) Swelling on the scalp due to a bruise or cephalhaematoma.

    (d) Skin lesions; bite marks, scratches, cigarette burns, excoriations, scalds.

    (e) Abdominal distension, bile-stained vomiting or shock, may indicate rupture or haematoma of a viscus.

    (f) Vomiting and bulging fontanelle in infants suggest subdural haematoma.

ACTION ON SUSPECTING NON-ACCIDENTAL INJURY

(a) Admission to hospital

The child is admitted at once to hospital for observation and investigation. This is rarely resisted by the parents at this stage since they are usually glad of the resulting relief of emotional tension. If the parents are unwilling to have the child admitted voluntarily a Place of Safety Order can be obtained at any hour through a magistrate (Justice of the Peace) on application by a local authority social worker, an officer of the National Society for the Prevention of Cruelty to Children (N.S.P.C.C.) or, in exceptional cases, a police officer; all these agencies have someone 'on-call' at all times. Normally the hospital ward will be the designated place of safety; the order expires after 28 days (8 days if on police application) but can be renewed for a further 28 days (Interim Order) through another application to a Juvenile Court.

While a Place of Safety or Interim Order is in operation the parents cannot remove the child, and the police will if necessary provide enforcement of the order.

(b) Talking to the parents

As soon as possible after admission the parents should be seen by the consultant, usually a paediatrician. No accusations should be made but every effort should be made to gain their confidence and to work with them towards an understanding of what has happened. This does not mean acting as an amateur detective. The parents should be seen by the hospital social worker who will also gather information from other sources about the family. Many of the affected families are already known to one or more social agencies or to the police. A doctor is considered to be within his rights in relation to confidentiality in giving all necessary information to safeguard the child, without having to obtain the permission of the parents (*Annual Report of the Medical Defence Union*, 1972).

(c) Physical examination and investigation

(*i*) *Evidence of other injuries*   A meticulous physical examination should be made, with accurate descriptions of all injuries and sketches in the notes. An estimate of the age of each injury should be given. The state of cleanliness (or otherwise) of the hair, skin and clothing is also important. An assessment of the child's behaviour and response to adults (apathetic, frightened, withdrawn, etc.) should also be included, and the approximate level of psychomotor achievements. In all cases the height, weight, and head circumference should be recorded and the retinae examined for haemorrhages after dilating the pupils. The mouth should be inspected for tears of the frenum of the upper lip or other evidence of trauma. The time, date and place of the examination must be recorded and signed legibly, with the doctor's name printed below the signature. Whenever practicable, photographs of the injury should be taken, preferably in colour.

(*ii*) *Differential diagnosis*   On the clinical findings this should include bleeding disorders, coagulation defects, capillary fragility, scurvy, Mongolian blue spot. In Vietnam, Malaysia and other countries in the Far East, 'coin-rubbing' produces linear petechial or purpuric lesions which may be mistaken for strap-marks (Golden and Duster, 1977).

(*iii*) *Special investigations*   A radiographic examination of the whole skeleton should be made (skeletal survey) to detect the bony involvement in known injuries and any previous or unsuspected injury. The characteristic radiographic findings in non-accidental injury are multiple injuries of different ages, obvious fracture of the forearm, ribs or skull, chip fractures of the metaphyses, displaced epiphyses, calcified subperiosteal haematoma, and new bone formation in the mandible.

The differential diagnosis of the radiographic findings includes, infantile cortical hyperostosis (Caffey's disease), osteogenesis imperfecta (fragilitas ossium), scurvy, syphilis, the severe renal osteodystrophy and rickets sometimes seen in cystinosis (cystine storage disease), hypophosphatasia (often associated with subdural haematoma).

Haematological investigations should include platelet count, prothrombin time, partial thromboplastin time, and a cuff (Hess') test for capillary fragility.

(*d*) *Psychiatric examination*

A psychiatric assessment of the pre-school or school child may provide useful baseline observations, but more important is an assessment of the parents. This is aimed at discovering any unrecognized condition such as depression, where treatment could alter the whole situation and make it possible to return the child to his parents without fear of further injury. The psychiatrist can usually give a prognosis for response to treatment or case work. Psychosis (rare) and psychopathic personality (common) have a poor prognosis for normal family life. Borderline subnormality or definite subnormality is common, particularly in the mothers, and a criminal trend is found in about 10 per cent of the mothers and 30 per cent of the fathers (Smith, Hanson and Noble, 1973).

(*e*) *Case conference*

If at all possible this should be called within 48 hours of admitting the child to hospital and should involve the paediatrician, pyschiatrist, any other specialist involved (e.g. orthopaedic surgeon), hospital and local authority social workers, the worker originally involved in bringing the child to hospital, and any others with recent or relevant knowledge of the family. The conference may include the very important family doctor, health visitor, probation officer, N.S.P.C.C. representative, school teacher, education welfare officer, school nurse and the police.

Even though many helpers may be called in, a small group requires less organization and reaches a decision more quickly, and one person (often the paediatrician) should guide the discussion.

The objects of a case conference are:

(i) To correlate all relevant information.

(ii) To obtain an agreed plan of action.

(iii) To nominate one person in particular to work with the parents, to prevent a multiplicity of visits, to avoid contradictory statements, and to establish a good relationship.

(f) Long-term planning

This is outside the scope of this chapter, but should involve an attempt to improve the attitudes of the parents in order that the child can, at some time, return safely to the family.

References

Annual Report of the Medical Defence Union, (1972). p.21

Golden, S. M. and Duster, M. C. (1977). Hazards of misdiagnosis due to Vietnamese folk medicine. *Clin. Pediat.* **16**, 949

Smith, S. M., Hanson, R. and Noble, S. (1973). Parents of battered babies. A controlled study. *Br. med. J.* **4**, 388

GENERAL REFERENCES

Helfer, R. E. and Kempe, C. H. (1973). *The Battered Child*, 2nd ed. University of Chicago

Kempe, C. H. and Helfer, R. E. (1972), *Helping the Battered Child and his Family*. Philadelphia: J. B. Lippincott

Schmitt, B. D. and Kempe, C. H. (1975). Management and prevention of the Battered Child syndrome. *Folia Traumatologica. Geigy*. Basle: Ciba-Geigy Ltd.

CHAPTER 54

Sudden Infant Death

(Cot death; Sudden Infant Death syndrome)

J. R. Oakley

In the United Kingdom, approximately 1 in 400 of all apparently normal and well-formed infants die unexpectedly at home, and provide roughly half of all the deaths between the ages of 1 week and 2 years. Much research has been carried out to try to discover a single, but as yet unidentified, disease process causing these deaths. It is now generally accepted that these unexpected deaths have a variety of causes (*British Medical Journal,* 1975) and that many are due to recognizable and potentially treatable conditions (McWeeny and Emery, 1975). These treatable conditions are mainly infective illnesses, particularly bronchopneumonia, gastroenteritis with dehydration, meningitis, septicaemia and tracheobronchitis. Deaths from these diseases are potentially avoidable. Unfortunately, at least a quarter of the unexpected deaths remain unexplained, even after extensive necropsy.

RECOGNITION

The classic history initially obtained is of an infant who has been apparently well when put to bed, and who had later simply been found dead. (Later investigations usually reveal the presence of signs or symptoms of disease in the infant before death (McWeeny and Emery, 1975)). A doctor becomes involved either by being called to the infant's home, or by receiving the infant at a Casualty Department. Often, the parents will be attempting to revive the infant by 'mouth to mouth' resuscitation, even though the infant may obviously have been dead for some time. Occasionally a moribund infant will be seen, who will need vigorous resuscitation (by endotracheal intubation and inflation of the lungs, external cardiac massage or IPPV).

The only important differential diagnosis is that of infanticide, which is rare, and usually made obvious by clinical evidence of excessive ill-treatment.

MANAGEMENT

(a) The infant

Initial physical examination should certify that death has occurred (fixed dilated pupils, absent heart sounds, absent respiration). The exact findings and time of day should be noted for medico-legal purposes. It is rare to find clinical indications of the cause of death, but the purpura of meningococcal septicaemia, and signs of ill treatment such as excessive or unusual bruising, should be looked for and documented. If meningococcal infection is suspected, prophylactic treatment of the family and medical personnel in contact with the infant should begin, using sulphonamides, after throat and nasal swabs have been taken from the infant and contacts.

As the majority of the unexpected deaths are found to have recognizable causes at necropsy, it is not for the doctor who certifies that death has occurred to give a cause of death. All unexpected deaths should be reported to the Coroner, who will arrange a necropsy, and subsequently issue a cause of death. The Coroner will expect an account of the clinical findings when death was certified, and a brief history of the infant's last 48 hours of life, including the amount and type of feeds taken, medical consultations and medicaments, the time of the last feed, the time the infant was last seen alive, and the time the infant was discovered, and by whom.

If the infant is certified dead at home, arrangements should be made to transfer the body to the town mortuary. Otherwise, the body should be transferred to the hospital mortuary.

(b) The parents

Most doctors fortunately encounter a 'cot death' only rarely, but the management of the bereaved parents is of the utmost importance, and often inadequate. The parents are bewildered and devastated by the inexplicable death of their infant, often experiencing much unfounded guilt and self-reproach. Accordingly, history-taking should not be lengthy and interrogative, but brief and sympathetic.

Many doctors dealing with bereaved parents feel themselves ill at ease, the feeling being accentuated by being asked questions about the infant's death which they are ill-equipped to answer. It is wise to admit that the cause of death is unknown, and as such a 'post-mortem' is necessary, which may reveal not only the cause of death, but also provide information to help research into the causes and prevention of other similar unexpected deaths.

To allay fears that they may be under suspicion of infanticide, the parents should be warned that the Coroner is involved in all cases of unexplained death at any age (and, as such, parental permission for necropsy is not required), and that in the United Kingdom the police are required to take a statement concerning the facts of death. The parents should be referred to the Coroner's Officer or to the hospital mortuary attendant for advice concerning interment of the body; a personal introduction is a kindly action.

Following the initial explanatory counselling, the bereaved parents will need subsequent support, preferably from someone interested in unexpected deaths locally to whom they can be referred. The family's general practitioner can play an important role, and should be informed of the death of the patient within a few hours at the latest, of the occurrence. Further help can be obtained from organizations founded by similarly bereaved parents. In the United Kingdom, an address for the parents to write to is:

The Secretary,
The Foundation for the Study of Infant Deaths,
23, St. Peter's Square,
LONDON W6 9NW
Tel: 01-748-7768

References

British Medical Journal. (1975). Risk of cot deaths. (Leading article). **3**, 664
McWeeny, P. M. and Emery, J. L. (1975). Unexpected postneonatal deaths (cot deaths) due to recognizable disease. *Archs Dis. Childh.* **50**, 191

Sexual Interference with Children

Alan Usher

Sexual interference with children is nearly always perpetrated by men—often middle-aged, or older men in positions of trust. It can be divided into two categories—major sexual interference, where the assailant makes a serious attempt to insert his penis into the child's vagina or anus and thus enjoy a form of coitus; and minor sexual interference, where he contents himself with some lesser degree of molestation.

Minor sexual interference

This shades almost imperceptibly from hugging and caressing children, through 'bottom-patting' to touching and fondling the child's private parts outside and inside the clothing, digital penetration of the vulva or anus, and frank masturbation. Sometimes the adult will persuade the child to handle him indecently (which constitutes a separate offence under the 1967 Sexual Offences Act) or will attempt to have oral sex or will indulge in intercrural intercourse either from behind or in front. These practices rarely result in physical harm, except that in very young girls the hymen, which is small and usually membranous, may be ruptured by even the passage of a finger through its hiatus, and occasionally there can be small tears of the vagina from jagged finger nails. The only physical traces of such acts apart from those noted above are likely to be some evanescent reddening of the labia (a not uncommon finding in young girls, anyway, from a variety of causes) and the inner aspects of the thighs together with the deposition of semen on thighs, buttocks, clothing or in the oral cavity according to where (and if) ejaculation has taken place. Such cases are generally classed as 'indecent assault' or 'indecency with children' by the police.

Major sexual interference

The first penetration of the vulva by the erect adult penis in an older co-operative girl (unlawful sexual intercourse) usually results in stretching and eventual rupture of the hymen in its posterior segment with transient pain and bleeding; the tear takes some ten days to heal. In a proportion of girls, those with a crenated distensible hymen, there is no tear even after several penetrations. The vaginal introitus merely distends and the hymen stretches. Eventually with repeated penetrations the hymen becomes deficient and largely disappears. In a younger, smaller child forcible penetration may result in serious injury with tearing of the hymen, the fourchette and even the perineum and rectum. The only real proof that penetration was due to a penis is the finding of semen in the vagina or the rectum. Where the act has been accomplished by force (rape) evidence of resistance is likely to be found in proportion to the age and size of the child; a 5-year-old girl may well be overcome by the sheer weight of her assailant on top of her and show little evidence of resistance, while a muscular 15-year-old may show bruises over the sacrum, shoulder blades, wrists and arms as well as between the knees and on the throat. She may also show scratches on her thighs, neck and vulva in addition to the signs of recent defloration.

Penile penetration of the anus (buggery), especially without the aid of lubricants produces initially a painful, bruised anus often with radial bleeding tears of the mucosa, and spasm of the anal sphincter which may last for several days. Swabs taken from inside the rectum as well as from the external anal margin may reveal the presence of semen and/or lubricants, as well as venereal disease. Gross damage to the anus, including complete tearing of the sphincter, may be caused in the small child thus abused.

Repeated acts of buggery produce in the passive partner epithelialization of the anus, often with radial fissures, a lax sphincter with loss of normal sphincteric reflex and ultimately loss of the ischiorectal pads of fat producing a 'funnel-shaped anus'.

EXAMINATION

The best person to examine a child thought to have been molested sexually is undoubtedly a trained police surgeon, who in the United Kingdom can always be contacted by the local police. If however, he is not available the most senior clinician available should be asked to do so. This doctor should be given all the information available concerning the incident and should see the parents, obtaining their formal consent to examination before interviewing the child, not only about this episode but where appropriate about any previous sexual experience. The examination should be carried out under the best conditions possible, even in the operating theatre should the child's condition merit this. Clothing worn at the time should be retained, each garment separately, in large (x-ray) envelopes labelled and listed. Swabs from the mouth, anus, vagina, rectum, vulva etc. should be sealed, labelled and listed as should 'universal bottles' containing nail clippings, head and pubic hair, stain scrapings etc. The extent of the examination will vary with the nature of the case but young children who cannot be relied upon to tell the whole story and cases of rape, where the signs of resistance are of vital importance, should always be examined from head to toe including the anus and the genitalia. Notes and diagrams must be made at the time or immediately afterwards while the facts are fresh in the mind, and retained personally by the examiner who may copy a summary into the case notes. Bacteriology specimens must be dealt with by a hospital laboratory, the rest of the labelled, dated and listed specimens should be handed over to a police officer for transmission to the nearest government forensic laboratory. The child's parents should be re-interviewed and told the results of the examination; they should be encouraged to 'play the matter down' as much as possible, unless in fact the child begins to display symptoms suggesting the need for referral to a child psychiatrist.

REPORT

The police are involved in a large proportion of these cases since parents are generally keen to bring this type of offender to book. The officer in the case will usually be glad to have an immediate verbal report from the doctor after his examination, stating whether or not the findings are consistent with what was alleged or suspected to have taken place. Later when laboratory examination of the specimens is complete, the examiner, using his notes, should write a full report in the form of a statement for use in court. This is in three parts, the first setting out the examiner's name, professional qualifications and position and stating when, where and how he came to make the examination, the second recounting the factual part of the examination, i.e. his observations, and a third part, his reasonable deductions from these facts.

Part XVI: Tropical and Subtropical Disorders

CHAPTER 56

Heat Illnesses and Hyperpyrexia

J. A. Black

The acute clinical states associated with exposure to excessive heat are described separately; but it should be realized that they rarely occur in a pure form and that various combinations can be expected. The main diagnostic points are given in Table 56.I.

Always look for a predisposing condition

Sunburn

This may be associated with pyrexia and occasionally with hyperpyrexia in heatstroke when a large area of the body surface is involved, with impaired sweating, or where there is concomitant water or salt depletion.

AT RISK
Infants left lying in the sun: fair skinned or red-haired individuals, albinos.

MANAGEMENT
See page 493.

Heat syncope

A typical syncopal attack occurring in the absence of water or salt depletion.

AT RISK
Older children coming to a hot climate, in whom acclimatization has not occurred.

TABLE 56.I
Differential diagnosis of heat illnesses

Diagnosis	Predisposing cause(s)	Symptoms	Temperature	Thirst	Urine vol.	Chlorides in urine	Plasma sodium
Heat syncope	Lack of acclimatization	Fainting	N	O	N	+	N
Heat cramps	Muscular work with sodium depletion + drinking water to relieve thirst	Cramps in muscles used.	N	O	N	O or reduced	Reduced
Heat exhaustion (water depletion)	Infants, ill or subnormal children unable to drink freely	Irritability in infants; giddiness or faintness in children: dry mouth	N or Raised	+ +	Reduced	+	Raised
Heat exhaustion (sodium depletion)	Any salt-losing state: sweating, cystic fibrosis, gastroenteritis	Apathy in infants. Weakness, lassitude in children	N	O	N	O	Reduced
Heatstroke	Environmental overheating, sodium depletion, impaired sweating (*Figure 56.1*)	Listlessness and headache leads to Sweating ceasing leads to Hyperpyrexia leads to Coma $\pm$ fits	Markedly raised	+	Reduced	O	N or Reduced

N = Normal; O = Absent; + = Present; + + = Marked increase

MANAGEMENT
Reassurance only, and advice on adaptation to heat.

Heat cramps

Painful muscle spasms due to excessive or prolonged work or exercise in conditions producing profuse sweating, and the resulting thirst being relieved by unsalted fluids.

AT RISK
Unacclimatized individuals are most likely to suffer, and the condition is rarely seen in its pure form in children. Either very high environmental temperature with low humidity, or lower temperatures with high humidity, can produce this condition.

RECOGNITION
The muscles affected are usually those involved in the muscular work. The general condition is good and there is no dehydration.

CONFIRMATION
The cramps can sometimes be reproduced by exposing affected muscles to cold or prolonged contraction. Depletion of sodium (sodium chloride) can be quickly confirmed by the absence of chloride in the urine* or by the finding of low plasma sodium and chloride levels.

MANAGEMENT
  (a) There may be a considerable sodium chloride deficit amounting to as much as 15 to 20 g (200–300 mmols) in adolescents. It may be difficult to persuade children to drink large quantities of normal saline without vomiting, though this can sometimes be avoided if the saline is flavoured with lime juice or other fruit drinks. Even using normal saline approximately 1500 ml will be required to replace 15 g of salt, and double this amount if half-strength saline is used. If normal saline is not available 1-g sodium chloride tablets can be used in the proportion of 1 g to 100 ml or $3\frac{1}{2}$ fluid ounces of water (1 teaspoonful of salt is equivalent roughly to 4 g of salt). The replenishment of salt stores is indicated by the reappearance of chloride in the urine.
  If there is vomiting, use IV normal 0.9 per cent sodium chloride in proportion to the estimated requirements.

Treat any coexistent condition

* Fantus' test: *see* Appendix 15

Heat exhaustion (Heat prostration)

Water-depletion heat exhaustion.

A state of water depletion (true dehydration) due to inadequate replacement of water lost from sweating and often accompanied by gastroenteritis or other febrile illness which may interfere with normal feeding.

AT RISK

Any child who cannot indicate its need for additional water or who is unable to obtain extra water independently.

Infants, mentally subnormal children, or those suffering from cerebral palsy or other chronic neurological disorder.

This condition is most likely to occur in sudden heat-waves in areas unaccustomed to coping with excessive heat.

RECOGNITION

(*a*) *Infants*   Irritability, dry mouth, refusal of normal feeds but avid acceptance of water, small hard stools, oliguria or anuria (dry nappy). If a hyperosmolar (hypertonic or hypernatraemic) state has developed there will be peripheral cyanosis and a doughy or firm feel to the skin. Fits, hyperpyrexia or heatstroke may complicate severe cases.

(*b*) *Older children*   Thirst, fatigue, giddiness, oliguria. In both age groups, chloride will be present in the urine.

CONFIRMATION

(*a*) *Infants*   If urine is passed it is small in amount and of high osmolality (specific gravity); plasma sodium is usually above 140 mmol per litre and urea above 25.0 mmol per litre (150 mg%).

(*b*) *Older children*   Except in the mentally subnormal or those with chronic neurological disease the plasma sodium is unlikely to be much above 140 mmol per litre. Oliguria is present and the urine will be of high osmolality (specific gravity).

MANAGEMENT

(*a*) *Infants*   If the plasma sodium is 150 mmol per litre or above special treatment will be needed to prevent intractable fits and brain damage, or cerebral oedema resulting from a too rapid reduction of intracellular fluid sodium concentration (*see* page 130).

In the absence of hypernatraemia, replacement of fluids can normally be done by giving extra water (equivalent to the volume of the child's usual feed) between feeds and diluting the usual feeds to half-strength by the addition of water. If intravenous fluids are required because of severe illness without hypernatraemia, or because of vomiting or refusal of feeds, 0.18 per cent sodium chloride in 4 per cent glucose (N/5 saline) should be used; completely salt-free solutions such as 5 per cent or 10 per cent glucose may cause water intoxication (*see* page 130).

(*b*) *Older children*   Except in the mentally subnormal or those with neurological disease the replacement of fluid should be by mouth in quantities dictated by thirst or the re-establishment of a normal urine flow, if communication is difficult.

Treat any coexistent condition

Salt-depletion heat exhaustion

A state of sodium depletion with hypovolaemia and reduced extracellular fluid due to excessive losses of sodium and water in the sweat. Other febrile illnesses or gastroenteritis may precipitate symptoms.

AT RISK
Unacclimatized individuals; children with cystic fibrosis or other salt-losing states and those on salt-restricted diets.

RECOGNITION

(*a*) *Infants*   Apathy, reluctance to feed, sunken appearance, loss of skin elasticity, depressed fontanelle.

(*b*) *Children*   Weakness, lassitude, apathy, faintness, syncope, nausea and vomiting, diarrhoea and abdominal pain.

CONFIRMATION
(a) Skin: pale and cold with or without peripheral cyanosis:
(b) *Sweating present*
(c) *No thirst*
(d) *Normal urine output: chlorides absent from urine* (unless there is a renal salt-losing state or adrenal insufficiency).
(e) BP usually low: tachycardia
(f) Plasma and urine-sodium levels low

MANAGEMENT

    (a) Acutely ill: IV normal (0.9 per cent sodium chloride (normal saline) initially at 20 to 30 ml per kg per hour (for details *see* page 100).

    (b) Less acutely ill with normal peripheral circulation: (*see* Heat Cramps) give additional fluids with salt added.

Treat any coexistent condition

Heatstroke (Sunstroke)

A condition in which the body temperature rises to a level at which cellular damage occurs. Cerebral damage may be permanent. The term heatstroke implies the presence of hyperpyrexia with cerebral symptoms; and the rectal temperature is above 40.5°C (105°F).

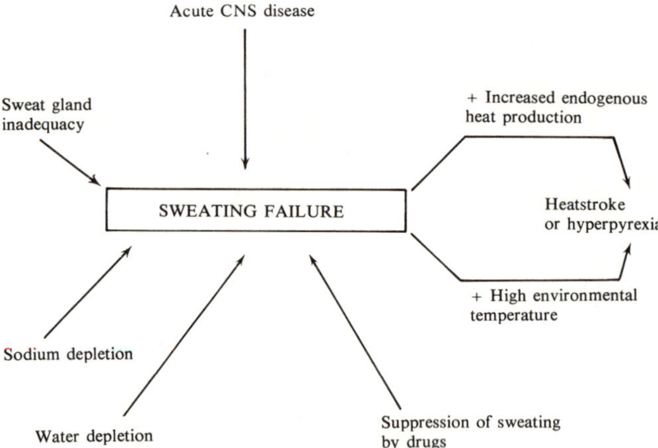

Figure 56.1. Pathogenesis of heatstroke and hyperpyrexia. Heatstroke or hyperpyrexia is caused by a failure of heat loss (lack of sweating) combined with increased heat production (infection; or muscular work as in status epilepticus) with or without high environmental temperature

AT RISK

    (a) Newborn infants, especially pre-term infants: overheating in faulty incubators, by hot-water bottles, or proximity to a hot radiator.

    (b) Infants: in hot environmental temperatures; especially in sudden heat-waves, failure to supply extra fluids, coexistent gastroenteritis or other febrile illnesses; inadvertent exposure to heat when left in direct sun, or in a closed car; overheated ship's cabin; overclothing in hot weather.

(c) Children with cystic fibrosis: sodium depletion from excessive losses in sweat.

(d) Epileptics: tendency to status epilepticus.

(e) Children with congenitally-impaired sweating as in anhidrotic ectodermal dysplasia and congenital icthyosis (*see* page 493).

(f) Acquired skin conditions with impaired sweating; extensive sunburn or thermal burns, eczema, psoriasis and anhidrotic heat exhaustion (miliaria profunda).

(g) Asthmatics: overheating of oxygen, mist or steam tents, drugs which suppress sweating (*see* (h) *below*).

(h) Children treated with drugs which suppress sweating.

  (i) Asthma and eczema: the antihistamine group.
  (ii) Migraine; phenothiazines.
  (iii) Anorexia nervosa, juvenile schizophrenia; phenothiazines.
  (iv) Motion sickness; atropine, hyoscine group.
  (v) Eye conditions: atropine or homatropine preparations.
  (vi) Vomiting (pyloric stenosis) atropine methyl nitrate (Eumydrin).
  (vii) Nocturnal enuresis: belladonna preparations.
  (viii) Whooping cough: Eumydrin (*see above*).

(i) Children in whom normal heat losses are impaired: extensive burns with occlusive dressings.

(j) Unacclimatized children undergoing unaccustomed muscular activity.

RECOGNITION

Prodromal symptoms are important; they include listlessness, muscle weakness, headache, slight fever, *cessation of sweating about 48 hours before hyperpyrexia.*

(a) Presenting symptoms are likely to be those of hyperpyrexia accompanied by: disorientation, delirium, hallucinations, ataxia, photophobia, convulsions (focal or generalized), stupor, coma, decerebrate rigidity.

(b) Skin: red, hot, dry: prickly heat (miliaria rubra) or anhidrotic miliaria (profunda) may be present. Blotchy cyanosis of head and face, and conjunctivae may be red. In infants, doughy skin.

(c) *Rectal temperature 40.5°C (105°F) or more.*

(d) Tachycardia: pulse initially fast, later feeble.

(e) Blood pressure: initially slightly raised or normal, later low.

(f) Respiration irregular or Cheyne–Stokes in type.

(g) Oliguria.

(h) Ecchymoses, petechiae, oozing from injection or venepunctures indicate DIC (*see* page 482).

CONFIRMATION

(1) *Take the rectal temperature.*

(2) Test the urine for chlorides: chlorides are usually reduced or absent in heatstroke.

(3) *Consider cerebral malaria* (p. 557) *if this possibility exists,* (endemic area or recent passage through or residence in an endemic area. Infants are not always given suppressive treatment).

(4) Consider other possible diagnoses such as meningitis, encephalitis.

LABORATORY INVESTIGATIONS

(a) Plasma urea and electrolytes: the urea is usually raised, plasma sodium normal or low except in infants in whom a level of 150 mmol per litre or more requires special treatment (*see* page 98).

(b) Acid-base state: there is usually a metabolic acidosis.

(c) Thick and thin films for MT (Plasmodium falciparum) malaria, where and when appropriate (*see also* page 554).

(d) Lumbar puncture to exclude meningitis. In heatstroke the pressure may be normal or slightly raised with a slight increase in red cells or protein.

(e) White-cell count usually shows a leucocytosis which does not necessarily indicate an infection.

(f) Thrombocytopenia indicates probable DIC (*see* page 482).

(g) Liver function tests; bilirubin and transaminases are usually slightly raised.

MANAGEMENT

(1) Give oxygen by mask.

(2) Reduction of body temperature: remove to a cool room (18°C; 65°F) preferably with low humidity: take *rectal temperature* half-hourly.

(3) Cool by putting in bath filled with ice chips until *rectal temperature falls to 39°C (102°F).*

(4) Control shivering if necessary by i.m. chlorpromazine (1 mg per kg during the first year; 10 mg at 1 year; 25 mg at 7 years; and up to 50 mg at 14 years). At 39°C (102°F) remove from the ice.

(5) Alternatively, sponge with tepid water or wrap in a wet sheet and play fans on to the surface of sheet, or apply spirit to skin and evaporate by fans. Stop when rectal temperature reaches 39°C (102°F).

(6) Correct dehydration, electrolyte and acid-base disorders. Take particular care in infants with suspected hypernatraemia.
(7) Control convulsions with IV diazepam. Be prepared to intubate in the event of respiratory arrest.
(8) Stop any drugs which may have predisposed to heatstroke (*see above*).
(9) Treat any concomitant disease: treat for MT malaria (cerebral malaria) with parenteral chloroquinine (*see* page 554) if there is a strong possibility of this, even if it cannot be proved.
(10) Treat DIC (*see* page 482).

Hyperpyrexia

Hyperpyrexia is a symptom, not a diagnosis, and is defined on a RECTAL TEMPERATURE of 40.5°C (105°F) or more. If cerebral symptoms are present the diagnosis may be heatstroke (under appropriate conditions) or an infection of the CNS such as meningitis, cerebral malaria or encephalitis.

Hyperpyrexia may occur in severely ill children with cutaneous vasoconstriction from shock or dehydration and does not require suppression of sweating for the body temperature to rise. It may also be a complication of tetanus (p. 338) and polioencephalitis (p. 335).

RECOGNITION
Rectal temperature of 40.5°C (105°F) or more. Any of the conditions which cause heatstroke may cause hyperpyrexia, but hyperpyrexia is not uncommon in temperate climates. Hyperpyrexia in association with an anaesthetic or operation should suggest malignant hyperpyrexia (*see* page 195).

MANAGEMENT
Prompt treatment will prevent the development of heatstroke.
(1) Remove to cool room (18°C; 65°F); if oxygen has been previously given in an incubator or tent, continue to give it by mask.
(2) Take the rectal temperature half-hourly.
(3) Remove clothes and play fans on exposed body. If necessary sponge with tepid water or wrap in wet sheet and play fans on the sheet. Stop cooling when *rectal temperature* falls to 39°C (102°F).
(4) Control shivering by chlorpromazine (p. 44).
(5) Control fits if in status epilepticus (p. 318).
(6) When sufficiently improved, investigate for underlying disease.

DRUGS LIKELY TO REDUCE OR SUPPRESS SWEATING

Atropine group   Atropine, atropine methylnitrate (Eumydrin), belladonna, homatropine, hyoscine, scopolamine.

Antihistamine group having an atropine-like action on the sweat glands e.g. Chlorpheniramine (Piriton), diphenhydramine (Bendryl), promethazine (Phenergan).

Phenothiazines e.g. Chlorpromazine (Largactil), prochlorperazine (Stemetil), promethazine (Phenergan), thioridazine (Melleril), trifluoperazine (Stelazine).

CHAPTER 57

Venomous Bites and Stings

H. Alistair Reid

Venomous creatures can secrete venom in a gland or specialized cells, and can deliver this venom during biting or stinging. All venoms contain a complex mixture of toxins, but in man the important clinical effects may be arbitrarily classified as:

(a) Fright effects (often due to fear that rapid, painful death is inevitable).

(b) Venom effects which may be:

    (i) Local, mainly vasculotoxic (pain, swelling, necrosis).

    (ii) Systemic vasculotoxic (bleeding, shock).

    (iii) Systemic neurotoxic (autonomic effects; myoneural block of muscles for vision, swallowing, breathing).

    (iv) Less commonly, systemic cardiotoxic or myotoxic effects. If poisoning is severe, acute renal failure can occur in most types.

Although the effects in man of venomous bites and stings depend on what type and how toxic the venom is, a much more important factor is the AMOUNT of venom injected. Clinicians should realize that, although fatalities and serious poisoning *can* occur, more commonly (and fortunately) little or no envenoming results from venomous bites and stings in man. In the latter cases, fear often dominates the clinical picture.

Venomous bites and stings in the sea

Fish stings

RECOGNITION

Venomous fish have bony spines covered by venom-secreting tissues; they include dogfish, stingrays, catfish, weeverfish and scorpionfish.

Stings cause intense, often agonizing pain. Local necrosis sometimes occurs with scorpionfish stings.

MANAGEMENT
The most effective treatment is immersion in water as hot as the patient can bear, removal to avoid blistering, and re-immersion until pain no longer recurs (usually about half an hour). Alternatively, the puncture wound can be infiltrated with 2 to 5 ml of 1 per cent lignocaine hydrochloride.

Jellyfish stings

RECOGNITION
Jellyfish have many microscopic stinging capsules called nematocysts on their tentacles. When touched, these capsules extrude a sting which can eject venom. However, only a small number of jellyfish have stings which can penetrate intact human skin. The most dangerous jellyfish, the cubomedusan or box jellyfish, sometimes called sea-wasp, is confined to tropical waters. After contact, the jellyfish can usually tear itself away from the victim leaving strings of tentacles adhering and resembling greyish or pinkish earthworms. Several deaths following stings by the box jellyfish, *Chironex fleckeri,* have been recorded in Australian waters. The victim screams in agony and rapidly loses consciousness, to die often before the shore is reached. These rapid deaths appear to be more due to heart failure than to respiratory failure. If the victim survives for 30 minutes death does not occur, but the parts stung become swollen and, later, necrosis along the weals can ensue. Stings by *Physalia* (Portuguese man-o'-war) and by most jellyfish other than sea-wasps cause only immediate pain and wealing, usually lasting a few hours. Weals may be single or multiple, of varying width, sometimes zig-zagging. Often there is an interrupted pattern of papules since only 10 to 20 per cent of the nematocysts discharge their stings and venom.

MANAGEMENT
Methylated spirits (or any other alcohol) should be applied to the stung parts to kill the undischarged nematocysts. If no alcohol is available, dry sand or any dry powder should be thrown on the sting and then the tentacles and slime should be scraped off. Dry sand is better than wet sand. The sting should NOT be rubbed with wet hands, cloth etc., as this will spread and aggravate the sting. After the spirits have dried, calamine lotion is a suitable local application. In severe cases, with rapid collapse, the victim should be placed on his back, methylated spirits poured on the sting, and tourniquets put on affected limbs. If breathing stops, mouth-to-nose artificial respiration should be given; if

the heart stops, closed-chest cardiac massage should be carried out. A potent sea-wasp antivenom has recently been available from the Commonwealth Serum Laboratories, Melbourne, Australia. Its administration has resulted in dramatic recovery from severe poisoning by *Chironex fleckeri* stings.

Sea-snake bites

RECOGNITION

Sea-snakes have short (3 to 4-mm) fixed fangs and flattened tails; common only in Asian and western Pacific coastal waters, they are not found in the Atlantic ocean or the Mediterranean. Most victims are fishermen bitten at their work; occasionally bathers and skin divers are bitten if they tread on or handle sea-snakes. Although their venom is extremely toxic, sea-snakes rarely inject venom when they bite man. In a series of 103 patients with unequivocal sea-snake bite, 80 per cent had trivial or no poisoning. But, when poisoning did occur the mortality rate was 50 per cent until effective antivenom became available. It is thus very important to distinguish sea-snake bite from sea-snake bite poisoning.

CLINICAL PICTURE

Sea-snake bites have no important local effects—there is no swelling or pain and the pinprick marks of the bite may be difficult or even impossible to make out. If venom *is* injected, characteristic generalized myalgic pains start 30 to 60 minutes after the bite, followed in a few hours by the red-brown colour of myoglobin in the urine. In severe poisoning, the myalgic pains merge into paresis with inability to move the eyes, open the mouth, protrude the tongue or swallow. Respiratory insufficiency and hyperkalaemia follow (tall, peaked T waves in chest leads of the electrocardiogram). Fatal respiratory failure may occur within a few hours of the bite from inhalation of secretions or vomit. In other cases, where respiratory failure is due to weakness of respiratory muscles, death is usually 12 to 24 hours after the bite. In the absence of effective antivenom, the myotoxic effects are prolonged and full recovery may take several months. In such cases, acute renal failure is the rule.

MANAGEMENT

Adequate reassurance is most important and a placebo injection should be given promptly unless clear signs of poisoning are already evident; in this event effective antivenom should be given. If used correctly antivenom can be effective even though not given until hours after the bite. Both tiger-snake antivenom and sea-snake antivenom (Commonwealth Serum Laboratories, Melbourne, Australia) are effective. Anti-venom (1000 to 10 000 units) should always be given by intravenous infusion, which is the most effective and safest route. Treatment of respiratory or renal failure is similar to that for elapid snake bite poisoning (*see below*).

Venomous bites and stings on land

Scorpion stings and spider bites

RECOGNITION
Scorpions have a poisonous sting at the end of their tail which is bent forward over the body to inject venom. Spiders have fangs similar to those of venomous snakes. Some spiders, even large ones, are harmless to man; perhaps the most dangerous is *Latrodectus,* the black-widow spider. The effects of scorpion stings and spider bites are similar. If venom is injected, there is local pain which can be severe and may last some hours, even 1 to 2 days. Local necrosis may follow bites by spiders of the *Loxosceles* genus. Systemic effects are unusual but include rapid breathing, salivation, sweating, vomiting, abdominal and generalized pains, and, in very severe poisoning, falling blood pressure and pulmonary oedema probably due to cardiotoxic effects. The latter can be fatal in children.

MANAGEMENT
If local pain is severe, the area should be infiltrated with lignocaine hydrochloride. Local injection of emetine hydrochloride has been reported as successful in relieving pain but is not recommended because it sometimes causes local necrosis. For systemic symptoms, scorpion or spider antivenom should be given if available; if not, general supportive treatment is indicated; atropine and calcium gluconate have been recommended for poisoning by scorpion stings. There are no adequate controlled trials to support the somewhat anecdotal clinical accounts claiming benefit from these two drugs. Calcium is recom-mended because of its effect on cell-membrane potential and permeabil-ity. Morphine and paraldehyde should not be necessary in scorpion stings. Pethidine and/or local infiltration of the area should be perfectly adequate in relieving pain.

Bee, wasp and hornet stings

RECOGNITION
Honey bees (*Apis mellifera*) have a barbed sting which is left behind

together with the venom sac. Wasp and hornet (*Vespa* species and others) stings are not barbed and are therefore not left behind. Local pain is the commonest clinical feature of these stings but, with multiple stings, general symptoms with haemoglobinuria or myoglobinuria and acute renal failure may develop. Deaths have been reported after only 30 to 60 stings by the honey bee, but usually 400 to 500 stings are necessary to produce death in an adult; and survival after 2242 stings has been recorded.

ALLERGIC OR ANAPHYLACTIC REACTIONS

In the United States and Britain, there are more deaths from anaphylaxis following wasp or bee stings than from all other venomous bites or stings combined together. In very susceptible patients, symptoms start after a few seconds with tingling of the scalp, vasodilatation, hypotension, and death within 1 to 2 minutes. In most patients, however, the reaction begins in 1 to 2 minutes with generalized urticaria, followed during the next hour by oedema of the glottis, bronchoconstriction, hypotension, and coma. Once an immediate reaction has occurred, the response to further stings starts progressively sooner and the severity of the shock increases. Delayed allergic reactions may also occur, coming on 1 to 7 days after the sting, such as fever, urticaria, enlarged lymph nodes, joint pains and leucocytosis. These episodes usually last 1 to 2 weeks.

MANAGEMENT (*See also* sections on Ear, Nose and Throat Emergencies and Anaphylaxis)

The bee sting should be removed. It is a tiny black shaft with the white poison sac attached to its free end. It should not be grasped by forceps or fingers as this can express more venom from the sac. The sting should be scraped from the flesh with the fingernail or the blade of a knife. Local antiseptic is then applied. Pethidine may be needed for pain.

Adrenaline is indicated for anaphylactic reactions, either by injection or by inhalation. Inhalation of an adrenaline aerosol from a pressurized can similar to that used for asthma is more rapid than giving an injection. Five inhalations of the aerosol described in the reference quoted (*British Medical Journal,* 1969) are equivalent in effect to 0.5 ml of injected 1:1000 adrenaline, but instructions for these medihalers vary: the Riker Medihaler, EPI, delivers 0.5 ml in two inhalations. The instructions should be carefully followed. People who are known to be allergic to bee or wasp stings should always carry such a can. Hyposensitization can be induced but this is usually temporary unless maintenance hyposensitizing injections every 1 to 4 months are continued indefinitely.

Land-snake bites

RECOGNITION

(a) *Elapids* (cobras, mambas, kraits, coral snakes, all the Australian venomous snakes) have short, fixed fangs.

(b) *Vipers* have long, moveable fangs; subdivided into pit vipers (crotaline) with heat-sensitive pits between eye and nose, and viperine vipers, which do not have these pits.

(c) Identification: seeing the fangs usually involves handling the snake; and fangs are normally covered by a gum-fold, so can be very difficult to see, especially in elapids. Vipers have vertically elliptical pupils (but so do some non-poisonous snakes). The European adder, *Vipera berus,* has a zig-zag mark along its back, often enabling identification in Britain. But specimens can be so dark as to obscure this characteristic. Thus, amateurs are advised to 'leave snakes well alone'.

(d) Snake bite is a rural and occupational hazard most common in the tropics; but nowhere in the world does the danger of snake bite approach that of road accidents.

(e) Viper bites of man are generally much more common than elapid bites except in the Pacific/Australian area, where vipers do not naturally occur.

(f) Viper venoms are mainly vasculotoxic in man, elapid venom neurotoxic; but there are notable exceptions to this generalization. In viper bites about one-third of the human victims escape with trivial or no poisoning, in elapid bites about one-half.

(g) On the other hand, *if* sufficient venom is injected to cause serious poisoning, mortality can be high when adequate medical treatment is not given. Therefore, careful observation of all snake bite victims is most important.

IMMEDIATE EFFECTS

(i) Fright is usual and can cause collapse with feeble pulse within minutes of the injury.

(ii) Collapse due to envenoming rarely appears until half to one hour after the bite, but there are exceptions. For example, in bites by the European adder, *Vipera berus,* early collapse with hypotension, vomiting and abdominal pain and diarrhoea can follow within a few minutes, and it is not due to fright. This early collapse usually resolves spontaneously within half to one hour.

(iii) Local pain is very variable and of no diagnostic clinical value.

(iv) Local swelling starts within a few minutes of a viper bite after venom is injected. It is a very valuable clinical sign because if swelling is absent and one knows the biting snake was a viper, then poisoning can be immediately excluded.

(v) Local swelling is also a feature of poisoning in bites by Asian cobras and the African spitting cobra, *Naja nigricollis,* though it may not appear for one to two hours.

EARLY SYSTEMIC SIGNS

(i) There are three important non-specific early signs of systemic envenoming: (a) vomiting (sometimes of emotional origin but more often denoting systemic poisoning); (b) hypotension; (c) polymorph leucocytosis.

(ii) Viperine systemic poisoning: (a) bleeding; (b) non-clotting blood. (a) and (b) may start within 15 minutes of the bite, but may be delayed for a few hours.

(iii) Abnormal bleeding may cause one or more of: oozing from bite or injection site; blood in spit, from the gums, in vomit or stool; discoid ecchymoses; positive tourniquet test.

(iv) Some, though not all, viper venoms cause consumption of fibrinogen resulting in non-clotting blood which is a simple and extremely sensitive bedside test of systemic envenoming. Also, non-clotting blood can differentiate envenoming by one type of viper from that of another (for example, in Africa envenoming by the carpet viper, *Echis carinatus,* causes non-clotting blood whereas the puff adder, *Bitis arietans,* does not).

(v) Elapid systemic poisoning: ptosis and glossopharyngeal palsy; may be delayed up to even 10 hours after the bite.

LATER EFFECTS

(i) Blisters extending up the limb often precede necrosis in bites by Asian cobras, and some vipers (such as the African puff adder).

(ii) Necrosis becomes evident a few days after the bite and is shown by darkening of the skin together with an offensive 'putrid' smell, which is particularly marked in cobra-bite necrosis. Necrosis can be extensive but it is usually superficial; involvement of tendons, muscle and bones is exceptional. Bacterial infection follows necrosis and may spread to joints. But in the absence of necrosis or meddlesome local measures such as incision, application of dressings, etc., bacterial infection virtually never occurs.

(iii) Haemorrhage into a vital organ, especially the brain, can be delayed until at least a week after a viper bite if effective antivenom is not given and is often, though not inevitably, fatal.

(iv) Shock in viper and in cobra bite envenoming is shown by prostration, sweating, cold extremities, tachycardia. hypotension, and sometimes electrocardiographic and serum-enzyme abnormalities.

(v) In severe elapid bite poisoning, respiratory failure is shown by confusion and stupor, shallow breathing, rise in pulse and respiratory rate and blood pressure, increased sweating, and cyanosis of finger tips. At any time during this phase of respiratory failure, obstruction by inhaled vomitus or secretions can result in sudden death. Otherwise, deepening coma, non-reactive dilated pupils, twitchings and convulsions presage death.

PROGNOSIS

(i) Viperine poisoning is severe if, within 1 to 2 hours of the bite, swelling reaches above knee or elbow, shock is evident, or haemorrhagic signs are profuse.

(ii) Elapid poisoning is severe if neurotoxic signs start within 1 hour or less of the bite and rapidly progress to respiratory failure.

(iii) The average death time in viper bites is 2 to 3 days after the bite; in elapid bites, about 6 to 20 hours after the bite.

(iv) Swelling in viper bites usually resolves completely in a few days to weeks, but local necrosis following viper and cobra bites may take months to heal and can result in permanent disability.

(v) In patients who recover without receiving specific antivenom, systemic symptoms generally subside within a week, but in bites by some vipers coagulation changes may persist for 2 to 3 weeks or even longer if specific antivenom is not given.

MANAGEMENT

First-aid treatment

'Measures taken by the victim or associates prior to receiving medical treatment'. Recommendations for first-aid treatment should be short, simple, practicable and should do more good than harm.

Reassurance is most important   If available, aspirin and alcohol in moderation are helpful, for their calming effects.

Wipe the site of the bite and *cover* with a handkerchief or dressing. DO NOT INCISE THE BITE as this may delay recovery, introduce infection or aggravate bleeding.

Tourniquet   The purpose is to compress the tissues above the bite and delay systemic absorption during transit to hospital. If *Hospital* treatment is available within 30 minutes, no tourniquet is needed. Otherwise, a firm, but not tight, ligature should be applied just above the bite, using cloth, grass, etc. The ligature should not be released during transit.

The snake   If killed, the snake should be taken to hospital for identification, otherwise, it should be left alone, since attempts to find or kill it often result in further bites. On no account should the snake be directly handled, even if dead. Decapitated head reactions can persist for up to one hour.

Hospital   All victims should be taken to hospital. The bitten limb should be moved as little as possible (because movement spreads the venom even when a tourniquet has been applied). If retching or vomiting occur, turn the victim onto the side to prevent vomit being inhaled.

Antivenom   Some publications on first-aid for snake bite mention the use of antivenom. It is therefore emphasized that *antivenom wrongly used can be more dangerous than snake bite.* Antivenom is specific *medical* treatment which is needed only in severe cases. It should be given only in hospital by a doctor as an intravenous infusion.

Management

   (a) DO NOT PANIC—there is abundant time to administer anti-venom *if* indicated; but do not dismiss as trivial without observation. Fatalities have occurred because the victim, on admission, was thought to have only slight poisoning.
   (b) Adequate reassurance is most important, so tetanus toxoid or a placebo injection should be promptly given unless antivenom is already indicated.
   (c) Except for cases in which there is no possibility of significant poisoning ensuing, the patient should be admitted and carefully observed, preferably in an intensive care unit, at least until the next day.
   (d) The following should be monitored and charted:
      (i) Hourly blood pressure, respiration rate, and differential white blood-cell count.
      (ii) Electrocardiogram and creatine phosphokinase or SGOT, at least twice daily (more often if hypotension persists).
      (iii) Urine-protein output, specific gravity, blood urea.
      (iv) Local necrosis, if relevant (extent of blisters and skin darkening, putrid smell).
   (e) Additionally, in viper bites: abnormal bleeding (injection sites, gums, etc.), blood coagulability (positive or negative), haemoglobin, swelling (circumferences compared with unbitten limb).

In elapid bites: ptosis, difficulty in talking and swallowing, vomiting, breathing.

General measures

(a) If a tourniquet has been applied it should be released. After cleansing (if necessary), the site of the bite should be left alone.

(b) Cryotherapy is harmful, causing or aggravating local necrosis. Antibiotics are NOT indicated unless and until there is clinical evidence of local necrosis.

(c) Local dressings should not be applied at this stage as they greatly increase the incidence of secondary bacterial infection. For the same reason blisters should be left strictly alone; they will then break spontaneously and will quickly heal without infection provided there is no underlying necrosis.

(d) But as soon as local necrosis is obvious, sloughs should be excised. At this stage, systemic antibiotics and tetanus antiserum may be helpful, and skin grafting should be carried out early rather than late, even if infection is still evident.

(e) Pain is rarely a problem once the patient has received an injection (placebo or antivenom).

(f) Heparin therapy is contra-indicated in snake bite as it can seriously aggravate haemorrhage from vasculotoxic damage.

(g) Blood transfusion helps in viperine shock, especially if the victim was anaemic before the bite, but specific antivenom is usually dramatically successful in viperine shock if given intravenously in adequate dosage.

(h) Steroids benefit neither local nor systemic poisoning, but are useful for delayed serum reactions. Steroids may delay the appearance of local necrosis in cobra bites but do not lessen the final severity.

(i) Some cobra species in Africa and Asia are able to 'spit' from the fang tips whose venom-duct exits are directed forwards instead of downwards. These cobras can eject venom up to two metres and on rare occasions venom has entered the eyes of victims. Conjunctivitis results; such venom is not absorbed systemically. The treatment is *prompt* irrigation of the eyes with saline.

(j) Patients with glossopharyngeal palsy in elapid or sea-snake bite poisoning should be nursed in the prone position to minimize the risk of inhaling vomit or secretions or both. The onset of confusion, stupor, and other signs of acute respiratory failure urgently indicate the need for tracheostomy. Artificial respiration may also be required.

(k) Acute renal failure due to snake bite will usually resolve with conservative treatment, with limited intake of fluids and electrolytes; otherwise peritoneal dialysis or haemodialysis would be needed. In such cases, it is important to avoid tetracycline, which can aggravate renal failure; sulphadimidine or penicillins are safe.

Antivenom

(a) The main indication for antivenom is *systemic poisoning*. For this, it is the most important therapeutic agent available.

(b) If used correctly, antivenom can effectively reverse systemic poisoning, even if it is not given until hours or even days after the bite.

(c) It is therefore not only safe but highly desirable to wait for clear clinical evidence of systemic poisoning before giving antivenom. It should NOT be given as a routine in all cases of suspected snake bite because antivenom is expensive (important in many tropical countries) and it can cause adverse reactions.

(d) Severe immediate reactions occur in about 3 per cent and on very rare occasions have been fatal.

(e) A second and less certain indication for giving antivenom is in bites by snakes known to cause local necrosis, if there are signs of local envenoming such as swelling and the patient presents within 2 hours of the bite. In these cases, the object is to prevent or to minimize local necrosis. If antivenom cannot be given until more than 2 hours after the bite, it is unlikely to benefit local necrosis (but will of course help systemic features).

(f) *Type of antivenom*

    (i) To be effective, antivenom must, generally speaking, be specific although some antivenoms have sufficient para-specific activity as to warrant the term 'broad-spectrum' antivenom. Thus, tiger snake (*Notechis scutatus*) antivenom (*see* list) is effective against poisoning both by sea-snakes and by most elapids, excepting mamba bite poisoning. *Vipera ammodytes* (long-nosed viper) antivenom is very effective in envenoming by the European adder, (*Vipera berus*).

    (ii) In contrast, monospecific *Echis carinatus* antivenom made in India, although effective against *Echis carinatus* envenoming by Indian species, is not effective against envenoming by African species of *Echis carinatus*. In Africa, non-clotting blood is very useful in differentiating *Echis* poisoning from poisoning by other vipers such as the puff adder.

Non-clotting blood also occurs in taipan (*Oxyuranus scutellatus*) envenoming whereas coagulation is normal in death adder (*Acanthophis antarcticus*) envenoming.

(iii) Neurotoxic features of elapid bites are easily distinguished from the haemorrhagic features of viper bites, but in many countries, distinctions are academic as regards choice of antivenom because only polyvalent antivenom is available.

(iv) Recent work indicates that liquid antivenom kept at ordinary refrigerator temperature (4°C) retains potency almost indefinitely. Any potency loss is preceded by opacity of antivenom. It therefore follows that clear antivenom is fully efficacious regardless of the date of manufacture.

(g) A known 'allergic' history contra-indicates antivenom, unless it seems likely the victim will die from envenoming. Such cases are very rare but if it were decided to proceed with antivenom administration, two intravenous drips of isotonic saline should be set up, one containing the antivenom and the other adrenaline. Small amounts of the adrenaline are infused first, followed by antivenom. The patient is closely observed for anaphylaxis and, according to progress, alternate amounts of antivenom are increased, adrenaline decreased.

If antivenom is indicated either for systemic or for local effects, a serum sensitivity test is not advocated. In treating several hundred patients with antivenom, sensitivity tests (subcutaneous injection and observation for 30 minutes for reaction) were misleading. When the antivenom was infused, reactions sometimes occurred despite negative test results, and in some severe cases with a positive test reaction intravenous antivenom was subsequently infused without any reaction. When immediate reactions occurred adrenaline was invariably successful, provided it was promptly injected. Adrenaline should be available in the syringe before antivenom infusion is started.

(h) Antivenom should always be given by intravenous infusion—the most effective and the safest route. The intravenous drip is started slowly (15 drops per minute). If a reaction occurs, the drip should be temporarily stopped, and 0.5 ml adrenaline 1:1000 solution should be injected subcutaneously. If adrenaline is injected at the first sign of anaphylaxis it is almost always quickly effective and usually the drip can be cautiously restarted. In some cases, several injections of adrenaline are needed.

(i) Depending on the potency of the antivenom being used, 20 to

50 ml, more often 100 ml (usually contained in 10 ampoules), is suitably diluted in 2 to 3 volumes of isotonic saline.

(j) The speed of administration is progressively increased so that the infusion is completed within about an hour. If, by then there has been little significant improvement, further antivenom should be given. This is specially important in neurotoxic poisoning, because polyvalent antivenoms are usually less potent against elapid than against viper venoms.

(k) In viper envenoming, antivenom may promptly and effectively alleviate shock and haemorrhage, and rectify clot-quality, and yet in rare cases, haemorrhage can recur a day or so later. Further antivenom may then be needed. Early warning of such a recurrence is given by continuing the clot-quality test daily for several days. A return of non-clotting blood precedes recurrence of bleeding.

Some institutes making antivenoms

AFRICA

South African Institute for Medical Research, P.O. Box 1038, Johannesburg, South Africa. *Bitis*-mamba-cobra polyvalent antivenom; *Echis* monovalent antivenom; spider (*Latrodectus*) antivenom; scorpion (*Parabuthus*) antivenom.

AMERICAS

Instituto Butantan, Caixa Postal 65, São Paulo, Brazil.
Wyeth Inc., Box 8616, Philadelphia 19101, Pa., USA.
Both supply polyvalent viper antivenom, and coral-snake antivenom. Instituto Butantan supplies scorpion (*Tityus*) antivenom and spider antivenoms.

ASIA AND AUSTRALIA

Commonwealth Serum Laboratories, Parkville, Melbourne, Australia. Sea-snake antivenom; monovalent antivenoms against black snake (*Pseudechis australis*), brown snake (*Demansia textilis*), death adder, taipan, tiger snake; Australian-New Guinea polyvalent antivenom; sea-wasp, spider and stone-fish antivenoms. Tiger snake antivenom is very effective against sea-snake and most Afro-Asian elapid venoms, except mamba.

Haffkine Institute, Parel, Bombay 12, India. *Echis-Russelli*-cobra-krait polyvalent antivenom.

Queen Saovabha Memorial Institute, Bangkok, Thailand. Monovalent antivenoms against *Naja,* king cobra (*Ophiophagus hannah*), krait (*Bungarus fasciatus*), Russell's viper, Malayan pit-viper (*Agkistrodon rhodostoma*), and green pit-viper (*Trimeresurus popeorum*).

EUROPE

Institute of Immunology, Rockefellerova 2, Zagreb, Yugoslavia. *Vipera ammodytes* antivenom: very effective also against *Vipera berus* venom.

Behringwerke AG, Postfach 167, 355 Marburg, Germany. *Bitis*-mamba-cobra polyvalent antivenom ('Central Africa' antiserum); 'North and West Africa' antiserum is claimed effective against *Echis, Bitis* and cobra (but not mamba).

MAIN ANTIVENOM CENTRES IN BRITAIN

A comprehensive stock of antivenoms for bites by foreign snakes is held at the two main Antivenom Centres:

   (i) Walton Hospital, Rice Lane, Liverpool L9 1EA. (*tel.* 051-525 3611), in conjunction with Liverpool School of Tropical Medicine, Pembroke Place, Liverpool L3 5QA. (*tel.* 051-708 9393).
  (ii) The National Poisons Information Centre, New Cross Hospital, Avonley Road, London SE14 5ER. (*tel.* 01-407 7600)

Advice on management of bites by foreign venomous snakes is available from the Liverpool School of Tropical Medicine (out of office hours; Walton Hospital, *tel.* 051-525 3611).

References

British Medical Journal (1969). Any Questions? **3**, 703
Reid, H. A., (1976). Adder bites in Britain. *Br. Med. J.* **2**, 153
Reid, H. A., (1978). Bites by foreign venomous snakes in Britain. *Br. Med. J.* **1**, 1598
Reid, H. A., (1978). Venomous bites and stings. *Medicine,* 3rd series, pp. 341–346
Theakston, R. D. G. and Reid, H. A., (1976). Effectiveness of Zagreb antivenom against envenoming by the adder, *Vipera berus. Lancet,* **2**, 121

CHAPTER 58

Malaria

J. Paget Stanfield

Malaria is among the major worldwide causes of mortality and morbidity in children.

With the resurgence of malaria in many areas from which it had been almost eradicated, and children frequently travelling from non-malarious areas into endemic areas, malarial illness is occurring at all ages and in unlikely places where the index of suspicion is low.

RECOGNITION

Plasmodium (*P.*) *falciparum* is the most virulent ('malignant tertian malaria'); *P. vivax, malariae* and *ovale* have much less severe effects.

Malarial infection during pregnancy may produce:
(a) Fetal death.
(b) Premature delivery.
(c) Small-for-dates infant.
(d) A combination of (b) and (c).
(e) Intrauterine infection in an infected neonate; this is rare.

Emergency treatment is necessary in three groups of children:
(a) Infection, usually falciparum, in the infant and young child with waning or absent maternally-transferred immunity.
(b) Infection, usually falciparum, in the older non-immune child. This may occur in children visiting endemic malarious areas from malaria-free countries who have omitted prophylaxis or are infected with a resistant strain. It is increasingly a risk in indigenous children who suddenly stop taking prophylaxis after the first two or three years of life. Falciparum infection in non-immune children should always be regarded as an emergency.
(c) Infection in malnourished, anaemic, or otherwise sick or infected children.

The usual acute presentation is with fever, vomiting and convulsions and one or more of the acute 'complications'. These syndromes are (with considerable overlap):

    (a) The acute neurological syndrome.
    (b) Hyperpyrexia.
    (c) Collapse, or 'algid' malaria.
    (d) Severe haemolytic anaemia.
    (e) The gastrointestinal syndrome.
    (f) The acute renal syndromes.

All or any of these could be the result of other acute diseases, but malaria must never be forgotten. The younger the child the less specific will be the symptoms, and the more difficult to distinguish from other possible acute infections.

Uncomplicated acute malaria causes no specific physical signs. The spleen and liver enlarge but such enlargement is not limited to malarial infection.

Attributing the findings in a severely ill infant or child to malaria should be easy, by means of a blood film. However, difficulties may arise:

    (a) The density of the parasitaemia may not correspond with the severity of the symptoms. The number of parasites in the blood not only indicates severity but also the degree of immunity and the duration and efficacy of any previous antimalarial therapy or chemoprophylaxis.

    (b) A non-immune child, or one who has received a parenteral dose of antimalarial drug shortly before admission, may be severely ill from malaria and yet have very few parasites in the blood film. On the other hand a heavy parasitaemia may be present in an immune older child in a hyperendemic area in whom symptoms are slight.

    (c) Parasitaemia may mask another underlying infection. The presence of parasites in the blood of children from endemic areas is so common that they may well be evident where the primary cause of the symptoms, such as a severe meningococcal septicaemia, is entirely different.

    (d) A mild attack of malaria may precipitate severe symptoms of an underlying disease, such as a crisis in a child with sickle-cell anaemia.

    (e) Previous treatment may complicate the diagnosis:
        (i) by reducing the parasitaemia without immediately altering the symptoms, as in cerebral malaria;
        (ii) by inducing toxic effects, such as the haemolysis in glucose-6-phosphate dehydrogenase (G-6PD) deficiency by the 8-amino quinoline drugs or the sudden collapse and death produced by too large a dose of parenteral chloroquine.

Toxic effects also result from home or herbal remedies which may produce gastrointestinal or hepatic symptoms unrelated to the malarial infection; bizarre symptoms should raise this suspicion. The induction of blackwater fever by quinine following repeated inadequate courses of the drug has never been adequately explained and has recently been largely discounted.

The child may be so severely ill that there may seem to be no time to take a blood film and examine it, but it is very important before starting any antimalarial therapy, particularly parenteral therapy, on suspicion, to collect a thick and thin film for examination as soon as possible. It is recognized that in certain situations the diagnosis of the contribution of malaria in an acute illness requiring emergency antimalarial therapy may well have to depend retrospectively on the response.

MANAGEMENT

Initial emergency treatment of malaria aims to suppress the asexual cycle of the parasite within the red cells. Such suppressive schizonticides must be highly active against *P. falciparum* and need to be capable of being given parenterally to obtain an immediate effect.

(a) Chloroquine (a 4-amino quinoline) and quinine are the two common drugs in present use, though if the oral route is considered possible amodiaquine can replace chloroquine with its very similar action. Recent powerful schizonticides, such as mefloquine, are being developed to use in combination with or actually to replace quinine in chloroquine-resistant falciparum malaria. Outside a few foci in South East Asia and Central and South America falciparum malaria is sensitive to chloroquine.

Chloroquine is available in variously named commercial preparations for use both orally (tablet and syrup) and parenterally. It is important to make certain of the content of chloroquine base in each tablet or ampoule before use. The usual preparations contain 150 mg of chloroquine base per tablet and 40 mg of chloroquine base per ml of injectable solution.

(b) Amodiaquine is usually prepared with 150 mg of the drug in each tablet.

(c) Quinine is formulated as a solution containing 100 mg per 3.5 ml or in tablets containing 300 mg.

All these preparations have a bitter taste.

Chloroquine therapy

(a) Immediate treatment

In severe infection chloroquine is given intramuscularly in a dose of

5 mg per kg body weight. A second similar dose can be given between 12 and 24 hours after the first but the total amount over 24 hours must not exceed these two doses. In very ill, collapsed children chloroquine can be given intravenously; 5 mg per kg is given slowly over 6 hours in an approprate amount of fluid. If a 'bolus' dose has to be given this should be no more than one-fifth of the initial dose (1 mg per kg), through as large a syringe as slowly as possible; the remainder can then be given intramuscularly. Parenteral choloroquine in higher doses exposes the child to the risk of sudden death. It is therefore necessary to make careful notes of the amount of parenteral chloroquine administered to any infant or child. These should be attached in some inseparable manner to the patient if transferred to a more central unit.

(b) Oral treatment

As soon as possible oral therapy should be commenced though it may, rarely, be necessary to continue parenteral chloroquine (5 mg per kg per 24 hours) for up to the next two 24-hour periods if the child is severely collapsed, comatose or vomiting. Oral therapy is given by nasogastric tube or in crushed tablet or syrup form by spoon depending on the state of consciousness. The dose must be repeated if obviously vomited within the next half hour.

> (i) *For infants under one year* the dose is 75 mg (half a 150-mg tablet) twice in the first day initially ($\frac{1}{2}$ tablet as a loading dose followed by a further $\frac{1}{2}$ tablet in 6 to 8 hours). This is followed by 37 to 75 mg ($\frac{1}{4}$ to $\frac{1}{2}$ tablet) daily for the next two to three days.
>
> (ii) For children from 1 to 3 years these doses should be doubled (2 tablets in the first 24 hours as loading dose followed by $\frac{1}{2}$ to 1 tablet daily).
>
> (iii) For children over 3 years the loading dose should be 2 tablets followed by 1 tablet daily for three days.
>
> The loading oral dose is omitted if parenteral therapy has been given.

Quinine therapy

In areas of chloroquine resistance quinine replaces chloroquine. The initial dose of quinine is 10 mg per kg to a maximum of 20 mg per kg per 24 hours, and is best given intravenously slowly over 4 to 6 hours in a solution of 0.5 to 1 mg quinine per ml. Intramuscular quinine produces tissue necrosis and abscesses unless given deeply and diffusely and should be avoided especially in small children.

Oral quinine 20 mg per kg per day should replace parenteral therapy as soon as possible. Like chloroquine the taste is very bitter and it will have to be given determinedly and skilfully, preferably by nasogastric tube.

Complications

(a) The acute neurological syndromes

RECOGNITION

The distinction between 'cerebral malaria', falciparum malaria with febrile convulsions and encephalitic syndromes with parasites in the blood smear is difficult. Cerebral malaria is never associated with other than *P. falciparum* and so can be ruled out if the parasites are all clearly vivax. For an excellent review of recent research on its pathophysiology *see* Yoeli (1976).

The infant of child presents with convulsions or coma with initial fever of varying degree. There is a parasitaemia, usually heavy, and the cerebrospinal fluid is clear with or without slight pleocytosis and slightly raised protein.

Diagnosis is not easy and treatment must be directed to the treatable condition, i.e. malaria. *An unconscious or convulsing child with malarial parasites in the blood, especially if they are recognized to be falciparum, ought to be treated as if the diagnosis is cerebral malaria until proved otherwise by virtue of rapid recovery, or by evidence indicating some other cause for the symptoms.*

MANAGEMENT

(a) Specific parenteral antimalarial therapy is started immediately either intravenously or intramuscularly or both as above.

(b) Convulsions must be controlled by IV diazepam or a combination of i.m. phenobarbitone followed by i.m. paraldehyde (*see* page 319).

If coma persists for longer than 24 hours, reduction of cerebral oedema may be attempted by mannitol or dexamethasone (p. 323). There is no clear evidence of the efficacy of anticoagulant and fibrinolytic drugs. In such cases recovery if it occurs is often slow, even after total elimination of circulating parasites, and may never be complete.

(c) In addition to the specific therapy of convulsions and coma, adequate hydration and nutrition must be maintained either by nasogastric tube or, if vomiting is severe, by intravenous infusion. Hypoglycaemia and acidosis should be kept in mind. Rectal temperature must be taken regularly 6-hourly, because hyperpyrexia increases the risk of further convulsions or brain damage. In prolonged coma intragastric milk feeding will be necessary.

(b) Acute hyperpyrexia

See page 537 for description.

MANAGEMENT

See page 537 for treatment of hyperpyrexia. A swinging recurrent fever is usually characteristic of malaria and care must be taken not to let the temperature fall below normal especially in infants. The fever will also tend to fall after convulsions are controlled with diazepam or paraldehyde. Once the antimalarial therapy has begun to reduce the parasitaemia the spiking temperature will fall.

(c) The collapsed child or 'algid' malaria

This may be the terminal phase of severe falciparum malaria, but can appear rapidly with a short history of fever, diarrhoea and vomiting, or may follow an overdose of parenteral chloroquine.

RECOGNITION

The child is pale, with cold extremities and a weak rapid pulse. Rectal temperature may be very high or low. The condition resembles shock, due to a combination of fluid and electrolyte loss, anaemia, hyperpyrexia and toxaemia.

MANAGEMENT

Severely collapsed children will need all the resuscitative measures available. This is the condition 'par excellence' requiring intravenous antimalarial therapy, followed or accompanied by plasma or blood if there is severe anaemia. Not more than 20 ml per kg should be given. 5 ml per kg rapidly and the remainder slowly. The rate and amount of blood given should be monitored by regular pulse, blood pressure and venous pressure measurements. Intravenous or intramuscular hydrocortisone (50 to 100 mg per dose) can also be used.

(d) Severe haemolytic anaemia syndrome

RECOGNITION

Pallor and slight-to-moderate jaundice develop in the course of a febrile illness. Splenomegaly may be considerable. Tachypnoea, cardiac and hepatic enlargement, pulmonary oedema and neck-vein engorgement indicate a 'high-output' cardiac failure. This is a fairly common presentation in infants of non-immune status, and may be superimposed on an already anaemic state such as iron deficiency or sickle-cell anaemia. G-6PD deficiency may be present, with haemoglobinaemia and haemoglobinuria.

MANAGEMENT
Control the parasitaemia as rapidly as possible.

A slow blood transfusion, preferably of packed or sedimented red cells, is indicated if the haemoglobin is below 5 g per 100 ml (though haemoglobinaemia may mask the full reduction of red cells available), or if there is any indication of cardiac failure not responding to bed-rest. Cardiomegaly and moderately increased venous pressure are often indicators of a haemodynamic adaptation to a low haemoglobin, and digoxin and diuretics given in such circumstances can interfere with this adaptation.

During the blood transfusion, which should not exceed 20 ml per kg given over not less than 6 hours, careful watch should be kept for increasing hepatic enlargement or neck-vein engorgement. Diuretics (frusemide 2 to 5 mg) can be given in the transfusion or separately during transfusion intramuscularly either as a routine or in the presence of increasing venous congestion. A limited exchange transfusion has proved life-saving. Some workers give 10 ml per kg blood intravenously to restore an immediate quantity of non-parasitized red cells and give the remaining 10 ml per kg intraperitoneally.

(e) The gastrointestinal syndrome

RECOGNITION
Malaria is often present in the infant with gastrointestinal symptoms. Vomiting is a major feature, the diarrhoea is rarely as copious and watery as in primary gastroenteritis.

MANAGEMENT
In any febrile infant with diarrhoea a blood slide should be taken and chloroquine given if in any doubt. Vomiting usually stops dramatically after antimalarial therapy. Intragastric glucose-electrolyte solution (page 404) is usually all that is required for rehydration with chlorpromazine (1 mg per kg per dose) if vomiting is severe. Intravenous fluid and electrolyte replacement may be necessary initially until the antimalarial therapy becomes effective, and as a vehicle for intravenous antimalarials.

(f) The acute renal syndrome

The kidney may be affected by severe haemolysis, dehydration, electrolyte disturbances, and toxaemia.

RECOGNITION

(i) Prerenal azotaemia may occur in infants in whom fever, vomiting and diarrhoea have occurred without adequate rehydration. Adequate rehydration should be accomplished during antimalarial therapy.

(ii) In algid malaria or during an acute haemolytic episode, oliguria may develop, progressing to anuria; the urine may be red or dark brown due to haemoglobin ('black water fever'). Uraemia ensues rapidly with vomiting, acidosis and hyperkalaemia.

Tubular obstruction is probably not the cause of the renal failure; but partial or total cortical necrosis certainly occurs, and DIC probably occurs in some cases. The haemoglobin casts are probably a measure of the acuteness and degree of haemolysis and haemoglobinaemia.

MANAGEMENT

Antimalarial therapy must be started immediately, and then with care, if anuria supervenes. Management of the renal failure will depend on the glomerular and tubular function, measured most simply by urine flow and level of blood urea. An in-dwelling catheter may be necessary to assess urine output, though some prefer intermittent bladder puncture.

If urine flow is maintained and blood urea and serum potassium are not rising rapidly, the fluid intake orally or intravenously will be adjusted to the urine output. A rapidly rising urea and serum potassium with falling urine output or anuria are indications for peritoneal dialysis or subsequent haemodialysis.

References for further reading

Bruce-Chwatt, L. J. (1978). Malaria. In *Diseases of Children in the Subtropics and Tropics*. 3rd ed. Ed. D. B. Jelliffe and J. P. Stanfield. London: Edward Arnold

Gilles, H. M. (1966). Malaria in children. *Br. med. J.* **3**, 1375

Gilles, H. M. (1972–74) Malaria. *Medicine* **26**, 1522

Hall, A. P. (1976). The treatment of malaria. *Br. med. J.* **1**, 323

Ransome-Kuti, O. (1972). Malaria in childhood. *Adv. Paediat.* **19**, 319

Yoeli, M. (1976). Cerebral malaria—the quest for suitable experimental models in parasitic diseases of man. *Trans. R. Soc. Trop. Med. Hyg.* **70**, 24

CHAPTER 59

Cholera

H. A. Reid

Cholera is an acute endemic or epidemic gastroenteritis caused by pathogenic vibrios. In the most recent pandemic, which started in 1961, the causal organism has usually been *Vibrio cholerae El Tor*. Cholera is currently endemic in many parts of Africa and Asia; in endemic zones, adults have some immunity and cholera predominates in children. Cholera has been imported into almost every country during recent years. Most infections are symptomless; in those who do have symptoms there is a clinical spectrum ranging from mild diarrhoea to a fulminating illness killing the victim within 2 hours of the onset.

PATHOPHYSIOLOGY
Cholera vibrios do not penetrate the gut wall but release an exotoxin which stimulates excessive secretion of isotonic, protein-poor fluid. All the important clinical features of severe cholera are due to the loss of the fluid and its contents, mainly water and sodium chloride, potassium and bicarbonate. Compared with adults, children lose more potassium (stool concentration about 30 mmol per litre) and less sodium (stool concentration about 105 mmol per litre); children differ also in a tendency to hypoglycaemia producing stupor or coma. Loss of water and sodium is shown clinically by tissue shrinkage and hypovolaemic effects; potassium loss by limb weakness, paralytic ileus, cardiac arrhythmias, and renal insufficiency. Bicarbonate loss is variable; the resulting acidosis is shown clinically by mental confusion and rapid deep breathing. If intravenous saline is given without simultaneously rectifying the acidosis, signs of pulmonary oedema develop and may be wrongly interpreted as indicating 'overhydration'.

ASSESSMENT OF SEVERITY
It follows that the important signs for clinical assessment are the level of consciousness, the general appearance (especially the face), the skin turgor, the pulse volume, the blood pressure, and the type of breathing.

T

Plasma levels of sodium and potassium are usually normal and do not help the clinician, but the arterial H⁺ concentration (pH) is useful in assessing acidosis. Absent peripheral pulses indicate a fluid deficit exceeding 10 per cent of body weight.

MANAGEMENT

In epidemics, special treatment centres are often needed but simple arrangements using tents or huts can be completely successful. Elaborate isolation techniques are unnecessary; the most important precaution for staff is to wash the hands after any and every contact with infected material. The child should be weighed and placed on a cot with a central hole under the buttocks so that the stools are guided into a measuring bucket through a sleeve from the waterproof sheet covering the cot. Stool volume, urinary volume and specific gravity should be charted. A rectal swab is taken and a rapid clinical assessment is made as outlined.

In symptomatic cholera, the rectal swab can be examined directly by dark-field microscopy; in detecting carriers, the rectal swab should be incubated for a few hours in a selective medium such as alkaline peptone broth at pH 9.2. Dark-field microscopy clearly shows the motile vibrios which can be confirmed as pathogenic by adding specific antiserum which immobilizes the vibrios within 3 to 5 minutes.

(*a*) *Initial rehydration* (*See also* Appendix 7 for oral electrolyte solutions)

Oral rehydration suffices for moderate cholera, but for severe cholera intravenous infusion is essential initially. The deficit should be rectified rapidly, and *preferably within 1 hour of admission*. A single infusing solution is useful in epidemics and an effective example for use with children is equal volumes of isotonic sodium chloride, sodium acetate (or lactate) and glucose (5 per cent); 1 g potassium chloride is added to each litre of the mixture which then approximately provides in mmol per litre: sodium 100, chloride 50, potassium 13, acetate 50, glucose 93 (1.7 per cent). The intravenous route is established, sometimes using the internal jugular or subclavian vein for the first 10 minutes. When the peripheral veins have expanded they can be used for the remaining initial rehydration which may require over 120 ml per kg, depending on fluid loss during the rehydration. The amount needed is judged by the clinical assessment features. Over-hydration is rare but may be reflected by facial oedema.

(*b*) *Oral maintenance rehydration* (*See also* page 404 and Appendix 7)

A suitable fluid is potassium citrate 1.5 g, sodium chloride 3.5 g, sodium bicarbonate 2.5 g, glucose 20 g, water 1 litre (in mmol per litre: Na 90, K 20, Cl 80, HCO₃ 30). The amounts needed are assessed by the clinical features and measured losses. Vomiting is rarely a problem after adequate initial rehydration. A nasogastric tube may be used to facilitate sleep. Milk, fruit juice and bananas can be added after a few hours. If tetany occurs, it can be relieved by intravenous calcium gluconate with due precautions (p. 143).

(c) Antibiotic treatment

Tetracycline or chloramphenicol by mouth lessens the volume and duration of diarrhoea and thus reduces the amount of intravenous therapy needed. Tetracycline is the drug of choice. Vibrios are quickly eradicated. The dose is 250 mg 6-hourly for 48 hours (under 1 year, half the dose). This regimen produces a 'clinical cure' in 95 per cent of severe cases. But follow-up reveals that about one-quarter will have a bacteriological relapse, vibrios reappearing in the stool. Doubling the dose and continuing antibiotic treatment for 96 hours has not significantly improved results. If tetracycline or chloramphenicol administration were prolonged to a 10-day course it is possible that bacteriological relapses would be prevented. But when an epidemic is raging such a prolonged course as a routine is rarely feasible. However, in the small number of patients who still have diarrhoea after 48 hours it would be advisable to continue antibiotic treatment until diarrhoea stops. With modern treatment, children with severe cholera can usually be discharged after less than 72 hours in hospital.

(d) Vaccination and immunity

(i) Controlled field trials indicate that currently used vaccines can reduce the incidence of clinical cholera by 50 to 60 per cent, but this protection declines rapidly after three months. (ii) Vaccination does not reduce the severity of symptomatic cholera; does not limit the spread of cholera; does not prevent asymptomatic infections; and does not prevent the establishment of the carrier state in household contacts. (iii) Children under 5-years-old do not possess a 'natural' basic immunity and therefore a single inoculation is ineffective. (iv) It is not known whether recent immunization of the mother confers passive immunity in the newborn child, but in endemic areas clinical disease is rare in infants under 1 year of age although they are commonly found to be infected. (v) Almost certainly, re-infection of children must occur commonly in order to build up immunity to the high levels seen in adults in endemic areas.

Reference

Barua, D. and Burrows, W. (Eds). 1974. *Cholera*. Philadelphia: W. B. Saunders
World Health Organisation (1976). *Treatment and Prevention of Dehydration in Diarrhoeal Disease. A Guide for Use at Primary Level.* Geneva: WHO.

CHAPTER 60

Typhoid Fever

Joan N. Scragg

Aspects of typhoid fever in children which require urgent consideration are: awareness of the disease in the very young; severe febrile-toxic state; atypical presentation and complications.

Typhoid fever in the very young

All age groups are involved, even the newly-born due to transplacental infection. Acute awareness that typhoid fever can occur at a very early age is especially necessary in endemic areas. In infants the onset is frequently abrupt, with diarrhoea and vomiting dominating the picture, so misdiagnosis is likely. In childhood the majority of deaths from typhoid fever occur in infants in whom the correct diagnosis has not been made and appropriate therapy has not been given.

Severe febrile-toxic state

Deaths can occur from typhoid fever where no catastrophe such as peritonitis or intestinal haemorrhage is demonstrated. Such patients have invariably been severely ill, febrile and toxic. Infants and children exhibiting severe manifestations should be regarded as emergencies. Appropriate drug therapy should be started without delay. It is unwise to await blood culture confirmation of diagnosis.

Atypical presentation and complications

Typhoid fever, a septicaemic illness, involves practically every organ and tissue in the body. Presentation with encephalopathy, hepatitis, nephritis, myocarditis, etc. may direct attention to the system(s) affected and delay in diagnosis results. In endemic areas a high index of suspicion for this great mimicker is important.

Neurological complications

Confusion exists over what should be regarded as frequent neurological manifestations in typhoid fever and those that would be better classified as neurological complications.

RECOGNITION
  (a) In children, delirium, stupor or meningism occurs frequently at the onset, the clinical picture resembling encephalitis or meningitis.
  (b) There is a variety of neurological complications. Convulsions, ataxia, aphasia, nystagmus, clonus, cranial-nerve palsies, etc. with or without cerebrospinal fluid changes, are common in typhoid fever in children. Recognition of the possible aetiology is urgent.
  (c) Typhoid meningitis, though very rare, carries a high mortality. Recovery depends on early recognition.

Intestinal perforation

The incidence varies in children in different areas but is probably about 3 to 5 per cent. There is variation in the reported mortality rate which, in children, is high.

RECOGNITION
  (a) Early recognition offers the only hope of survival.
  (b) Perforation occurring in patients who seem well on the way to recovery raises no difficulty in diagnosis as classic signs of perforation are likely to be apparent and surgical management without delay is justified.
  (c) Definitive diagnosis may be extremely difficult in a patient who for many days has had a distended tender abdomen with infrequent bowel sounds.
  (d) Transition from a state of threatened to actual perforation may not be shown by a dramatic change in the patient's condition.
  (e) In all who are seriously ill constant observation is essential.
  (f) Increasing tachycardia, restlessness and apprehension should alert one to the possibility of peritonitis.
  (g) Vomiting is not a striking feature in typhoid except in infants. Its occurrence late in the disease should be regarded as a danger sign.

Intestinal haemorrhage

This complication in children is fortunately rare ($\pm$ 2 per cent) but an alertness for it is ever necessary, as blood transfusion can be life-saving.

RECOGNITION
- (a) The first sign may be the passage of a moderate amount of blood from the bowel.
- (b) Despite absence of external evidence of haemorrhage an increasing amount of blood may accumulate in the bowel lumen for some hours before the catastrophe is made apparent by collapse and the passage of a massive quantity of blood.
- (c) Increasing pallor, restlessness, poor pulse and a fall in temperature should arouse suspicion of this complication.

Hepatitis

Typhoid hepatitis is not the rare complication that many reports on this disease suggest.

RECOGNITION
With this complication patients are usually seriously ill and appropriate drug and supportive therapy are urgently required. It is unusual for viral or toxic hepatitis to be accompanied by a high swinging temperature; the presence of this should alert one to the likelihood of typhoid fever.

Cardiovascular complications

RECOGNITION
- (a) Congestive cardiac failure is sometimes the presenting picture.
- (b) Profound anaemia may be the likely explanation in some instances.
- (c) Clinical and electrocardiographic findings will support a diagnosis of myocarditis in others.
- (d) Management will depend on the results of investigations.
- (e) Blood transfusion, with caution regarding amount and speed, may be all that is necessary.
- (f) If there is evidence of myocarditis management will be the same as for myocarditis of other aetiology with the addition of appropriate drug therapy.

Nephritis

Typhoid nephritis has been recognized since the early writings on the disease. Although infrequent ($\pm$ 4 per cent) an awareness of this complication is necessary.

RECOGNITION

The clinical picture is indistinguishable from acute post-streptococcal nephritis but it is unusual for the latter to be accompanied by a high swinging temperature. The usual management of nephritis with appropriate drug therapy results in rapid improvement.

Management

For well over 20 years the treatment of choice has been chloramphenicol and it remains so in most parts of the world despite serious drawbacks. *In view of the emergence of strains of* Salmonella typhi *resistant to chloramphenicol in certain parts of the world the need for an alternative drug has become urgent.*

A new semi-synthetic penicillin (α-amino-p-hydroxybenzyl penicillin: amoxycillin: 'Amoxyl') is now regarded by some (Scragg and Rubidge, 1975; Scragg, 1976) as the treatment of choice and by others (Pillay, Adams and North-Coombes, 1975) as a safe alternative to chloramphenicol.

(a) CHLORAMPHENICOL

(i) For the average case of moderate severity 50 mg per kg per 24 hours in divided doses is sufficient.

(ii) In those severely ill and toxic or in the presence of complications the dose should be 100 mg per kg per 24 hours until improvement is obvious, when it may be reduced.

(iii) It is advisable to continue therapy for 21 days in order to keep relapse and carrier rates at a low level.

(iv) If oral medication is not possible because of vomiting or where continuous gastric suction is necessary, chloramphenicol is given intramuscularly.

(v) A difference of opinion exists about the management of peritonitis. Where there is clear-cut evidence of acute perforation surgical treatment is justified. However, the majority in whom threatened or actual peritonitis is present are probably best managed conservatively by continuous gastric suction, intravenous fluids and parenteral chloramphenicol. This regime should continue with careful attention to electrolyte balance until the clinical state indicates improvement and cautious return to oral feeding and medication is possible. If undoubted peritonitis has occurred additional antibiotic therapy against bacterial contamination of the peritoneal cavity is wise.

(b) AMOXYCILLIN

(i) The recommended dose of amoxycillin in children is 100 mg per kg per 24 hours in divided doses.

(ii) The duration of therapy should be 21 days.

(c) CORTICOSTEROIDS

Corticosteroids dramatically shorten the febrile-toxic stage. Their use does not result in a higher incidence of complications and does not alter the relapse or carrier rates.

> (i) Their use should be reserved for those children who are critically ill with severe febrile-toxic manifestations.
> (ii) Prednisolone in the dose of 2 mg per kg per 24 hours may be given for not more than 3 days.
> (iii) Prednisolone should not be used alone, but in combination with antibiotic therapy.

(d) SUPPORTIVE THERAPY

> (i) Severe anaemia of infection may require correction by blood transfusion.
> (ii) In the presence of intestinal haemorrhage blood transfusion without delay is all that can be offered, as surgery has no part to play in its management.
> (iii) Fluid and electrolyte replacement may be urgently required in the early febrile-toxic stage in those in coma or where gastro-intestinal complications exist.

References

Pillay, N., Adams, E. B. and North-Coombes, D., (1975). Comparative trial of amoxycillin and chloramphenicol in the treatment of typhoid fever in adults. *Lancet* (2), 333

Scragg, J. N. (1976). Further experience with amoxycillin in typhoid fever in children. *Br. med. J.* 2, 1031

Scragg, J. N., and Rubidge, C. J. (1975). Amoxycillin in the treatment of typhoid fever in children. *Am. J. Trop. Med. Hyg.* 24, 860

CHAPTER 61

Amoebiasis

Joan N. Scragg

Emergencies arising in children suffering from amoebiasis are:
  (a) Severe amoebic colitis.
  (b) Local complications of intestinal amoebiasis—peritonitis, intussusception, haemorrhage.
  (c) Hepatic amoebiasis.

Severe amoebic colitis

Extensive destruction of the bowel wall extending from caecum to rectum accounts for most of the deaths in children with amoebiasis. Early recognition and appreciation that the fulminant case is a medical emergency is of paramount importance, as correct management may be life-saving. It is wise to regard such cases as threatened peritonitis.

RECOGNITION
  (a) A history of bloody diarrhoea is invariably obtained.
  (b) Patients appear critically ill, febrile, toxic and usually dehydrated.
  (c) Vomiting is common.
  (d) Abdominal palpation elicits generalized tenderness.
  (e) Unless the process is checked at this stage ileus soon follows, with increasing abdominal distension.
  (f) Proctoscopy undertaken gently will invariably reveal typical large ulcers covered by greyish sloughs. Careful removal of some of this material, which is then placed in a drop of saline under a cover-slip, will confirm the diagnosis, as usually haematophagous *Entamoeba histolytica* will be found on examination.

MANAGEMENT
  (a) Rehydration and electrolyte replacement by intravenous fluids.
  (b) Assessment of daily fluid and electrolyte needs.
  (c) Blood or plasma are indicated if shock is present.
  (d) Efficient gastric suction is essential if abdominal distension is present and should continue until distension is reduced, when intermittent suction is advisable for a further 24 hours.
  (e) Oral fluids may then be given. If there is no return of distension intravenous fluids may be discontinued.

DRUG TREATMENT
  (a) Oxytetracycline 10 to 15 mg per kg per 24 hours added to the intravenous fluids.
  (b) Emetine hydrochloride 1 mg per kg per 24 hours or dehydro-emetine in double this dose by intramuscular injection. This dose of emetine should not be exceeded and should not continue beyond 10 days. Emetine is an excellent tissue amoebicide, but when used alone is inadequate therapy for intestinal amoebiasis. Thus, once oral medication is possible, the following treatment is recommended:
   (i) Oxytetracycline 25 to 50 mg per kg per 24 hours given 6-hourly to complete a 5-day course.
   (ii) Metronidazole (Flagyl) 50 mg per kg per 24 hours in divided doses for 5 days or tinidazole 60 mg per kg in a single daily dose for 3 days.

Local complications of intestinal amoebiasis

(a) Peritonitis

Prognosis of this serious complication is determined by the stage at which adequate therapy is started.

RECOGNITION
All patients with severe amoebic colitis need close observation in order to detect the onset of vomiting and abdominal distension, however mild. Localized perforation in relatively healthy bowel is unusual. If signs of perforation occur suddenly in a patient on treatment who is only moderately ill, immediate laparotomy is advisable. However, amoebic peritonitis is usually slow of onset, occurring in patients with severe fulminating colitis with extensive ulceration of the bowel, which is extremely friable. Surgery has no part in its management.

MANAGEMENT AND DRUG TREATMENT
This is the same as that for severe amoebic colitis.

(b) Intussusception

This rare complication, when it does occur, has a grave outcome unless diagnosis is made early.

RECOGNITION
   (i) It is usually caecocolic.
  (ii) A complaint of colic more severe than is usual in amoebiasis, or, in infants, the observation of screaming attacks should arouse suspicion.
 (iii) Diagnosis is confirmed by palpation of an elongated mass in the line of the colon and a relatively 'empty' right-iliac fossa. Spontaneous reduction may occur. Barium enema could confirm the diagnosis but is an unwise procedure in the presence of a friable bowel.

MANAGEMENT
   (i) Laparotomy without delay is essential. Undue delay may necessitate resection, with an unfavourable outcome.
  (ii) Intravenous fluids and electrolytes.
 (iii) Drug treatment is the same as that for severe amoebic colitis.

(c) Haemorrhage

RECOGNITION
Severe haemorrhage due to erosion of a vessel by amoebic ulceration is uncommon, but it carries a high mortality. Sudden collapse, pallor and shock with the passage of much fresh blood will suggest the diagnosis.

MANAGEMENT
Apart from immediate blood transfusion and adequate amoebicides no other form of treatment can be offered. Surgical intervention is not practicable.

Hepatic amoebiasis

RECOGNITION

  (a) The peak incidence is from 1 to 2 years. It may occur as early as 4 weeks of age.

(b) Tender hepatomegaly is the most important sign. In all cases of hepatomegaly in endemic areas, amoebiasis should be considered, even in the absence of a palpable mass or a history of dysentery. (Antecedent or concomitant dysentery is likely in only 55 per cent)

(c) Radiological changes when present aid the diagnosis but their absence does not exclude it.

(d) Anaemia is an important diagnostic feature; it may be severe.

(e) The gel-diffusion precipitin test is a useful aid, as it is positive in 97 per cent of cases. However, 2 to 3 days elapse before the result is available.

MANAGEMENT OF UNCOMPLICATED LIVER ABSCESS

(a) Immediate aspiration is required; this should be done directly at a point of maximum bulge, fluctuation or tenderness, or transcostally in the presence of diaphragmatic elevation. Successful evacuation relieves pain, makes rupture or extension less likely and hastens recovery. There is no place for diagnostic needle aspiration. Aspiration should be thorough and viewed as part of treatment. The number of aspirations necessary is dictated by the clinical response.

(b) Metronidazole (Flagyl) or tinidazole in the dosage indicated above should be started without delay. Any anatomically adjacent structure may be involved by extension or rupture of an amoebic liver abscess. If rupture occurs into a hollow viscus pus is usually efficiently drained. However, involvement in certain situations is life-threatening.

MANAGEMENT OF COMPLICATED LIVER ABSCESS

(a) Pleuropulmonary rupture

RECOGNITION

With extension upwards there is likelihood of rupture with:

(i) Amoebic empyema which calls for immediate, thorough and usually repeated, aspiration.

(ii) Hepatobronchial fistula formation. The abscess contents are usually coughed up with a satisfactory outcome. Only an adequate course of amoebicides is necessary.

(b) Amoebic pericarditis

RECOGNITION

Acute awareness of the danger of left lobe abscesses involving the pericardium is necessary. Adequate aspiration of abscesses in this situation may prevent rupture into the pericardium or limit such involvement to presuppurative pericarditis. Sudden rupture into the pericardium may cause severe shock and rapid death. More commonly the onset is less abrupt, with:

    (i) Retrosternal pain.

    (ii) Dyspnoea.

    (iii) Increasing signs of pericardial effusion.

    (iv) Electrocardiographic changes.

    (v) Radiological changes.

MANAGEMENT

    (i) In the presence of cardiac tamponade thorough aspiration of the liver abscess and pericardium is of extreme urgency. If pus is not obtained surgical drainage without delay is imperative.

    (ii) Pericardial aspiration should be done under electrocardiographic control with a wide-bore needle introduced beneath and slightly to the left of the xiphisternum and directed towards the cardiac apex.

    (iii) The need for re-aspiration will be indicated by returning signs of tamponade.

    Conservative management results in slow improvement, and resolution without constriction is possible.

    (iv) In-dwelling drainage tubes should be avoided because of the serious hazard of bacterial infection.

    (v) Drug therapy: emetine as indicated above; metronidazole or tinidazole as indicated above; prophylactic antibiotic cover is wise if re-aspiration is needed or surgical drainage is undertaken.

(c) Intraperitoneal rupture

RECOGNITION

    (i) Rupture may be sudden, with severe shock and death.

    (ii) Occasionally localized peritonitis results from a slowly leaking abscess.

    (iii) More commonly, however, there is a gradual leak with chronic generalized peritonitis.

MANAGEMENT

Most cases of localized peritonitis will respond to conservative management and adequate amoebicides. A difference of opinion exists with regard to the management of generalized peritonitis. Some prefer surgical drainage while others advocate conservative treatment. With concomitant dysentery there may be extreme difficulty in determining whether peritonitis is due to extension from the bowel lesion or from the liver abscess. In these circumstances management should be:

(i) Conservative with supportive measures.

(ii) Amoebicides as indicated under severe amoebic colitis.

(iii) Antibiotic coverage against possible bacterial contamination of the peritoneal cavity.

CHAPTER 62

Haemorrhagic Fever (Dengue)

Wong Hock Boon

About 5 per cent of dengue haemorrhagic fever (DHF) develop the shock syndrome, which constitutes one of the most important paediatric emergencies in South East Asia.

RECOGNITION
Because DHF occurs in outbreaks, it can easily be diagnosed clinically, by the following features:
  (a) Fever lasting 3 to 10 days, usually low or medium grade.
  (b) Presence of the DHF rash on the third or fourth day. The rash starts on the trunk and spreads centrifugally; it may be macular or diffuse, and/or petechial.
  (c) Spleen usually palpable in affected children.
  (d) Leucopenia with mild thrombocytopenia.
  (e) Confirmation of diagnosis is serological, and rapid methods are now available.
  However, the main problem is shock; but since 95 per cent are not in shock, it is important to recognize the pre-shock state in a predisposed patient and to start anti-shock measures early.

Pre-shock or shock

Common manifestations:
  (a) Shock, if it occurs, develops from 3rd to 7th day of the illness.
  (b) The patient complains of abdominal pain and vomiting.
  (c) There is restlessness with clouding of the sensorium.
  (d) There is associated massive gastrointestinal bleeding.
  (e) The development of hypotension, ascites, pleural effusion (usually on the right).
  (f) Investigations may show:
    (i) A leucocytosis instead of leucopenia.

(ii) The platelets reduced to 50 000 per mm^3 or less.

(iii) Signs of myocarditis in the ECG.

(iv) Hyponatraemia.

PATHOPHYSIOLOGY OF DHF SHOCK

This may occur in the first or primary infection when the virus causes a direct vasculitis with exudation of fluid out of the intravascular space, and consequent shock. However, the majority of cases are secondary (i.e. have had a previous infection) as shown by the high serological titres found in DHF shock. Complement studies have shown that serum levels are inversely proportional to the severity of the illness, demonstrating that immunological mechanisms play a large part in DHF shock.

The shock state may be made worse by the development of disseminated intravascular coagulation (DIC, p. 482). However, DIC plays a secondary rather than a primary rôle.

Whatever is the real cause of DHF shock, the important thing is that it evolves rapidly, and the patient can reach an irreversible stage in a short time.

MANAGEMENT

It is even more important to identify those patients who are going into shock rather than those who are already in shock. The chances of saving the former are much better than those of saving the latter.

(a) Intravenous fluids 0.45 per cent NaCl in 2.5 or 5 per cent glucose should be given immediately at the rate of 40 ml per kg in the first 1 to 2 hours then at 10 ml per kg per hour depending on the state of the patient. Care must be taken not to overload the circulation (0.45 per cent NaCl in 2.5 per cent glucose has been shown to be more effective in DHF than the 'standard' 0.9 per cent NaCl in 5 per cent glucose).

(b) Observations to be made and recorded during treatment.

(i) Pulse rate.

(ii) Blood pressure.

(iii) Central venous pressure (CVP); IV fluids can be given if the CVP is less than 10 cm of water.

(iv) Respiration rate.

(v) Chest x-ray (for pleural effusion).

(vi) Intake-output chart.

(vii) Haematocrit, WBC count, platelets.

(viii) Plasma sodium, potassium, bicarbonate, chloride, urea.

If facilities are available:

(i) Blood gases and acid-base state.

(ii) Blood clotting studies and fibrin breakdown products (p. 482).

(c) Further intravenous treatment.

(i) Blood transfusion need only be given if there is considerable loss of blood.

(ii) Plasma* is sometimes useful but may initiate shock lung syndrome and is therefore of doubtful value.

(iii) Platelet transfusions may be useful if bleeding cannot be controlled.

(iv) Intravenous fluids and electrolytes should be given according to the results of serial electrolyte estimations.

(d) Later progress.

If the patient is going to respond, improvement usually occurs within 24 to 48 hours, when emergency measures may be relaxed. Over-treatment may be hazardous. Corticosteroids, antibiotics and heparin are of no proven value.

---

* Plasma-protein fraction is replacing pooled plasma.

CHAPTER 63

Smallpox

Ian W. Pinkerton

The disease has now apparently been confined to Ethiopia and Somalia in East Africa*. The speed and volume of international air travel however maintain the possibility of recurrence and importation in any area of the world and requires the continuing vigilance of doctors.

The causative agent belongs to the pox virus group and exists in two types; the highly virulent variola major and the less severe variola minor or alastrim.

Transmission of infection is from the mucous membranes and skin lesions of a case. Patients are infectious from the onset of symptoms until the last crust has separated, but infectivity is greatest at the end of the prodromal period and at the onset of the rash. The virus can survive in dust and on clothing for several months so that remote spread of infection is a possibility, although it is uncommon.

RECOGNITION

After an incubation period of 10 to 16 days (commonly 12 days) the onset of illness is sudden with fever, headache, backache and vomiting. A fleeting erythematous rash may be present at this time. This prodromal illness lasts about 3 to 4 days and is followed by the appearance of the true rash. This takes the form at first of round macules, a few millimetres in diameter, on the face and forearms, soon enlarging and spreading to the rest of the body but maintaining a centrifugal distribution with lesions more densely concentrated on the face and extremities than on the trunk. The rash is often more profuse on areas of skin pressure or irritation and is more marked over prominences and on extensor surfaces. Lesions in the mouth are common. The rash passes through successive stages of papules, vesicles and pustules during the first few days. Pustules continue to enlarge until at about 10 days they begin to dry into crusts which are gradually shed during the following 2

*Possibly completely eradicated

to 3 weeks leaving temporarily depigmented areas. Survivors of the disease often show pock marks on the face.

Mortality among unvaccinated subjects is around 50 per cent, death usually occurring during the first week of illness. About 3 per cent of variola major cases experience a fulminating illness with haemorrhage into the skin and mucous membranes. Such cases are rapidly fatal and since the characteristic rash does not develop they may be confused with other haemorrhagic conditions such as leukaemia and meningococcal infection.

In previously vaccinated persons the rash may be considerably modified to the extent that only a few atypical lesions are present. Such cases have often been the source of outbreaks in non-endemic areas.

DIAGNOSIS

Before the rash, diagnosis is impossible unless there is a known exposure to infection.

Other vesicular or pustular conditions which must be distinguished include chickenpox, generalized vaccinia, Stevens–Johnson syndrome, herpes simplex and Hand, Foot and Mouth disease which is a Coxsackie virus infection causing vesicles on the extremities with minimal systemic upset.

Chickenpox is the most important differential diagnosis but can usually be distinguished by consideration of possibility of contact, incubation period (14 to 21 days), brief duration of prodromal illness, period of maturation and distribution of the rash. The rash of chickenpox, mainly concentrated on the face and trunk, appears in successive crops over a few days and is completely crusted within a week. The vaccination history of the suspect or a reliable history of previous chickenpox may be of diagnostic importance.

LABORATORY TESTS

The taking of adequate specimens for laboratory examination is an important duty in this disease and should include as appropriate:

(a) Throat swab from early cases.
(b) Smears on microscope slides of fluid from the base of several papules or pustules.
(c) Fluid from vesicles in a tuberculin syringe.
(d) Several crusts in a sterile container.
(e) 10 ml of clotted blood.

Specimens should be sent to an appropriate virus laboratory in a sealed metal container.

Electron microscopy of fluids or smears is the most rapid definitive investigation, allowing morphological differentiation of pox virus (smallpox and vaccinia) from herpesvirus (chickenpox and herpes simplex).

Culture of the virus on fertile hens' eggs is the most important and reliable test but takes 3 days to give a result.

Direct microscopy of vesicular fluid may show multinucleated giant cells highly suggestive of chickenpox. Fluid or scrapings may be used for antigen detection by gel diffusion and serve to distinguish pox virus from herpesvirus. Variola antibody may be measured in the blood.

MANAGEMENT
As early as possible, on suspicion of the diagnosis, the patient should be isolated in an appropriate hospital where the safety of the staff has been secured by regular vaccination and the community can be protected by safe decontamination and disposal arrangements. There is no specific treatment for the disease.

PREVENTIVE AND PUBLIC HEALTH MEASURES
The appropriate Public Health Authority responsible for prevention and outbreak control must be informed immediately. Close contacts, particularly those in the family, at hospital or in school should be identified, vaccinated immediately and kept under daily surveillance for 16 days. Human antivaccinial immunoglobulin (0.3 ml per kg i.m.) provides some passive immunity to smallpox if given in the first half of the incubation period and should be given to previously unvaccinated close contacts and to those whose immune status is uncertain.

Contacts who develop any untoward symptoms should be isolated and particular attention directed to disinfection of clothing, personal effects and premises.

CHAPTER 64

Rabies

D. R. Bell

Rabies is an enzootic infection, usually transmitted by the saliva of an infected animal during biting or the licking of an abrasion. Inhalation of virus can infect people exploring caves which harbour infected bats. Most human infections come from the bite of the domestic dog, and may occur in children. Ideally all cases of rabies in man and animals should be notified in accordance with the recommendations of the World Health Organization. Rabies is now a notifiable disease in Britain and many other countries but there is no uniformity of procedure.

DISTRIBUTION AND EPIDEMIOLOGY

Wild animal or domestic dog reservoirs of rabies are found in most parts of the tropics, subtropics, the Americas and large parts of Europe. Man is not often affected directly from a rabid wild animal, although bat-transmitted outbreaks have occurred. Rabies in the European fox has spread into France and is at present moving south, and it is the fox-transmitted infection of a dog or cat smuggled into Britain that presents the greatest danger to the British Isles.

Recognition

(a) CLINICAL

The diagnosis of human rabies during life is usually clinical. After an incubation period of from 2 weeks to more than a year, the onset is rapid. Early symptoms are fever, malaise, anxiety and sometimes pain at the site of the original bite. Then follows reflex hyperexcitability of the nervous system, most typically manifest as painful cramps of the throat muscles when attempting to swallow, giving the disease the name 'hydrophobia'.

The reflex spasms, often accompanied by apnoea, become more and more frequent over the course of a day or two. Between spasms, the patient is conscious, and can often talk rationally. Restlessness, pruritus and excessive salivation are common, and the patient typically spits abundant ropy saliva.

Hyperexcitability is often followed by progressive paralysis and the appearance of bizarre focal neurological signs. Death usually occurs within 7 days of the onset, preceded by respiratory irregularities and cardiac arrhythmias.

(b) SPECIFIC DIAGNOSIS

More specific diagnosis can be confirmed by specific immunofluorescent staining of corneal impression smears, but a negative result is indecisive, as the test is negative in more than 50 per cent of confirmed cases. Advice on the technique should be obtained from the Virus Reference Laboratory, Central Public Health Laboratory, Colindale Avenue, London NW9 5HT or from similar centres in other countries.

Management

(a) TREATMENT OF ESTABLISHED RABIES

Once rabies is diagnosed, treatment should be symptomatic. The single well-documented case of claimed survival from rabies (Hattick *et al.,* 1972) lacks the vital evidence of virus isolation, and could have been an atypical 'post-vaccinial encephalitis', as vaccine had been given. Rabies is an agonizing disease, and treatment with full doses of diamorphine, chlorpromazine and amylobarbitone together is effective. Conventional dosage must be exceeded if symptoms are not controlled. Whether heroic supportive measures are justified is a matter for the individual physician, but even in the most optimistic view, the prospects for recovery are infinitesimal.

(b) PROTECTION OF STAFF IN CONTACT WITH RABID PATIENT

Staff in contact with rabies must be protected by gowns, gloves, goggles and masks, and cautioned about the special danger of saliva. Preexposure immunization is feasible now that human diploid cell vaccine is available.

(c) POST-EXPOSURE PREVENTION OF RABIES AFTER THE BITE

(*i*) *Indications for post-exposure protection*

When a child is seen who might have been exposed to rabies, the decision on what to do is often difficult, but detailed advice is given in the World Health Organization Report (1973). In general, if an animal is *well* 5 days after inflicting a bite, or *alive* 10 days later, it is extremely unlikely that it was infective at the time of biting. This information should always be sought. Where a bite was received in an area where rabies is endemic and there is no information about the animal (as in the case of one that attacks and then runs off) one must assume that exposure occurred. Factors which increase the likelihood of infection are: severe bites, proximal bites and bites from wild animals. The incubation period is also shortened by all these factors, and with increasing youth.

(ii) Local treatment

If the child is seen within 12 hours of exposure, local treatment might be effective, although proof of this is confined to delays of up to 3 hours. Irrigation of superficial wounds or swabbing of deep puncture wounds with 1 per cent benzalkonium chloride or 20 per cent soft soap solution is recommended. Débridement and delayed primary suture are used when surgery is needed.

(iii) Antirabies serum

Passive immunity can be provided by injecting antirabies serum pre pared from various animals, most commonly the horse. The dose is 40 iu. per kg for heterologous, or 20 iu. per kg for the scarce and costly human serum. One-half of the dose can be infiltrated into the wound site, the remainder given intramuscularly. The usual precautions with serum must be observed. In practice, serum is given where the risk of exposure is high and the incubation period likely to be short. Vaccine alone protects against mild exposure, and a difficult balance must be struck between risk and possible benefit. Up to 50 per cent of patients receiving horse serum will develop serum sickness. Serum is given at the same time as the first dose of vaccine, but at a different site.

(iv) Vaccination and its complications

Vaccination is started as soon as it is decided that exposure to rabies might have occurred. Duck embryo vaccine and the Semple type vaccines which are derived from the nervous tissue of infected animals, have both been superseded by the new human diploid cell vaccine manufactured by the Merieux Institute of Lyons. The only disadvantage of the new vaccine is its expense; its great advantages are its lack of side-effects and its extreme effectiveness in raising antibody levels in the vaccines.

The normal regime for post-exposure vaccination is by 1-ml doses of reconstituted vaccine given by the deep subcutaneous route. Because of the small dose of the vaccine, it is no longer necessary to use the subcutaneous tissues of the abdomen. The normal regime is to give injections on days 0, 3, 7 and 14, followed by booster doses on days 30 and 90. It is usual for antibodies to be detectable after the first two doses of vaccine have been given.

If a patient has been vaccinated previously within the last 12 months, and is re-exposed to rabies, it is normally only necessary to give one booster dose. If previous vaccination was more than one year previously, then two or three booster doses should be given at intervals such as days 0, 3 and 7.

Pre-exposure vaccination can be offered to those at special risk of rabies infection, such as veterinary surgeons and others at special risk in endemic areas. Effective levels of antibody are produced after two injections one month apart and the levels are increased by giving a booster dose one year later. Subsequent booster doses can be given every three to five years according to the risk of exposure.

So far, there have been no reports of neuroanaphylactic accidents with the human diploid cell vaccine. The only complication of diploid cell vaccine normally encountered is that the site of injection may become somewhat red and indurated. This is by no means as severe as the reaction that used to be produced by Semple vaccines or by the duck embryo vaccine.

To conclude: there is no stringent evidence that treatment of established rabies is effective. Aggressive therapy should be concentrated on efforts to produce effective immunity as soon as possible after exposure, and these efforts should not be relaxed just because there has been a long delay. The quickest way of doing this is by a combination of active and passive immunization.

With the advent of human diploid cell vaccine, pre-exposure vaccination of children is feasible now.

Centres where rabies vaccine and antiserum is available

England   Virus Reference Laboratory,
Central Public Health Laboratory,
Colindale Avenue, LONDON,
NW9 5HT   *tel.* 205 7041
Public Health Laboratory,
East Birmingham Hospital,
Bordesley Green East,   *tel.* 772 4311
BIRMINGHAM, B9 5ST   ext 680
Public Health Laboratory,
Church Lane,
Heavitree
EXETER, EX2 5AD   *tel.* 77833

	Public Health Laboratory, Bridle Path, York Road, LEEDS, LS15 7TR	*tel.* 645011
	Public Health Laboratory, Fazakerley Hospital, Lower Lane, LIVERPOOL, L9 7AL	*tel.* 525 2323
	Public Health Laboratory, Institute of Pathology, General Hospital, Westgate Road, NEWCASTLE UPON TYNE, NE4 6BE	*tel.* 38811 ext 297
Wales	Public Health Laboratory, University Hospital of Wales, Heath Park CARDIFF, CF4 4XW	*tel.* 755944
Scotland	King's Cross Hospital, Clepington Road, DUNDEE, DN3 8EA	*tel.* 85241
	Central Microbiological Labs, Western General Hospital, Crewe Road South, EDINBURGH EH4 2XU	*tel.* 332 1311
	Glasgow Royal Infirmary, GLASGOW, G4 0SF	*tel.* 552 3535
	Ruchill Hospital, Bilsland Drive, GLASGOW	*tel.* 946 6491
	Raigmore Hospital, INVERNESS	*tel.* 34151
Northern Ireland	Belfast City Hospital, Lisburn Road, BELFAST	*tel.* 29241

For further advice in Britain ring: Liverpool School of Tropical Medicine (*tel.* 051-709 7611), Ward 17, Sefton General Hospital (*tel.* 051-733 4020), or London School of Hygiene and Tropical Medicine (*tel.* 01-636 8636).

References

Hattick, M. A., Weis, T. T., Stechschulte, J., Baer, G. M. and Gregg, M. B. (1972). Recovery from rabies; a case report. *Ann. internal Med.* **76**, 931

World Health Organization Expert Committee on Rabies. (1973). *W.H.O. Tech. Rep. Ser.* 523

CHAPTER 65

Lassa Fever

H. Alistair Reid

Lassa fever, a serious viral disease, was first described in a nurse from the town of Lassa in north-eastern Nigeria in 1969. Epidemics have been observed in Nigeria, Liberia, and Sierra Leone with high mortality rates (36 to 67 per cent) although recent studies suggest that symptomless infections may be widespread in parts of Africa. Lassa virus is designated an Arenavirus, similar to the virus of lymphocytic choriomeningitis; the natural host and reservoir is *Mastomys natalensis,* a rat widely distributed in Africa south of the Sahara. Infection is probably through direct contact with an infected rat or its excreta, or through person-to-person transmission, especially within the hospital environment. Lassa virus has been isolated from both the serum and the pharynx of patients 19 days after the onset of illness, and from the urine 32 days after onset. Serum generally contains higher virus concentrations than urine or pharynx. It is not yet known if persons with symptomless infections or in the incubation period (3 to 17 days, usually 7 to 10 days) can transmit the virus. There is no epidemiological evidence to indicate that Lassa fever is an arthropod-borne infection.

RECOGNITION
Symptomatology is non-specific. There is an insidious onset of fever, malaise, and sore throat. Other features, variably present, include vomiting, diarrhoea, lymphadenopathy, and in more severe cases, increasing toxicity, serous effusions, ecchymoses, petechiae, encephalopathy, oliguria and shock. Death generally occurs in the second week of illness. In survivors, the illness resolves gradually between the second and fourth week.

MANAGEMENT
The danger of importing Lassa fever is obvious. The problem is twofold when a person, recently in Africa, presents with fever: (a) For the individual, the possibility of Lassa fever may influence the clinician to overlook diseases for which specific treatment is available, particularly

malaria and typhoid. (b) For the community, overlooking Lassa fever might result in further cases. Laboratory diagnosis is of very limited help—facilities are confined to centres such as the Microbiological Research Establishment, Porton, Wilts., and the Center for Disease Control, Atlanta, U.S.A. Viral isolation takes *several days* and complement fixation tests provide only retrospective diagnosis. Initially, therefore, the diagnosis is clinical. Lassa fever can be excluded if:

(i) The patient has not been in west or central Africa during the 3 weeks before the onset.

(ii) Fever has lasted more than 1 month.

(iii) Blood film and clinical features are positive for malaria.

On the other hand, Lassa fever is suggested if:

(i) The patient has been in west or central Africa during 3 weeks or less of the onset, *particularly* if the patient has had hospital contact there.

(ii) Insidious onset and/or fever lasts over 4 days (streptococcal pharyngitis and many other viral illnesses having a briefer course).

(iii) Sore throat occurs.

(iv) Examination shows one or more of the following: temperature over 39°C (102°F), prostration, cervical adenopathy, ulcerative pharyngitis, abnormal bleeding, hypotension.

The strictest barrier nursing is essential; it should be realized that both blood and urine are highly infective.

Convalescent serum has been used in a few cases of Lassa fever but is not of proven value, and the amount of 'immunity' in the serum is quite unknown. Furthermore, the predicament is as follows: diagnosis of Lassa fever has to be clinical in the early stages. Convalescent serum is only likely to be of benefit if given in the early stages and may in fact contain the virus. Therefore convalescent serum might cause Lassa fever in a patient who did not originally have it.

If Lassa fever is considered to be a possibility, the patient should be immediately admitted to a high-security isolation unit specifically organized for such cases by consultants in tropical medicine and in infectious disease.

NOTE: Lassa fever is now a notifiable disease in the United Kingdom. Transport to hospital must be in a special ambulance.

References

Bulletin of the World Health Organization. (1978). Ebola haemorrhagic fever in Sudan 1976, **56**, 247.

Bulletin of the World Health Organization. (1978). Ebola haemorrhagic fever in Zaire 1976, **56**, 271.

Department of Health and Social Security and the Welsh Office. (1976). *Memorandum on Lassa fever.* London: H.M.S.O.

Monath, T. P. (1975). In International Symposium on Arenaviral Infections of Public Health Importance. *Bull. W.H.O.* **52**, 577 (*See also* other relevant articles *ibid.*).

CHAPTER 66

Acute Metabolic Disorders in Protein-Energy Malnutrition

(Kwashiorkor, Protein-Calorie Malnutrition PCM)

B. Heyworth

In children severe Protein-Energy Malnutrition (PEM) should be regarded as a medical emergency. The mortality in PEM tends to be very high in the first week after admission to hospital and particularly high in the first 48 hours.

Septicaemia, especially with Gram-negative bacteria, severe anaemia, shock secondary to dehydration, and disseminated intravascular coagulopathy may all occur, requiring urgent detection and appropriate treatment in every new patient seen.

At the same time the following metabolic derangements, singly or in combination are frequently encountered and must be treated promptly:

(a) Hypothermia
(b) Hypoglycaemia } Often in combination

(c) Hyponatraemia
(d) Hypokalaemia
(e) Hypomagnesaemia
(f) Acute cardiac failure } In varying degrees, often in combination

Hypothermia

In some countries 20 per cent of children with severe PEM have a rectal temperature at or below 35°C (95°F).

The child who has had to travel far, who may be in a fasting state, or who is exposed to the cool night air, will have a lower rectal temperature. Hypothermia may coexist with an infection.

MANAGEMENT
Unnecessary washing or exposure should be avoided. The child is

wrapped in a blanket, but rapid heating with hot water bottles should be avoided. Bodily contact with the mother will be very helpful. Aluminium foil wrapped around the blanket will further conserve body heat.

It is important to give calories especially around midnight, ideally in the early hours of the morning.

Hypoglycaemia

This is often associated with hypothermia and may be the presenting feature on admission following a long journey, and is also associated with overnight fasting or infection. Symptoms include drowsiness or coma, but sweating, tremors or convulsions caused by hypoglycaemia are not usually evident in PEM.

MANAGEMENT

If a Dextrostix shows a blood glucose of < 2.5 mmol per litre (< 45 mg%), confirmed if possible by the laboratory, even in the absence of symptoms, oral glucose feeds are necessary. If symptoms occur an immediate intravenous injection of 25 to 50 per cent glucose at a dose of 1 g per kg should be given, followed by 10 per cent glucose by continuous drip to prevent rebound hypoglycaemia. These solutions are hyperosmolar and should be given slowly.

Only in the very severe case, with a tendency to persistence of the hypoglycaemia or comatose state, should hydrocortisone be given. In these cases blood for culture should be taken and antibiotics started, and the child can then be given hydrocortisone 50 mg IV followed by predisone or prednisolone 0.5 mg per kg 6-hourly.

Electrolyte disturbances are largely the result of chronic diarrhoea, but secondary hyperaldosteronism may also contribute (*See* Acute cardiac failure *below*).

Hyponatraemia (*See also* page 100)

The total body sodium is usually increased but hyponatraemia is common. Unless the serum sodium is $\leqslant 115$ mmol per litre, sodium supplements should be avoided because of the risk of heart failure. The serum sodium will often rise when hypokalaemia is corrected.

MANAGEMENT

If the illness is associated with peripheral circulatory failure, IV therapy is given carefully with half-strength plasma (or PPF), 20 ml per kg per hour for 1 to 2 hours, then 0.45 per cent saline in 2.5 per cent glucose at 6 ml per kg per hour for 4 to 8 hours. The child should be examined frequently for signs of cardiac failure.

Hypokalaemia (*See also* page 136)

Total body potassium is usually grossly depleted in PEM, particularly in the presence of diarrhoea, but the serum potassium may be normal or only slightly reduced.

MANAGEMENT

Potassium should be given by mouth, if possible, when up to 10 mmol per kg per 24 hours can be given in divided doses. A solution of potassium *for oral use* containing 1 mmol per ml can be made up by dissolving 7.5 g KCl in 100 ml of water.

Potassium can be given by *slow* IV infusion once the child is passing urine; the rate should be not more than 20 mmol per hour at a concentration of 40 mmol per litre.

Hypomagnesaemia (*See also* page 145)

Because magnesium is mainly an intracellular ion, serum levels on admission may be relatively normal, but hypomagnesaemia is made worse when the high protein, phosphate, calcium and potassium diet is started.

RECOGNITION

Clinical evidence may not appear for a few days after admission. The signs and symptoms are irritability, carpopedal spasm, increased muscle tone, hyper-reflexia and later, coarse tremors and convulsions. Opposition of the thumb within a clenched fist is often an early sign of hypomagnesaemia in PEM. The Chvostek's sign is often negative. If an ECG is available, shortening of the P–R interval and TV_5 depression are said to be specific. The serum magnesium is often low ($\leqslant 0.7$ mmol per litre).

MANAGEMENT

Treatment consists of intramuscular magnesium sulphate 7 mg per kg immediately and half this amount daily for 3 to 4 days. This would be 1 ml 50 per cent $MgSO_4$. $7H_2O$ (2 mmol of magnesium) immediately and 0.5 ml magnesium sulphate daily, for a 7-kg infant.

Even in the presence of diarrhoea, magnesium hydroxide mixture (milk of magnesia) 10 ml 3 or 4 times daily (41–54 mmol daily) can be given orally after the first 3 or 4 days of intramuscular treatment. The usual preparation of magnesium hydroxide is an 8 per cent solution containing 6.8 mmol of magnesium in 5 ml.

Acute cardiac failure

There is an excess of water in the body and in some cases an increased plasma volume, particularly in the presence of anaemia. Anaemia (Hb $<$ 7 g per 100 ml) and a sodium intake of $>$ 1 mmol per kg per 24 hours increase the risk of heart failure. As oedema is lost there is a rapid shift of fluid from the tissues to the plasma. There may also be difficulty in excreting sodium at this stage. In some cases of PEM the serum aldosterone level is raised (author's unpublished observation). All of these factors contribute to heart failure.

Impending cardiac failure must be suspected in a child losing peripheral oedema without losing weight. Increasing tachypnoea and increasing liver size are important signs.

MANAGEMENT
  (a) Frusemide 5 to 10 mg IV may be given.
  (b) Spironolactone 12.5 mg three times daily may help to remove oedema fluid without precipitating heart failure (unpublished observation). It may also help to prevent urinary loss of potassium.
  (c) Oxygen should be given.
  (d) Digoxin 0.04 mg per kg i.m. followed by 0.015 mg per kg 6 and 12 hours later can be given, with a maintenance dose of 0.02 mg per 24 hours, providing that the child is receiving potassium. There is danger of digoxin toxicity because of the low serum potassium which is especially liable to occur when oedema fluid is lost and potassium moves back into the cells. The pulse rate and rhythm must be recorded carefully.

Evidence of hepatic damage

Elevation of serum alanine aminotransferase and other liver enzymes and bilirubin have been described, probably related more to enzyme leakage from the liver cells than to true hepatic necrosis. If drowsiness occurs which is not related to hypoglycaemia, electrolyte disturbances, septicaemia or meningitis, it will probably respond to rest and the normal diet for PEM.

References

Staff, T. H. E. (1968). Treatment of severe kwashiorkor and marasmus in hospital. *E. Afr. med. J.* **45**, 399

Whitehead, R. G. and Alleyne, G. A. O. (1972). Pathophysiological factors of importance in protein-calorie malnutrition. *Br. med. Bull.* **28**, 72

CHAPTER 67

Infantile Beri-Beri

Wong Hock Boon

Infantile beri-beri is different in its presentation from thiamine-deficient cardiomyopathy in adults, the latter being often associated with alcoholism. The infantile form occurs in areas of the world where there is still gross malnutrition both in adults and children. In those areas, lactating mothers subsist on a low-thiamine diet, and many of the affected babies are breast-fed. However, infantile beri-beri can occur also in artificially-fed babies.

RECOGNITION

This is of great importance because the diagnosis can be missed unless the paediatrician is familiar with its presentation. Moreover, it is an extremely satisfying disease to treat because thiamine injections are specifically curative, and an apparently dying baby becomes almost normal within $\frac{1}{2}$ to 1 hour after the injection.

(a) The baby is usually aged 1 to 6 months, and may appear well-nourished.

(b) There may be prodromal symptoms of refusal of feeds and vomiting a few days before the onset of acute symptoms.

(c) There is restlessness, excessive crying or drowsiness.

(d) The onset is associated with dyspnoea which is usually severe. At this stage, clinical examination will show cardiac failure with raised jugular venous pressure and an enlarged liver. There is tachycardia with a tic-tac rhythm. The pulmonary second sound is usually loud, and a gallop rhythm is not uncommon. Oedema may or may not be present. Cyanosis may be present with signs of hypotension due to cardiac decompensation.

(e) Obviously, other causes of cardiac failure should be excluded, especially congenital heart disease and acute myocarditis. The ECG shows a right heart preponderance in addition to the tachycardia.

(f) However, in association with the cardiac failure, the baby with infantile beri-beri may show certain specific signs:
    (i) Hoarseness of voice or aphonia due to oedema of the larynx. The baby may have grunting or sighing respirations.
    (ii) The tendon reflexes are absent.
    (iii) There may be fits, with meningism.
(g) If the baby is breast fed, examination of the mother may give a clue. She may have oedema and signs of thiamine deficiency, such as peripheral neuritis.

PATHOLOGY

The signs and symptoms are due to acute right-heart failure more than left failure. Thiamine is necessary for the metabolism of cardiac muscle. Similarly, the nervous system tissue needs thiamine to function normally, and a peripheral neuritis may occur.

MANAGEMENT

(a) Specific treatment consists of i.m. injection of thiamine in a dose as little as 25 mg. This in itself is a diagnostic therapeutic test, as the condition of the baby becomes totally different within $\frac{1}{2}$ to 1 hour. Intravenous thiamine (5 to 10 mg) can also be given, followed by the i.m. injection.
(b) Oxygen may be given intranasally.
(c) Secondary chest infections should be treated with antibiotics. A chest infection may tip the balance in the marginally deficient baby, culminating in cardiac failure.
(d) After the baby has settled down, it is usual to carry on thiamine treatment for a few days more.
(e) However, it is very important also:
    (i) to treat the mother, and other members of the family who often suffer from thiamine deficiency and malnutrition;
    (ii) to ensure that the diet of the baby is not thiamine-deficient after discharge.

U

CHAPTER 68

Acute Toxic Hypoglycaemia (Ackee Poisoning)

E. H. Back

The ackee was introduced into Jamaica from Africa in the 18th century: however, in other parts of the West Indies and in Africa it is regarded as a poison and is not eaten. The fruit resembles a small pear which when ripe splits into three at the end. It is the flesh supporting the seed which is cooked. If this is cooked before the fruit is ripe, or cooked with the seeds, severe hypoglycaemia occurs. Now that tinned ackees are available and are exported the possibility of symptoms arising in other countries from the use of unripe ackees in canning must be considered. The toxic substance in the unripe ackee is hypoglycin, an amino acid with a structure similar to that of leucine. Hypoglycin is thought to cause hypoglycaemia by interfering with fatty-acid oxidation (Senior and Sherratt, 1968; Senior, Robson and Sherratt, 1968); recently Milner and Wirdnam (1977) have shown that it also stimulates insulin secretion, but the clinical significance of this latter finding is as yet uncertain.

RECOGNITION

Young and malnourished children are the group most likely to eat the unripe fruit and are also the most likely to suffer severe symptoms, or even to die, whereas older children and adults are less severely affected. The onset is sudden, either with fits or coma; often the child cannot be roused in the morning, having eaten ackees for supper. Vomiting is not a constant feature and may be absent, but the history of vomiting followed by coma is highly suggestive. A typical patient is comatose (the level of coma often fluctuating) and afebrile; clinical examination is essentially negative. Signs of meningitis are absent but a similar clinical picture can be found in pyogenic meningitis, which is the most important differential diagnosis. Viral encephalitis, intracranial tumour and other acute poisonings should also be considered.

The symptoms are due to profound hypoglycaemia, blood-glucose levels frequently being unrecordable. If coma lasts for longer than 6 hours brain damage may result.

MANAGEMENT

Prompt treatment is life-saving. Blood is taken for glucose estimation, and immediately, without waiting for the result 50 ml of 50 per cent glucose solution are injected intravenously. Usually the child regains consciousness and sits up during the injection. When consciousness is regained the injection can be stopped and the child can be given glucose drinks by mouth. Observation for twenty-four hours is necessary because the hypoglycaemia may recur. If hypoglycaemia has been prolonged, recovery of consciousness may be delayed. Under these circumstances 10 per cent glucose should be given by intravenous drip followed by nasogastric feeding. The level of blood glucose should be monitored. A few patients show evidence of temporary damage to the nervous system.

If there is any suspicion of meningitis, a lumbar puncture should be done as soon as the intravenous glucose has been given so that proper antibiotic treatment is not delayed. The cerebrospinal-fluid-glucose level is very low or unrecordable in acute toxic hypoglycaemia.

References

Milner, R. D. G. and Wirdnam, P. K. (1977). Hypoglycin stimulates insulin secretions. *Diabetologia* **13**, 637

Senior, A. E. and Sherratt, H. S. A. (1968). Biochemical effects of the hypoglycaemic compound pent-4-enoic acid and related non-hypoglycaemic fatty acids. *Biochem. J.* **110**, 499, 521

Senior, A. E., Robson, B. and Sherratt, H. S. A. (1968). *Biochem. J.* **110**, 511

Part XVII: Neonatal Emergencies

CHAPTER 69

Resuscitation of the Newborn

J. A. Black

(For older children, *see under* Acute Respiratory Failure, Cardiac Arrest, Shock and Dehydration, *also* Drowning and Near-Drowning).

Adequate resuscitation of the apnoeic or hypoxic infant is the most important and most urgent of all neonatal emergencies. Failure to act immediately and correctly may cause death or permanent cerebral damage.

Effective resuscitation requires:
- (a) Intelligent anticipation that an infant requiring resuscitation may be delivered.
- (b) The presence at all 'at risk' deliveries of someone capable of intubation and other resuscitation procedures.
- (c) Adequate resuscitation facilities in working order.
- (d) Good co-operation between the obstetrician and the paediatrician at all levels.

Apparatus (*see* Appendix 19 for list of recommended equipment). Basic requirements are:
- (a) A satisfactory working surface.
- (b) A safe source of oxygen, suction and radiant heat.
- (c) Equipment for delivery of oxygen by mask or endotracheal tube.
- (d) Appropriate drugs immediately accessible.

Conditions requiring intubation

Severe hypoxia or apnoea at delivery ('White Asphyxia')

RECOGNITION

It should be recognized that with complete apnoea the oxygen content of the blood falls to zero within 3 to 4 minutes; the pCO_2 rises at 2.6 kPa (20 mm Hg) per minute and the H^+ concentration rises by 10 to 12 nmol per litre (falls by 0.1 pH units) per minute (Swyer, 1975).

In most cases fetal hypoxia ('fetal distress') will have been recognized before delivery.

(a) Appearance

Such infants are:
   Pale
   Limp
   Unresponsive
   Apnoeic
The heart rate is likely to be <60 per minute or inaudible.

(b) Other causes of pallor at delivery (See Table 78.II page 653)

(i) Shock from fetal blood loss; these infants are not apnoeic.
(ii) Severe chronic anaemia with heart failure (hydrops) usually due to Rhesus isoimmunization.

MANAGEMENT (*Figure 69.1*)
(*See below* for methods)
(1) Start the clock on the resuscitation trolley.
(2) Transfer the infant to the resuscitation surface under radiant heat.
(3) Examine the larynx under direct vision and suck out any obstructing material above and below the larynx.
(4) Pass an endotracheal tube.
(5) Inflate the lungs with intermittent positive pressure (IPPV).
(6) Start external cardiac massage if the apex beat is <40 per minute, or if it is inaudible, but the fetal heart was heard during the second stage of labour.
(7) Inject (over 1 to 5 minutes) 5 ml of 8.4 per cent $NaHCO_3$ into the umbilical vein, avoiding direct puncture of the umbilical vein (*see* page 606 for technique).
   Dose: 5 ml is a safe partial correction for a baby of 3 to 3.5 kg: for other weights use 1.5 ml (1.5 mmol) of 8.4 per cent $NaHCO_3$ per kg.
(8) If there is a strong probability of depression by the morphia group of drugs give naloxone (Narcan) or nalorphine (Lethidrone) into the umbilical vein (p. 604).
(9) At 5 minutes if there is still apnoea, repeat the dose of $NaHCO_3$ *.

* *Dose of NaHCO₃:* a number of different strengths of $NaHCO_3$ are in use. If the 5 per cent solution is used, give twice (actually 1.7 ×) the dose specified for the 8.4 per cent solution.

(10) At 10 minutes, if there is still apnoea and no apex beat inject 1 to
     2 ml of *1 in 10 000* adrenaline into the heart or umbilical vein,
     followed by 0.1 mg of atropine.
(11) At 30 minutes:
     (a) If there is no respiration or apex beat and the pupils are dilated
         and fixed, IPPV should cease.
     (b) If there is no respiration but the beat is >60 with a good
         colour and peripheral circulation, and the pupils are of nor-
         mal size, IPPR should continue while the Astrup is checked.
         (Correction of a severe metabolic acidosis may initiate spon-
         taneous respiration.)
     (c) If there is no respiration with IV NaHCO$_3$ but the infant's
         condition is otherwise satisfactory (*see* (b) *above*), transfer it
         to a ventilator.

Delayed onset of respiration

Delayed respiration may be caused by:
  (a) Severe hypoxia (*see above*).
  (b) Drug depression, usually from the morphia, pethidine (meperi-
      dine) codeine (diamorphine) group, occasionally due to a pro-
      longed general anaesthesia or by heavy maternal sedation with
      barbiturates. There is no specific treatment for the infant de-
      pressed after maternal general anaesthesia and it is rare for this
      to be a cause of apnoea.
  (c) No obvious reason.

Drug depression (Morphia group)

RECOGNITION

It is generally agreed that some degree of depression of the infant's
respiration is likely if the mother has received one of this group of drugs
within 4 hours of delivery. Such an infant is normally in good condition
at delivery but does not breathe immediately.

MANAGEMENT

(1) If the probability of morphia group drug depression is high a
    specific antagonist should be given either prophylactically (i.e.
    immediately after delivery) or after a predetermined period of
    apnoea under close observation; normally after 30 seconds (by the
    clock) of apnoea.

    Nalorphine (Lethidrone) has been used until recently but has the
    disadvantage that it may itself have a depressant effect on respira-
    tion if given when there is in fact no existing drug effect.

FIG. 69.1
RESUSCITATION: PAEDIATRICIAN
Start clock for all deliveries
ACTION
& TIME

Apgar	Appearance	0 Min immediate	2 Min	5 Min	10 Min	30 Min +
0–2	Pale/Grey Limp Apnoea Heart <100	(1) Suck out (too vigorous sucking may cause bradycardia) (2) IPPV (intubation) (3) Na HCO$_3$ 8.4% (5 ml IV over 1–5 min; 2–2.5 ml for Baby <1.5 kg) (4) Score 0: ECM (*See* Note 3)	(1) Continue IPPV (2) Naloxone if previous opiate (Note 2) 0.04 mg IV ($\frac{1}{2}$ dose if baby <2.5 kg) (3) *Regular respiration for 2 min* Remove tube Apnoea ·········→	(1) Continue IPPV (2) Repeat NaHCO$_3$ over 5–10 min (Dose as for 0 min) (3) Glucose 10% (3 ml IV over 1 min) (4) *Regular respiration for 2 min* Remove tube Apnoea ·········→	(1) Continue IPPV (2) Adrenaline 1 in 10 000:1–2 ml into heart or umbilical vein (3) Atropine (0.1 mg IV) (4) *Regular respiration for 2 min* Remove tube Apnoea ·········→	*Apnoea* No circulation cease IPPV *Apnoea* Good circulation correct acidosis ventilator *Regular respiration* after 2 min Remove tube Apnoea ·········→
3–6	Blue/Grey Respiration Gasping Weak Irregular Tone ± Response ±	(1) Suck out and wipe down (2) Insert airway (3) Oxygen: bag and mask	(1) IPPV (intubation) (2) NaHCO$_3$ 5% (2 ml IV) (3) Naloxone if previous opiate 0.04 mg ($\frac{1}{2}$ dose if baby <2.5 kg) IV or i.m. No change or apnoea ·····→	(1) Continue IPPV (2) Repeat NaHCO$_3$ over 5–10 min (2 ml IV) (3) Glucose 10% (3 ml IV over 1 min) No change or apnoea ·····→	(1) Ventilator (2) Astrup NaHCO$_3$ as indicated No change or apnoea ·····→	

7–10	Pink Active Crying Regular Resp. at <1 min	Suck out and wipe down →	*Regular respiration* *for 2 min* warm towel mother or cot	*Regular respiration* *for 2 min* (1) Remove tube (2) Warm towel mother or cot	*Regular respiration* *for 2 min* (1) Remove tube (2) Incubator
Good condition at birth but apnoea at 1 min or stops breathing	*0 Min* Suck out and wipe down	*1 Min* (1) Insert airway (2) Oxygen bag & mask (3) Naloxone if previous opiate (0.04 mg ½ dose if baby <2.5 kg IV or i.m.	(1) IPPV (2) NaHCO$_3$ 8.4% (5 ml IV 2–2.5 ml if <1.5 kg over 1–5 min) Apnoea · · · · · · · · · · · →	As for Apgar 3–6 (above) Apnoea · · · · · · · · · · · →	As for Apgar 3–6 (above) Apnoea · · · · · · · · · · · →

· · · · · · · → Deterioration or no change
————————→ Improvement

(1) Failure to go pink after IPPV for 1 min. Consider:
   (a) Tube: oesophagus   (d) Bronchi blocked
   (b) Tube: right main bronchus   (e) ?Lung condition
   (c) Tube: blocked   ? Heart condition

(2) Previous opiates: mother has received at < 4 hours before delivery: pethidine, codein, heroin, (diamorphine)
(3) External cardiac massage: use with IPPV if fetal heart was heard during second stage

Dose: 0.25 mg; 0.125 mg under 2.5 kg: double dose if given i.m.
Route: IV (umbilical vein) or i.m. (*see below* for method).
NOTE: the paediatric ampoules should be used; these contain 1 mg per 1 ml. AMPOULES FOR ADULTS CONTAIN 10 mg PER 1 ml.

Recently, naloxone (Narcan) has been shown to be a better antagonist without depressant side-effects.
Dose: either 0.01 mg per kg; or as a standard dose of 0.04 mg (2 ml) for term infants and half this dose for infants <2.5 kg. The dose can be repeated if necessary after 1 hour.
Route: as for nalorphine.
NOTE: the paediatric ampoules should be used; these contain 0.02 mg per 1 ml (ampoules contain 2 ml).
ADULT AMPOULES CONTAIN 0.4 mg PER 1 ml.
(2) Failure to breathe at 1 minute (i.e. 30 seconds after giving the antagonist): proceed as for the severely asphyxiated group, and intubate.

Delayed onset of respiration for no obvious reason

Whatever the Apgar score, if respiration does not start immediately after routine aspiration of the nose and mouth:
(1) Oxygen should be given by mask and bag until 30 seconds after delivery.
(2) If there is no respiratory effort at 1 minute after delivery, the infant should be intubated and treated as for the severely asphyxiated group.

Meconium aspiration

RECOGNITION
It is not always possible to predict whether aspiration of meconium has occurred, even if the infant is covered with meconium at delivery, or there is meconium stained liquor. If respiration is obviously difficult, with tachypnoea, in-drawing and recession, aspiration of meconium is certain. Staining of the cord, nails, and skin occur after contact with meconium for 4 to 6 hours (Fujikura and Klionsky, 1975); obviously the longer the interval between the passage of meconium and delivery, the greater the possibility of inhalation.

Fetal hypoxia (fetal distress) in the pre-term infant very rarely causes the passage of meconium.

MANAGEMENT
(a) If meconium stained fluid has been draining before delivery, an

attempt should be made to clear the nose, mouth and upper air passages *before* the first breath, using direct laryngoscopy and suction.

(b) If the membranes have been ruptured for longer than 48 hours, or the amniotic fluid is smelly, or the mother is febrile, the infant should be given a 5-day course of antibiotics, normally gentamicin and penicillin.

(c) If there is severe respiratory distress, with tachypnoea and pallor, cyanosis, the umbilical artery should be catheterized for subsequent monitoring of oxygen concentration. Oxygen should be given initially in a concentration of 50 to 60 per cent and the pO_2 should then be measured.

(d) For later management and complications *see* page 275.

Methods
(For apparatus *see* Appendix 19)

(a) INTUBATION
  (i) Flex the infant's neck and extend the head ('sniffing a flower') by putting one towel under the neck.
  (ii) A straight-bladed infant laryngoscope should be used, with gentle suction available. An endotracheal tube of appropriate size (FG 10, 12 or 14) is passed. The tube is secured and connected to a source of humidified oxygen with a satisfactory safety blow-off at 30 cm (12 in) of water. The rate of flow should be 0.5 to 1.0 litres per minute and rate of inflation approximately 30 to 40 per minute.
  Occasionally expansion of the lungs can only be obtained by using an *initial* pressure of 60 to 70 cm (24–28 in) of water, but this pressure should not be sustained.

(b) BAG AND MASK
This method can be used initially if intubation is not immediately required, or in the infant with weak and gasping respiration.

A suitably fitting mask with re-breathing bag and stopcock is used; the valve should be open but the stopcock shut. The same type of oxygen connection should be used as for the intubated infant.

It is important to make sure that the chest moves with pressure on the bag, and that the head is kept extended. The procedure is made more effective if an infant oropharyngeal airway is used.

(c) MOUTH-TO-MOUTH INFLATION
This is indicated only when no other method is available.

The head is kept extended. The nose should be covered by the operator's mouth, or pinched during inflation if an oropharyngeal airway is used. Inflationary pressure should be applied by the cheeks, NOT the chest, at 30 to 40 times per minute.

(d) EXTERNAL CARDIAC MASSAGE

The infant is placed on a firm, flat surface; the middle of the sternum is depressed sharply (1 to 1.5 cm, $\frac{1}{2}$ in) by the index and middle fingers at 100 to 120 times per minute. Alternatively, the infant's chest is grasped by the operator's hands with the fingers at the back of the chest, the thumbs in the middle of the sternum; the sternum is then depressed sharply by squeezing between the thumbs and fingers.

(e) INJECTION OF DRUGS INTO THE UMBILICAL VEIN

There are a number of dangers if an incorrect technique is used.

    (i) A haematoma, and possibly injection into the artery.

    (ii) The drug cannot be washed into the circulation and may therefore be ineffective.

    (iii) The intima of the vein may be damaged by a hyperosmolar solution, causing thrombosis.

The correct method is as follows. An umbilical catheter is attached to a 5- or 10-ml syringe; the catheter and half the syringe are filled with sterile 0.9 per cent NaCl; the catheter is then inserted into the umbilical vein for about 5 to 7 cm (2–3 in) until blood can be freely withdrawn. The catheter is then firmly pinched, the syringe is detached. The drug to be injected is aspirated into the syringe which now contains the drug diluted with 0.9 per cent NaCl. The syringe is re-attached to the catheter and all air bubbles are now removed. Blood is now aspirated to fill the rest of the syringe and the whole contents are slowly injected. No drug should be injected more rapidly than over a period of 1 minute.

References

Fujikura, T. and Klionsky, B. (1975). The significance of meconium staining. *Am. J. Obstet. Gynec.* **121**, 45

Swyer, P. R. (1975). *The Intensive Care of the Newly Born* p. 36. Basle: S. Karger

CHAPTER 70

Birth Trauma and Accidents Related to Delivery

J. A. Black

An accurate knowledge of the complications of the various types of delivery will assist early diagnosis and treatment. Only complications requiring urgent treatment are considered here.

(a) Precipitate vertex delivery

Lack of moulding and stretching of the tissues causes tearing of the venous sinuses in the tentorium cerebelli or falx cerebri, with a resulting acute subdural haemorrhage.

(b) Breech delivery

(i) Rapid delivery of the unprotected head may cause a tear of tentorium or falx, as described above.

(ii) Brachial plexus injury is common in difficult breech deliveries but only constitutes an emergency when injury to the phrenic nerve causes diaphragmatic paralysis (*see* page 278).

(iii) A fracture of the clavicle, humerus or femur may also result from a difficult breech delivery.

(iv) Shock may occasionally develop from massive bleeding into the soft tissues of the buttocks (*see* page 666).

(c) Face delivery

(i) A goitre may be the cause of the malpresentation and the neck should be carefully examined in every case; there is a danger of respiratory obstruction from tracheal compression (*see* page 460).

(ii) Direct pressure of the larynx against the symphysis pubis may occasionally cause oedema of the glottis or dislocation of the cricothyroid or cricoarytenoid articulations (*see also under* Stridor, page 647).

(*d*) *Brow delivery*

As for face delivery, except that fetal hypoxia may result from a prolonged labour and difficult delivery.

(*e*) *Forceps delivery*

(i) In very difficult or traumatic deliveries an acute subdural haemorrhage may result from rupture of communicating veins or from a torn venous sinus.

(ii) Cephalhaematoma is commoner in forceps deliveries than in normal deliveries.

(iii) In rare cases a supaponeurotic haemorrhage develops. Unaccountably this is commoner in infants of African race; or it may be the first indication of a coagulation defect.

(iv) Direct trauma to the nose, eye or ear may result from misapplication of the blade.

(*f*) *Vacuum (ventouse) extraction*

A supaponeurotic haemorrhage may occur, as above.

(*g*) *Caesarian section*

(i) The majority of emergencies in caesarian section are related to the condition for which the section was done (e.g. a hypoxic infant in a section for fetal distress).

(ii) Acute fetal haemorrhage, which is easily overlooked at operation, may be due to:
Fetal bleeding in addition to maternal bleeding in placenta praevia or accidental haemorrhage.
Incision of a fetal vessel at operation.
Bleeding from an incision into the scalp or elsewhere.
Draining blood out of the infant into the placenta by holding the infant above the placenta without first clamping the cord.

(*h*) *Twins and multiple pregnancy*

Difficult or obstructed labour is relatively common, and an undiagnosed twin may be severely hypoxic when finally delivered. Respiratory distress syndrome is commoner or may be more severe in the second of twins. Other conditions which may require urgent attention are:

(i) Entanglement of the cords in a monoamniotic pregnancy; fortunately this is rare since death of one or both twins is common; but severe fetal distress may be detected in time for effective action.

(ii) Fetofetal (twin-to-twin) transfusion; this occurs only in monozygotic twins (*see also* page 658).

(*i*) *Antepartum haemorrhage*

Fetal bleeding from placenta praevia (*see also under* Caesarian section).

(*j*) *Accidental haemorrhage (Abruptio placentae)*

The infant may be severely hypoxic but additional complications may be:

(i) Haemorrhagic shock, as for antepartum haemorrhage.

(ii) Inhalation of blood or meconium due to premature onset of respiration.

(iii) Vomiting or passage in the stools of swallowed maternal blood (*see* page 399).

(*k*) *Prolapsed cord*

In addition to severe hypoxia the infant may inhale meconium (*see above*).

(*l*) *Local (regional) anaesthesia*

The fetus may be affected:

(i) Indirectly: due to maternal hypotension in spinal or epidural anaesthesia, or convulsions and hypoxia due to overdosage. In either case a severely hypoxic infant will result.

(ii) Directly: the fetus may be adversely affected by high blood levels of local anaesthetic (not necessarily with maternal symptoms of overdosage) in paracervical, caudal or perineal block. Direct injection into the fetal scalp or brain has been described in both paracervical and caudal block.

(*m*) *Fetal scalp electrodes and blood sampling*

Apart from subsequent infection of the puncture site. bleeding may occur.

Recognition and management of the emergencies

Acute fetal haemorrhage for any cause
(See page 652)

Acute subdural haemorrhage

RECOGNITION

The infant becomes shocked within a few hours of delivery with apnoeic attacks or fits and a tense or bulging fontanelle. Small tears and collections of blood on the surface of the cortex or cerebellum are common at post mortem but are probably only incidental findings.

MANAGEMENT

Rapidly developing collection of blood large enough to cause acute symptoms may be fatal but nevertheless an attempt should be made to aspirate blood by subdural taps at the lateral angles of the anterior fontanelle.

Supaponeurotic haemorrhage

RECOGNITION

An obvious swelling of the head usually develops at 24 to 36 hours after delivery, occasionally as early as 12 hours. The head is deformed (turban-shaped) by a tense swelling with pitting oedema of the scalp. Blood may track backwards as far as the attachment of the aponeurosis to the superior nuchal line, or forwards into the frontal region and may be visible in the upper lids, or laterally as far as the zygoma. The swelling of the sides of the face may be mistaken for enlargement of the parotid gland.

MANAGEMENT

As much as 150 ml of blood may be lost and acute shock may develop; urgent blood transfusion may therefore be required (p. 654). Vitamin K_1 (1 mg) should be given i.m., or IV if a coagulation disorder is suspected. In every case the infant should be investigated for thrombocytopenia and coagulation defects.

Fetal scalp haemorrhage

RECOGNITION

This may be difficult until after delivery; blood may collect in the oedematous tissues of the caput.

MANAGEMENT

In some cases blood transfusion is required. Investigation should be as for subaponeurotic haemorrhage (*see above*).

Direct injury to the larynx

See page 648.

Diaphragmatic paralysis with brachial plexus injury

See page 278.

Effects of local anaesthesia

RECOGNITION

Fetal bradycardia followed by the delivery of a depressed and possibly apnoeic infant following local anaesthesia (particularly paracervical. caudal, perineal, or pudendal block) should suggest the possibility of the effect of high fetal-blood levels of the local anaesthetic. Convulsions occur in severely affected infants.

MANAGEMENT

The apnoeic or hypoxic infant should be resuscitated in the usual way (p. 599). A metabolic acidosis is common and should be corrected with intravenous $NaHCO_3$ (p. 126). Convulsions should be treated with diazepam (p. 689). Severely affected infants who show no improvement on the treatment described above may require an exchange transfusion (p. 677) or a ventilator (p. 616).

Rupture of liver, spleen

See page 655

Adrenal haemorrhage

See page 455

Renal vein thrombosis

See page 656

Acute intraventricular haemorrhage

See page 655

CHAPTER 71

Transport of the Sick Neonate

M. F. Whitfield

With the growing complexity of neonatal intensive care, its requirements for expensive equipment, a high specialist staff/patient ratio, and the better survival statistics obtained by larger well-equipped and well-staffed units, the transport of sick or at risk infants for specialist treatment from the Special Care Baby Units (SCBU) of District General Hospitals to Regional Neonatal Intensive Care Units (NICU) with their concentration of staffing and equipment, is of crucial importance.

Whenever possible an infant anticipated to be at risk (e.g. because of premature delivery, severe Rhesus disease, poorly controlled maternal diabetes) should be delivered in the obstetric unit of the hospital containing the regional NICU. For a variety of reasons this frequently is not possible, and the infant is born in a unit where full intensive care facilities which may be required by the infant are not available.

The decision to transfer the infant lies with the senior staff of the referring SCBU, a decision made in consultation with the staff of the receiving NICU.

The arrangement for transport must be the responsibility of the NICU, which provides the necessary equipment and staff to collect the infant and to ensure that it remains in the best possible condition during transit.

Facilities required for optimal transport of the sick neonate

The neonatal intensive care transport facility, be it a modified ambulance or modified transport incubator, acts as an extension of the NICU, intensive care of the infant beginning with the arrival of the transport facility and NICU staff at the referring SCBU.

The transport facility must provide:

(a) Adequate temperature homeostasis. Usually this involves a transport incubator which can be run off 240V ac. or 12V dc. The infant should be wrapped in Gamgee tissue and this covered with a 'silver swaddler' or piece of kitchen aluminium foil.

(b) Self-contained infant ventilator and oxygen supply.

(c) Continuous monitoring facilities for heart rate, body temperature (by thermometer probe) and inspired oxygen concentration.

(d) Equipment for resuscitation, connection to ventilator, intravascular infusion, chest drains and chest drain valves, Dextrostix.

   Intravascular infusion should be controlled by a battery-powered infusion pump as drop-counting in a moving ambulance is impossible.

(e) Drugs: sodium bicarbonate, digoxin, antibiotics, anticonvulsants, 20 per cent glucose, IV infusion fluid.

Three staff are necessary: two nurses and one doctor or two doctors and one nurse. All must be familiar with the location of equipment and be experienced members of the NICU staff.

Transfer of sick small infants accompanied by one junior nurse without knowledge and facilities for intensive care intervention is a recipe for disaster.

Indications for transfer

The majority of infants requiring transfer are small pre-term infants with developing or already serious respiratory problems. The remainder are term infants with other illnesses requiring specialist care and investigation and possibly neonatal surgery. The stage in an infant's illness when transfer is required depends on the facilities, staff numbers and their training, and laboratory facilities of the referring SCBU.

It is not possible or desirable to give fixed indications for transfer. It is, however, possible to provide a list of situations where the infant and its further management and possible transfer should be discussed by the doctor in charge of the infant's care at SCBU with NICU staff.

Indications for initiation of a discussion between SCBU and NICU staff

(a) (i) Birth weight less than 2 kg.
     (ii) Gestation less than 35 weeeks.

(b) (i) Administration of more than F_1O_2 0.35 (35 per cent inspired oxygen) to abolish cyanosis if blood gas analysis is not readily available.
     (ii) PaO_2 less than 8.0 kPa (60 mm Hg) in F_1O_2 0.6 (60 per cent inspired oxygen) at atmospheric pressure if blood gas analy-

sis is available and reliable. (The use of Continuous Distending Pressure (CDP, CPAP*) should not be embarked upon at SCBU level in view of the risks of pneumothorax and possible graduation to IPPV).

(c) Suspected systemic infection.
(d) Severe intrapartum hypoxia with neurological abnormality, however slight.
(e) Apnoeic attacks.
(f) Jaundice other than mild 'physiological' jaundice.
(g) Serious congenital abnormality, somatic or metabolic.
(h) Neonatal convulsions.
(i) Sustained hypoglycaemia.
(j) A sick infant presenting diagnostic problems.
(k) An infant whom referring doctor is anxious about and feels unable to cope with.

A decision about the best management of the infant should then be made mutually and, if transfer to NICU is decided upon, advice about treatment to be given to the infant by SCBU staff while the team is in transit to the SCBU can be given (e.g. administration of bicarbonate or glucose).

On arrival at SCBU the Intensive Care team assess the infant and transfer it to the transport incubator monitoring systems and ventilation if required.

The mother must see the infant being collected by the NICU staff and be assured about early access to the infant and full details of the baby's progress once in the intensive care unit. All details regarding pregnancy and delivery must be copied from the mother's notes, and the baby's notes, x-rays, fluid-balance records etc. transferred with the baby. 10 ml of the mother's blood should be taken for subsequent crossmatching if blood has to be given to the infant. In transit the baby may well improve with adequate oxygenation and body-temperature homeostasis, and correction of acidosis and hypoglycaemia.

On arrival at NICU the baby is moved from the transport to the Intensive Care Area and the neonatal intensive care already started is continued and consolidated.

Further reading

Swyer, P. R. (1975). *Intensive Care of the Newly Born*. Chapter 8. Basle: S. Karger
Blake, A. M., McIntosh, N., Reynolds, E. O. R. and Andrew, D. (1975). Transport of newborn infants for intensive care. *Br. med. J.* **4**, 13
Cunningham, M. D. and Smith, F. R. (1973). Stabilization and transport of the severely ill infant. *Pediat. Clin. N. Am.* **20**, 359
Swyer, P. R. (1970). The Regional Organisation of Special Care of the Neonate. *Pediat. Clins. N. Am.* **17 (4)**, 761

*CPAP = Continuous Positive Airway Pressure

CHAPTER 72

Care of the Infant of Very Low Birth Weight (under 1.5 kg)

M. F. Whitfield

A large proportion of deaths in childhood occur in small immature infants in the first few days of life. With increasing understanding of neonatal physiology and development of techniques of neonatal intensive care, the mortality and morbidity rates of these small infants have improved dramatically. With a high standard of care a high proportion of these infants grow into normal children and adults, with a consequent reduction in the numbers of surviving brain-damaged children.

An infant's birth weight may be less than 1.5 kg because he is:
(a) born early: probably less than 32 weeks completed gestation, or
(b) subjected to intrauterine malnutrition due to 'placental failure' producing an infant who is small-for-gestational-age, or
(c) born early *and* undernourished *in utero*.

Some infants with congenital or metabolic abnormalities associated with reduced growth potential are born with birth weights less than 1.5 kg and may have super-added placental failure and short gestation.

An infant anticipated to be of very low birth weight antenatally should, if possible, be born in the maternity unit serving the Regional Neonatal Intensive Care Unit so that all available neonatal expertise and equipment are available from birth. Frequently, however, premature labour is far advanced on arrival of the mother at the local maternity unit and the infant has to be delivered there. A very small infant born in a neonatal unit with less than neonatal care facilities should be transferred to a larger, better equipped and better staffed unit.

RECOGNITION

(*a*) *Size* The infant's small size is obvious, but this must be accurately documented by measurements of weight, length and head circumference shortly after birth before the infant becomes irremovable from the incubator due to drips, monitoring leads, etc.

(*b*) *Gestational age*   This may be assessed by a combination of:
  (i)   Obstetric dates.
  (ii) Physical characteristics assessed in the light of experience.
  (iii) Scoring system for neurological and physical characteristics (e.g. Dubowitz' scheme).

(*c*) *Growth parameters in relation to gestational age*   These may be assessed by plotting them on a standard chart (e.g. Gairdner and Pearson (1971)). The 'small-for-gestational-age infant' is defined as having a weight lying below the 10th percentile for gestational age. The greater maturity and exposure to 'intrauterine stress' make the small-for-gestational-age infant less liable to severe respiratory distress syndrome than a more immature infant of the same weight but more liable to brain damage, hypoglycaemia, meconium aspiration syndrome and reduced intelligence and ultimate stature.

MANAGEMENT

Life support of three separate kinds is required in the first 48 hours by the low-birth-weight infant, due to immaturity of the infant's organs and homeostatic mechanisms. These are: respiratory support; temperature homeostasis; nutrition and fluid balance.

Respiratory support

Any infant of 1.5 kg or less can be expected to develop some degree of ventilatory failure in the first 24 hours of life due to respiratory distress syndrome. Blood gas estimations on arterial blood or free-flowing capillary blood are essential, providing the only objective way of assessing adequacy of ventilation, if harmful degrees of hypoxia, acidaemia or oxygen toxicity are to be avoided. An umbilical arterial catheter provides ready access to arterial blood with minimal disturbance of the infant.

The aim is to maintain the infant's arterial PO_2 between 6.7 to 11.0 kPa (50–85 mm Hg) and an H^+ concentration less than 65 nmol per litre (pH > 7.20) by administration of oxygen, ventilatory assistance as CPAP or IPPV and administration of bicarbonate. Avoidance of hypoxia, hypoglycaemia, acidaemia and hypothermia keep the baby in the best possible condition, favouring optimal surfactant synthesis.

Temperature homeostasis

Small immature infants lose heat very rapidly due to their large surface area: mass ratio, deficiency of brown fat, and slow response of thermoregulatory mechanisms to temperature drop.

A small infant covered by a perspex heat shield nursed in an incubator for ease of observation requires an air temperature of around 35°C (95°F) to maintain core temperature above 36°C (97°F). A skin temperature more than 0.5°C (1°F) below core temperature suggests that the infant is at the lower end of the thermoneutral zone and is having to catabolize metabolic fuel to maintain his body temperature. Drop in core temperature below 36°C (97°F) for more than a few hours is associated with general deterioration of the infant and poorer survival. The newer infrared overhead-heated intensive care tables maintain the infant's temperature but may double insensible water loss (to over 100 ml/kg/24 hours) in very immature infants. At the present time the most suitable equipment in which to nurse a low-birth-weight infant is a proportional servocontrolled incubator providing at least 70 per cent humidity with some kind of heat shield, of aluminium foil, or of a perspex semicylindrical type.

Nutrition and fluid balance

Delayed gastric emptying, ileus, and immature sucking reflex make feeding of small infants hazardous, and gastrointestinal absorption at best unreliable. Hypoxia, acidaemia, electrolyte disturbances and possibly the presence of an umbilical arterial catheter delay the appearance of normal gastrointestinal motility. Fluid and calorie requirements may have to be given totally by the parenteral route. A low-birth-weight infant needs around 65 ml per kg in the first 24 hours but this may be as much as doubled by phototherapy, tachypnoea, pyrexia and unhumidified ambient oxygen–air mixture. A urine osmolality of 200 milliosmoles per kg or less indicates adequate hydration. 10 per cent glucose by peripheral vein or via umbilical arterial catheter usually provides the bulk of the infant's fluid requirements over the first 48 hours although small volumes (1 to 2 ml per hour, increasing) of expressed human milk may be tolerated by intermittent or continuous nasogastric infusion with frequent aspiration of the stomach to prevent inhalation of gastric contents. 10 per cent glucose orally delays gastric emptying and is tolerated less well than human milk if aspirated into the lungs.

65 ml per kg per 24 hours of 10 per cent glucose provides between $\frac{1}{3}$ and $\frac{1}{2}$ of the infant's calorie requirement and must be supplemented by parenteral nutrition after 48 hours if significant amounts of milk are not

being tolerated. Inadequate hydration and nutrition in the first few days of life produce brain damage or suboptimal brain growth. However an extremely cautious approach to feeding low-birth-weight infants with respiratory problems in the first few days of life decreases the incidence of apnoeic attacks and serious aspiration episodes. Continuous nasojejunal feeding may in the future prove to be a considerable advance.

Timetable for management of low-birth-weight infant

Aim to maintain the infant in the best possible respiratory, blood-gas, thermal, metabolic and nutritional condition at all times.

(1) BEFORE BIRTH
Preparation; liaison with obstetric staff; possibility of fetal therapy.

Doctors

Close liaison with obstetric staff is a necessity, to be aware of antenatal problems, intrauterine growth, possibility of caesarian section, progress in labour. Results of recent biparietal diameters of the fetus and lecithin:sphingomyelin ratio (L:S ratio) may be available.

Low L:S ($<2:1$) and maturity under 34 weeks suggest possibility of administration of dexamethazone (6 mg twice daily) to the mother and attempting to delay delivery for 24 to 48 hours to induce fetal pulmonary enzyme maturity. Paediatricians and mother should meet before delivery.

Nurses

Assemble and check the equipment likely to be used, in a warm intensive care cubicle:
    Proportional servocontrolled incubator.
    Maximum humidity, prewarmed.
    Heat shield.
    Cardiopulmonary monitoring equipment.
    Oxygen analyser.
    Check oxygen cylinders if not piped O_2.
    Tray for umbilical catheterization.
    Resuscitation equipment and laryngoscope (check light).
    Ventilator/CPAP system.
    Oxygen hood.
    Pneumothorax drain kit.
    Anglepoise light.

(2) BIRTH TO 2 HOURS

Birth; resuscitation; transfer to SCBU/NICU; phase of acute adaptation to extrauterine life.

Doctors

Adequate prompt resuscitation with low threshold for intervention: baby may need glucose (3 ml of 20 per cent) and sodium bicarbonate (2 to 2.5 mmol) via umbilical vein.

Dry infant all over with a towel early in resuscitation to prevent heat loss. Resuscitation must be done under an overhead heater.

When infant is breathing spontaneously he should be transferred as soon as possible to *NICU/SCBU having first been shown to the mother*.

Nurses

The infant requires the full attention of an experienced neonatal nurse. The baby should be transferred to incubator and connected to monitoring equipment after first being *measured and weighed*.

30 per cent oxygen if cyanosed.

Dextrostix. Heat shield in place.

$\frac{1}{4}$-hourly recordings of heart rate.

Respiratory rate, colour, temperature and the appearance of signs of respiratory distress syndrome (e.g. nostril flaring, grunting, chest recession).

Infant once settled must be handled as little as possible and be in a good light so that any change in colour can be readily appreciated.

Suck out mouth if mucousy.

Call doctor if patient is deteriorating or if cyanosed in 30 to 35 per cent O_2 before 1 to $1\frac{1}{2}$ hours of age.

Doctors

Reassess after 1 to $1\frac{1}{2}$ hours.

Is the baby getting better or worse on the basis of:

Colour.

Oxygen requirement.

Development of signs of RDS.

Air entry on auscultation.

Stability of observations?

If there are signs of RDS and a requirement for more than 30 per cent O_2 the baby needs:

(a) Umbilical arterial catheter. (Open-ended Argyle PVC catheter with x-ray opaque tracer 3.5 FG or 5 FG).

(b) Chest x-ray including most of abdomen.
    (i) for signs of RDS;
    (ii) to define position of arterial catheter. (Should be just above
        aortic bifurcation)
(c) Blood gases.
(d) 10 per cent glucose drip via umbilical catheter.
(e) Nasogastric tube to aspirate stomach contents.

(3) 2 TO 12 HOURS—DEVELOPING RESPIRATORY FAILURE, FLUID AND CALORIE PROVISION

If respiratory problems are evident based on assessment at 1 to $1\frac{1}{2}$ hours of life the baby needs:

(a) 4-hourly blood gases and Dextrostix.
(b) Action, if necessary, to maintain blood-gas status by ventilatory assistance (CPAP or IPPV) and buffer therapy, and to maintain Dextrostix 1.4 mmol per litre (25 mg%) or greater.
(c) Monitoring of urine passed for:
Sugar—as an index of glucose overload and osmotic diuresis.
Osmolality—as an index of adequacy of hydration.

If the infant does not have RDS and does not require an umbilical arterial catheter, continuous nasogastric or nasojejunal feeds should be started beginning at 1 to 2 ml per hour with 3-hourly nasogastric aspiration and check of Dextrostix. Intermittent, small, frequent nasogastric feeds are a suitable alternative.

(4) 12 TO 48 HOURS

Stabilization; fluid, calorie and electrolyte balance; possibility of apnoeic attacks.

Doctors

Check on and assess:

(*a*) *Fluid intake and urine osmolality*   Fluid requirement is about 90 ml per kg per 24 hours by 48 hours. If the infant does not have an umbilical arterial catheter, supplementary parenteral fluids must be provided by peripheral-vein drip unless the nasogastric intake is adequate.

(*b*) *Nutrition*   Use of a supplementary parenteral nutrition schedule at this stage may be indicated if calorie and protein intakes nasogastrically are inadequate. Nasojejunal infusion of isotonic milk frequently can provide an adequate fluid and calorie intake when nasogastric feeding is not well tolerated.

(*c*) *Temperature homeostasis.*

(*d*) *Blood gas status* Oxygen requirement, adequacy of respiratory support.

(*e*) *Neurological state of infant*

(*f*) *Chest x-ray*

(*g*) *Can the arterial catheter be removed?*

Nurses

Infants who have previously done well may get apnoeic attacks at this stage due to excessive damping in blood gas : respiratory drive feedback mechanism due to central nervous system immaturity. Most respond to stimulation but facilities for IPPV by mask (e.g. Ambu bag) must be available in the incubator. Infants requiring ventilation mechanically for apnoeic attacks generally do well. Infants requiring ventilation since the first few hours of life frequently begin to have more copious tracheal secretions by 48 hours and require much more intensive tracheal toilet.

The further management of the small pre-term infant becomes progressively more diverse and complex the longer intensive care is required and is outside the scope of this book.

Further reading

Swyer, P. R. (1975). *Intensive Care of the Newly Born.* Basle: S. Karger
Dubowitz, L. M. S., Dubowitz, V. and Goldberg, C. (1970). Clinical assessment of gestational age in the newborn infant. *J. Pediat.* **77**, 1
Gairdner, D. and Pearson, J. (1971). A growth chart for premature and other infants. *Archs Dis. Childh,* **46**, 783.
Gamsu, H. R. (1972). The low-birth-weight infant. *Br. J. Hosp. Med.* **8**, 29
Hey, E. N. (1972). Thermal regulation in the newborn. *Br. J. Hosp. Med.* **8**, 51

CHAPTER 73

Sudden Collapse in the Newborn

J. A. Black

(a) If there is no evidence of a respiratory or abdominal emergency, an acute infection should be considered and a complete infection screen should be done (blood culture, lumbar puncture, swabs from nose, umbilicus, axillae, anus and any septic lesions, urine culture, chest x-ray).

(b) In infants with *either* respiratory or abdominal symptoms (or both) an x-ray of *both* chest and abdomen should be done since it is not always possible to distinguish whether the disease is above or below the diaphragm.

(c) The most common biochemical cause of acute collapse is hypoglycaemia.

TABLE 73.I

Abdominal conditions	Possible clues	Diagnostic investigation
Rupture of the liver (p. 655)	Large infant, 36–72 hours after delivery. Shock	X-ray of abdomen upright. Aspiration of peritoneal cavity
Rupture of the spleen (p. 656)	Rhesus isoimmunization, shock.	As above
Rupture of umbilical vein (p. 652)	During exchange transfusion	As above
Adrenal haemorrhage (p. 455)	Lumbar mass or masses	IVP
Necrotizing enterocolitis (p. 380)	Usually pre-term; related to umbilical vessel catheterization. Distension; blood in the stool. Usually 4th–7th day of life	X-ray of abdomen upright and supine
Gastric perforation	Sudden collapse and distension. Usually 1st–5th day of life	X-ray of abdomen upright shows free air outlining the falciform ligament

TABLE 73.I (*continued*)

Abdominal conditions	Possible clues	Diagnostic investigation
Acute intestinal bleeding (p. 399)	4th–7th day. Shock	Blood in stool or on rectal examination
Intrathoracic conditions		
Tension pneumothorax (p. 271)	Meconium aspiration, Respiratory Distress Syndrome. Hypoplastic lung. IPPV	Needle in the chest, x-ray of chest
Pneumomediastinum Pneumopericardium	Usually complicating pneumothorax	X-ray of chest
Oesophageal perforation	Pre-term infants; spontaneous or related to tube feed	X-ray of chest may show pneumothorax or displaced tube
Massive pulmonary haemorrhage (p. 272)	Usually pre-term infants. Dyspnoea, frothy blood in the mouth	X-ray of chest
Acute pneumonia (p. 276)	Numerous; especially sudden deterioration on IPPV	X-ray of chest
Cardiovascular conditions		
Arrhythmia (p. 682)	Exchange transfusion	ECG
Air-embolus (p. 682)	Exchange transfusion	None
Paroxysmal tachycardia (p. 291)	Tachycardia	ECG
Cardiac failure	Tachycardia, murmur, cyanosis	X-ray of chest. ECG
Neurological conditions		
Intraventricular haemorrhage (p. 655)	Respiratory distress syndrome	Lumbar puncture: sudden fall in Hb level or PCV
Biochemical conditions		
Hypoglycaemia (p. 445)	Infant of diabetic mother. Small-for-date infants. Pale, unconscious with or without fits	Dextrostix

CHAPTER 74

Acute Infections

J. A. Black

The fetus may become infected during pregnancy and occasionally during labour, while the infant may become infected during delivery, or postnatally. Only infections requiring urgent attention are considered here.

Infections during pregnancy (transplacental infections)

These are all intrauterine infections which are secondary to a maternal infection involving the placenta.

RECOGNITION AND DIFFERENTIAL DIAGNOSIS
(a) Infants with CMV disease, rubella, syphilis, toxoplasmosis and trypanosomiasis may have a similar appearance at delivery, and may be mistaken for infants with severe Rhesus isoimmunization (*See* Table 74.II).
(b) Trypanosomiasis (Chagas' disease) is an important intrauterine infection in South America. Affected infants are pre-term or small-for-dates. Jaundice if present is usually due to unconjugated bilirubin. Tremors and convulsions indicate a meningoencephalitis (Bittencourt, 1976).
(c) Diagnostic tests: the level of IgM in the infant is usually raised but is non-specific. Estimation of specific IgM may however be diagnostic.
 (i) CMV infections: fresh urine should be examined, and urine and throat swabs cultured. Specific IgM is present.
 (ii) Malaria: the parasite can be identified in blood films from mother and infant. Specific IgM is present.
 (iii) Rubella: urine and throat swabs can be cultured. Specific IgM is present but in a few cases is normal or very low.

TABLE 74.I
Infections during pregnancy *

Disease or organism	Maternal infection obvious clinically	Clinical findings in the newborn
Viral infections		
Cytomegalovirus (CMV)	No	*See* Table 74.II
Herpesvirus hominis (HVH)	Primary lesion which is easily missed	Transplacental infection is rare
Rubella	Easily missed, especially in dark-skinned people	*See* Table 74.II
Bacterial infections		
Listeria	No	Transplacental infection probably rare: *see* page 631 for clinical findings
Tuberculosis	Usually obvious, either clinically or radiologically	Hepatosplenomegaly with or without miliary spread
Other organisms		
Malaria (usually MT falciparum)	Usually, but is easily missed. Mainly in non-immune mothers	Anaemia, high fever, hepatosplenomegaly
Syphilis	Not obvious: maternal infection may be acquired *after* routine WR in early pregnancy	*See* Table 74.II
Toxoplasmosis	Not obvious: occasionally an illness like infectious mononucleosis	*See* Table 74.II
Trypanosomiasis† (South American type Chagas' disease)	Not always	*See* Table 74.II

* For a more complete list of infections acquired transplacentally *see* Davies (1972).
† For further information *see* page 628.

Metaphyseal lesions may be found on x-ray of the long bones.

(iv) Syphilis: scrapings from the placenta and skin lesions should be examined under dark-ground illumination. Specific IgM is present. WR in the infant is unreliable. Periostitis may be seen on x-ray of long bones.

(v) Toxoplasmosis: the parasite may be identified in the CSF using special methods. Serial serological testing may be necessary, but specific IgM is present.

(vi) Trypanosomiasis: the parasite may be identified in a blood film or thick drop preparation. Specific IgM is present. Other special tests are also available (Bittencourt, 1976).

TABLE 74.II
Differential diagnosis of infants with anaemia, jaundice and hepatosplenomegaly

Disease	Anaemia	Jaundice	Hepatosplenomegaly	Skin lesions	Other features
Rhesus isoimmunization	++	++ within 1–4 hours of delivery	++	Skin haemorrhages, nodular lesions, petechiae	Coombs' test +
CMV	+	Sometimes	++	Purpura, petechiae	Microcephaly, retinitis, cerebral calcification
Rubella	±	Sometimes	+	Purpura, nodules, petechiae	Cardiac lesions, cataract, glaucoma
Syphilis	+	Rare	+	Mucocutaneous lesions, vesicles	Periostitis, lymphadenopathy
Toxoplasmosis	+	Sometimes	++	Purpura, petechiae	Hydrocephalus, retinitis, cerebral calcification
Trypanosomiasis (*see* (b) p. 624)	+	+	++	Petechiae, necrotic or haemorrhagic skin lesions	

(vii) Tuberculosis: immediate identification of the bacilli from
the infant is rarely possible but a positive sputum from the
mother is diagnostic in the presence of a pulmonary lesion. The infant may have miliary tuberculosis on chest x-
ray, or meningitis (p. 356).

MANAGEMENT
See Tables 74.IV, 74.V for dosage

(*a*) *Anaemia and jaundice*

Transfusion with packed cells may be required if the Hb is < 10 g% and
an exchange transfusion if there is a rising unconjugated bilirubin level,
using the standard criteria (p. 677). Since the unconjugated bilirubin
may also be raised, both fractions should be estimated.

(*b*) *Thrombocytopenia and DIC*

Thrombocytopenia may occur alone and may require treatment with
platelet transfusions. If there is evidence of DIC, this should also be
treated (p. 482), but prompt and effective treatment of the underlying
infection will correct the DIC if it has not progressed too far.

(*c*) *Infectivity*

(i) Infants with rubella are highly infective but the risk is only to
pregnant staff.
(ii) Infants with syphilis should be isolated and those handling the
infant should wear gloves.

(*d*) *Specific treatment*

(*See* Table 74.V for dosage)
(i) CMV: Davies *et al* (1972a) have suggested idoxuridine by continuous IV drip for 5 days; cytosine or adenine arabinoside
should also be considered but the efficacy of either drug is uncertain. (*See* Appendix 9 Table A9.VI for methods of
administration.)
(ii) Malaria: chloroquine base should be given i.m. for 5 days (Davies *et al.*, 1972b). (*See also* Appendix 9 Table A9.VI for methods
of administration.)
(iii) Rubella: there is at present no effective antiviral treatment.
(iv) Syphilis: 150 000 units of procaine penicillin can be given in a
single injection daily for 15 days, or divided into 3 doses of
50 000 units of benzylpenicillin.
(v) Toxoplasmosis: a combination of sulphadiazine and pyrimeth-
amine should be used.

(vi) Trypanosomiasis: Alvarez and Cob Sosa (1976) suggest treatment with nifurtimox (Lampit, Bayer) orally in a dose of 15 mg per kg per day for 3 months, and metronidazole 20 mg per kg per day orally for one month, but the best combination of drugs and effectiveness in the neonatal period is uncertain. (Bittencourt, 1976). *See also* Appendix 9 Table A9.V.

(vii) Tuberculosis: isoniazid should be used; resistant organisms should be treated with streptomycin.

Infection acquired during labour

Two routes are possible:

(a) Transplacental infection during a maternal bacteraemia or septicaemia, e.g. during an untreated attack of pyelonephritis. The infecting organism is a Gram-negative bacillus, commonly *E. coli* or *Proteus*.

(b) An ascending infection after rupture of the membranes: the risk is greatly increased when the membranes have been ruptured for longer than 48 hours. However the possibility of infection of the amniotic fluid should be considered earlier if the mother becomes febrile.

RECOGNITION

(a) Transplacental infection

The fetus may develop a septicaemia with or without meningitis. Cultures should be taken from the mother's blood and urine, and from the blood, CSF and urine of the infant.

(b) Ascending infection

This type of infection is commonly due to Gram-negative bacilli from the mother's intestinal tract, but may also be due to Listeria. Group B haemolytic streptococci (p. 635) and possibly Herpesvirus hominis (HVH) from a lesion of the maternal genitalia (p. 630). An intrapartum pneumonia with or without a septicaemia is likely with infection with Gram-negative bacilli, and a pneumonia or septicaemia with Group B streptococci. In HVH infection the clinical picture is the same as that acquired during delivery itself (p. 630).

If an infection is suspected, the amniotic fluid should be cultured, also the blood, CSF, urine and gastric aspirate of the infant. Other less acute infections acquired by the ascending route are described by Davies (1972).

MANAGEMENT
Since it is often (unless organisms can be seen on a Gram film of the
CSF) impossible to know the type of organism until it has been
cultured, initial treatment should be with i.m. benzylpenicillin and
gentamicin, with the addition of IT gentamicin if meningitis is present.

Infections acquired during delivery

Not all such infections cause an acute illness, but the following require
special attention.

Gonococcal conjunctivitis (ophthalmia) (Fong, 1978)

RECOGNITION
This condition should be suspected in any severe purulent conjunctivitis, unilateral or bilateral, developing within the first week (usually 2 to
5 days) after delivery.

Immediately the diagnosis is suspected a Gram film of the pus should
be examined for Gram negative diplococci, and the pus should be
cultured in appropriate media. *This examination is an emergency and
the swab should be taken to the laboratory by a doctor personally, to
ensure immediate examination. On no account should swabs or other
specimens from suspected gonococcal infections be allowed to take the
more leisurely routine route to the laboratory.*

MANAGEMENT
   (a) Treatment with benzylpenicillin 200 000 units should be given
       4-hourly i.m. and continued until there is no further purulent
       discharge and the swelling has subsided. Local irrigation with
       penicillin drops (20 000 units per ml) should also be started,
       given at $\frac{1}{2}$-hourly intervals for the first 12 hours, *but it is unsafe to
       rely on this route alone since the swelling may make separation of
       the lids extremely difficult.* All cases should be seen by an
       Ophthalmologist as soon as possible and the local Venereologist
       should be asked about the possibility of a penicillin-resistant
       strain.
   (b) If there is no clinical improvement within 24 to 48 hours the
       possibility of a penicillin-resistant organism should be consid-
       ered; by this time laboratory confirmation of the sensitivity
       pattern may also be available. Alternative antibiotics at present
       available are: kanamycin i.m. or erythromycin stearate suspen-
       sion (100 mg per 5 ml) in a dose of 50 mg orally 6-hourly for 4
       days and 1 per cent chlortetracycline ointment applied locally
       every 2 hours for the first 24 hours and 6-hourly for 3 to 5 days;

spectinomycin (Trobicin *Upjohn*) requires further evaluation before it can be recommended for parenteral use in the newborn.

(c) The mother should be investigated for gonococcal infection and blood should be taken from the mother and infant for a WR.

Chlamydial conjunctivitis (Fong, 1978)

This infection (previously known as inclusion body conjunctivitis), which is becoming increasingly common, is acquired in the same way as is the gonococcal infection, and may cause conjunctival scarring if inadequately treated.

RECOGNITION

The conjunctivitis usually develops between 5 and 10 days after birth and is less severe than the gonococcal infection. Smears should be made from the pus and stained with Giemsa. Special cell culture media are required for chlamydia which can be identified by staining the cultured cells with Giemsa or by direct immunofluorescent techniques.

MANAGEMENT

1 per cent chlortetracycline ophthalmic ointment should be applied 4 times daily for 2 weeks and a suspension of erythromycin stearate should be given orally in a dose of 20 mg 4 times daily, also for 2 weeks.

Herpesvirus hominis (HVH) infection

This is a potentially fatal condition which can be acquired from maternal genital herpes (Type 2 virus). If the condition is recognized in the mother before delivery the infant should be delivered by caesarian section to avoid infection by contact.

RECOGNITION

(a) The disseminated form develops about one week after delivery with a generalized illness with irritability and fits. Respiratory distress, jaundice, petechiae, skin haemorrhages or a vesicular rash may be present. Sudden shock is a rare presentation. In infants with CNS involvement the CSF shows a moderate increase in cells (up to 200 per mm^3) and a disproportionately high protein content of 5 to 10 g per litre (500–1000 mg%).

(b) In less severe cases the infection may be limited to a vesicular eruption in clusters.

(c) Direct identification of the virus may be possible by immuno-fluorescent methods, and it can be easily cultured.

MANAGEMENT

(a) Treatment is as for CMV infection with idoxuridine or cytosine or adenine arabinoside but the results in infants with CNS involvement have been very poor. The reduction of cerebral oedema by dexamethasone (p. 324) is the most urgent consideration.

(b) The possibility of infection of staff or other infants via the staff should be considered, but the risk does not appear to be great.

Listeria infection

RECOGNITION

There is good evidence that this infection may be acquired transplacentally, by the ascending route, or more commonly during delivery.

(a) Transplacental: the infant becomes hypothermic and lethargic; in some cases there is hepatosplenomegaly and, in a few cases, small reddish or grey papules on the trunk. X-ray of the chest may show patchy areas of infiltration.

(b) In infections by the ascending route or acquired during delivery the infant develops a septicaemic illness at the age of one week. Tachypnoea is sometimes present without radiological changes in the lung fields. Meningitis is common.

MANAGEMENT

See under Listeria meningitis, page 353.

Pneumonia

Inhalation of infected material from the mother's genital tract may cause pneumonia; this is more likely to occur in hypoxic infants which have gasped before delivery of the head.

RECOGNITION AND MANAGEMENT

See page 277

Exposure of the infant to the infective mother

Though the infective mother poses the greatest difficulties, a similar risk is present when an infant has been exposed to any infective individual. The commoner situations are considered in Table 74.III.

TABLE 74.III
Management of the infective mother

Disease or organism	Management
Viruses	
Herpesvirus hominis (genital lesion)	Deliver by caesarian section (p. 630); if delivered vaginally give γ-globulin
Poliomyelitis	γ-globulin
Varicella	Immune Zoster globulin (p. 475)
Variola	Specific immunoglobulin (p. 580)
Bacteria	
Diphtheria	γ-globulin and benzylpenicillin i.m. for 5 days
Enteropathogenic *E. coli*	Oral gentamicin or colistin for 5 days as a prophylactic
Meningococcal infections	Benzylpenicillin i.m. for 5 days
Pertussis	Ampicillin, amoxycillin or erythromycin orally for 5 days
Salmonella (typhoid, paratyphoid)	Amoxycillin orally, 5 days
Salmonella (typhimurium and related species)	As above
Shigella species	Ampicillin or amoxycillin orally, 5 days
Tuberculosis	BCG
Other organisms	
Amoebiasis (Axton, 1972)	Observe closely; treat only if symptoms develop (p. 571)
Hookworm (Hollander *et al.*, 1973) *See* Table A9.VII for dosage	As above (p. 640)

In all cases the infant should be separated from the mother (or other infective individual) until she is non-infective.

Acute postnatal infections

The possibility of septicaemia should always be considered in investigating and treating acute illnesses in the newborn. A septicaemia may arise in three possible ways.

(a) As an acute initial illness without localized disease.

(b) As a septicaemic illness complicated by a coexisting infection elsewhere, e.g. meningitis, pyelonephritis or osteitis.

(c) As a septicaemia which follows a primary localized infection, or a gastrointestinal infection with shigella or salmonella organisms.

Acute septicaemic illnesses

Since localizing symptoms or signs are uncommon in the newborn, particularly in the pre-term infant, the early symptoms are usually non-specific.

RECOGNITION

Symptoms which require immediate investigation are:
 (a) A sudden change in behaviour or appearance, such as pallor, grey colour, decreased activity, reluctance to feed. These are more likely to be noticed by the mother or nurse.
 (b) A rise or fall in temperature.
 (c) Apnoeic attacks, tachypnoea, dyspnoea or cyanosis.
 (d) Abdominal distension.
 (e) Sudden jaundice with or without hepatosplenomegaly.
 (f) Sudden diarrhoea or vomiting.
 (g) Sudden shock.
 (h) Bleeding, or oozing from the puncture sites (possibility of DIC).

It should be remembered however that similar symptoms, including jaundice (e.g. in galactosaemia and fructose intolerance) may also be due to various inborn errors of metabolism, which are considered on pages 697–705.

INVESTIGATION: THE INFECTION SCREEN

A standard plan of investigation should be used in all cases ('infection screen') and should be completed even after one of the investigations is found to be abnormal.
 (a) Blood culture: blood should not be taken from umbilical catheters because of the likelihood of contamination.
 (b) Lumbar puncture (*see also* page 726): if the CSF shows clear evidence of meningitis a Gram film indicating the type of organism can be used as a guide to the initial choice of antibiotics. Even in the absence of a raised cell count, a Gram film should still be examined and the fluid should be sent for culture.
 (c) Urine: specimens obtained from collecting bags are often contaminated by faecal or skin organisms, and by vaginal cells in female infants. Two or three specimens may have to be cultured before a definite answer can be obtained. In acutely ill infants the fresh urine should be examined under the microscope; the presence of >10 cells per high power field (uncentrifuged specimen) is suggestive of an infection, and this is more probable if numerous organisms are seen. If a specimen is required urgently, before starting antibiotics, a suprapubic bladder puncture should be done (p. 724). A count of $>10^5$ organisms (the same organism) per ml on culture indicates an infection.
 (d) Chest x-ray: this should always be included in the 'infection screen'.
 (e) Swabs from various sites (nose, umbilicus, rectum, minor skin lesions) are helpful in indicating the organisms which have colonized the infant and may have also caused an actual infec-

tion. A rectal swab (or preferably stool culture) may indicate a gastrointestinal infection with a septicaemia (salmonella) and is sometimes positive in systemic infections with Listeria or Group B haemolytic streptococci.

MANAGEMENT OF INFECTIONS IN GENERAL

(a) Shock: this may occur in any septicaemic illness and is most likely in infections due to Gram-negative bacilli but may also occur in Group B streptococcal infections.

Moderate degrees of shock may respond to IV fluids (initially 0.9 per cent NaCl in 5 per cent glucose) but severe shock should be treated with IV plasma* (20 ml per kg) and hydrocortisone (50 to 100 mg IV initially, repeated at 3- to 6-hourly intervals); *see also* pages 107–109.

(b) Thrombocytopenia and/or evidence of DIC require specific investigation and treatment (p. 482); in early DIC the most effective treatment is control of the infection.

(c) Antibiotics

(i) The initial choice of antibiotics must be made without knowing the bacterial sensitivities and in many cases without any indication of the type of organism. A combination of two antibiotics is therefore required to cover the two main groups of pathogenic bacteria. With the antibiotics at present available, gentamicin should be used to cover the Gram-negative bacilli and benzylpenicillin for the Gram-positive cocci. If there is a possibility of infection with a penicillin-resistant staphylococcus, cloxacillin should be given *in addition* to benzylpenicillin. In meningitis, the initial choice of antibiotics should normally be chloramphenicol and gentamicin but the choice may be influenced by the identification of the type of organism on a Gram film of the CSF (*See* Chapter 36).

(ii) Second choice: this will be governed by the bacterial sensitivity.

Infections requiring special attention

Meningitis (p. 347).
Pneumonia (p. 276).
Skin infections (p. 489).

---

* Plasma-Protein Fraction is replacing pooled plasma.

Group B β-haemolytic streptococcal infections

This infection is usually acquired from a symptomless maternal colonization of the genital tract but may also spread within a hospital or special care unit.

RECOGNITION
The infection may occur in various forms.
(a) An acute septicaemic illness developing within the first 12 to 24 hours but occasionally presenting at birth or shortly afterwards. Apart from signs of shock, respiratory distress with attacks of apnoea or cyanosis is common, and a chest x-ray may show an aspiration type of picture with patchy or streaky opacities; jaundice may also develop early. This condition may easily be mistaken for respiratory distress syndrome (IRDS) (p. 264).
(b) A late infection with meningitis with an onset at 1 to 12 weeks of age.
(c) Other less common manifestations of Group B streptococcal infections are, septic arthritis, osteitis, pneumonia with empyema, cellulitis, and ethmoiditis.
(d) Diagnosis is by culture of blood and CSF or pus from localized infection.

MANAGEMENT
(a) Shock, if present, should be treated with IV 0.9 per cent NaCl in 5 per cent glucose or if severe with plasma (p. 108). There is no indication that corticosteroids are useful in this form of septic shock.
(b) Antibiotic treatment with i.m. (or IV because of the large volume of injection) benzylpenicillin in high dosage (250 000 units per kg per 24 hours) for the newborn should be given for a week followed by the same dose orally for a further 2 weeks, but gentamicin i.m. should be used in addition for 5 to 7 days. Antibiotics should be given in all cases of apparent IRDS in which there is *any* possibility of Group B streptococcal infection.

Osteitis (osteomyelitis)

Osteitis in the newborn differs from osteitis in other age groups in four ways.
(a) Infection of the upper metaphysis of the humerus or femur may involve the shoulder and hip joints, respectively, causing a septic arthritis.
(b) More than one bone may be involved.

(c) Unusual sites may be infected (e.g. the maxilla or premaxilla).

(d) Numerous organisms may cause osteitis, the commonest being the staphylococcus; less commonly, osteitis may be due to Gram-negative bacilli, streptococci, pneumococci, gonococci and meningococci.

RECOGNITION

(a) The initial symptoms may be those of a septicaemia and evidence of bone involvement may only become apparent later. When osteitis is suspected a complete x-ray skeletal survey should be done.

(b) Localizing symptoms are those of swelling and loss of movement, or crying when the affected area is touched or moved.

(c) Infection of the shaft of the long bones is usually obvious because of the swelling, but infection of the upper end of the humerus or femur is less obvious since swelling occurs later. It should be remembered that infection of the femoral head or hip joint may be a complication of femoral-vein puncture.

(d) Confirmation of the diagnosis may be provided by aspiration and culture of pus from an obvious swelling, or from blood culture. Aspiration of the shoulder or hip joint should be done by an orthopaedic surgeon.

Osteitis at special sites

(a) Sites which are difficult to detect

(i) The vertebrae: osteitis of the vertebrae is particularly difficult to detect clinically. Infection of a cervical vertebra may cause torticollis in an infant, with or without a swelling due to the development of an abscess.

(ii) Sacrum or sacroiliac joint: infection may only become obvious at a very late stage unless it is included in a skeletal survey as part of a search for osteitis.

(b) Osteitis of the maxilla

This infection is rarely seen outside the neonatal period. It may present with swelling of the cheek, with periorbital oedema, proptosis, or chemosis of the conjunctiva. Pus may be discharged at the inner or outer canthus of the eye, the mid-point of the lower lid, the outer surface of the alveolar margin near the site of the first molar, through the hard palate, or through the nose on the affected side. The condition may be mistaken for orbital cellulitis. Radiography is rarely helpful, but culture of the blood or pus usually yields a growth of staphylococcus.

Early diagnosis and treatment will avoid damage to the first dentition and facial asymmetry.

(c) Osteitis of the premaxilla

This causes similar symptoms but the first sign is swelling of the upper alveolar margin near the midline. Infection is usually confined to the premaxilla but may spread to the maxillary sinus.

Investigation is as for maxillary osteitis.

MANAGEMENT

(a) In the absence of contrary evidence it should be assumed that the infection is a staphylococcal one. An orthopaedic surgeon should be asked to see infections involving the long bones or joints, and a dental surgeon to see infections of the maxilla and premaxilla.

(b) Antibiotics: treatment should be started with cloxacillin with gentamicin in addition if the organism is not known. There is no justification in using benzylpenicillin initially since the likelihood of a penicillinase producing staphylococcal infection is high. In staphylococcal infections which do not respond to cloxacillin, erythromycin, fusidic acid (Fucidin), lincomycin or clindamycin may have to be considered.

(c) Duration of treatment: antibiotic treatment should be continued for a minimum of 2 weeks after all signs of activity (return of WBC count and ESR to normal) have disappeared and in any case for not less than 4 weeks. There is no need to continue treatment until the x-ray appearance is normal.

Pyelonephritis

Acute pyelonephritis in the newborn may develop in two ways:

(a) As part of a septicaemic illness in which infection of the renal tissue occurs as part of the septicaemia. Subsequent investigation of the renal tract usually shows a normal result.

(b) As a primary infection in an abnormal tract, often with a *secondary* septicaemia. In either case jaundice may be the presenting feature.

RECOGNITION

Unless there is a palpable renal mass, hypertrophied and palpable bladder, or an obviously defective urinary stream, it is often impossible to distinguish clinically between (a) and (b) (above). The urine should be examined by microscopy and both blood and urine should be cultured. Since the infection is usually a generalized septicaemia a full 'infection screen', including lumbar puncture, should be done.

MANAGEMENT
    (a) When it has been established that the urine is infected the plasma urea and electrolytes should be estimated. Even with a normal renal tract the plasma-urea level is usually slightly raised during the acute phase of the illness. An initially high plasma urea (>16 mmol per litre, 100 mg%) which remains high after adequate treatment suggests an abnormal tract.
    (b) Antibiotics: gentamicin (reduced dose with a raised blood urea (p. 806)) and benzylpenicillin should be used in the treatment of an initial septicaemic illness without meningitis, and ampicillin should be used in an infection confined to the renal tract. A course of treatment should be continued for 2 weeks.
    (c) All infants should have an IVP after recovery: a micturating cystogram may also be required.
    (d) Infants with an anatomical abnormality of the renal tract should be treated with a maintenance dose of an appropriate antibiotic while the possibility of surgical correction is being considered.

Acute gastrointestinal infections

These may be acquired at delivery (p. 632) or postnatally.

Acute infective gastroenteritis

This may be due to serologically distinguishable types of enteropathogenic *E. coli*, organisms of the shigella or salmonella group or a virus, and occasionally an intestinal staphylococcal infection.

RECOGNITION
The possibility of infective gastroenteritis should always be considered with the sudden onset of frequent loose stools with vomiting or refusal of feeds. Blood and mucus in the stool do not occur in viral gastroenteritis, are rare in *E. coli* infections, but are common in shigella infections and rather less common in salmonellosis. Other conditions which must also be considered are:
    (a) Severe underfeeding, causing vomiting, possibly due to air-swallowing, and *small* fluid olive-green stools. The hunger of the underfed infant is in marked contrast to the refusal to feed of the infant with gastroenteritis.
    (b) Profuse diarrhoea within a few hours of starting milk (human or

cow's) feeds may be due to congenital lactose intolerance; vomiting and abdominal distension or ileus may also occur.

(c) Blood and mucus in the stool may be due to necrotizing entero-colitis (p. 380), or to an intussusception, which is rare in the newborn.

(d) Diarrhoea with abdominal distension, usually preceded by de-layed passage of meconium may be due to Hirschsprung's disease.

(e) Acute adrenal failure due to congenital adrenal hypoplasia or hyperplasia may cause vomiting with loose watery stools (p. 454).

(f) Some drugs when given orally cause loose or frequent stools: penicillin, ampicillin, ferrous sulphate, calcium gluconate.

(g) Incarceration of an inguinal hernia, with vomiting, crying and an occasional watery stool may easily be mistaken for gastroenteri-tis if the infant is not properly examined; incarceration is particularly common in pre-term infants.

(h) A septicaemic illness may present with abdominal distension and diarrhoea.

MANAGEMENT

(a) At the first suspicion of gastroenteritis the infant should be isolated (*see below*) and a stool or rectal swab should be sent for culture. If there is a raised temperature, sudden hypothermia, or blood and mucus in the stool a blood culture should also be done.

(b) IV fluids should be given, if there is moderate to severe dehydra-tion with a loss of 10 per cent or more of body weight (*see* page 96 for signs of dehydration), if there is persistent vomiting or refusal of clear fluids, and in all pre-term infants or any infant already ill from another condition.

(c) Oral replacement of fluids can be attempted (p. 401) in term infants who show mild dehydration (5 per cent loss of body weight or less) and who are able to retain oral feeds by bottle, teaspoon or nasogastric tube, and in whom the diarrhoea is not profuse.

(d) Choice of oral fluids: in early cases such as are usually encoun-tered in the newborn one of the standard oral glucose-electrolyte solutions can be used (p. 764); alternatively 0.45 per cent NaCl (sodium 77 mmol per litre) in 2.5 per cent glucose or Darrow's solution diluted with an equal volume of 5 per cent glucose (composition in mmol per litre: sodium 61, potassium 18, chloride 51, bicarbonate as lactate, 25 mmol, and glucose 2.5 per cent) can be used.

(e) *Antibiotics:*

(i) In (presumed) viral gastroenteritis there is of course no indication for antibiotics, nor from the therapeutic point of view is there any reason to give them in proved infections due to enteropathogenic *E. coli.* There is little evidence that the infectivity or duration of carriage of specific *E. coli* organisms is reduced by giving oral antibiotics but this may be indicated to prevent further infection in an SCBU or to reduce the number of infective infants if the spread of infection appears to have got out of control. In an exceptionally severe outbreak of *E. coli 0114*, infants given gentamicin or colistin orally had a slightly reduced mortality compared with those who did not receive this treatment, but the results were inconclusive (Jacobs *et al.*, 1970). It is possible that oral antibiotics reduced the amount of bacterial toxin which was the probable cause of hepatic damage in this *0114* outbreak. Neomycin and streptomycin should not be used orally because of the risk of inducing lactose intolerance. Other drugs traditionally used for diarrhoea should not be used as they are ineffective or dangerous (p. 401).

(ii) In salmonella or shigella infections antibiotics should however be given because of the frequency of septicaemia in the newborn. In salmonella infections amoxycillin is the most effective antibiotic if oral treatment is possible; otherwise ampicillin should be used i.m. or IV; for shigellosis ampicillin parenterally or amoxycillin should be given (*see also* page 406).

Less common intestinal infections

Amoebiasis

RECOGNITION

This possibility should be considered in areas where amoebiasis is endemic, and particularly if the mother is known to be infective, though most infections are probably from asymptomatic carriers. The youngest recorded case developed symptoms at the age of two weeks (Axton, 1972).
Diagnosis and treatment are the same as in the older child (p. 569).

Hookworm infection

RECOGNITION
Massive intestinal haemorrhage due to the American hookworm (*Neca-*

tor americanus) has been described in an infant of $4\frac{1}{2}$ weeks (Hollander, Tabingo and Stankewick, 1973). Similar symptoms could also presumably occur with the ankylostoma duodenale.

MANAGEMENT

    (a) Transfusion may be required.

    (b) Tetrachlorethylene is widely used in a dose of 0.1 ml per kg, repeated after 2 weeks if the stools are still positive (Jung and Jelliffe, 1972), but may be less effective in infancy than bephenium (Alcopar, *Wellcome*) in a dose of 2.5 g by gastric tube daily for 3 days (Hollander, Tabingo and Stankewick, 1973).

Administrative aspects of infective gastroenteritis in a maternity unit

(a) Single cases

    (i) An infant developing sudden diarrhoea with or without vomiting should be regarded as infective and transferred to an isolation cubicle in the Special Care Baby Unit while non-infective conditions are being excluded (p. 638). Once this has been done the infant should be transferred to the isolation ward of the nearest paediatric unit. Only very small or ill infants whose survival depends upon intensive care in a SCBU should be retained and barrier-nursed.

    (ii) To identify the source of the infection, rectal swabs or stools should be cultured from all those in contact with the infant during the previous 10 days: this includes the mother, medical and nursing staff, and other infants. All infants, with or without symptoms, with a positive culture, should be isolated as in (i) above. All staff with a positive culture should be put off duty until they have produced three consecutive negative cultures. An infective mother should be isolated and sent home as quickly as possible.

    (iii) To discover whether the infected infant has transmitted the infection to other infants daily specimens should be sent from contacts for 10 days after the last contact. Symptomless infants who are ready to go home should be accompanied by a letter to the family doctor asking that the infant should be observed carefully for the next 10 days.

    (iv) In presumed viral infections a period of 10 days without symptoms in a contact should be regarded as evidence of non-infectivity, though it should be realized that an infant can acquire a pathogenic organism and remain asymptomatic.

(*b*) *More than one case occurring simultaneously*

This is likely to be due to infected feeds originating from a common source or to the spread of infection from an undetected case. In these circumstances closure of the hospital to further admission is essential until the source of the infection has been discovered and all infective patients have been discharged and infective staff are clear of infection.

Antibiotics policy in the newborn

(a) Local applications should not contain any antibiotic which could be used for a systemic infection, because of the risk of inducing resistant organisms.

(b) Certain antibiotics are *contra-indicated* in the newborn unless there are very specific indications. These are: bacitracin, cotrimoxazole (Septrin, Bactrim) neomycin, novobiocin, polymyxin, tetracyclines, tobramycin; sulphonamides in the presence of jaundice. Chloramphenicol should normally be used only for the treatment of meningitis due to Gram-negative bacilli. Tobramycin may be useful in infections, particularly with *Pseudomonas aeruginosa* which is resistant to gentamicin but there is no intrathecal preparation of tobramycin, and little is known about its ototoxic effects.

(c) In all special care units a continuous record should be kept of all organisms isolated (and their sensitivities) from routine nose, umbilical and rectal swabs, and from minor septic lesions of the skin. This gives an up-to-date picture of the pattern of bacterial infections in the unit and their sensitivities. A high incidence of resident penicillin-resistant staphylococci will indicate the use of cloxacillin instead of benzylpenicillin.

(d) More than one aminoglycoside antibiotic should not be used together; the commonly available aminoglycosides are streptomycin, neomycin, gentamicin, kanamycin, tobramycin: colistin is a polymyxin, not an aminoglycoside.

Antimicrobial drug dosage

(a) Antibiotics.
The dosage should be related both to the age and weight of the infant. Davies (1975) gives the usually accepted dosage (Table 74.IV).

(b) The dosage of the less commonly used antimicrobial drugs are as given in Table 74.V.

TABLE 74.IV

Neonatal dosage of intramuscular antibacterial drugs†. (After Davies (1975). Reproduced by kind permission)

Drug	Single intramuscular dose	Frequency of dose for all antibiotics given i.m.
Ampicillin	50 mg/kg	*For term infants*
Benzylpenicillin	25 000 units/kg (15 mg/kg)	(>37 weeks gestation)
Carbenicillin	100 mg/kg	Give every 12 hours if in the
Chloramphenicol	12.5 mg/kg (the maximum daily dose should not exceed 25 mg/kg for the first week of life in term babies and the first 4 weeks in pre-term infants)	first 48 hours of life, 8-hourly between 3 days and 2 weeks, and 6-hourly if over 2 weeks unless otherwise indicated *For pre-term infants*
Gentamicin	2.5 mg/kg*	(<37 weeks gestation)
Kanamycin	7.5 mg/kg**	Give every 12 hours if the first week of life, 8-hourly if between
Methicillin (or Cloxacillin)	50 mg/kg	1 and 4 weeks and 6-hourly if over 4 weeks unless otherwise indicated.

* Need not be given more often than 8-hourly.
** Need not be given more often than 12-hourly.
† For intrathecal dosage see page 351. For other antibiotics *see* Appendix 9.

TABLE 74.V

Neonatal dosage and route of some antimicrobial drugs*. (After Davies (1975). Reproduced by kind permission)

Infection	Drug	Dose and route
Candidiasis (disseminated)	Amphotericin B	0.25–0.5 mg/kg/day IV; 0.05 mg in 2 ml distilled water intrathecally if indicated
	Flucytosine	100–150 mg/kg/day orally, 6-hourly
Herpesvirus hominis (HVH)	Idoxuridine	50–100 mg/kg/day IV, total dosage not exceeding 300–400 mg/kg
Malaria	Chloroquine	10 mg/day i.m. as chloroquine base (Nivaquine) injection
Toxoplasmosis	Sulphadiazine	150 mg/kg/day orally, 6-hourly
	Pyrimethamine	1.0 mg/kg/day, orally, 12-hourly
	Spiramycin	50 mg/kg/day orally, 6-hourly
Trichomonas vaginalis	Metronidazole	50 mg/kg/day orally, 8-hourly
Tuberculosis	Isoniazid	10–20 mg/kg/day orally, 6-hourly

* *See* Appendix 9 for methods of administration and available preparation.

References

Alvarez, R. and Cob Sosa, C. (1976). Enfermedades parasitarias. In *Conceptos Clinicos de Infectiologia* 3rd edn., p. 454. Ed. E. Calderón Jaimes and M. Salas Alvarado. Mexico: Publishers Mendez Cervantes

Axton, J. H. M. (1972). Amoebic proctocolitis and liver abscess in a neonate. *S. Afr. Med. J.* **46**, 258

Bittencourt, A. L. (1976). Congenital Chagas' disease. *Am. J. Dis. Child.* **130**, 97

Davies, P. A. (1972). Infection in embryo, fetus and newborn. *Br. J. Hosp. Med.* **8**, 13

Davies, P. A. (1975). Antimicrobial therapy in the neonatal period. *Br. J. Hosp. Med.* **14**, 517

Davies, P. A., Robinson, R. J., Scopes, J. W., Tizard, J. P. M. and Wigglesworth, J. S. (1972). Medical care of newborn babies. (a) 172; (b) 171. London: Heinemann

Fong, R. (1978). The modern management of ophthalmia neonatorum. *J. Maternal Child Care* **3**, 62

Hollander, M., Tabingo, R. and Stankewick, W. R. (1923). Successful treatment of massive intestinal haemorrhage due to hookworm infection in a neonate. *J. Pediat.* **82**, 332

Jacobs, S. I., Holzel, A., Wolman, B., Keen, J. H., Miller, V., Taylor, J. and Gross, R. J. (1970). Outbreak of infantile gastroenteritis caused by *Escherichia coli 0114*. *Archs Dis. Childh.* **45**, 656

Jung, R. C. and Jelliffe, D. B. (1972). Intestinal helminths. In *Diseases of Children in the Subtropics and Tropics*. 2nd edn., p. 459. Ed. D. B. Jelliffe. London: Edward Arnold

CHAPTER 75

Cyanosis in the Newborn

(*See* Chapter 26 for cyanotic spells or attacks)

J. A. Black

RECOGNITION

Persistent cyanosis in the newborn requires urgent investigation.

Peripheral cyanosis

(a) Traumatic cyanosis is usually seen in the face and head, due to the cord around the neck or delay in delivery of the shoulders, and occasionally in a limb which has prolapsed during delivery. No treatment is required apart from reassurance to the mother.
(b) Peripheral cyanosis in a vigorous infant with warm extremities is of no consequence and usually disappears after 2 to 3 days. It may also occur transiently due to the moderate chilling which occurs after delivery.
(c) Peripheral cyanosis may also occur in shock from any cause (p. 91) or in hypothermia (p. 694).

Central cyanosis

Central cyanosis may be due to a variety of causes of which cardiac and respiratory abnormalities are the commonest. In the absence of demonstrable cardiac (p. 289) or respiratory distress (p. 264), the following causes should be considered:

(a) Severe metabolic acidosis (p. 123).
(b) Severe hypoglycaemia (p. 446).
(c) Intracranial haemorrhage (p. 655).
(d) Congenital or acquired methaemoglobinaemia in which the blood has a chocolate-brown colour and fails to turn red when exposed to air (oxygen) by placing a drop on a piece of filter paper: final confirmation is of course obtained by spectroscopy.

MANAGEMENT OF CYANOSIS

The management of the commoner causes of cyanosis is considered under the various causes. Methaemoglobinaemia can be abolished (temporarily in the congenital forms) by the IV injection of 1 per cent (10 mg per 1 ml) methylene blue in a dose of 1 to 2 mg per kg. Ascorbic acid 100 mg 3 to 4 times daily can be given orally; it acts more slowly, but can be used as maintenance treatment.

CHAPTER 76

Stridor in the Newborn

J. A. Black

RECOGNITION

The noise made by an infant with stridor may be loud and rasping or it may be a loud wheeze or a soft purr like a vibration. In making a preliminary assessment it is necessary to determine: (a) the probable site of obstruction; (b) the severity.

(a) The site

(i) Inspiratory stridor alone is invariably due to an obstruction in or near the larynx.

(ii) A hoarse or absent cry indicates involvement of the vocal cords. An exception is severe subglottic stenosis in which the expiratory flow is insufficient to produce a cry.

(iii) Inspiratory and expiratory ('to-and-fro') stridor indicates tracheal obstruction.

(iv) Stridor which varies with position, particularly if reduced or absent in the prone position, indicates either an 'infantile' larynx (as in congenital laryngeal stridor) or obstruction due to the tongue falling back, in the supine position or upper respiratory infection.

(v) Stridor accompanied by extension of the head may be due to a goitre, tracheal compression by a vascular ring, or (rarely) injury to the larynx in the course of a face delivery: the extension of the head after face delivery is merely a persistence of the intrauterine position.

(vi) Expiratory stridor alone is likely to be due to bronchial obstruction, as in lobar emphysema, or lung cyst, or mediastinal displacement.

(*b*) *Severity*
>   (i) Stridor which is intermittently present or is absent during quiet
>   breathing usually indicates a mild degree of obstruction.
>   (ii) Continued stridor with marked in-drawing and recession indi-
>   cates a moderate-to-severe obstruction.
> (iii) Stridor with cyanosis or pallor and restlessness requires immed-
>   iate relief.

MANAGEMENT OF SEVERE OBSTRUCTION WITH STRIDOR
Urgent direct laryngoscopy in the theatre by an experienced ENT
surgeon is necessary; facilities for intubation or tracheostomy must be
available.

(*a*) *Inspiratory stridor with normal cry*

This may be due to:
>   (i) 'Congenital laryngeal stridor', or the Pierre–Robin syndrome:
>   nursing in the prone position is usually all that is required (*see*
>   page 279).
>   (ii) Where change in posture makes no difference, the cause may be
>   a goitre (*see* page 460), subglottic stenosis or haemangioma.

(*b*) *Inspiratory stridor with weak, hoarse or absent cry*

This may be due to:
>   (i) Traumatic injury to the cords during resuscitation, or post-
>   intubation oedema.
>   (ii) Cyst, haemangioma of the cords, or laryngeal web.
> (iii) Unilateral or bilateral recurrent laryngeal palsy (rare).
>   (iv) Direct injury to the larynx at delivery (rare).

In (i), relief of the obstruction is usually unnecessary; a short course of
corticosteroids (*see* page 221) may reduce the oedema, or in some cases
re-intubation with a loosely fitting endotracheal tube may be necessary.

In (ii), tracheostomy is usually required, followed by appropriate
treatment of the obstruction at the time of tracheostomy or later.

In (iii), a bilateral cord paralysis may require tracheostomy, but a
unilateral paralysis seldom needs it.

(*c*) *Inspiratory and expiratory stridor*

This is rarely an emergency in the immediate neonatal period, though
obstruction may suddenly increase later, possibly due to oedema from
an upper respiratory infection. All cases should be thoroughly investigated *before* the obstruction becomes severe.

(*d*) *Expiratory stridor*

Chest x-ray may indicate the probable cause of the bronchial obstruction; bronchoscopy may be required. For management of lobar emphysema, or lung cyst *see* page 279.

CHAPTER 77

Nasal and Nasopharyngeal Obstruction in the Newborn

J. A. Black

Unilateral nasal or nasopharyngeal obstruction does not cause severe symptoms and may not be recognized until a mucopurulent nasal discharge develops on the affected side.

Bilateral nasal obstruction in the obligatory nose-breathing newborn causes severe symptoms which can be fatal if not recognized and treated.

RECOGNITION

   (i) Complete bilateral obstruction causes severe inspiratory indrawing and recession with cyanosis, but *without stridor*; the symptoms are instantly relieved when crying causes the infant to breathe through the mouth, or by the insertion of an oropharyngeal airway. The commonest cause is choanal atresia (*see* page 280).

   (ii) Incomplete or intermittent nasal obstruction, particularly if it varies with position, is likely to be due to a nasopharyngeal tumour or nasal encephalocele. If the obstruction is incomplete, inspiration is likely to be accompanied by a snoring or snorting noise. These tumours are often pedunculated and asymmetrically placed, so that obstruction is incomplete, or inconstant.

   (iii) Mild nasal obstruction developing after birth is usually due to an upper respiratory infection, to oedema and infection from an in-dwelling nasogastric tube or from the nasal catheters used in the treatment of respiratory distress syndrome.

MANAGEMENT

Bilateral choanal atresia is an emergency which requires experienced operative intervention. Fortunately temporary relief can be obtained by the insertion of an oropharyngeal airway; this may have to be fixed with adhesive tape to prevent rejection by the infant. Suspected tumours may require similar management and should be seen by or referred to a specialist as an emergency.

The obstruction due to nasopharyngitis can usually be relieved by giving vasoconstrictor drops; crusts should be softened by cotton wool soaked in warm, sterile normal saline.

If there is interference with feeding this may be improved by giving nasal drops (0.5 per cent ephedrine in 0.9 per cent NaCl, NOT oily drops) 10 minutes before each feed, but this treatment should not be continued for longer than 7 to 10 days.

CHAPTER 78

Acute Blood Loss at or after Delivery

J. A. Black

Acute blood loss in the newborn may occur during pregnancy, during labour, during delivery or after delivery. If blood loss has occurred before the infant was delivered, shock may be present at birth and this must be distinguished from hypoxia (asphyxia).

TABLE 78.I
Acute blood loss up to delivery

Time	Cause	Diagnostic investigation
During pregnancy	Fetomaternal bleed (acute)	Kleihauer on maternal blood
	Fetofetal bleed (acute) in twins	Hb on both twins: appearance of twins and placenta
	Injury at amniocentesis or intrauterine transfusion	Blood-stained amniotic fluid
	Fetal bleeding in placenta praevia or accidental haemorrhage	Clinical features
During labour or delivery	Injury to fetal vessels at caesarian section, rupture of fetal vessels in vasa praevia, velamentous insertions, accessory lobe of placenta	Examination of placenta and fetal vessels
	Puncture or tear by monitor electrode or fetal-blood sampling	Examination of the infant
During delivery	Rupture of umbilical vessels from: short or entangled cord, cord round the neck, or precipitate or unattended delivery	Appearance of cord
	Draining blood into placenta at caesarian section	

Acute blood loss up to delivery

RECOGNITION

Fetal tachycardia or bradycardia already recognized during labour may be attributed to hypoxia (fetal distress). However, *shock from haemorrhage does not usually cause apnoea* (Table 78.II). In shock from haemorrhage, attempts at conventional resuscitation are unlikely to produce any clinical improvement. The infant appears pale and hypotonic, with cool greyish-blue extremities, is unresponsive to stimuli and may be semiconscious, with rolling eyes. The cord is collapsed, with weak or absent pulsation. The brachial pulse is rapid and feeble or impalpable and the heart sounds are weak: the heart rate is rapid (>160) or slow (<60) in a preterminal (but recoverable) state. Respiration is shallow and irregular, or gasping. (*See* Table 78.II for differential diagnosis of pallor at delivery.)

TABLE 78.II
Pallor at delivery: differential diagnosis

	Severe hypoxia	*Acute blood loss*	*Severe chronic anaemia**
Fetal tachycardia	+	Depends on the cause	May occur
Apnoea	+	No	Only in hydrops
Pallor	+	+	+ +
Cyanosis	+ +	+ +	No
Cord	Collapsed	Collapsed	Distended
Cord pulsation	Feeble or absent	Feeble or absent	Normal
Heart rate	Slow	Rapid to slow	Rapid
Brachial pulse	Feeble or impalpable	Feeble or impalpable	Normal
Hypotonia	+ +	+	No
Abdomen	Normal	Normal	Distended
Skin haemorrhage	No	No	In severe Rhesus isoimmunization

* Severe Rhesus isoimmunization, or chronic fetomaternal or fetofetal bleeding

MANAGEMENT

Restoration of the plasma volume is the most urgent consideration, and should precede attempts to discover the cause of the blood loss. In nearly every case, when bleeding has occurred before or during delivery, the blood loss will have ceased as soon as the cord has been clamped. An Hb level estimated during early shock may give a misleadingly normal or near normal level; nevertheless blood should of course be taken from the infant for Hb (base-line) and grouping and from the mother for crossmatching.

(a) Extreme urgency, (i.e. the infant appears likely to die within the next few minutes). An IV drip should be set up immediately, using the umbilical vein and taking a blood sample at the same time.

  (i) Any of the immediately available IV fluids or plasma expanders* can be used provided that the fluid is NOT cold from refrigeration, since this may produce arrhythmias. The IV fluid should be given at a rate of 20 to 30 ml per kg *per hour* until emergency crossmatched blood becomes available; this should be possible within 20 to 30 minutes of its request; at the same time a formal crossmatching should be set up, taking between 1 and 2 hours.

  (ii) Blood when available should NOT be given cold (*see above*); a warming coil should be used, as for an exchange transfusion (p. 679). It should be assumed that an infant has lost 20 to 30 ml per kg of blood (i.e. about 25 to 30 per cent of its blood volume). Undertransfusion is a more likely error than overtransfusion. The newborn infant in any case is very tolerant of large additions to its blood volume (as in the placental transfusion in delayed clamping of the cord) but is intolerant of blood loss.

  Rate of transfusion:
  0 to 30 minutes: (electrolyte solution or plasma expander): 10 ml per kg.
  30 to 60 minutes: blood, 10 ml per kg.
  60 minutes onwards: blood, 10 to 20 ml per kg *per hour* until shock is relieved.

(b) In less urgent cases, all preparation should be made for transfusion through the umbilical vein, but the actual transfusion can be delayed until grouped and crossmatched blood is available. If the infant begins to deteriorate during this period, an IV drip should be started as in (a) above. The respiration rate and heart rate should be monitored continuously while waiting for the blood.

(c) If the infant appears shocked but the diagnosis of blood loss is uncertain it is safer to give blood empirically as in (a) or (b) according to the degree of urgency.

Acute blood loss after delivery

The commoner causes of acute postnatal bleeding are given in Table 78.III. The reabsorption of blood from an enclosed cavity or damaged tissues may contribute to the development of hyperbilirubinaemia, particularly in the pre-term infant.

*Including ORh negative blood.

TABLE 78.III
Acute blood loss after delivery: commoner causes

0–24 hours	24–36 hours	36–72 hours	2–7 days	At any time
Fetal scalp-sampling site	Rupture of liver	Adrenal haemorrhage	Haemorrhagic disease	Renal-vein thrombosis
Cord haemorrhage	Rupture of spleen (Rh cases only)	Intracranial haemorrhage	Intracranial haemorrhage in RDS	Bleeding into giant haemangioma with thrombo-cytopenia
Cephalhaematoma	Subaponeurotic haemorrhage	Bleeding into the mesentery of the intestine		
	Muscle and soft-tissue bleeding (breech)			
	Pulmonary haemorrhage			

RECOGNITION

(a) Intracranial haemorrhage

(i) Intraventricular haemorrhage: this occurs mainly in pre-term infants with respiratory distress syndrome and is indicated by fits, or apnoeic spells, with or without a bulging fontanelle. The CSF is heavily blood-stained. This type of bleed is frequently fatal.

(ii) Acute subdural haematoma (*see* page 610).

(iii) Subarachnoid haemorrhage: this occurs mainly in term infants or may accompany a bacterial meningitis (*see* page 348).

(b) Cephalhaematoma

Shock or anaemia requiring transfusion are rare and reabsorption of blood is so slow that it very rarely contributes to the development of hyperbilirubinaemia.

(c) Subaponeurotic haemorrhage

(*See* page 610).

(d) Massive pulmonary haemorrhage

(*See* page 272).

(e) Intraperitoneal haemorrhage

(i) Rupture of the liver: this occurs more commonly in large term infants after a latent period of 24 to 36 hours. A definite diagnosis is difficult to make but should be suspected in any infant developing sudden shock (symptoms as described on page

653); there may be slight abdominal distension and an erect x-ray of the abdomen may show a fluid level of blood in the pelvis, with the bowel above it. Confirmation of intraperitoneal bleeding is by aspiration of blood from the peritoneal cavity on the introduction of a wide-bore needle into the left flank.

(ii) Rupture of the spleen: this is only likely to occur in Rhesus isoimmunization. The symptoms and signs are the same as in rupture of the liver.

(f) Retroperitoneal haemorrhage

(i) Renal-vein thrombosis produces a massive accumulation of blood into one or both kidneys; there is a large mass in the flank, usually with obvious or microscopic haematuria. (*See* Table 78.IV for distinction from massive adrenal haemorrhage.)

(ii) Adrenal haemorrhage: the physical signs are similar to those of renal-vein thrombosis, but shock is severe if both adrenals are involved (*see* Table 78.IV and page 455).

TABLE 78.IV
Adrenal haemorrhage and renal-vein thrombosis: differential diagnosis

	Adrenal haemorrhage	*Renal-vein thrombosis*
Predisposing maternal conditions	Anticoagulant treatment except heparin. Drugs causing thrombocytopenia	None: maternal diabetes
Age of onset	36–72 hours	Any time in infancy
Septicaemia	Common	Rare
Shock	Usually	Sometimes
Anaemia	Always	Sometimes
Haematuria	None or a few RBCs	Usually obvious
Proteinuria	None or trace	Marked
IVP	Kidney on affected side displaced downwards, with flattening of the upper calyces	Affected kidney does not excrete

(g) Gastrointestinal haemorrhage

(i) For haematemesis and the effects of swallowed maternal blood *see* page 399.

(ii) Haemorrhagic disease: *see* pages 397 and 663.

(iii) Bleeding into the mesentery of the intestine produces a mobile mass in the abdomen. An x-ray may show the intestines to be displaced laterally.

(*h*) *Bleeding into a giant haemangioma*

(*See* page 496).

(*i*) *Soft-tissue haemorrhage in a breech delivery*

(*See* pages 607, 666).

MANAGEMENT
  (a) Investigation: if there is any possibility of DIC, coagulation disorder or thrombocytopenia, the appropriate investigations should be done (p. 482).
  (b) If an exploratory laparotomy (e.g. for a ruptured liver) is required, Vitamin K_1 (phytomenadione) should be given i.m. (or IV if a coagulation defect is present) in a dose of 1 to 2 mg.
  (c) Shock: the treatment is as described on page 654.

X

CHAPTER 79

Anaemia in the Newborn

J. A. Black

Acute anaemia is considered under Acute Blood Loss, page 652. Severe chronic anaemia in the newborn results from a continued blood loss or haemolysis. Either of these may occur before or after delivery but haemolysis may continue after delivery. A clinical picture similar to that of chronic anaemia is also produced by a number of intrauterine infections (p. 624).

At delivery

Continued blood loss

(*a*) *Fetomaternal haemorrhage*

The acute form may cause shock (p. 652); more commonly the bleeding occurs slowly or recurrently.

RECOGNITION
The infant is pale, with hepatosplenomegaly (occasionally hydropic) and closely resembles an infant with severe Rhesus isoimmunization, except that jaundice does not develop within 1 to 4 hours of delivery. The Hb level is usually at 7 to 10 g per 100 ml, with numerous nucleated cells in the blood film. Confirmation of the diagnosis is made by a Kleihauer test on the mother's blood.

(*b*) *Fetofetal ('twin-to-twin') haemorrhage*

This may also occur in an acute form (p. 652), but more commonly as a severe anaemia in one twin and plethora in the other.

RECOGNITION

The anaemic twin has the same appearance as in fetomaternal haemor-rhage; the plethoric twin has a reddish-blue appearance, often with cyanosed extremities. The difference between their Hb levels is at least 3 g per 100 ml, and often more.

Continued haemolysis

This is almost invariably due to Rhesus isoimmunization, but may be due to other blood group incompatibilities. ABO incompatibility very rarely causes anaemia during fetal life. (*See* page 673 for Rhesus isoimmunization, etc.)

Severe haemoglobinopathy

Homozygous α-thalassaemia (Chinese and Far Eastern races) causes hydrops in the newborn which appears to be incompatible with sur-vival. Very rarely, homozygous sickle-cell disease presents in the neonatal period, with jaundice and anaemia (Hegyi *et al.*, 1977).

Intrauterine infection

A number of chronic intrauterine infections cause moderate anaemia with hepatosplenomegaly and rapidly developing jaundice, with or without thrombocytopenia, and may be mistaken for some form of blood group incompatibility. For further consideration of these condi-tions (syphilis, toxoplasmosis, cytomegalovirus infection, rubella, ma-laria, Chagas' disease) *see* pages 624–628.

Malignancy

Very rarely, congenital leukaemia or neuroblastoma may present with severe anaemia.

MANAGEMENT

(*a*) *Rhesus and ABO haemolytic disease*

See page 673.

(*b*) *Fetomaternal and fetofetal bleeding*

Infants in a state of hydrops (cardiac failure with ascites and pleural effusion) and an Hb of <7 g per 100 ml require a partial exchange transfusion (p. 684) as described under Rhesus isoimmunization.

Infants with an Hb of 7–10 g per 100 ml without hydrops should be transfused by slow drip with packed or concentrated red cells.

(i) Volume of packed or concentrated cells: *see* page 484 for calculation.

(ii) Duration of transfusion: normally this should be given *slowly*, over at least 4 hours. A careful watch should be kept on the respiration and heart rate and the size of the liver. Dyspnoea and tachypnoea with rapid enlargement of the liver indicate cardiac failure; the transfusion should be temporarily stopped and frusemide should be given IV or i.m. The transfusion can be restarted or completed when the infant has recovered.

(c) The piethoric twin in fetofetal bleeding

Normally no treatment is required, though the development of cardiac failure with a raised venous pressure may require a venesection of 10 ml per kg. Frusemide should NOT be given because of the danger of thrombosis. The serum bilirubin should be estimated at least daily until it is clear that there is no risk from hyperbilirubinaemia. A reversed exchange transfusion using plasma has been used to lower the haematocrit if there is considered to be a risk of cerebral or renal-vein thrombosis from hyperviscosity. The critical level for thrombosis appears to be a haematocrit of >70 per cent; an exchange transfusion of 15 ml per kg using plasma as the donor fluid should lower the haematocrit to 60 per cent.

Anaemia developing postnatally

This may be due to:

(a) Missed Rhesus or ABO haemolysis (p. 673).
(b) Missed fetomaternal haemorrhage (p. 658).
(c) Congenital haemolytic anaemias (p. 468).
(d) Intrauterine infections (p. 624).
(e) Congenital hypoplastic anaemia (p. 468).
(f) Early or late anaemia of prematurity.
(g) β-thalassaemia at 3 to 4 months (p. 468) or homozygous sickle-cell disease (*see above*).

Anaemia of prematurity

(a) Early anaemia

A slowly developing anaemia may develop in very low-birth-weight infants (<1.5 kg) in the first 6 to 8 weeks.

(*b*) *Iron deficiency anaemia*

Iron deficiency anaemia may develop at 4 to 5 months which may be so severe (before recognition) that the Hb is 4 to 5 g per 100 ml.

MANAGEMENT

(*a*) *Early anaemia*

A transfusion should be given when the Hb falls below 8 g per 100 ml, using concentrated cells.

(*b*) *Late anaemia*

Normally this does not constitute an emergency and can be treated with oral iron preparation. A transfusion is indicated at Hb levels of <7 g per 100 ml, if the infant is not thriving, or to expedite return home.

Reference

Hegyi, T., Delphin, E. S., Bank, A., Polin, R. A. and Blanc, W. A. (1977). Sickle-cell anaemia in the newborn. *Pediatrics* **60**, 213

CHAPTER 80

The Bleeding Neonate

Judith M. Chessells

Haemorrhage in the newborn infant may be due to local causes (e.g. slipped cord clamp) or to a generalized bleeding disorder. Bleeding from one site can be due to a bleeding disorder. In management of the bleeding newborn infant three problems must be faced:

(a) Emergency treatment of acute blood loss (p. 652).
(b) In case of gastrointestinal loss, could this be maternal blood? Do the Apt test (p. 399).
(c) Is the bleeding a manifestation of haemostatic failure? Blood is taken for Hb, PCV, film, platelet count and screening tests of coagulation (PT, PTTK, TT) before transfusion. If the baby has not received vitamin K give 1 mg IV or i.m. phytomenadione. If DIC is suspected be sure to take sample for FDP into EACA or other fibrinolytic inhibitor.

Normal values in the neonatal period

In pre-term and mature infants the platelet count and factors V, VIII and fibrinogen are in the normal adult range. Prothrombin and factors II, VII, IX and X are low at birth (so the PT and PTTK may be prolonged even in a normal newborn) and drop further at 3 to 4 days *unless* the baby is given vitamin K. The thrombin time is moderately prolonged but should not exceed twice that of the control.

Clinical clues to the type of bleeding disorder

(*a*) *The baby* Breast- or bottle-fed. Has vitamin K been given? Is there evidence of respiratory distress, hypothermia, infection, or hepatosplenomegaly? If so, this suggests DIC. Has the bleeding followed trauma, e.g. circumcision in a well baby? If so consider haemophilia or Christmas disease. Late cord bleeding is seen in the (very rare) deficiencies of fibrinogen or factor XIII. Extensive purpura in an otherwise well baby suggests immune thrombocytopenia. Presence of congenital anomalies may indicate a genetically determined thrombocytopenia.

(*b*) *The mother* History of bruising or drugs which may cause thrombocytopenia (rare, e.g. quinidine, thiazides) or affect platelet function (common, e.g. aspirin). The WR result should be checked. Blood is taken for platelet count and film.

By assessment of these points and results of screening tests (*see* Tables 80.I, 80.II) a diagnosis may be made.

Management of individual disorders

THROMBOCYTOPENIA WITH NO CLOTTING DEFECT

Immune thrombocytopenia is most likely; for other rare causes *see* Table 80.II. Problems in immune thrombocytopenia are most likely in the first few hours of life. If bruising is the only problem no treatment is needed. If bleeding is severe, platelet concentrate (from one unit of blood is sufficient) should be given but may not be effective. Exchange transfusion should be considered using fresh heparinized blood to remove antibody and (in isoimmunization) subsequent infusion of washed maternal platelets.

VITAMIN K DEFICIENCY

See Table 80.I. This is manifest by bleeding usually on days 3 or 4 in breast fed babies who have not received vitamin K, and it may also

TABLE 80.I
Screening tests of haemostasis in the newborn

Disorder	Platelets	PT	PTTK	TT***
Immune thrombocytopenia*	ABN	N	N	N
Disseminated intravascular coagulation	ABN	ABN	ABN	ABN
Vitamin-K deficiency	N	ABN	ABN	N
Afibrinogenaemia	N	ABN	ABN	ABN
Factor XIII deficiency**	N	N	N	N
Haemophilia	N	N	ABN	N
Liver disease	N	ABN	ABN	ABN

* *See* Table 80.II.
** Special screening test needed
*** *See* page 482, Table 50.V, for key to abbreviations.
N = normal result. ABN = result usually abnormal.
See text for normal values in the newborn and influence of vitamin K.

TABLE 80.II
Thrombocytopenia in the newborn

Mechanism	Examples
Platelet production decreased or abnormal	Thrombocytopenia with absent radius. Wiskott–Aldrich syndrome. Infections.
Immune thrombocytopenia	
Passive	Maternal ITP. Maternal systemic lupus erythematosus. Maternal drug ingestion.
Active	Isoimmune neonatal thrombocytopenia.
Intravascular coagulation	
Generalized	Asphyxiated, hypothermic, acidotic infants. Erythroblastosis fetalis (Rhesus isoimmunization). Respiratory distress syndrome. Congenital infections: syphilis, rubella cytomegalovirus, herpes simplex. Acquired infections.
Localized	Cavernous haemangioma. Renal-vein thrombosis. Catheter thrombus.

exacerbate subaponeurotic haemorrhage after vacuum extraction. It may also occur in infants of mothers on anticonvulsants. This is the *only* condition in which vitamin K stops bleeding and restores normal clotting factors. If vitamin K does not work the diagnosis should be reconsidered, e.g. liver disease or DIC.

FAILURE OF SYNTHESIS OF CLOTTING FACTORS
This can occur in neonatal hepatitis, galactosaemia or fructose intolerance. The cause should be found and treated where possible. Fresh frozen plasma 10 to 15 ml per kg will replace clotting factors.

CONGENITAL CLOTTING-FACTOR DEFICIENCIES
Replacement therapy as detailed on page 485.

DISSEMINATED INTRAVASCULAR COAGULATION (p. 482)
For common causes in the newborn *see* Table 80.II. The cause should be found and treated: DIC in the newborn is often self-limiting. If bleeding is a continuing problem, platelet concentrates must be given and FFP as detailed above; heparin is rarely indicated except when thrombosis is the main problem. The dose of heparin is as on page 483.

IDENTIFICATION OF GROUPS AT RISK AND PREVENTION OF HAEMORRHAGE
Routine administration of vitamin K$_1$ (phytomenadione) to all babies at

birth will prevent vitamin-K-responsive bleeding. Prompt correction of neonatal hypoxia, shock and hypothermia, and treatment of infection, will help in prevention of DIC.

CHAPTER 81

Jaundice

J. A. Black

This may present as an emergency in three ways:
   (i) In the management of a haemolytic anaemia of known cause, e.g. Rhesus or ABO isoimmunization, G-6PD deficiency (*see* pages 673, 470).
   (ii) Jaundice developing in the first 24 hours after delivery.
   (iii) Rapidly increasing jaundice of unknown cause.

(a) DANGERS OF HYPERBILIRUBINAEMIA
   (i) Kernicterus, irrespective of the cause of the jaundice, apart from obstructive jaundice.
   (ii) Unrecognized septicaemia (*see below*).
   (iii) Unrecognized metabolic disorder (*see below*).

(b) FACTORS WHICH MAY CONTRIBUTE TO HYPERBILIRUBINAEMIA
Particularly in the pre-term infant severe hyperbilirubinaemia may result from the summation of a number of factors, each one alone being unlikely to cause more than a moderate degree of jaundice.
   The commonest contributory factors are:
   (i) Pre-term delivery.
   (ii) Enclosed haemorrhage or soft-tissue bruising.
   (iii) Infection.
   (iv) Haemolysis from any cause (e.g. hereditary spherocytosis, pyruvate kinase or G-6PD deficiency, isoimmunization and rarely homozygous sickle-cell disease, *see* page 659).
   (v) Respiratory distress syndrome.
   (vi) Infant of the diabetic mother.
   (vii) Dehydration and metabolic acidosis.
   (viii) High Hb level (e.g. in the plethoric infant in fetofetal transfusion).

(ix) Breast milk in certain mothers.
 (x) Hypothyroidism.

(c) DIFFICULTIES IN ESTIMATING
Difficulties in estimating clinically the degree of jaundice are increased:
   (i) In artificial light.
  (ii) In pre-term infants with red skin.
 (iii) In dark-skinned infants.
  (iv) After phototherapy.

Jaundice developing in the first 24 hours after delivery

The probable causes are:
   (a) Missed Rhesus isoimmunization which may result from:
       (i) Inadequate antenatal screening.
      (ii) The development of Rhesus antibodies late in pregnancy,
           though this rarely causes a severely affected infant.
     (iii) Failure to test the Rhesus-negative woman in her *first*
           successful pregnancy; a number of women develop antibod-
           ies after a spontaneous or induced abortion, or after
           amniocentesis.
      (iv) The development of antibodies in a Rhesus-positive
           woman;
               This is most likely to occur after transfusion for a post-
               partum haemorrhage, with antibodies to E, e, or c.
   (b) Severe ABO incompatibility.
   (c) Isoimmunization against rare blood groups. Duffy, Kell etc.
   (d) Chronic intrauterine infections (*see* page 624).

RECOGNITION
   (a) If there is skin pallor due to anaemia the early development of
       jaundice is easily recognized.
   (b) Blood should be taken from the infant (preferably via the
       umbilical vein, making the specimen more comparable to a cord-
       blood specimen) for Hb, ABO and Rhesus grouping, Coombs'
       test and where appropriate circulating immune anti-A or anti-B
       in the infant's serum and on the red cells. Blood is taken from the
       mother for ABO and Rhesus grouping, antibody screening and
       specific antibody titre, and where appropriate immune anti-A or
       anti-B in the serum. Sufficient blood should be retained for
       crossmatching against the maternal serum.
           If there is no evidence of isoimmunization and the cause of the
       jaundice is obscure, 10 to 20 ml of blood should be taken for
       subsequent investigation at the beginning of an exchange trans-
       fusion if this proves to be necessary.

MANAGEMENT
  (a) The main concern is the prevention of kernicterus, the critical
       level of bilirubin depending on the gestational age of the infant
       (p. 677).
  (b) Even in the absence of a diagnosis a serum bilirubin increasing at
       >8.5 μmol per litre (>0.5 mg%) per hour will probably necessi-
       tate an exchange transfusion, and the standard criteria for this
       should be used (pp. 677, 678).
  (c) Phototherapy should be used on the standard indications (p.
       671).

Rapidly increasing jaundice of unknown cause (excluding the first 24 hours)

The same causes may be operating as in jaundice in the first 24 hours.
   However, other possibilities which should be considered are:
   (a) Septicaemia.
   (b) Metabolic disorders.
   (c) Chronic intrauterine infection.
   (d) Haemolytic anaemia due to a genetically determined red cell
        abnormality.

Septicaemia

RECOGNITION
  (a) The infant appears ill; signs of meningitis or other infection may
       be obvious. The liver is often moderately enlarged and firm.
       Though the jaundice is due mainly to an increase in the unconju-
       gated bilirubin, the conjugated fraction is usually somewhat
       increased also.
  (b) A complete investigation for sepsis should be done (blood
       culture, lumbar puncture, urine microscopy and culture, chest x-
       ray). Immediate positive evidence of infection may be obvious
       from an abnormal CSF or urine.

Metabolic disorders

RECOGNITION
The two most important metabolic conditions to be excluded are
galactosaemia and fructose intolerance.

(a) Galactosaemia

The liver is usually much enlarged and both fractions of bilirubin may be increased. In the severely ill infant there may be skin haemorrhage or oozing from the umbilicus or puncture sites. Confirmation of the diagnosis is made by the detection of galactose in the urine (Clinitest-positive, Clinistix-negative, with laboratory confirmation of galactose) and blood and a positive screening test on the red cells. At times the plasma glucose may reach hypoglycaemic levels. It is important to realize that galactose will not be detected if the infant is on IV fluids, and also that *both* glucose and galactose may be present in the urine at the same time, so that a positive Clinistix or other glucose-specific test does NOT exclude the diagnosis. (*See also* page 702).

(b) *Fructose intolerance*

Clinically the condition is similar to galactosaemia, but symptoms cannot occur until the infant has received sucrose (ordinary sugar) or fructose (sucrose is immediately converted into fructose). In theory the diagnosis can be excluded if it is known that the infant has been exclusively breast-fed, but in practice many infants receive occasional unrecorded bottle feeds during the night. The urine should be tested with Clinitest and Clinistix (*see* page 702 (Galactosaemia) for possibility of errors in interpretation), and any reducing sugar or sugars identified by the laboratory; plasma fructose levels should also be estimated. As with galactosaemia, hypoglycaemia is probable. There is no simple test for fructose intolerance and confirmation of the diagnosis should be delayed until empirical treatment has improved the infant's condition.

Chronic intrauterine infection

RECOGNITION
Hepatosplenomegaly is usually marked, with moderate anaemia. Both fractions of the bilirubin are likely to be increased. Petechial skin haemorrhages are common. The infant's IgM will be increased in any chronic infection. The clinical picture and diagnostic tests are described in more detail on pages 624–628.

Haemolytic anaemia due to a red cell abnormality

RECOGNITION
    (a) A full history should include:
        (i) A family history with special reference to jaundice, anaemia and splenectomy.
        (ii) Drugs recently given to the mother and infant.
    (b) Anaemia is usually present though not always obvious clinically.

(c) Splenomegaly is not common at this age.

(d) The conditions which should be considered are:
Hereditary spherocytosis.
G-6PD deficiency.
Rarer genetically determined red cell abnormalities, e.g. pyruvate-kinase deficiency.
Homozygous sickle-cell disease (very rare) (*see* page 659).

(e) A reticulocyte count is the most important investigation, but will not distinguish between a haemolytic anaemia due to isoimmunization and red cell abnormalities; a reticulocyte count of >5 per cent in the presence of jaundice indicates haemolysis.

(f) Spherocytosis is inherited as a dominant though the affected parent may not have been detected. The blood film shows numerous microspherocytes (these are often seen in ABO incompatibility also), and there is increased osmotic fragility.

(g) G-6PD deficiency (*see also* page 470) should be considered in infants of the following racial groups or origins:
African origin*.
Mediterranean basin.**
Chinese**, especially from South China (Canton, Kwangtung) and Hong Kong (Chan, Dodd and Tso, 1976).
Thailand.**
Hawaii.**
Israel.*

(h) Clinically haemolysis due to G-6PD deficiency in the newborn has the following characteristics:
(i) The maximum bilirubin levels usually occur between the second and fifth day of life, but may be as late as the second week.
(ii) During the first week the Hb level may be normal or as low as 7 to 8 g%.
(iii) Occasionally the Hb level and reticulocyte count are normal.
(iv) Fragmented red cells may be seen on the blood film.

(i) Blood-group isoimmunization should be excluded (as described above).

MANAGEMENT

(a) An exchange transfusion may be necessary irrespective of the diagnosis.

(b) It may occasionally be impossible to exclude the simultaneous

* Spontaneous haemolysis (i.e. haemolysis occurring without drugs) appears *not* to occur in these groups, though there is a high incidence of hyperbilirubinaemia in G-6PD-deficient *pre-term* infants of African origin (Oski, 1975).
** These forms have spontaneous haemolysis in the neonatal period.

presence of septicaemia and a metabolic disorder. If both are suspected, antibiotics should be given combined with exclusion of the suspected sugar or sugars.

(c) Septicaemia; if this is proved or suspected, appropriate antibiotics should be given by injection (*see* page 634).

(d) Metabolic disorder; if the diagnosis is uncertain all sugars metabolized to galactose or fructose should be excluded (i.e. lactose, sucrose, fructose itself). Initially an IV drip should be given of either 0.18 per cent NaCl with 4 per cent glucose, or 10 per cent glucose alone depending on the plasma glucose levels.

Feeds should then be started on a synthetic milk containing no lactose, sucrose or fructose. If the diagnosis can be proved or is reasonably certain, oral feeds can be started using an appropriate milk.

(e) Chronic intrauterine infections require specific management.

(f) Haemolysis due to red cell abnormality:

(i) In G-6PD deficiency all drugs likely to induce haemolysis should be avoided (Table 50.II). If vitamin K is indicated, K_1 (phytomenadione) should be used in a dose not greater than 1.0 mg.

(ii) In hereditary spherocytosis and other red cell abnormalities jaundice is most severe in the pre-term infants in the immediate postnatal period and it is in this group that exchange transfusion may be required. In more mature infants phototherapy may be useful.

Phototherapy

The indication for this form of treatment is a mild degree of jaundice which is increasing slowly and which is not due to infection, severe haemolysis or an identified metabolic disorder. Its main use is in the pre-term infant in whom an exchange transfusion might be required if the serum bilirubin were to continue to increase. Phototherapy is no substitute for exchange transfusion, but its use after an exchange transfusion may prevent the necessity for a second or subsequent one.

The usual indication, based upon serum bilirubin (unconjugated only) is to start at a level of bilirubin 85 mmol per litre (5 mg%) below that at which exchange transfusion would be indicated:

At term, start at $255\,\mu$mol per litre (15 mg%).
At 36 weeks, start at $220\,\mu$mol per litre (13 mg%).
At 34 weeeks, start at $188\,\mu$mol per litre (11 mg%).
At 32 weeks, start at $154\,\mu$mol per litre (9 mg%).
28 to 32 weeks, start at $120\,\mu$mol per litre (7 mg%).

MANAGEMENT

(a) All diagnostic investigations must be completed before starting phototherapy.
(b) The procedure should be explained to the mother before phototherapy is started.
(c) A safe and effective eye shield should be used.
(d) The infant's temperature should be recorded every 4 hours.
(e) An additional 10 per cent of extra fluid should be given and the infant should be weighed every 12 hours.
(f) Serum-bilirubin levels should be estimated at 12-hourly intervals.
(g) Phototherapy should normally be used for 18 out of every 24 hours.

References

Chan, T. K., Dodd, D. and Tso, S. C. (1976). Drug-induced haemolysis in glucose-6-phosphate dehydrogenase deficiency. *Br. med. J.* (**ii**), 1227
Oski, F. A. (1975). Haematologic problems. In *Neonatology*, p. 393. Ed. G. B. Avery. Philadelphia: J. B. Lippincott

CHAPTER 82

Rhesus and Other Forms of Isoimmunization

J. A. Black

Rhesus incompatibility

RECOGNITION

(a) Antenatal diagnosis

With repeated testing for antibody titre and amniocentesis in selected cases the affected fetus should have been identified before delivery, and a prediction of the severity of the haemolytic process should have been made.

(b) At delivery

(i) The severely affected infant.
There is extreme pallor with the abdomen distended from hepatosplenomegaly; blotchy or nodular skin haemorrhages and occasionally petechiae may be present. In the hydropic infant there is ascites, with or without pleural effusions, and cardiac failure.

(ii) The infant who is apparently normal at birth.
Even if the severity of the haemolysis has already been predicted on amniocentesis the cord blood will give a more accurate prediction of those infants requiring exchange transfusion.

(c) Confirmation of the diagnosis and prediction of severity by the cord blood

Table 82.I gives the normally accepted criteria for exchange transfusion in term infants. In pre-term infants or where there is an additional factor contributing to the hyperbilirubinaemia (p. 666) exchange transfusion may be required when this would not have been predicted on the cord blood results, but this decision is made by repeating the serum bilirubin estimations at frequent intervals.

TABLE 82.I
Classification of infants by means of cord-blood results

Rhesus group	Coombs' test	Hb in g%	Serum bilirubin in μmol/litre (mg%)	Category	Treatment
Negative	Negative	Not required	Not required	Unaffected	None
Positive	Negative	Not required	Not required	Unaffected	None
Positive	Positive	>14, and	50 (3) or less	Mild	Observe and repeat bilirubin at 4 hours and at intervals if jaundice develops
Positive	Positive	7–14 and	>50 (>3)	Moderate to severe	Exchange transfusion within 4–6 hours
Positive	Positive	<7 or clinically hydropic	≥50 (≥3)	Very severe	Modified exchange

(d) Difficulties and errors in the interpretation of cord blood results

(i) Errors in technique in taking the blood cause haemolysis which may interfere with the estimation of serum bilirubin, or cause clots which give a falsely low Hb reading.

(ii) In severely affected cases a Rhesus-positive infant may give a false Rhesus-negative result, and the direct Coombs' test may also show a false negative. In such cases the tests should be repeated but management is based on the clinical condition of the infant and cord Hb and serum-bilirubin levels.

(iii) If the infant has had an intrauterine transfusion the results on the cord blood may reflect the characteristics of the donor blood, with a negative Coombs' test and Rhesus-negative cells with ABO group of the donor blood; the serum bilirubin is however >50 μmol per litre (>3 mg%) usually with >17 μmol per litre (>1 mg%) of conjugated bilirubin.

(e) Assessment of an affected infant when cord blood is not available.

(i) A venous sample can usually be taken from the umbilical vein if it can be cannulated, in which case the results are more or less comparable to Hb levels in the cord blood.

(ii) However, a capillary sample may only be available. It should be recognized that a capillary Hb level is usually (not invariably) 3 g per cent higher than a venous sample.

(iii) Since there is no base-line (cord blood) level for serum bilirubin, the necessity for exchange transfusion must be based upon the rate of rise, the chart of Diamond, or the absolute level of a single estimation, according to circumstances (*see* pages 677–678).

(*f*) *Phototherapy*

This should never be relied on to control the rise of serum bilirubin in severe Rhesus isoimmunization, but it may be useful in mildly affected cases. (*See* page 671 for criteria and method.)

ABO incompatibility

There are a number of differences between Rhesus and ABO isoimmunization which are summarized in Table 82.II.

TABLE 82.II

Summary of differences between Rhesus and ABO incompatibility

	Rhesus	*ABO*
Prediction from antenatal testing	Yes	Neither practicable nor necessary
First infant affected	Very rarely	Often
Subsequent infants affected	Yes	Infants affected randomly without relation to birth order
Clinically more severe in subsequent pregnancies	Often	No
Intrauterine death or hydrops	Yes	Very rare
Anaemia at delivery	Common	No
Direct Coombs' test (infant's red cells)	Positive	Weakly positive or negative
Severity of jaundice	All grades up to kernicterus	Rarely necessitates exchange transfusion except in pre-term infants

RECOGNITION

Early jaundice in the first 24 hours of life due to ABO incompatibility is not common, but does occur, especially in pre-term infants: usually the jaundice develops in the 3rd or 4th day, or later and presents as a moderately severe jaundice. ABO appears to be relatively common and more severe in the West Indies. Confirmation of the diagnosis is shown by:

   (a) The mother's group is usually O and the infant A or B, though other combinations occur.

   (b) A mild anaemia with a reticulocytosis and microspherocytosis.

   (c) The presence of a high titre of immune anti-A or anti-B in the mother's serum; the antibody should be eluted off the infants' red cells and tested against adult cells.

MANAGEMENT

   (a) Phototherapy is effective in the majority of cases. (*See* page 671 for instructions.)

   (b) Exchange transfusion may be required in severely affected infants or those of very low birth weight. (*See* page 677 for indications.)

   (c) If an exchange transfusion is required, the donor blood should be of the same Rhesus group as the infant, but of group O only. Some centres wash the donor cells and resuspend them in a plasma containing no agglutinins; this requires an additional 2 hours, which should be allowed for in planning the transfusion. If available, group O blood with low titre anti-A and anti-B can be used.

CHAPTER 83

Exchange Transfusion

J. A. Black

An exchange transfusion should be done only by someone experienced in the technique; in inexperienced hands there will be a high morbidity and mortality.

Although the usual indication for exchange transfusion is for predicted or actual hyperbilirubinaemia from any cause, it may be required in severe anaemia, acute poisoning (p. 73), potentially lethal electrolyte disorders (p. 149), and in certain inborn errors of metabolism (p. 699).

Indications in hyperbilirubinaemia

(a) Rhesus isoimmunization, based on cord blood predictions (p. 674).

(b) On postnatal blood samples, based upon a rate of rise of 8.5 µmol per litre (>0.5 mg%) per hour, from the chart (*Figure 83.1*) of Allen and Diamond (1958) or on absolute critical values, or the prediction that critical values will be reached within 4 hours. The critical values which show that there is a danger of kernicterus vary with the gestational maturity of the infant; commonly accepted levels (Swyer, 1975) are as follows:

      At term   = 340 µmol per litre (20 mg%)*
      At 36 weeks   = 306 µmol per litre (18 mg%)*
      At 34 weeks   = 272 µmol per litre (16 mg%)*
      At 32 weeks   = 238 µmol per litre (14 mg%)*
      At 28 to 32 weeks = 205 µmol per litre (12 mg%)*

(c) Clinical evidence of kernicterus, irrespective of the level of serum bilirubin.

* Unconjugated bilirubin only: it can normally be assumed in haemolytic conditions and in hepatic immaturity that the total bilirubin measured is wholly unconjugated.

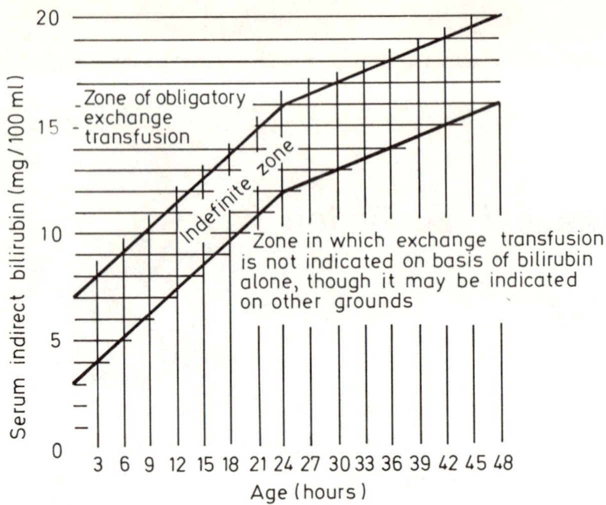

Figure 83.1. Guide to the use of serum-indirect bilirubin as the sole criterion for exchange transfusion in mature infants. Note: 20 mg/100 ml = 340 μmol/litre. (Allen and Diamond, 1958. Reproduced by kind permission)

Contra-indications

A full exchange transfusion should not be done in hydropic infants or those which are severely anaemic (cord Hb <7.0 g%) with a central venous pressure of >12 cm (4.8 in). In such cases a partial exchange should be done (p. 684).

REQUIREMENTS

(a) *Blood.* Acid-citrate-dextrose (ACD) stored blood or heparinized blood can be used. Heparinized blood must be used within 24 hours of collection and should be used with care in severely ill infants in whom 1.0 mg of protamine should be given for every 100 ml of blood exchanged (Maisels, 1972). ACD blood has the disadvantages of a high glucose content, a high acid load, the binding of calcium and magnesium with the citrate, and the possibility of a high plasma potassium level (*see below*).

(b) *Whole, concentrated or packed blood.* For routine purposes concentrated red cells are given, the supernatant plasma being removed just before use.

(c) *Age of the blood.* To avoid the risk of hyperkalaemia the blood should be <5 days old.

(d) *Blood group.* Ideally the blood used should be of the same ABO group as the infant and Rhesus negative in all cases of Rhesus isoimmunization and Rhesus-negative infants requiring exchange for other reasons. The donor cells should always be crossmatched against the mother's serum. If a severely affected Rhesus infant is expected a number of bottles of different ABO group can be crossmatched against the mother's serum and the final selection made when the infant's ABO group is known. In emergencies Rhesus negative group O blood can be used irrespective of the infant's ABO group, provided that crossmatching is satisfactory.

(e) *Preparation of the blood.* Blood should *never* be given to the infant straight from the refrigerator, as this will induce arrhythmia. Blood should *never* be warmed under a hot tap or by standing in hot water, as this is likely to damage or destroy the red cells and produce a dangerously high potassium level in the plasma.

    Blood should be warmed by passage through a heating coil in a waterbath at 37°C (98.6°F).

(f) *Volume of blood to be exchanged.* Normally 180 ml per kg should be exchanged, with a minimum of 160 ml per kg. However, in any ill infant or where the procedure is poorly tolerated, it should be remembered that the first 100 ml per kg is often adequate to arrest or slow down haemolysis.

The actual transfusion

(*See* Appendix 20 for complete list of apparatus required).

(a) *Assistance.* At least one assistant should be present to record the progress of the exchange, heart rate etc.

(b) *The infant's body temperature* must be maintained within the normal range by using a radiant heat shield, or by keeping the infant in an incubator.

(c) *Immobilization.* Some immobilization or restraint may be necessary, but the limbs should not be bandaged to a crucifix splint, since this will obstruct the venous return and reduce the efficiency of the exchange.

(d) *Feeds and oral drugs.* No feeds or oral drugs should be given during the 4 hours before the exchange. The stomach should be aspirated before starting the transfusion, but there is no need to retain the gastric tube unless there is repeated vomiting.

(e) *Heparinized saline (0.9 per cent NaCl).* This should be available to wash out the tubing and syringes if there is clotting. Heparin, 2 ml of a 1000 units per ml solution, should be added to every 250 ml of saline.

(f) *Apparatus.* The disposable sets are the safest and most convenient to use; the risk of clotting and leakage from joints is much less than with a 'home-made' set. Leakage is particularly dangerous in an exchange transfusion since it may cause a cumulative imbalance of volumes in either direction.

Technique

Though a number of techniques are available, the standard method using the umbilical vein is safe and simple to use. Alternative techniques are described on page 681.

(1) A graduated catheter (FG5 or 8) is inserted into the umbilical vein which has been cut at about 2.5 cm (1 in) from the abdominal wall. The catheter is pushed into the vein until it is thought to be in the inferior vena cava above the diaphragm. The actual position of the tip should be checked by x-ray and screening. A tape is tied around the cord and is tightened when the catheter is correctly placed. Blood should be aspirated from time to time during the insertion of the catheter and a free flow of partly oxygenated blood should be obtained. A catheter should *never* be passed without its end connected to a 10-ml syringe full of saline, to avoid the possibility of air embolism. When the position of the catheter is satisfactory a thread marker should be tied round it at the point of entry into the vein to detect any displacement.

In all severely ill infants the central venous pressure (CVP) should be measured at the beginning of the transfusion. Great care should be used to avoid air embolus; fluctuations in the pressure should be visible if the catheter is correctly placed. If the pressure is within 5 to 8 cm (2–3 in) it is safe to start the tranfusion; pressures above or below this level require a partial transfusion (p. 684).

(2) Size of syringes. A 10-ml rather than a 20-ml syringe is preferable since the volume and pressure variation in the right atrium are less, and the use of a smaller syringe reduces the temptation to proceed too fast.

(3) An initial blood sample (10 ml) should be retained for Hb, serum bilirubin and any other investigations.

(4) Blood pH. If the initial pH is >65 nmol per litre (<7.20) the acidosis, which can be assumed to be metabolic unless there is respiratory distress from any cause, should be partly corrected by injection of 5 mmol of $NaHCO_3$ (8.5 ml of 5 per cent solution or 5 ml of 8.4 per cent solution) and the pH estimation should be repeated after 15 minutes. It is safe to start the transfusion if the H^+ (pH) is < 50 nmol per litre (>7.30). Further estimations of pH and correction can be made if necessary and should be done if the infant's condition deteriorates during the transfusion.

(5) Drugs.
  (a) Calcium gluconate. There is no evidence that this has a useful
      or lasting effect on the level of ionized calcium in the infant's
      blood. This is a potentially dangerous drug, capable of causing
      arrest or damage to the vascular endothelium; its routine use is
      no longer recommended (*see also* page 143).
  (b) Digoxin. There are no indications for digoxin.
  (c) Frusemide. This should be given in hydropic infants or those
      with a high CVP. Dose 1 mg per kg IV or i.m.
(6) Duration of procedure. An exchange transfusion should not be
    completed in under 1 to $1\frac{1}{2}$ hours, stopping if necessary if there is
    deterioration in the infant's condition. In sick or very small infants
    the procedure should take up to 2 hours, or is done in two stages.
(7) Complications during exchange transfusion. These are listed in
    Table 83.I.
(8) At the end of the transfusion the vein or artery should be occluded
    by a purse-string suture round the base of the cord. If the cord, for
    ease of access to the vein, has had to be cut flush with the abdominal
    wall, both vessels should be crushed flat with an artery forceps and
    the skin should be sewn over the umbilical site with sutures on
    either side of the umbilicus. The catheter tip should be cut off and
    sent for culture.

Alternative routes for exchange transfusion

  (a) If the umbilical vein cannot be catheterized, an attempt should be
      made to catheterize the artery and to use this in the same way as
      the umbilical vein (for technique *see* page 714).
  (b) Difficulty in passing the catheter past the umbilical 'ring'. This
      may be due to clots in the vein which can sometimes be sucked
      out by the syringe on the end of the catheter. Difficulty may also
      be due to narrowing or folding of the vein: if this is so the vein
      can usually be entered just before it passes upwards to the liver.
      There are two approaches:
    (i) A vertical incision is made at 12 o'clock (head end) of the
        funnel of fibrous tissue at the base of the cord and the cut is
        extended upwards for 2 to 3 cm (1 in) into the skin of the
        abdomen. With gentle traction of the cord the vein in its
        upward course usually becomes obvious. The vein is dis-
        sected free at its uppermost part and a 45° incision is made
        with fine-pointed scissors. A catheter can usually be passed
        upwards without any difficulty.
    (ii) A crescentic incision is made about 1 to 2 cm ($\frac{1}{2}$—$\frac{3}{4}$ in)
         above the umbilicus and the underlying fascia is dissected

TABLE 83.I
Complications during exchange transfusion

Symptoms	Cause	Treatment
Vomiting, retching, crying, grunting respiration, restlessness, aspirated blood becoming blue	Too rapid rate of exchange, or circulatory overload	Slow down or stop for 15–30 minutes
Cyanosis or pallor	Too rapid rate: volume imbalance especially overload	(i) Check balance sheet. (ii) ECG for peaked P waves in overload. (iii) Readjust imbalance
Bradycardia	Hyperkalaemia (blood >5 days old or red cells damaged by heating)	(i) Stop transfusion. (ii) ECG for evidence of hyperkalaemia (*Figure 13.4*). (iii) Check the infant's serum level of potassium; if >7 mmol per litre use specific treatment (p. 13.8)
Air embolism (air seen entering umbilical vein)	(i) Leaking apparatus. (ii) Air entering umbilical vein during pressure measurement	(i) Hold infant with head downwards. (ii) If there is cardiovascular collapse, attempt aspiration of air from left ventricle
Convulsion	(i) Hypocalcaemia or hypomagnesaemia. (ii) Possibly blood clot or air embolism	(i) Stop transfusion. (ii) If prolonged or repeated control with IV or i.m. diazepam
Cardiac arrest or arrhythmia	(i) Hyperkalaemia. (ii) Cold blood	(i) Stop transfusion. (ii) External cardiac massage if arrhythmia is causing cardiovascular collapse
Sudden collapse with shock	(i) Air embolus. (ii) Arrhythmia. (iii) Perforation of intra-abdominal umbilical vein	(i) Air embolus, arrhythmia *see above.* (ii) Suspected perforation of umbilical vein. Stop transfusion; confirm intraperitoneal blood by aspiration in left flank to avoid the liver; give blood by peripheral vein or umbilical artery

until the vein is identified. This dissection is not easy since the peritoneum lies immediately beneath the vein and may be opened inadvertently. However, it can be sutured easily without appealing for surgical aid.

(c) Use of the saphenous vein. This should only be used when all approaches on the umbilical vessels have failed, or in the older child in whom the umbilical vessels are not available. A horizontal incision is made parallel to, but about 1 cm ($\frac{1}{2}$ in) below the inguinal fold, medial to the femoral artery. The vein passes through the fascia at this point, to join the femoral vein. The saphenous vein is very small and a smaller than usual size of catheter may be required. The catheter should be passed up into the inferior vena cava in the usual way. Swelling of the leg is not uncommon after this procedure but appears to resolve without any evidence of permanent venous obstruction.

Care after exchange transfusion

(a) Post-exchange levels of Hb and serum bilirubin will indicate the effectiveness of the exchange and it can be expected that the post-exchange level will be half the pre-exchange level. However, there is invariably a 'rebound' rise at about 4 hours, which may be followed by a slow fall or by a continued rise.

(b) In the ill or severely affected Rhesus infant, hypoglycaemia may occur after the exchange transfusion. The recognition and management are described on page 445.

(c) Repeat exchange transfusion may be required, according to the rate of rise of the serum bilirubin. In severely affected infants obstructive jaundice may develop and the amount of conjugated bilirubin should be measured in addition to the total amount; the level of conjugated bilirubin must then be taken into account (by subtraction from the total bilirubin concentration) when deciding on further exchange transfusion.

(d) Follow-up should include weekly Hb levels, and folic acid and oral iron from 5 weeks of age onwards.

Late complications of exchange transfusion

Sepsis: this is more likely to result from prolonged retention of an umbilical catheter in the vein than the exchange transfusion itself. Repeated exchanges increase the risk. Evidence of infection is generally seen 12 to 24 hours after the exchange: the infant becomes pale, with episodes of high temperature and sweating. A maculopapular rash may develop and the liver and spleen may be enlarged, and obstructive jaundice may develop.

MANAGEMENT OF SEPSIS

(i) Blood cultures should be done: also cultures from the umbilical vein.

(ii) Antibiotics should be given for at least two weeks initially. Cytomegalovirus disease may be produced by infected blood (p. 624).

(iii) Portal thrombosis. This may be a complication of septic throm-
bophlebitis of the portal vein, or it may occur without obvious
infection. The infant's spleen is found to be enlarged; this may
be preceded by an illness with prolonged obstructive jaundice
with moderate hepatomegaly. If sepsis is thought to be a
possibility, two weeks treatment on antibiotics should be given.

Necrotizing enterocolitis

For the infant's survival this must be recognized early, before perforation has occurred. The first sign is usually the passage of blood *per
rectum* at 4 to 12 hours (occasionally up to 4 days) after the exchange
transfusion.

The other symptoms, signs and management are described on pages
380–381.

Partial exchange transfusion

INDICATIONS
  (a) Hydrops; in a severely ill infant with chronic anaemia (from any
cause) with a high CVP.
  (b) Infants with plethora and a packed cell volume >70 per cent,
which is the critical level above which the increased blood
viscosity may predispose to thrombosis. This can occur from
fetofetal transfusion or from delayed clamping of the cord, with
a large placental transfusion.

MANAGEMENT

(a) Hydropic and anaemic infants

Concentrated or packed cells should be used of the same ABO group as
the infant; Rhesus-negative blood should be used in Rhesus isoimmunization, in Rhesus negative infants with other conditions, or in
an extreme emergency after a rapid crossmatch.
  (i) Continuous oxygen should be given by face-mask or other
means.
  (ii) If there is apnoea, dyspnoea or grunting respiration the infant
should be intubated and given IPPR.
  (iii) If there is abdominal distension, as much ascitic fluid should be
removed as possible by aspiration of the peritoneal cavity in the
left iliac fossa to avoid the liver.
  (iv) Both pleural cavities should be tapped using a posterior approach just below the angle of the scapula.

(v) If the CVP is >12 cm (4.8 in) the initial pressure should be recorded, and frusemide should be given IV or i.m. The transfusion is then started by the removal of 20 ml of blood and its replacement by 10 ml of donor blood. The venous pressure is then measured again. This 20 ml 'out' and 10 ml 'in' is continued until the CVP is between 5 and 8 cm (2–3 in), and a cumulative deficit of 40 to 80 ml of blood has been achieved. The infant is then put into an incubator, slightly propped up, and allowed to recover. A conventional exchange transfusion should be left until the infant's condition has improved or until a rising serum bilirubin makes an exchange necessary.

(vi) If the CVP is <5 cm (2 in), the procedure should be reversed and 10 ml of blood is removed and replaced by 20 ml of donor blood. This is continued until the CVP is between 5 and 8 cm (2–3 in). There is no indication for frusemide. An exchange transfusion is delayed as described above.

(b) Plethora

The infant's blood should be replaced by plasma in order to reduce the packed cell volume (PCV). To reduce the PCV from 70 per cent to 60 per cent, a one-to-one exchange of 15 ml per kg is required.

Religious objections to transfusion and refusal of consent

Though a consent form is not usually requested for transfusion of any sort, the parents should always be asked for their verbal consent for an exchange transfusion. On the rare occasions when this is refused, this possibility will usually have been forseen by knowledge of the parents' religious affiliation.

The formal legal procedure of making the infant a Ward of Court usually takes too long to be useful, particularly when an exchange transfusion is required. It is therefore necessary for the consultant to take the responsibility for the decision to transfuse and to discuss this with the parents. If, in spite of further discussion the parents still refuse consent the consultant should write his (signed) opinion in the case notes and obtain a similar signed opinion from a colleague. The parents may or may not wish to sign a statement of their refusal. In most cases the legal adviser to the consultants' employing authority should be informed. In the unlikely event of the parents wanting to remove their child from hospital in order to prevent the transfusion taking place, it should be possible to obtain a Place of Safety Order under the Children's Act (1969), as for children who are neglected or injured by their parents.

References

Allen, F. H. and Diamond, L. K. (1958). *Erythroblastosis Foetalis, Including Exchange Transfusion Technique*. Boston: Little, Brown

Maisels, M. J. (1972). Bilirubin: on understanding and influencing its metabolism in the newborn infant. *Pediat. Clins N. Am.* **19**, (No. 2), 447

Swyer, P. R. (1975). *Intensive Care of the Newly Born.* p. 147. Basle: S. Karger

CHAPTER 84

Convulsions in the Newborn

J. A. Black

RECOGNITION
(a) Normally it is easy to recognize a fit, but difficulty may arise in distinguishing between tonic fits with resulting cyanosis and a prolonged apnoeic attack with a resulting posthypoxic fit.

The sequence of events in these situations is as follows:

Fit: tonic phase → cyanosis → ± clonic phase.

Apnoeic attack: apnoea → cyanosis → tonic ± clonic fit.

Jitteriness may be mistaken for a fit; this is a state of hyperexcitability in which even slight stimuli will provoke symmetrical rhythmical jerking of the limbs, usually more marked in the arms. The random single jerking of an arm or leg in the very small pre-term infant ($<$30 weeks) must also be distinguished from a convulsion.

(b) A number of possible causes may be operating simultaneously (i.e. hypoxia, hypoglycaemia, and hypocalcaemia) and it is necessary to investigate each infant in a systematic manner in order not to miss a serious condition, such as intracranial haemorrhage or meningitis, in which there may be coexistent hypoglycaemia or hypocalcaemia.

(c) The type of fit offers little clue to its cause though, in general, focal fits, particularly those of multicentric origin (i.e. changing from one side to another or involving a different part of the body at each fit), are more likely to be due to hypoglycaemia or hypocalcaemia, whereas tonic fits more usually indicate serious intracranial disease such as hypoxic damage.

CAUSES OF FITS

Though this should not be used as an excuse for omitting thorough investigation, it is often possible to arrive at the probable cause of a fit from the perinatal history and from the interval between delivery and the first fit.

(*a*) *During the first 48 hours*

   (i) After severe perinatal hypoxia (posthypoxic state with presumed cerebral oedema); the infant is abnormal from birth with hypotonia or hypertonia.

  (ii) Mechanically difficult or precipitate delivery: acute subdural haemorrhage from a ruptured venous sinus should be suspected (p. 610).

 (iii) Hypoglycaemia in small-for-dates infants, smaller of twins, the infant of a diabetic mother (IDM). In an ill infant hypoglycaemia may be associated with the posthypoxic state.

 (iv) Early hypocalcaemia* in a well infant. This may be due to maternal hyperparathyroidism, primary or secondary (p. 140), or in an ill infant, with the posthypoxia state (*see* (i) *above*).

  (v) Drug withdrawal, from drug dependence in the mother (p. 709).

 (vi) Pyridoxine dependence (rare); this may have an onset *in utero*, or later, after the first 48 hours. Fits are usually frequent and are resistant to anticonvulsants, but respond to pyridoxine.

 (vii) Early meningitis (rare); this is due to a transplacental infection by Gram-negative bacilli.

(viii) Intrauterine infection from cytomegalovirus, toxoplasmosis, rubella.

(*b*) *3 to 4 days after delivery*

 (i) In an infant with RDS intraventricular haemorrhage is the most likely cause.

(ii) Hypocalcaemia* in the IDM.

(*c*) *4 days onwards*

 (i) Meningitis.

(ii) Late hypocalcaemia* (4 to 7 days), in infants fed on unmodified cow's milk.

INVESTIGATIONS

With the exceptions mentioned below *all* newborn infants should have a lumbar puncture after the first fit.

(*a*) *Lumbar puncture* It should be possible to make an immediate diagnosis of meningitis or intracranial haemorrhage; an abnormal CSF may also be due to intrauterine infection (p. 624). A low CSF glucose

---

* This may be accompanied by hypomagnesaemia (p. 145).

in an otherwise normal CSF may indicate past or present hypoglycaemia, which should be investigated.

(*b*) *Blood/plasma glucose*   As a screening test the Dextrostix papers should be used: a level >2.5 mmol per litre (>45 mg%) excludes hypoglycaemia; a level of <2.5 mmol per litre (<45 mg%) should be confirmed by the laboratory.

(*c*) *Additional investigations*   Investigations which should be done in all ill infants or in those in which lumbar puncture and plasma-glucose levels have failed to show the cause of the fits are:
(i) Plasma calcium and magnesium.
(ii) Test the urine for reducing substances (Clinitest).

(*d*) *Continued fits resistant to anticonvulsants*   The following investigations should be done:
(i) X-ray and transillumination of the head (for intracranial calcification and hydroanencephaly).
(ii) Injection of a test dose of pyridoxine (25 mg) IV or i.m. (pyridoxine dependence).
(iii) Amino-acid chromatography of the urine.
(iv) Examination of the infant's blood for raised IgM indicating an intrauterine infection.

MANAGEMENT
(*a*) *Prolonged or frequently recurring tonic fits*   (These are unlikely to be due to hypoglycaemia or hypocalcaemia):
(i) The airway must be maintained by suction, maintenance in the semiprone position, and if necessary, by the insertion of an oropharyngeal airway. Oxygen should be given by bag and mask; or if there is prolonged interruption of respiration, the infant should be intubated and oxygen given with IPPR.
(ii) The fits should be controlled, using diazepam (0.25 to 1.0 mg per kg) IV slowly, with IPPV immediately available in case of apnoea.

(*b*) *Posthypoxic state*   If cerebral oedema is likely (a bulging fontanelle is rarely present) the oedema should be reduced by:
(i) High potency steroids (p. 324).
or (ii) Mannitol (20 per cent); in a dose of 1 to 2 g per kg IV over 45 to 90 minutes, preceded by a test dose of 1 ml per kg IV over 5 minutes (Swyer, 1975).

(*c*) *Focal fits, infrequent tonic fits, or after the control of severe fits*   If

Y

these are not due to hypoglycaemia or hypocalcaemia, anticonvulsants should be used. Any *one* of the following drugs should be used:

    (i) Phenobarbitone i.m. initially, then orally, in a dose of 5 mg per kg per 24 hours, divided into 4 doses at 6-hourly intervals.

or (ii) Phenytoin, orally, in a dose of 4 mg per kg per 24 hours, divided into 4 doses at 6-hourly intervals (a parenteral preparation is also available containing 50 mg per 1 ml).

(*d*) *Hypoglycaemic fits*   (*See* page 445).

(*e*) *Hypocalcaemic fits*   (*See* page 139).

(*f*) *Meningitis*   (*See* page 347).

(*g*) *Intracranial haemorrhage*   (*See* page 655).

References

Swyer, P. R. (1975). *The Intensive Care of the Newly Born.* p. 152. Basle: S. Karger

CHAPTER 85

Infant of the Diabetic Mother

(See also under Hypoglycaemia)

J. A. Black

The infant of the diabetic mother (IDM) has a tendency to hypoglycaemia, which may be asymptomatic during the first few hours after delivery. In general, the better the control of the mother's diabetes the more nearly does the infant's weight approach the normal weight for its gestational age and the less severe is the postnatal hypoglycaemia. However, the infant of the prediabetic mother may also develop hypoglycaemia, but this condition may not be suspected before delivery; infants with a birth weight >4.5 kg, or with the typical appearance of IDM, irrespective of birth weight should be managed in the same way as the IDM.

RECOGNITION

There are four distinct groups of IDM each requiring different management.

(a) The IDM of typical appearance, often delivered at 38 weeks or less by induction or caesarian section.

(b) The IDM with a normal appearance and a birth weight appropriate to its gestational age.

(c) The small-for-dates IDM. The mother may have suffered from severe toxaemia necessitating delivery early (<37 weeks). Hypoglycaemia is likely to be severe, probably from a combination of hyperinsulinism and lack of liver glycogen. These infants must be distinguished from those with normal birth weight.

(d) The infant whose mother has received an oral hypoglycaemic drug (usually chlorpropamide or a related drug) up till delivery. Hypoglycaemia is likely to be more severe and to last longer (3 to 4 days) than in the other groups.

MANAGEMENT

(*a*) *Asymptomatic infants*

    (i) Plasma-glucose levels or Dextrostix estimations. These should be measured repeatedly using the cord blood level as a base-line. In all groups of IDM the levels should be measured at $\frac{1}{2}$ and 1 hour after delivery and estimations should be repeated at hourly intervals, then at increasing intervals until it is clear that oral feeding has been established with normal plasma-glucose levels without additional IV glucose. During oral feeding, the plasma-glucose level should be estimated immediately before feeds.

        Treatment is aimed at maintaining a plasma-glucose level above 1.7 mmol per litre (30 mg%) (Dextrostix: >1.4 mmol per litre) (>25 mg%). A Dextrostix level <1.4 mmol per litre (<25 mg%) requires immediate action but should be checked by a plasma-glucose estimation; at Dextrostix levels between 1.4 and 2.5 mmol per litre (25–45 mg%) a further estimation should be done after 1 hour.

   (ii) Oral feeds should be started as early as possible, normally within 6 hours of delivery, using bottle or tube feeding according to the maturity of the infant or its ability to feed by bottle. Standard milk feeds should be used (NOT glucose solutions). A rapid feeding schedule should be used, reaching 60 ml per kg in the first 24 hours, 90 ml per kg on the 2nd day, 120 ml per kg on the 3rd day and 150 ml per kg on the 4th day.

  (iii) Treatment of plasma levels of <1.7 mmol per litre (<30 mg%) Dextrostix 1.4 mmol per litre (<25 mg%). The most satisfactory method of controlling the plasma-glucose level is the use of a 10 per cent glucose solution IV, with an initial rate of infusion of 2 ml per kg per hour (50 ml per kg per 24 hours). If an infusion of 10 per cent glucose fails to maintain the plasma level above 1.7 mmol per litre (30 mg%) the rate can be increased to 4 ml per kg per hour (100 ml per kg per 24 hours) but the total fluid intake (oral and IV) should not exceed 150 ml per kg per 24 hours. It is usually preferable to increase the strength of glucose to 25 per cent and to maintain the same rate of infusion.

  (iv) Overlapping IV and oral intake. An IV infusion of glucose should never be stopped suddenly since this may cause a reactive hypoglycaemia. When the plasma-glucose levels are stable the IV drip should be gradually decreased and the oral feeds gradually increased over the next 24 hours.

   (v) Route for IV glucose. Normally a peripheral vein should be used, but the umbilical vein can be used in certain circumstances.

    (a) Severe hypoglycaemic symptoms.
    (b) Failure to find a suitable peripheral vein.
    (c) In a very ill child (e.g. with Respiratory Distress Syndrome) which will not withstand much handling.

(b) Symptomatic hypoglycaemia

If symptoms (p. 446) are considered to be due to hypoglycaemia the infant should be treated immediately by IV 10 per cent glucose; there is however usually time to confirm the clinical impression by using Dextrostix and by taking a blood sample for subsequent laboratory confirmation.

    (i) An immediate IV injection of 20 ml of 10 per cent glucose should be given over a period of 10 minutes, followed by a further Dextrostix and plasma-glucose level to confirm that an adequate rise has occurred. A maintenance dose of 10 per cent glucose should then be started, as described above.

    (ii) As an alternative, glucagon can be given IV or i.m. in a dose of 0.3 mg (300 μg) per kg; however, the effect does not last longer than 2 to 3 hours and there is evidence that repeated doses may act as a stimulant to further production of insulin, (one single dose should not exceed 1 mg). In the small-for-dates IDM glucagon would be ineffective owing to depletion of liver glycogen.

(c) Hypocalcaemia

Hypocalcaemia (plasma calcium <1.9 mmol per litre <7.5 mg%) is common in IDM and is likely to be responsible for symptoms which are similar to those of hypocalcaemia but which occur later and at a stage when the plasma glucose has stabilized at normal levels. Treatment is described on page 141.

(d) Other complications

    (i) Respiratory Distress Syndrome; this is commoner in IDM than would be expected for the infant's gestational age. The management is described on pages 264–272.

    (ii) Hyperbilirubinaemia is relatively common in IDM (*see* pages 668–672 for management).

    (iii) Renal-vein thrombosis, congenital cardiac lesions and sacral agenesis all appear to have a slightly increased incidence in IDM.

CHAPTER 86

Hypothermia

J. A. Black

Transient or primary hypothermia after delivery

Even in normal infants delivered into a warm environment the rectal temperature may drop by as much as 1 to 2°C (2–4°F). A normal stable body temperature may not be achieved until 4 to 8 hours after delivery. Situations associated with hypothermia after delivery are:
  (a) Pre-term delivery.
  (b) Hypoxia and prolonged resuscitation.
  (c) Delivery into a cold environment.
  (d) Delay in wrapping the infant after delivery.
  (e) Bathing the infant within 4 hours of delivery.
  (f) Morphia or related drugs given to the mother before delivery.

RECOGNITION
In mild hypothermia the hands and feet are blue and cool, but the face may be pink and the trunk is pink and warm; in more severe hypothermia the trunk is also cool.

MANAGEMENT
The rectal temperature (low-reading thermometer) should be taken if hypothermia is suspected. If the rectal temperature is <35°C (95°F) the infant should be warmed up quickly by wrapping in a warm towel or by being placed in an incubator at 29 to 35°C (84–95°F).
  In severe hypothermia, especially if the infant appears ill and fails to respond to re-warming, the possibility of secondary hypothermia should be considered (*see below*).

Secondary hypothermia

A fall in temperature may occur, due to some condition other than the transient factors described above; these are:
  (a) Acute infection, especially septicaemia.
  (b) Respiratory distress syndrome, complicated by hypoxia, hypo-glycaemia, or intraventricular haemorrhage.
  (c) Intracranial haemorrhage of any type.
  (d) Exchange transfusion.
  (e) Severe cardiac failure.
  (f) Small-for-dates infants with hypoglycaemia.

MANAGEMENT

The infant is put into an incubator at 35°C (95°F) and is investigated and treated according to the suspected primary condition; in nearly every instance hypoglycaemia may coexist and should be treated.

Severe acute hypothermia

When an infant is exposed to a cold environmental temperature for up to 6 hours there is a rapid fall in body temperature; this is most likely to occur in:
  (a) Unattended delivery at home or in an ambulance, especially in cold weather.
  (b) Delivery into a lavatory.
  (c) Failure of incubator heating.

RECOGNITION

The infant appears sluggish and apathetic, with slow respiration and heart rate. Both trunk and extremities feel cold and may have a blotchy white and blue appearance. The rectal temperature is usually below 29°C (84°F).

MANAGEMENT

Exposure to cold for not more than 6 hours is unlikely to cause cold injury and therefore rapid re-warming should be safe. The infant is placed in an incubator at 32 to 35°C (90–95°F).

Cold injury

This is the most serious form of hypothermia and is usually confined to the first month of life, though older children, especially those with Protein-Energy Malnutrition, may also develop cold injury.

RECOGNITION
Cold injury results from slow cooling over a long period and poor
socio-economic conditions are often a contributary factor; in Great
Britain it is usually seen in term infants born at home during cold
weather or sudden cold spells. Pre-term infants usually escape cold
injury, probably because they are usually born in hospital, or if born at
home, are rapidly transferred to hospital.

Apart from inadequate heating, particularly at night, infection and
undernutrition are important predisposing causes. Clinically the infant
has a misleadingly healthy appearance, with bright pink extremities and
tip of the nose. There is little spontaneous movement and the face is
expressionless. The diagnosis is obvious as soon as the frog-like
coldness of the trunk and limbs are felt. Both heart and respiration rate
are slow. The diagnosis should be confirmed by a low-reading
thermometer.

MANAGEMENT
  (a) Slow warming is still regarded as being safer than rapid warm-
      ing. The environmental temperature should be maintained at
      1°C (2°F) above the rectal temperature and this should be
      raised by 1°C every 4 hours.
  (b) During re-warming the plasma glucose level should be measured
      at hourly intervals; 10 per cent glucose should be given IV at
      approximately half the normal rate (3 ml per kg per hour).
  (c) The presence of infection should be assumed, but colistin and the
      aminoglycosides gentamicin, kanamicin, tobramycin, and ami-
      kacin should not be used because of the impaired renal function.
      Ampicillin and cloxacillin should be given IV or i.m.

CHAPTER 87

Acute Neonatal Illness in Inborn Errors of Metabolism

D. M. Danks

The diagnosis of an Inborn Error of Metabolism (IEM) in an acutely ill newborn infant depends upon constant alertness to this possibility, correct interpretation of the clinical course of the illness, and ready availability of effective investigation. Every neonatal unit should know the nearest centre where specimens, and if necessary the infant, can be sent. Even the best laboratory must receive some guidance from the paediatrician about appropriate investigation, in the form of adequate clinical information.

The number of IEM known to be capable of causing death, or irreversible brain damage, in the newborn period has increased steadily over the last 20 years. Diagnosis of those conditions for which effective treatment is available must take special priority. However, correct diagnosis is important even when treatment cannot be offered because the parents can be warned of the risk of further affected children and because intrauterine diagnosis may be possible in future pregnancies.

It is therefore important that neonatal paediatricians should remember these conditions and know how to look for them in the appropriate patients.

Infants at risk

(a) Symptomatic infants under investigation for an IEM which might explain their symptoms.
(b) Sibs of an infant known to have had a specific IEM.
(c) Sibs of infants which have died in the neonatal period without a satisfactory diagnosis or with symptoms which in retrospect suggest an IEM.
(d) Infants discovered to have an IEM on routine screening.

RECOGNITION

(a) The symptoms of IEM are mainly non-specific and may equally be due to more common causes such as in birth trauma, hypoxia and infection.

Suggestive symptoms are:

Refusal of feeds	Drowsiness	Respiratory failure	Jaundice
Vomiting	Unconsciousness	Tachypnoea	Haemorrhagic
Diarrhoea	Convulsions	(metabolic	tendency
		acidosis)	Pulmonary
			haemorrhage

(b) Absence of symptoms during the first 12 to 24 hours is more characteristic than the symptoms themselves. The majority of the treatable IEM, and many of those that cannot be treated, have little effect upon the fetus because placental haemodialysis is generally very efficient. Once symptoms do develop they usually increase progressively in the absence of effective treatment. By contrast, many of the non-genetic causes of acute neonatal illness produce symptoms at or very soon after birth, and the progression of symptoms is not so relentless.

(c) Symptoms are present at and before birth in a few IEM:

(i) Severe hypotonia in non-ketotic hyperglycinaemia.

(ii) Pyridoxine-dependant convulsions which may start *in utero* but nevertheless have a good outcome with early treatment.

(d) Improvement with treatment involving stopping oral feeds may be the first clue.

Clinical improvement may follow treatment instituted for a quite different reason which happens to have a beneficial effect on the IEM. For instance, a very sick baby with probable septicaemia may be taken off oral feedings and given intravenous fluid and antibiotics. Dramatic improvement may occur and may be attributed to the antibiotics and not to the incidental withdrawal of galactose. Some patients with galactosaemia present in this manner and may be re-fed milk with serious consequences (Oberklaid, Danks and Davies, 1976).

Expertise in the diagnosis of these conditions must be centralized in a small number of specialized metabolic units. Otherwise no-one will have the experience which is essential for the development of expertise. It is not just a matter of performing a number of laboratory tests. Correct interpretation of the results of these tests is vital. Specialized units need to be distributed within a country so that they are accessible to all patients. The initial tests must be performed on samples sent to a central laboratory where quick and efficient reporting of results is essential.

Three broad groups of tests are now employed to detect unusual metabolites or unusual amounts of normal metabolites:

(a) Colour reactions to recognize organic radicles—e.g. tests for ketone bodies, for ketoacids, for reducing substances, etc.

(b) Rapid methods of screening for amino acids in urine and serum, in high voltage electrophoresis (HVE) (Tippett and Danks, 1972) and thin-layer chromatography (TLC).

(c) Gas-liquid chromatography (GLC) for identification of organic acids (Tippett, Danks and Dimech, 1973).

(d) Gas chromatography–mass spectrometry (GC–MS) is a method of identifying a compound which has been detected by GLC (Jellum, Stokke and Eldjarn, 1972).

It has been usual to apply these techniques to urine and serum. Testing of CSF by the same techniques has not been used very widely and may warrant further exploration, especially in babies with neurological symptoms. For example, CSF glycine levels are increased in non-ketotic hyperglycinaemia, but are normal in ketotic hyperglycinaemia (Perry *et al.*, 1975).

MANAGEMENT

(a) Emergency treatment in suspected IEM

A newborn baby with acute dangerous symptoms must be treated empirically while awaiting laboratory results, or when attempts to make a diagnosis have been unsuccessful. Since most of the relevant conditions are caused by defects in catabolic pathways it is essential to prevent a catabolic state and if possible to initiate anabolism. This is certainly possible in some of the known defects, e.g. hyperammonaemia, and it is reasonable to treat unknown defects on this assumption.

(b) Empirical treatment with vitamins

Some of the acute IEM are vitamin responsive and there is some justification for blind use of massive doses of all water-soluble vitamins in the hope that the defect present may respond to one of them.

(c) Exchange transfusion

Exchange transfusion and/or peritoneal dialysis can have both therapeutic and diagnostic value. Most of the diseases concerned produce their effects through accumulation of a circulating metabolite and artificial removal of this metabolite may allow the baby to recover. Conversely a dramatic response to exchange transfusion or peritoneal dialysis may provide a clue to the existence of an IEM. It is even possible that these measures may allow a baby with an undiagnosed IEM to recover and that empirical dietary treatment may keep the baby alive in satisfactory condition.

DETAILED MANAGEMENT

(a) Termination of catabolism

This requires a high calorie intake and subsequently the provision of exactly the amounts of amino acids needed for growth.

The regime suggested involves feeding glucose plus glucose polymer (Caloreen, *Scientific Hospital Supplies*) orally or by intragastric tube to the maximum level of intestinal tolerance (generally a 5 per cent concentration of each) and/or feeding of a similar amount of glucose intravenously. If the sugar is given intravenously administration is monitored by repeated testing of urine for glucose and/or by intermittent measurement of blood glucose. If urine flow is adequate glucosuria will occur before dangerous levels of hyperglycaemia result. It is important to remember that hyperglycaemia can be dangerous through its osmotic effects.

It is very difficult to provide a sufficient caloric intake with glucose alone, and lipid must be added at a fairly early stage. Our own experience is confined to the administration of lipid by intragastric route and we have used either medium-chain triglyceride (MCT) oil or the more complex fats present in a commercially available powdered preparation which contains glucose, emulsified fat, minerals and vitamins (Nil Prote, *Mead Johnson*). Others have reported the use of intravenous lipids in this situation.

(b) Introduction of protein

If the baby improves on this type of regime it is important to introduce protein within two or three days to stimulate anabolism. The protein intake necessary to promote anabolism varies between 1 and 1.5 g per kg in different babies. This can be given as breast milk or as a humanized milk formula. There are some arguments for administering a mixture of essential amino acids and excluding the non-essential ones and this argument is particularly strong in hyperammonaemia. The use of the keto derivatives of essential amino acids may offer further advantage in hyperammonaemia. Their conversion to the corresponding amino acids should utilize ammonia rather than liberate it.

(c) Treatment of the infant diagnosed before symptoms

Finally, there are some circumstances in which it is possible to anticipate the birth of a baby with an IEM rather than having to treat a baby already very ill as a result of one of these conditions. This has been described elsewhere (Danks, 1974).

Specific diseases

Table 87.I lists the more important IEM which can present with acute neonatal symptoms and the reader is referred to larger texts for descriptions of most of these (Nyhan, 1974; Raine, 1975; Stanbury, Wyngaarden and Fredrickson, 1978).

TABLE 87.I

Some of the IEM which may cause severe illness in the newborn period

Disease	Methods of detection	Vitamin responsiveness in some cases	Inheritance
Carbamyl phosphate synthetase deficiency	Blood ammonia	Nil	AR
Ornithine transcarbamylase deficiency	Blood ammonia	Nil	XL
Citrullinaemia	Blood ammonia. HVE of urine or serum	Nil	AR
Other forms of hyperammonaemia	Blood ammonia	Nil	
Propionic acidaemia	Metabolic acidosis. GLC of urine	Biotin	AR
Methyl malonic acidaemia	Metabolic acidosis. GLC of urine	B_{12}	AR
Maple-syrup urine disease	Metabolic acidosis. HVE of urine or serum. GLC of urine	Thiamine*	AR
Isovaleric acidaemia	Metabolic acidosis. GLC of urine	Nil	AR
Non-ketotic hyperglycinaemia	Clinical features. HVE of urine and serum	Nil	AR
Galactosaemia	Clinical features. Glycosuria	Nil	AR
Hereditary fructose intolerance	Clinical features. Glycosuria	Nil	AR
Hereditary tyrosinaemia (French–Canadian variant)	Clinical features. HVE of urine and serum. GLC of urine	Nil	AR
Pyridoxine-dependent convulsions	Clinical features. Therapeutic response	Pyridoxine	AR
Congenital lactic acidosis	Metabolic acidosis. GLC of urine	Thiamine*	

* Noted only in mild cases presenting later in childhood

XL = X-linked; AR = Autosomal recessive; GLC = Gas-liquid chromatography; HVE = High-voltage electrophoresis

Galactosaemia

This is the most important IEM since it is one of the most easily treated and the diagnosis is simple; nevertheless it is frequently forgotten with tragic consequences (Oberklaid, Danks and Davies, 1975). Mass screening of newborn babies does not eliminate the clinical problem because the illness can start before the test is done or before the result is returned.

RECOGNITION

Vomiting, jaundice, drowsiness and convulsions are the most frequent symptoms. Onset is usually 24 to 28 hours after the start of milk feeding. Hepatomegaly is a constant finding and glycosuria (galactosuria) will be detected if the urine is tested with Clinitest, but all too often dip tapes of various types are used, which contain a reagent specific for glucose. The recent introduction of a strip specific for galactose (Galactostix, *Ames*) may help.

The illness may closely resemble septicaemia and in fact septicaemia commonly complicates the course of galactosaemia in the newborn period so that both diagnoses are correct. It is important to know that galactosuria may be minimal in some patients and certainly in some urine samples, especially if oral feeds have been stopped.

DIAGNOSIS

The assay of the red cell enzyme activity of galactose-1-phosphate uridyl transferase is now so simple that it should be applied in all patients with these symptoms. Misleading normal results may be obtained if the infant has been transfused.

MANAGEMENT

Dramatic improvement in a sick baby when intravenous therapy is initiated should make one think about the possibility of galactosaemia or one of the catabolic IEM, before giving full credit to antibiotics or other therapeutic agents.

Exchange transfusion is very valuable in critically ill patients with galactosaemia. A diet which excludes milk and milk products is then required.

Hereditary fructose intolerance

This condition is an exact parallel to galactosaemia and is equally easily treated (Froesch, 1975). However, it is much less common.

RECOGNITION

Symptoms are similar although even more acute. In many babies the diagnosis can be excluded merely by checking the feeding and showing that no fructose or sucrose has been ingested (e.g. in a fully breast-fed infant). However, it is easy to overlook one sucrose-containing feed given during the night when the mother was asleep.

DIAGNOSIS

Demonstration of fructosuria (fructose gives a positive reaction to Clinitest but requires laboratory identification) and a dramatic improvement after dietary exclusion of sucrose (i.e. cane or beet sugar, 'ordinary sugar') will support the diagnosis.

Absolute proof is more difficult and requires assay of fructose-1-P aldolase in a liver biopsy, or fructose tolerance test. The former assay is not widely available and the tolerance test must be performed with care, because serious hypoglycaemia may occur.

MANAGEMENT

Strict exclusion of fructose and sucrose-containing feeds: it should be noted that human milk and unaltered cow's milk do not contain either fructose or sucrose.

Hyperammonaemia

Defects of the first three steps of the urea cycle may cause very severe hyperammonaemia which may prove lethal in the first days after birth (Hsia, 1974).

RECOGNITION

Carbamyl-phosphate synthetase deficiency, ornithine transcarbamyl-ase (OTCase) deficiency and citrullinaemia all cause similar symptoms of drowsiness, loss of consciousness, convulsions, hypotonia and death. Breathlessness may also occur and sudden massive pulmonary haemor-rhage has been described in several babies (Sheffield *et al.*, 1976).

DIAGNOSIS

Diagnosis rests upon blood-ammonia estimation and HVE of urine amino acids. Levels of ammonia in excess of 500 μmol per litre (normal <100 μmol per litre in the newborn) are usual in unconscious patients with these conditions. Citrullinaemia can be diagnosed by HVE on urine or serum, but the other two conditions show no characteristic findings though glutamine levels are usually elevated and changes secondary to liver damage may appear. OTCase deficiency is X-linked in inheritance and affected males generally die in the neonatal period; females possessing the gene can be quite severely affected, but more often are not; however, they may suffer quite severe transient symptoms in the newborn period. Impaired ability of a heterozygous mother to metabolize ammonia may compound the fetal metabolic problem.

MANAGEMENT

Peritoneal dialysis is more efficient than exchange transfusion in removing ammonia and should be used immediately in any affected baby who is unconscious. Low-protein diet or a diet based on essential amino acids or keto derivatives of essential amino acids may be used.

Congenital lactic acidosis

The distinction between this condition and the lactic acidosis which may occur in septicaemia or in cardiac disease may be impossible to determine in a baby who dies rapidly. If the patient recovers, secondary lactic acidosis will clear over about 48 hours after restoration of good tissue perfusion and oxygenation. Persistence suggests that the lactic acidosis is primary.

A number of different enzyme defects can cause primary lactic acidosis and several are susceptible to effective treatment. Fructose 1,6-diphosphatase deficiency causes lactic acidosis and hypoglycaemia and can be controlled by a low-protein, low-fructose diet (Baerlocher *et al.*, 1971). A thiamine-dependent defect of pyruvate carboxylase has been described but did not present so acutely (Brunette *et al.*, 1972). The basic defect remains unknown in some patients (Tippett, Danks and Dimech, 1973).

Maple-syrup urine disease, propionic acidaemia, methylmalonic acidaemia, and isovaleric acidaemia

RECOGNITION

All these diseases involve defects in the catabolism of the branched-chain amino acids (leucine, isoleucine and valine) and all can cause acute neurological symptoms in the newborn period. Maple-syrup urine disease is easily diagnosed by elevations of all three amino acids in the urine and by excretion of the three corresponding ketoacids (detected by GLC). Hyperglycinuria and hyperglycinaemia may occur in propionic acidaemia or methylmalonic acidaemia (for unknown reasons) and these were originally described as ketotic hyperglycinaemia. However, the GLC pattern is the diagnostic test in these conditions and in isovaleric acidaemia (Gompertz, 1975). Staining of the region of the origin on the urine HVE with Fast Blue B provides a very sensitive method of detecting methylmalonic acid.

MANAGEMENT

A special diet is used in maple-syrup urine disease with restriction of the branched-chain amino acids. Low-protein diet is the mainstay of treatment of the other three conditions. Fortunately vitamin-dependent forms exist—vitamin-B_{12}-dependent methylmalonic acidaemia, biotin-dependent propionic acidaemia and a thiamine-dependent variant of maple-syrup urine disease.

Non-ketotic hyperglycinaemia

RECOGNITION

This condition has a very characteristic clinical presentation with extreme hypotonia. Few other conditions cause such a rag-doll type of baby. Respiratory inadequacy develops and is the cause of death. Cerebral depression is severe.

Diagnosis is very obvious on HVE of urine and serum. The absence of acidosis (other than that secondary to respiratory failure) distinguishes it from 'ketotic hyperglycinaemia'.

MANAGEMENT

Survival after repeated exchange transfusions and respiratory support has been reported, followed by a low-protein diet. No survivor has yet had normal intellect. Recent findings of a relationship between valine intake and symptoms may lead to new methods of dietary treatment.

References

Baerlocher, K., Gitzelmann, R., Nüsoli, R. and Dumermuth, G. (1971). Infantile lactic acidosis due to hereditary fructose 1,6-diphosphatase deficiency. *Helv. Paediat. Acta* **26**, 489

Brunette, M. G., Delvin, E., Hazel, B. and Scriver, C. R. (1972). Thiamine-responsive lactic acidosis in a patient with deficient low—K_m pyruvate carboxylase in the liver. *Pediatrics* **50**, 703

Danks, D. M. (1974). Management of newborn babies in whom serious metabolic illness is anticipated. *Archs Dis. Childh.* **49**, 576

Froesch, E. R. (1975). Hereditary fructose intolerance and fructose-1,6-diphosphatase deficiency. In *The Treatment of Inherited Metabolic Disease*. Ed. D. N. Raine. p. 151. New York: Elsevier—North Holland

Gompertz, D. (1975). Organic acidaemias. In *The Treatment of Inherited Metabolic Disease*. Ed. D. N. Raine. p. 191. New York: Elsevier—North Holland

Hsia, Y. E. (1974). Inherited hyperammonemic syndromes. *Gastroenterology* **67**, 347

Jellum, E., Stokke, O. and Eldjarn, L. (1972). Combined use of gas chromatography, mass spectrometry, and computer in diagnosis and studies of metabolic disorders. *Clin. Chem.* **18**, 800

Nyhan, W. L. (Ed.) (1974). *Heritable Disorders of Amino-Acid Metabolism: Patterns of Clinical Expression and Genetic Variation*. New York: Wiley

Oberklaid, F., Danks, D. M. and Davies, H. E. (1976). Problems encountered in the diagnosis of galactosaemia. *Austral. Paediat. J.* **12**, 14

Perry, T. L., Urquhart, N., MacLean, J., Evans, M. E., Hansen, S., Davidson, G. F., Applegarth, D. A., MacLeod, P. J. and Lock, J. E. (1975). Non-ketotic hyperglycinemia. Glycine accumulation due to absence of glycine cleavage in the brain. *New Engl. J. Med.* **292**, 1269

Raine, D. N. (Ed.) (1975). *The Treatment of Inherited Metabolic Disease*. New York: Elsevier—North Holland

Sheffield, L. J., Danks, D. M., Hammond, J. W. and Hoogenraad, N. H. (1976). Massive pulmonary haemorrhage as a presenting feature in congenital hyperammonemia. *J. Pediat.* **88**, 450

Stanbury, J. B., Wyngaarden, S. B. and Fredrickson, D. S. (Eds). (1978). *The Metabolic Basis of Inherited Disease.* (4th edn). New York: McGraw Hill

Tippett, P. A. and Danks, D. M. (1972). Screening for aminoaciduria: (i), a critical evaluation of 4 techniques; (ii), a survey of a mentally retarded population using high-voltage paper electrophoresis. *Austral. Paediat. J.* **8**, 255

Tippett, P. A., Danks, D. M. and Dimech, L. (1973). Detection of life threatening inborn errors of metabolism during infancy. *Austral. Paediat. J.* **9**, 297

CHAPTER 88

Maternal Drug Dependence

J. A. Black

There are four groups of drugs which are of importance: the narcotics (opiates), barbiturates, alcohol, and the hallucinogens. Those most likely to be encountered are listed in Table 88.I, though the pattern varies considerably in different countries. There is no evidence that maternal consumption of amphetamines, cocaine, or cannabis is associated with withdrawal symptoms in the newborn. However the continued taking of some of the minor tranquilizers (glutethimide, meprobamate, diazepam) by the mother has occasionally resulted in symptoms

TABLE 88.I
Drugs likely to cause withdrawal symptoms in the fetus or newborn

Narcotics (opiates)	Barbiturates	Alcohol	Hallucinogens
Dextromoramide (Palfrium)	Butobarbitone (Soneryl)	All forms	Lysergic acid diethylamide (LSD)
Dihydrocodeine (D.F.118)	Quinalbarbitone (Seconal)		
Dipipanone with cyclizine (Diconal)	Quinalbarbitone with amylobarbitone (Tuinal)		
Heroin (diamorphine)			
Morphine (all forms)			
Pentazocine (Fortral, Talwin)			
Pethidine (Meperidine, Demerol)			
Methadone (Physeptone)			

suggestive of withdrawal in the infant, though these are rarely severe (Neumann, 1973). Severe withdrawal symptoms in the narcotics and barbiturate group may cause the death of the infant if treatment is inadequate.

Non-specific effects on the fetus and newborn

(a) Due to a combination of poor maternal health and nutrition, and inadequate antenatal care, the perinatal mortality rate in the infants of drug users is high, and the infants tend to be small-for-dates.

(b) Maternal disease: there is a relatively high incidence of positive tests for syphilis and for hepatitis-B antigen, but biological false-positive tests for syphilis are exceptionally common in drug users. (Harris and Andrei, 1967). Although the hepatitis-B antigen is occasionally transmitted to the infant, there is little evidence that clinical hepatitis results.

Effects of withdrawal on the fetus

Naturally this only comes about from a planned or accidental reduction or withdrawal of the drug by the mother. There is evidence that abrupt withdrawal may cause fetal death; increased fetal movements and tachycardia have also been noted. Opinion appears divided on the advisability of attempting to withdraw the drug completely during pregnancy or continuing with a controlled maintenance programme throughout. If a withdrawal programme is planned during pregnancy it should be gradual and timed to be complete well before the onset of labour (Liu, Tylden and Tukel, 1976).

Withdrawal symptoms in the newborn

Both the incidence and severity of symptoms are so variable that it is generally best to await the development of symptoms before starting treatment. If the mother is known to be a drug user the infant should be kept under close supervision for a minimum of 7 days. If the mother is not known as a drug user, as is particularly likely with alcohol, the symptoms in the infant may be the first indication of the true situation.

Though the symptoms are likely to be similar, irrespective of the type of drug, there are certain differences:

(a) Narcotic group: gastrointestinal symptoms such as vomiting, and loose stools are relatively common.

(b) Barbiturates: in this group there is probably a higher risk of withdrawal convulsions.

RECOGNITION

Prompt recognition and adequate treatment are essential.

(*a*) *Age of onset*

In most cases symptoms develop within 24 hours of delivery but there may be a delay of up to 4 to 5 days.

(*b*) *Symptoms which may occur* (Zelson, Rubio and Wasserman, 1971)

 (i) Common:
  Coarse temors.
  Hyperactivity and hypertonicity.
  Irritability.
  Vomiting.
  Sneezing.
  Incessant high-pitched crying.
  Poor feeding.
 (ii) Less common:
  Loose stools.
  Yawning, lacrimation, sweating and salivation.
  Tachypnoea with hyperventilation.
  Fever.
  Convulsions.
  Hypothermia.
  Circulatory collapse.

MANAGEMENT

There is no general agreement on treatment, and it seems clear that mild symptoms can be successfully treated with a variety of drugs such as chloral, dichloralphenazone (Welldorm), diazepam, phenobarbitone, or chlorpromazine.

However it is obvious that no single drug can be used for all situations.

(*a*) *Narcotics*

The alternatives recommended are given in Table 88.II. Opinion

TABLE 88.II

Doses of drugs used in treatment of neonatal narcotic withdrawal. (After Neumann, 1973)

Phenobarbitone	8–10 mg per kg per 24 hours: in four divided doses: i.m. or oral
Chlorpromazine	2.5–4.5 mg per kg per 24 hours: in four divided doses: i.m. or oral
'Paregoric' (camphorated tincture of opium)*	1–3 drops per kg every 3–6 hours (may be increased if necessary)
Morphine	0.1–0.2 mg per kg per dose (emergencies only)

* The doses given apply to the United States Pharmacopoeia (*U.S.P.*) preparation which contains 4 per cent of tincture of opium: the British Pharmacopoeia preparation contains 5 per cent of tincture of opium.

appears divided on which drug is the most effective. Diazepam has also been used but has the disadvantage that it may predispose to kernicterus in infants with mild hyperbilirubinaemia. Morphia group antagonists (nalorphine, naloxone) should NOT be used in narcotic dependence.

(b) Barbiturate withdrawal

The morphia group of drugs is ineffective in treatment, and phenobarbitone in the dosage described is the most logical choice.

(c) Alcohol

Chlorpromazine appears to be the most useful drug using the lower of the dosages in Table 88.II.

(d) LSD

There is no evidence as yet of any specific symptoms in the newborn, but concern has mainly centred on the question of its possible teratogenic effect or the production of chromosomal abnormalities.

(e) Duration of treatment

In most instances full dosage is necessary for 7 to 10 days, after which the dose is gradually reduced every 2 to 3 days.
NOTE: This section is not based upon first-hand experience and the author has drawn heavily on a number of sources which are quoted below.

References

Harris, W. D. M. and Andrei, J. (1967). Serologic tests for syphilis among narcotic adults. *N.Y. Med. J.* **67**, 2967

Liu, D. T. Y., Tylden, E. and Tukel, S. H. (1976). Fetal response to drug withdrawal. *Lancet* (**ii**) 588

Neumann, L. L. (1973). In *Drugs and Youth*. Ed. E. Harms. Oxford and London: Pergamon Press

Zelson, C., Rubio, E. and Wasserman, E. (1971). Neonatal narcotic addiction; 10-year observation. *Pediatrics* **48**, 178

Part XVIII: Practical Procedures

CHAPTER 89

Practical Procedures

(*See* Appendix 17 for needle sizes in millimetres and inches)

Ian Shellshear

This section deals with procedures which involve penetration of the body tissues or cavities. There are a number of points which apply to all such procedures.

PREPARATION

For most procedures, local anaesthetic has little to offer, as it is painful in itself and obscures landmarks. The exceptions occur with large instruments, e.g. trocar and cannula, or with prolonged manipulation. Overhead heaters should be used for any prolonged procedure in the neonate. Sedation beforehand is often of value, particularly in young children. Trimeprazine (0.9 mg per kg i.m. or 3 to 4 mg per kg orally) or diazepam (1 mg per year, orally or i.m.) are useful to calm the child. Ketamine may also be used.

CORRECT DOSAGE

If drugs are to be inserted into a body cavity, it is the responsibility of the operator to ensure that he has the correct drug, the correct dose and the correct route. Unlabelled syringes offered by an assistant should never be accepted on the assumption that they are correct.

COMFORT

Success is in proportion to the comfort of the operator. The operator should be sitting and have an assistant, so that he is not attempting the procedure as well as restraining a patient.

INTRAVENOUS INFUSION

Intravenous or intra-arterial lines should always have a paediatric chamber between the infusing solution and the patient, to prevent accidental overload. Drip rates are best controlled by mechanical pumps, but if these are not available close supervision should be given. It should not be assumed that supervising staff know how to remove air from drip tubing, or other details of drip maintenance.

CATHETER SELECTION

Recent work on the irritant nature of catheters suggests a much lower incidence of thrombosis if silastic rather than polyvinylchloride catheters are used. The silastic catheters, however, have the disadvantage of being opaque and are less malleable.

Intravenous lines

INDICATIONS

To supply maintenance fluids, to replace lost fluids, to inject drugs or to insert monitoring devices. The site depends on these requirements and the age of the child.

Umbilical vessel catheterization (artery)

EQUIPMENT

Sterile procedure; intravenous cut-down set, vessel dilator (either a fine probe or a pair of iris forceps), $3\frac{1}{2}$ or 5F intravenous cannulae (sterile feeding tube with radio-opaque lines) or oxygen electrode, suture material.

PROCEDURE

The sooner after birth catheterization is attempted, the more likely it is to be successful. The umbilical vein is easier to cannulate than the umbilical arteries, but except for exchange transfusions, and in an emergency for blood transfusions or intravenous glucose, umbilical arteries are preferred (*see* exchange transfusion for venous cannulation, p. 680).

The umbilical cord is cut 1 to 2 cm ($\frac{1}{2}-\frac{3}{4}$ in) from the umbilicus and the lumen of one of the arteries dilated with a fine probe or one arm of a pair of iris forceps, care being taken not to strip between the intima and the media; if only the weight of the forceps is used, this is less likely. There are often obstructions to be found at 2 cm ($\frac{3}{4}$ in) (rectus sheath) or 5 cm (2 in) (the umbilical artery–internal-iliac artery junction). The first obstruction may be overcome by gentle pressure or by using a slightly larger catheter. It is helpful if the catheter is stored in a refrigerator as this makes it slightly stiffer. The second obstruction is more difficult but may be overcome by manipulation. The position of the catheter should be checked by x-ray and the femoral pulses palpated after insertion. If an oxygen electrode has been inserted, it will require standardization.

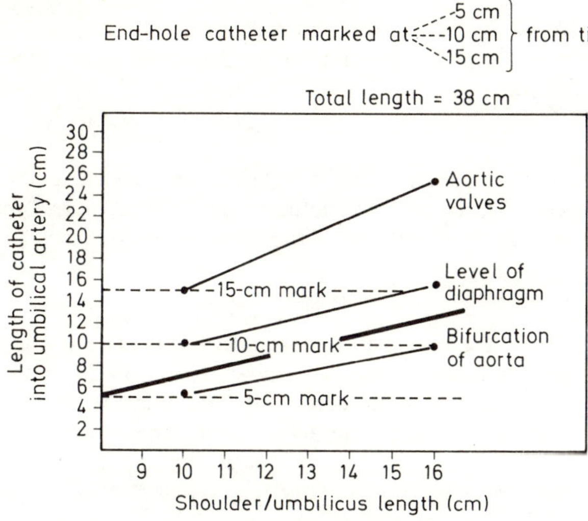

Figure 89.1. An umbilical artery catheterization guide is shown. The heavy black line indicates location of the tip of the catheter. Shoulder/umbilicus length is measured and the length of catheter to be introduced into the artery is read from the graph. For example, if the infant's shoulder/umbilicus length is 12.5 cm, the catheter is introduced to the 10-cm mark in order to position the tip at the bifurcation of the aorta. (From Swyer, 1975, modified from Dunn, 1966. Reproduced by kind permission)

COMPLICATIONS

Care should be taken to maintain body temperature, preferably by an overhead heater. Umbilical catheters should be left in place for the least possible time, preferably not longer than 36 to 48 hours, because of the risk of infection or thrombosis round the catheter. For this reason, if the neonate only requires fluid, a peripheral vein should be used. If this cannot be done, a catheter should be inserted in the umbilical vein and pushed in until blood is obtained on gentle aspiration.

Venepuncture

INDICATIONS

To take blood for investigation, inject drugs or place an intravenous line.

Blood specimens

The older child
The procedure using the antecubital fossa is the same as for adults. An

unhurried explanation should be given before approaching with a needle and syringe. Masks are frightening as well as unnecessary.

EQUIPMENT
A clean procedure, 5- or 10 ml syringe, 20–23-in × 1-in needle and specimen containers.

PROCEDURE
The venous return is obstructed by a cuff or an encircling hand. Care should be taken to have correct containers on hand as many laboratory procedures are rendered useless if the blood clots.

Infants

In small children, the external jugular vein is easier to use especially with a 21 or 23 butterfly needle, (*see Figure 89.2*). The vein is superficial and should be punctured as it runs over the sternomastoid. Deep punctures risk striking the apex of the lung.

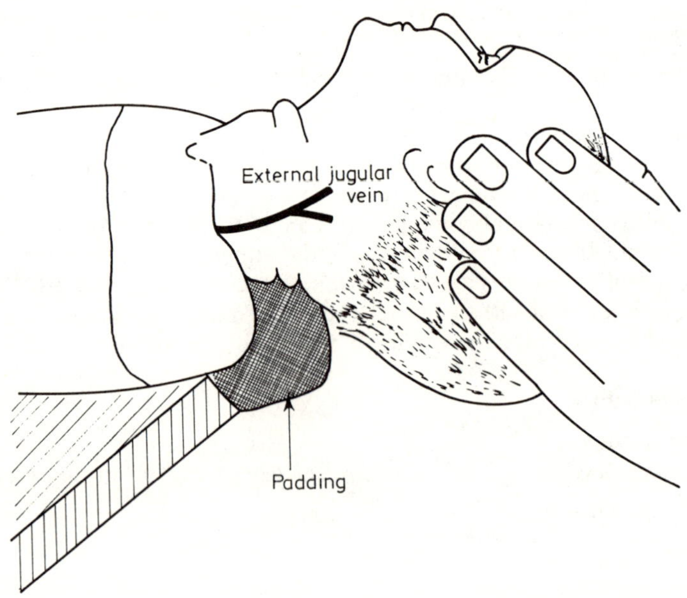

Figure 89.2. Venepuncture using the external jugular vein

Other sites

Blood may also be taken from the dorsum of the hands or feet and from the scalp veins. Puncture of the femoral vein should be avoided as it risks spasm of the femoral artery and injury or infection of the hip joint, producing aseptic necrosis of the femoral head or a septic arthritis. If femoral-vein puncture is necessary, the vein is found just medial to the artery and is best approached with the leg slightly flexed and abducted at the hips. In infants, the antecubital fossa is rarely considered, but the veins are often easily palpable, particularly in the pre-term or small-for-dates infant with little subcutaneous fat. It is essential that the infant is firmly held on a firm surface at a convenient height for the operator. The arm is fully extended by placing a folded towel under the elbow. The assistant holds the infant's palm flat to restrain movement of pronation and supination. The upper arm is occluded by firm pressure which need only be sufficient to obstruct the venous return. If the arm is held too tightly arterial flow is obstructed and venous distension will be reduced.

Scalp-vein technique

In neonates and infants, the scalp veins are easiest to use.

EQUIPMENT
Clean procedure, 21, 23 or 25 gauge butterfly needle, either strips of plaster of Paris or non-irritant strips of surgical tape. A large rubber band, intravenous tubing, paediatric chamber, intravenous fluids.

TECHNIQUE
The tubing should be primed with the infusing fluid before beginning. The infant may be restrained by a sheet, and the hands restrained by tube gauze with one end placed over the wrist, and held by tape, and the other end tied to the cot sides. A rubber band is placed around the head to obstruct the veins. Alternatively, the vein can be compressed with the finger. The frontal veins are particularly useful as the needle is less likely to be dislodged by movements of the head. The area is prepared with antiseptic. After insertion, needles are fixed either by plaster of Paris strips, or by surgical tape. Drip tubing should also be fixed at the side of the head so that an accidental sharp movement will not dislodge the needle. Accidental insertion of a needle into a scalp artery may cause distal skin necrosis. If this is suspected, the needle should be removed from the artery.

Older children

Clean procedure; 21, 23 or 25 butterfly needle, surgical tape, splints for the arms or legs, crêpe bandage, infusing fluid, paediatric chamber and drip tubing as before.

PROCEDURE
There are suitable veins on the dorsum of the hands, feet or forearm. Butterfly needles are preferable to plastic cannulae in most instances because of the ease of insertion, less pain and less long-term damage to veins. Packed cells can usually be run through a 23-gauge butterfly needle, and plasma can be run through a 25-gauge butterfly needle. Plastic cannulae if used, are more easily placed in the antecubital fossa, the anatomical 'snuff box' or the long saphenous vein in front of the ankle. The needle and tubing should be firmly fixed with surgical tape before splinting the limb lightly with a crêpe bandage.

Intravenous cut-down

INDICATION
A cut-down to a vein may be necessary in an emergency when peripheral veins are collapsed or cannot be found. The long saphenous vein is most easily approached but an arm vein gives the added advantage of being able to record central venous pressure (CVP).

EQUIPMENT
Sterile procedure, scalpel, two 10-cm (4-in) lengths of 00 catgut, 0000 catgut sutures, suture forceps, a pair of small scissors and three artery forceps. Local anaesthetic is required if the patient is conscious, preferably 1 per cent lignocaine without adrenaline.

PROCEDURE
The long saphenous vein is found most easily 1 to 2 cm ($\frac{1}{2}$–$\frac{3}{4}$ in) in front of the medial malleolus of the ankle. A horizontal incision 2 to 3 cm (1 in) long is made in front of the medial malleolus. The subcutaneous tissues are opened longitudinally with a pair of artery forceps or blunt scissors until the vein is exposed. Two 00 catgut threads are passed under the vein. One thread is used to tie off the distal end of the vein and the other to stretch the upper part of the vein. With fine scissors, the vein is cut halfway through at 45° towards the groin. The plastic cannula (5 or 8F) is inserted in the vein, care being taken not to strip the intima from the media. The upper thread is tied round the cannula and vein and the wound is sutured loosely. A cut-down in the arm is made anterior to the medial epicondyle, or across the front of the antecubital fossa, and the vein is cannulated in the same way as the saphenous vein; the tip of the catheter should be in the superior vena cava or the right atrium and its position should be checked by x-ray.

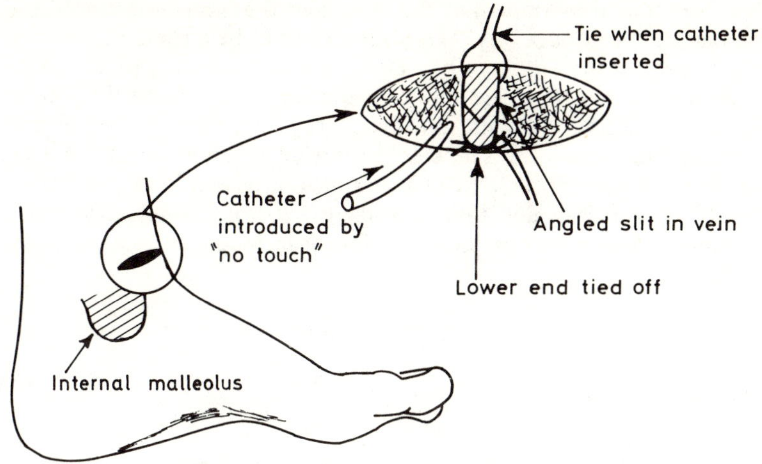

Figure 89.3. Cut-down to long saphenous vein

For CVP monitoring a three-way tap is inserted in the line and connected to a section of vertical glass tubing with a scale attached, ranging from -10 cm to $+15$ cm. Zero is set at a level of the manubrium sterni, and for reading the CVP the glass manometer is first primed with infusing fluid to $+15$ cm. The manometer is then connected to the patient and the CVP read from the scale. If the equipment is working correctly, the top of the column of fluid in the manometer reflects the respiratory cycle. The normal CVP is between $+5$ and $+10$ cm of water or saline. In an emergency, catheters may also be placed in other sites, using an intravenous needle and cannula. Possible sites are the right subclavian vein and the right internal jugular vein. The right subclavian vein is approached through the first intercostal space at the midclavicular point with the point of the needle aimed at the base of the sternal notch.

The internal jugular is approached between the two heads of the sternomastoid directed downwards and posteriorly. With both procedures there is a major risk of creating pneumothorax and of not being able to control bleeding on removal of the catheter. Introduction of infection or thrombosis of a major vein may occur and full aseptic technique should be used in the placement of catheters here.

Intravenous drugs
(*See also* Appendices 11, 12)

These may be injected into intravenous tubing or placed in the infusing chamber. It is important that the drug and the infusing solution are compatible (Appendix 12). There should never be a toxic quantity of drug in the chamber at any time. Drugs which are locally toxic should never be injected into a line which is not running satisfactorily. This is particularly important with cytotoxic drugs, calcium gluconate and hyperosmolar solutions. The sterile infusing solution should first be seen to run easily through the drip and then be used to clear the drip at the end of the drug injection. *See* page 790 for use of intravenous antibiotics; *see also* Appendix 11 for drug incompatibilities in IV fluids.

Arterial puncture

INDICATION
Arterial blood for estimation of blood gases or occasionally insertion of a cannula for blood oxygen or blood-pressure monitoring.

EQUIPMENT

Arterial sampling

Clean procedure; glass syringe 23 × 1 in needle, heparin solution.

Catheter insertion

Sterile procedure; intravenous cannula and needle, infusion solution and tubing, infusion pump.

PROCEDURE
Arterial sampling

The glass syringe is primed with heparin (5000 units per ml) by drawing a small quantity into the syringe and then expelling it, leaving a small amount of heparin in the needle. Local anaesthetic should be used throughout the procedure, although it may make palpation difficult.

(*a*) *Radial artery*　The radial artery is palpated between the index and middle fingers and the needle is inserted between them at an angle of 45° pointing towards the shoulder. When the artery is entered, blood will flow spontaneously into the glass syringe. If the plunger is withdrawn, there may be confusion between an arterial or venous source. When a sample has been withdrawn, the needle is removed and the site is compressed for 3 to 5 minutes. The site should be checked later for bleeding or distal ischaemia.

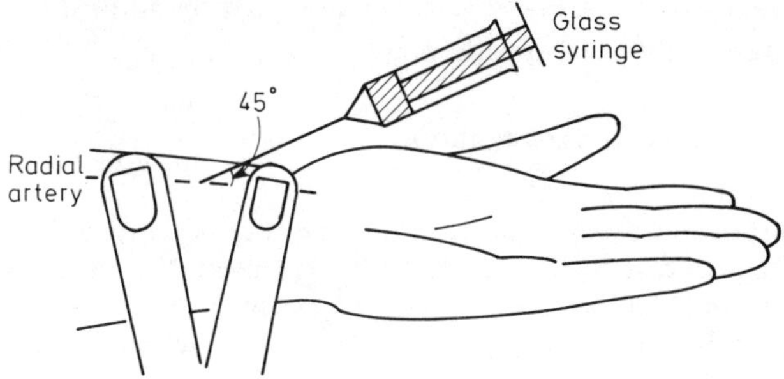

Figure 89.4. Radial artery puncture

(*b*) *Other sites*   These include femoral artery, temporal, brachial and dorsalis pedis arteries.

Catheter placement

A similar approach is used except that on obtaining arterial blood, the plastic sheath of the needle is advanced along the artery and the needle is withdrawn. Pressure should be maintained proximal to the cannula until the tubing is connected.

CONTRA-INDICATION
Arterial puncture should not be done if there is a coagulation disorder.

COMPLICATION
With catheter insertion, there is a risk of thrombosis or infection.

Aspiration of body cavities

With the exception of bladder aspiration (antiseptic procedure) these are usually sterile procedures requiring surgical gloves and drapes.

Aspiration of the chest

All procedures involving chest aspiration risk creating a pneumothorax and intrapulmonary haemorrhage. Local anaesthetic should be used. The chest should be examined clinically and x-rayed after the aspiration.

INDICATIONS
The diagnosis or treatment of intrapleural air, or effusion, pleural

z ⊦

biopsy or lung aspiration. The same approach is used for diagnostic procedures as for theraupeutic ones.

Aspiration of air in pneumothorax

EQUIPMENT
Sterile procedure, needle and catheter, underwater drain and seal. In an emergency intravenous cannulae may be used but these have the disadvantage of having a single-end hole and are too malleable. Suitable drainage catheters are of large bore, are stiff and have a number of side holes.

PROCEDURE
The needle should be inserted either through the second intercostal space in the midclavicular line, or in the 2nd or 3rd space posteriorly, medial to the border of the scapula. The catheter is connected to the underwater drain. Suction pumps should be avoided, and should not be used if air is unable to escape when the pump is not is use. Water in the drainage tubing should rise and fall with respiration. Absence of this movement indicates a probable block.

Pleural effusion (pus, blood, chyle, etc.)

EQUIPMENT
Sterile procedure, 30-ml syringe, three-way valve, $22 \times 1\frac{1}{2}$ in needle. If a pleural biopsy is required a Franklin–Silverman or Abrams needle will be required.

PROCEDURE
The needle is inserted in the lower chest where fluid has been demonstrated radiologically and at the highest space where the percussion note is still dull. This will usually be the lateral or posterior chest in the 6th to 9th intercostal spaces. A three-way tap is inserted between the syringe and the needle so that large effusions can be aspirated slowly and expelled from a side-arm without disconnecting the needle. Fluid should be sent for culture (including tubercle bacilli) cell count and cytology. If a pleural biopsy is required this should be done only when there is an effusion present. An Abrams needle is safer than a Franklin–Silverman needle.

COMPLICATIONS
If fluid is aspirated too rapidly there may be a mediasternal shift which is usually indicated by a hoarse cough. The aspiration procedure should be stopped temporarily. Pleural tears may be caused by inexperienced use of pleural biopsy needles.

Aspiration of the lung

INDICATION

When persistent consolidation is not responsive to normal therapy. The procedure is rarely indicated but may be necessary to establish a diagnosis, particularly if there is a possibility of pneumocystis infection.

EQUIPMENT

Sterile procedure, $2\frac{1}{2} \times 22$ in needle, syringe, sterile normal saline.

PROCEDURE

The aspiration procedure should be done as quickly as possible during one respiratory cycle. Good preparation including sedation is therefore essential. The needle is inserted in the area of lung thought to be suspicious radiologically. Sterile saline 1 to 2 ml is injected, provided aspiration has not drawn blood, and is then re-aspirated immediately. The needle is withdrawn and the aspiration fluid sent for culture, including tubercle bacilli. Special stains are necessary to demonstrate the presence of *Pneumocystis carinii*.

Pericardial aspiration

See section on Cardiac Emergencies, p. 296.

Peritoneal aspiration

INDICATIONS

To determine the nature of unexplained intraperitoneal fluid or to relieve tense ascites.

EQUIPMENT

Sterile procedure, 20-ml syringe, $22 \times 1\frac{1}{2}$ in needle, trocar and cannula if indicated.

PROCEDURE

If the effusion is large, it may be convenient to use a trocar and cannula under local anaesthetic, especially if large quantities of fluid are to be removed. Otherwise a $20 \times 1\frac{1}{2}$ in needle is inserted, with a 20-ml syringe attached, into either the right or left iliac fossa.

The fluid is aspirated and should be sent for cells, cytology and culture, including tubercle bacilli. For a trocar, a small incision is made in the skin under local anaesthetic. After completing the procedure, a butterfly tape or single suture is used to close the wound. Continuing leak of fluid may require careful re-suturing.

COMPLICATIONS
Particularly with trocar and cannula, there is a risk of puncture of the bowel.

Aspiration of the bladder

INDICATION
Definitive diagnosis of a urinary-tract infection when bag urines have been equivocal, especially in the newborn.

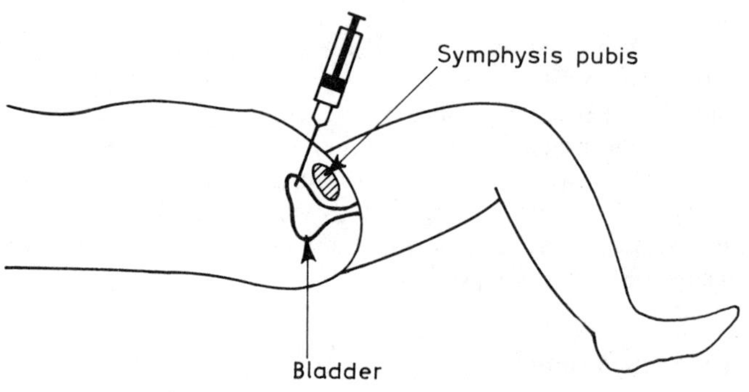

Figure 89.5. Bladder puncture

EQUIPMENT
Aseptic procedure, $22 \times 1\frac{1}{2}$ in needle, 10-ml syringe, cleaning solution and swabs.

PROCEDURE
If there is time, liberal or extra fluids should be given 1 to 2 hours before the puncture. The direction of insertion of the needle varies with age, as the bladder is an abdominal organ in infancy and a pelvic organ in the older child. In a neonate, the needle is inserted 1 cm ($\frac{1}{2}$ in) above the symphysis pubis in the midline and directed at 45° upwards. It is pushed in to a depth of 1 to 2.5 cm ($\frac{1}{2}$ to 1 in). In the older child, the needle is inserted just above the symphysis pubis inclined at 45° towards the pelvis and pushed in for 4 cm ($1\frac{1}{2}$ in) before aspirating. If no urine is aspirated, the procedure should be repeated once and if no urine is aspirated the procedure should be delayed until the patient has had further fluids.

COMPLICATION
There is often some haematuria afterwards but this should clear rapidly.

The bowel may be punctured and the urine contaminated with faeces. There is no danger to the child as the bowel appears to withstand this insult well but the urine sample is useless.

References

Dunn, P.M. (1966). Locality of the umbilical catheter in post-mortem measurement. *Archs Dis. Childh.* **41**, 69
Swyer, P.R. (1975). *The Intensive Care of the Newly Born.* p. 188. Basle: S. Karger

CHAPTER 90

Lumbar Puncture

J. A. Black

The technique in the older child is too well known to need description, but there are a number of difficulties in doing a lumbar puncture in the newborn infant.

Indications in acute conditions at any age

Diagnostic confirmation of meningitis, intracranial haemorrhage, encephalitis.

Lumbar puncture in the newborn

EQUIPMENT

A sterile procedure; stiletted spinal needles approximately 4 to 5 cm ($1\frac{1}{2}$–2 in) in length are suitable but No. 21 to 23 disposable injection needles or butterfly scalp-vein needles without stilettes are preferred by some (Greensher *et al*, 1971). In addition an antibiotic for intrathecal injection should be prepared beforehand if purulent fluid is expected. The ordinary manometer sets should not be used in the newborn, but the tubing attached to a butterfly scalp-vein set may be used instead. To remove fluid the tubing is simply lowered to allow it to drip out, or a sealed section of tubing containing fluid may be sent for analysis.

PROCEDURE

The same landmarks should be used as in other age groups, but failure to obtain fluid is not uncommon; a good flow of fluid can however sometimes be obtained by repeating the tap one space higher up.

The advantage of a needle without a stilette is that fluid is apparent as soon as the tip of the needle is in the right place, whereas the repeated removal and re-insertion of a stilette may cause displacement of the needle. With an acutely bevelled needle (as in scalp-vein or injection needles) the danger of introducing a piece of skin into the subarachnoid space is minimal.

Particularly in the newborn, the point of the needle is liable to slide off the interspinous ligament if the bevel is pointing towards the head.

A more satisfactory method is to maintain the bevel pointing laterally, which also reduces the possibility of cutting any spinal roots. If the flow is unsatisfactory after insertion, the needle should be rotated until the optimal flow is obtained.

If no flow is obtained with the needle correctly placed, the infant should be supported in the sitting position since low pressure may prevent an adequate flow of fluid in the usual lateral position. If thickly purulent fluid is expected but no fluid is obtained, gentle aspiration is safe.

Contra-indications (all ages)

(a) *Absolute contra-indications*

   (i) If there is evidence of 'coning' or brain herniation (neurological signs indicating compression from descent of the medulla into the foramen magnum or mid-brain compression from herniation through the tentorium), or if there are signs of incipient herniation (*see below*). Removal of fluid in these situations may cause irreversible medullary or mid-brain damage. PAPILLOE-DEMA IS PRESENT ONLY IN 50 PER CENT OF CASES WITH RAISED INTRACRANIAL PRESSURE (Brown, Ingram and Seshia, 1973).
   (ii) In the presence of a spinal block which is thought to be due to a tumour, removal of fluid from below the tumour may cause a paraplegia.

(b) *Relative contra-indications*

If it is absolutely essential to obtain lumbar CSF in the presence of known or suspected raised pressure, special precautions must be taken (*see below*).

Clinical signs of medullary or mid-brain compression due to herniation

   (a) The danger signs of early herniation, which are really those of incipient decerebrate or decorticate rigidity are as follows (Brown, Ingram and Seshia, 1973; Brown and Habel, 1975).
   Neck retraction.
   Squint.

Lessening of consciousness.

Cycling movements of the legs or 'dog-paddling' movement of the arms.*

Exaggeration of the tonic neck reflex.

Perez' reflex (extension of the spine, flexion of the legs and extension of the head on pressure on the dorsal spine).*

Trunk incurvation reflex.

Irregularities of respiration; tachypnoea or slowed respiration; Cheyne–Stokes respiration; laryngeal stridor.

(b) The signs of established herniation may be:

(i) Tonic decerebrate rigidity; extensor rigidity of the legs and inversion of the feet, extension at the elbows and pronation of the forearms. The wrists and fingers are flexed and the thumb is held across the palm.

or (ii) Decorticate rigidity; there is semi-flexion with adduction and internal rotation of the shoulders; the elbows are semi-flexed and the wrists and fingers are flexed.

In both states the abnormalities of respiration described above persist or become more marked. Slowing of respiration is more likely in foramen magnum herniation and hyperventilation or Cheyne–Stokes respiration in tentorial herniation (Brown and Habel 1975; Brown, 1976).

Lumbar puncture in the presence of known or suspected raised pressure

(a) This should be done only if there is no neurological evidence of brain herniation (*see above*).

(b) If a specimen of *lumbar* CSF is absolutely essential for diagnosis in spite of known or probable raised pressure, the following precautions should be taken (Brown, 1976).

(i) The procedure should be done gently, using a fine needle.

(ii) Preliminary sedation should be used; if it is done with a screaming, struggling child the risk of brain herniation is increased.

(iii) A syringe containing 1 to 2 ml of 0.9 per cent NaCl (without glucose) should be available to inject back into the theca if the pressure is very high or if there is a cardiorespiratory arrest or the sudden development of neurological signs of herniation.

(iv) Facilities for giving IV mannitol should be immediately available for use if evidence of herniation develops during or immediately after the lumbar puncture.

* May be absent in established hypertonus

(v) The stilette should be replaced after every 2 drops of CSF and 30 seconds should elapse before the removal of the next 2 drops. The stilette should always be removed slowly and on no account should the fluid be allowed to spurt out.

(vi) The minimum amount of CSF should be removed which is compatible with adéquate investigation.

(vii) Pressure measurements and the Queckenstedt manoeuvre should NOT be performed.

(c) If the examination of lumbar CSF is not absolutely essential diagnostically, other methods should be used to reach a diagnosis, or cortical subarachnoid or ventricular fluid should be examined after a tap through the anterior fontanelle or a burrhole. However it should be recognized that these fluids do not necessarily represent changes in the lumbar fluid, particularly in meningitis. If there is cerebral oedema the lateral ventricles may be obliterated and impossible to find.

Examination of CSF in patients with neurological evidence of brain herniation

(a) NEVER DO A LUMBAR PUNCTURE UNTIL THE INTRACRANIAL PRESSURE HAS BEEN REDUCED (*see below*) AND ALL NEUROLOGICAL SIGNS OF HERNIATION HAVE DISAPPEARED.

(b) The presence of neurological signs of herniation is more significant than papilloedema which may be absent.

(c) The intracranial pressure should be reduced by the following:

(i) 20 per cent Mannitol should be given IV over 20 to 30 minutes in a dose of 5 to 7 ml per kg (Brown and Habel, 1975).

(ii) Dexamethasone should be given IV or i.m. in a dose of 2 mg if under 1 year every 4 hours, and 4 to 6 mg at 4- to 6-hourly intervals if over 1 year.

(iii) If (i) and (ii) are unsuccessful a ventricular tap should be attempted through the anterior fontanelle or a burrhole, and 5 to 10 ml of fluid should be removed initially (*see* (c) *above*).

(iv) If (i), (ii) and (iii) are unsuccessful, hyperventilation with IPPV should be started.

(v) After reduction of the pressure, fluids should be restricted to 50 to 75 per cent of the normal requirements and electrolyte-free fluids should be avoided.

(d) Fluid for examination may be available from a ventricular tap (*see above*).

(e) Only when there is NO LONGER any evidence of brain herniation is it safe to do a lumbar puncture using the special precautions described above.

Lumbar puncture done in error in the presence of established brain herniation

(a) This may occur because:
  (i) Decerebrate or decorticate rigidity is mistaken for the neck
  and back stiffness of meningitis.
  (ii) The obtaining of lumbar CSF is *mistakenly* regarded as the
  first essential if meningitis is suspected in the presence of
  signs of brain herniation (*see also* page 359 for management of acute bacterial meningitis)
(b) In these circumstances the lumbar CSF pressure may be very
high or very low. If it is very low, this probably indicates
established 'plugging' of the foramen magnum by the medulla.
(c) As soon as the true situation is realized, immediate attempts
should be made to reduce the intracranial pressure and reverse
the herniation (*see above*, page 729).

Brain herniation precipitated by lumbar puncture

(a) This may occur during lumbar puncture, with the needle still *in
situ,* or a few mintutes or hours after the puncture.
(b) The indications that brain herniation has occurred are:
  (i) Sudden cardiorespiratory arrest (*see also under* Complications of lumbar puncture *below*)
  (ii) Development of neurological signs of mid-brain or medullary herniation (*see above*).
(c) If herniation occurs while the needle is still *in situ:*
  (i) 1 to 2 ml of 0.9 per cent NaCl should be injected into the
  theca.
  (ii) The child should be held upside-down.
  (iii) If the anterior fontanelle is open, a ventricular tap should be
  attempted, and 5 to 10 ml of fluid should be removed
  initially.
  (iv) If (i), (ii) and (iii) are unsuccessful, artificial ventilation and
  resuscitation should be started if there is cardiorespiratory
  arrest, with the other measures to reduce the pressure
  described above.
(d) If evidence of herniation develops *after* the lumbar puncture, the
measures, described in (c) on page 729 should be started
immediately.

Complications of lumbar puncture

(a) Brain herniation or cardiorespiratory arrest (*see above*).

(b) Cardiorespiratory arrest without raised pressure: occasionally this occurs in a child who is not acutely ill. It is a more likely complication if the procedure is done in a child acutely ill from cardiac or respiratory disease. In such cases a lumbar puncture should only be done on very clear indications, and great care should be taken not to cause an increased respiratory obstruction during this procedure.

(c) Increase in spinal block (*see under* Contra-indications, *above*).

(d) Lumbar puncture headache. This is relatively uncommon in children, and seems to bear no relation to the CSF pressure or to the amount of CSF removed. The headache may be quite severe with neck stiffness, opisthotonus, and irritability, and may last up to 5 days. The usual treatment is to keep the child lying flat, to give liberal fluids and analgesics as required. A second lumbar puncture may exacerbate the symptoms and should only be done if there is a definite possibility of meningitis which was not apparent at the first tap (*see below*).

(e) Other complications are:

    (i) Traumatic haemorrhage: this may confuse the picture at subsequent examination of the CSF, since red cells, xanthochromia (yellow colour from bilirubin derived from lysed red cells) and a slightly increased protein and cell count may all occur (*see also* page 348).

    (ii) Introduction of infection: this is rare except when the needle has to be introduced through an infected area, as in extensive burns.

    (iii) Development of meningitis after a lumbar puncture done during a septicaemia (Fischer *et al.*, 1975); this may be due to a natural progression of the disease or to the introduction of infected traumatic blood into the CSF.

    (iv) The seeding of leukaemic cells into the CSF during a lumbar puncture during an active phase ('blast' cells in the peripheral blood) of leukaemia.

    (v) Vertebral osteomyelitis.

    (vi) Puncture of an intervertebral disc causing acute localized back pain for a few days.

    (vii) Unexpected finding of a raised pressure at lumbar puncture. The child should be observed at 15-minute intervals for at least 6 hours after the puncture and the respiration rate should be counted and recorded for a complete minute (Brown, 1976). The development of *any* evidence of brain herniation requires immediate treatment, as described above.

References

Brown, J.K. (1976). Lumbar puncture and its hazards. *Devl. Med. Child Neurol.* **18**, 803

Brown, J.K. and Habel, A.H. (1975). Toxic encephalopathy and acute brain swelling in children. *Devl. Med. Child Neurol.* **17**, 659

Brown, J.K., Ingram, J.T.S. and Seshia, S.S. (1973). Patterns of decerebration in infants and children. *J. Neurol., Neurosurg.* **36**, 431

Fischer, G.W., Brenz, R.W., Alden, E.R. and Beckwith, J.B. (1975). Lumbar punctures and meningitis. *Am. J. Dis. Child.,* **129**, 590

Greensher, J., Mofenson, H.C. Borofsky, L.G. and Sharma R. (1971). Lumbar puncture in the neonate; a simplified technique. *J. Pediat.* **78**, 1034

CHAPTER 91

The Nervous System

Ian Shellshear

Subdural taps

See section on Neurological Emergencies (pp. 312, 363).

Ventricular tap

INDICATION
Investigation of an enlarging head or the diagnosis of ventriculitis.

EQUIPMENT
Sterile procedure, otherwise as for lumbar puncture using an 8-cm ($3\frac{1}{2}$-in) stiletted needle.

PROCEDURE
The child should be supine with the head resting to one side. The skin over the anterior fontanelle should be shaved and prepared with antiseptic solution. The needle is inserted in the lateral angle of the fontanelle 1 to 2 cm ($\frac{1}{2}-\frac{3}{4}$ in) from the mid-line. The needle is angled slightly anteriorly and parallel to the falx cerebri. The stilette is withdrawn every 0.5 cm ($\frac{1}{4}$ in) until fluid is obtained. This will give an indication of cortical thickness. The pressure is recorded with a glass manometer and CSF is taken for examination. The procedure may be supplemented by replacing 20 ml of CSF with 20 ml of air followed by x-rays to determine the extent of the hydrocephalus.

COMPLICATIONS
If the cerebrospinal fluid pressure is raised, this may cause dilatation of the needle track and creation of porencephalic cysts. Intracerebral bleeding may be produced or infection introduced.

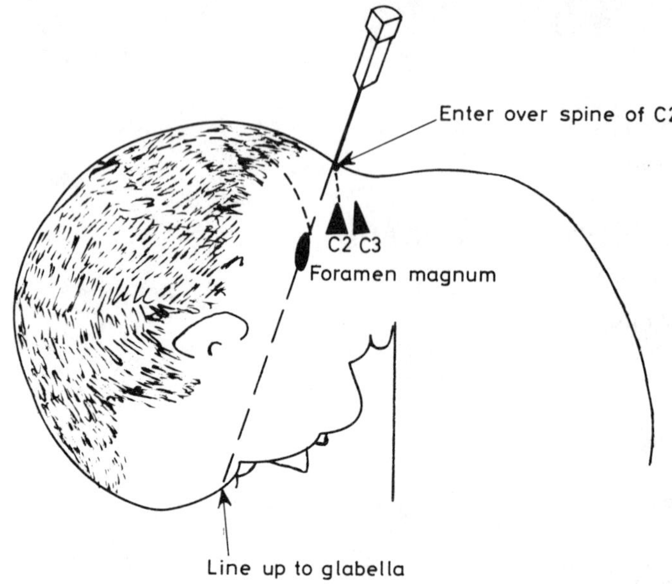

Figure 91.1. Cisternal tap

Cisternal tap

INDICATIONS
Where CSF cannot be obtained from the lumbar space because of a spinal block. This is a potentially dangerous procedure with the risk of damage to the medulla in addition to the risk of coning in the presence of raised intracranial pressure.

EQUIPMENT
Sterile procedure, 3 to 4 cm ($1-1\frac{1}{2}$ in) spinal needle, otherwise as for a lumbar puncture.

PROCEDURE
The patient should be sitting with the head slightly flexed. The back of the neck is shaved and prepared with an antiseptic solution. The needle is inserted over the spine of C2 and angled anteriorly towards the glabella in the mid-line. The needle should strike the posterior edge of the foramen magnum. The needle is then pulled back, then angled down slightly until the posterior edge of the foramen magnum is just cleared. A definite click is usually felt as the dura is penetrated, but this is not always so. The stilette is withdrawn every few millimetres until CSF

flows spontaneously. Fluid should never be aspirated as the tip of the needle is within millimetres of vital centres in the medulla.

COMPLICATIONS

Haemorrhage, introduction of infection, coning or puncture of the medulla.

Part XIX: Appendices

Weight, Height and Surface Area

(*See also* Appendix 8)

Weight has the advantage that it can be easily and accurately measured, but as a basis for calculation of dosage over the whole age range from infancy to adolescence it is unsatisfactory.

For example:

A 10-kg infant might be expected to require $\frac{1}{7}$ of the dose of a 70-kg adult, but this would be quite inadequate. In practice the correct amount would usually be about $\frac{1}{4}$ of the adult dose.

Surface area gives a more satisfactory basis for calculation, except in the neonatal period where a weight-based scale is preferable. This is because of the wide range of weights which are encountered over a narrow age range; and because surface area calculations are inaccurate in small infants, due to unsatisfactory data and the difficulty in measuring the infant's length.

Difficulties in the use of weights

(a) *Circumstances which prevent the child from being weighed*

These may arise because the child is too ill, is in a plaster cast or orthopaedic appliance, or because of refusal to be weighed. This difficulty can be got over in a number of ways.

   (i) The parents may have recent records of the child's weight; but only actual records should be accepted.

  (ii) The weight can be obtained from any standard series of figures giving weight-for-age. Before doing this it is necessary to confirm that the child is of average height, is not wasted and is of normal proportions.

 (iii) If the height can be measured the weight can be read off a height and weight curve obtained from normal children (*Figure A1.1*).

(b) *Excessively fat children*

For children above the 97th centile for weight the actual weight should not be used as a basis for calculation of drug dosage or surface area, since fat is relatively inactive metabolically and does not influence fluid

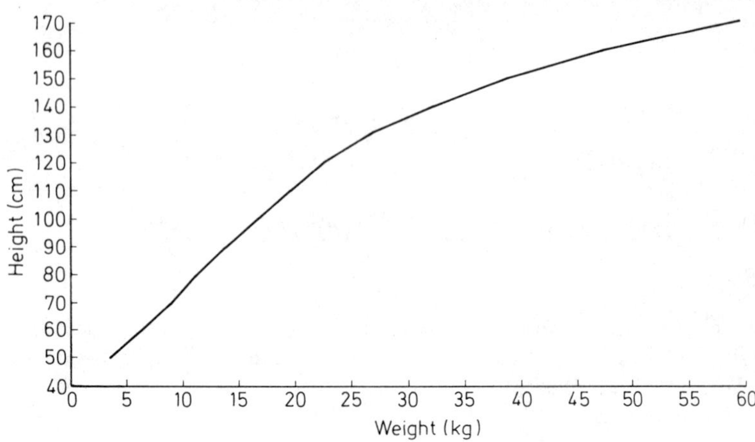

Figure A1.1 Weight-for-height. (Data from Tanner and Whitehouse charts using means of 50th centiles for boys and girls)

requirements or urine flow. In such circumstances the 'ideal' weight should be obtained from a height–weight chart, or from the standard centile charts, taking the same point on the weight chart as is shown by plotting the height.

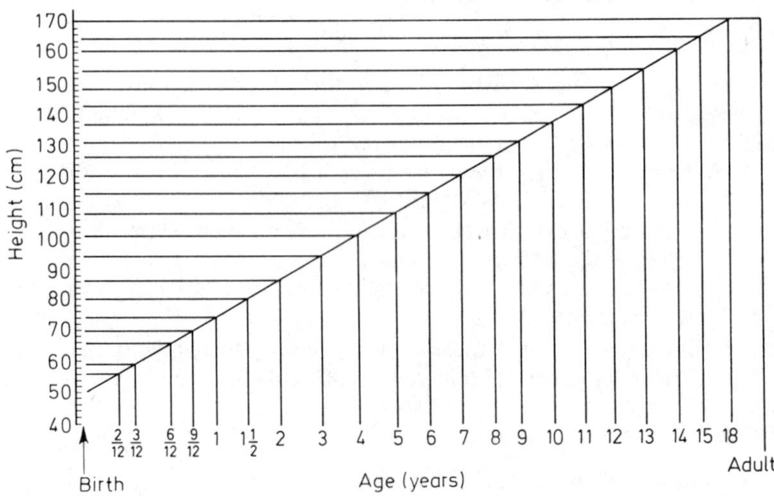

Figure A1.2. Height-for-age. 50th centiles means for boys and girls. (After Tanner, Whitehouse and Takaishi, 1966)

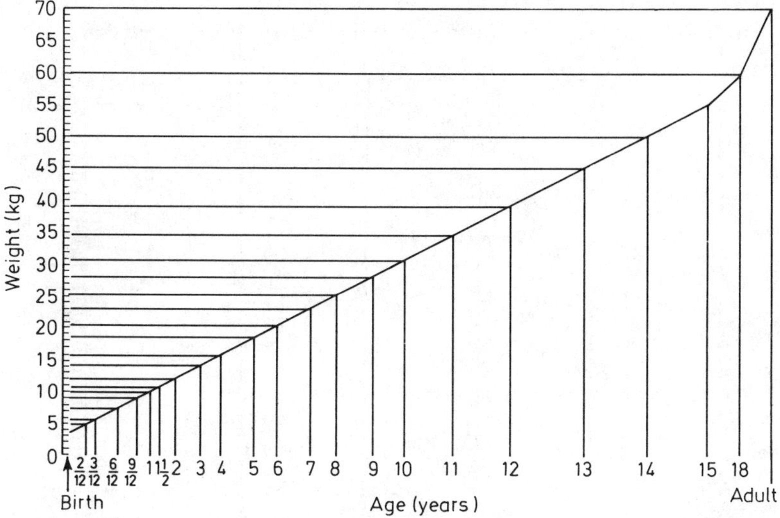

Figure A1.3. Weight-for-age. 50th centiles: means for boys and girls. (After Tanner, Whitehouse and Takaishi, 1966)

Determination of surface area (SA)

Both weight and height must be measured accurately, otherwise gross errors will occur. The standard nomograms can be used provided that the child has normal bodily proportions. Many of the published nomograms have a very compressed scale and can produce considerable errors if used carelessly. The nomograms given in *Figure A1.4* are the clearest available.

Though there are systems for calculating metabolic rate and fluid requirements using SA they are not wholly satisfactory. However SA is well suited for the calculation of drug dosage (p. 766) and for urine output (p. 754).

Calculation of surface area by formulae

(a) Costeff's (1966) formula can be used if a nomogram is not available or only the weight can be used.

$$SA, m^2 = \frac{4W + 7}{W + 90} : (W = weight, kg)$$

(b) Alternative method of calculating surface area (Vaughan, 1975).

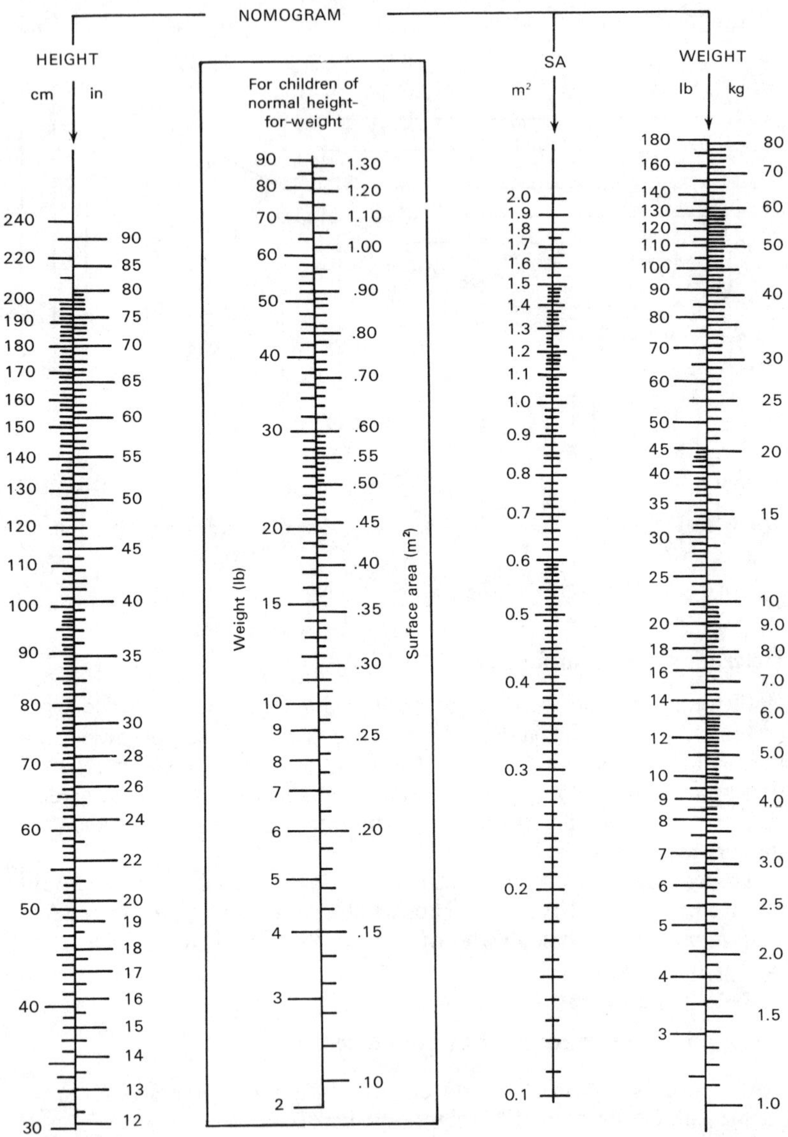

Figure A1.4. West nomogram for estimation of surface areas. The surface area is indicated where a straight line connecting the height and weight intersects the surface area (SA) column or, if the patient is roughly of normal proportion, from the weight alone (enclosed area). (Nomogram modified from data of E. Boyd by C. D. West. From Shirkey, 1975)

Weight range	Approximate SA (m^2)
1– 5 kg	$m^2 = 0.05 \times W^* + 0.05$
6–10 kg	$m^2 = 0.04 \times W + 0.10$
11–20 kg	$m^2 = 0.03 \times W + 0.20$
21–70 kg	$m^2 = 0.02 \times W + 0.40$

* W = weight (kg)

References

Costeff, H. (1966). A simple empirical formula for calculating approximate surface area in children. *Archs Dis. Childh.* **41**, 681

Shirkey, H. C. (1975). In *Pediatric Therapy*. Ed. H. C. Shirkey. 5th edn. p. 26. St. Louis: C. V. Mosby

Tanner, J. M., Whitehouse, R. H. and Takaishi, M. (1966). *Archs Dis. Childh.* **41**, 454

Vaughan, V. C. (1975). In *Textbook of Pediatrics*. Eds V. C. Vaughan and R. J. McKay. 10th edn. p. 37. London: W. B. Saunders

Metabolic (Energy) Requirements

The metabolic requirements can be considered under three headings:

(a) REQUIREMENT FOR NORMAL ACTIVITY
This figure should be used for calculating diets for diabetic children and other ambulant patients and for checking the adequacy of diets in general (*Figure A2.1* and Table A2.I).

(b) THE BASAL REQUIREMENT
This has little clinical significance but is sometimes used as a basis for calculating fluid requirements; it is approximately 50 per cent of (a).

(c) REQUIREMENTS FOR PATIENTS IN HOSPITAL
For infants under one year this can be assumed to be the same as (a). For all other ages the requirement of the hospital patient is about midway between (a) and (b) and is therefore approximately 75 per cent of the requirement for normal activity. Holliday and Segar (1957) have constructed a useful chart (*Figure A2.1*).

Rule of thumb calculation of normal requirement *

A commonly used method of calculation is to take the daily energy requirement at 1 year as 1000 kcalories (4200 joules) and to add 100 kcalories (420 joules) for each additional year (to 14 years) up to a maximum of 2500 kcalories (10 500 joules) for girls, and 2750 kcalories (11 500 joules) for boys. Calculations based upon surface area do not appear to have found general acceptance and are in any case probably unsuitable in infancy.

Example:
A 5-year-old child would require:
1000 + 400 kcalories = 1400 kcalories
4200 + 16 800 joules = 5880 joules

---

* The usual 'Calorie' in clinical medicine is actually a kilocalorie (kcalorie)
1 kcalorie (Calorie) = 4.2 joules

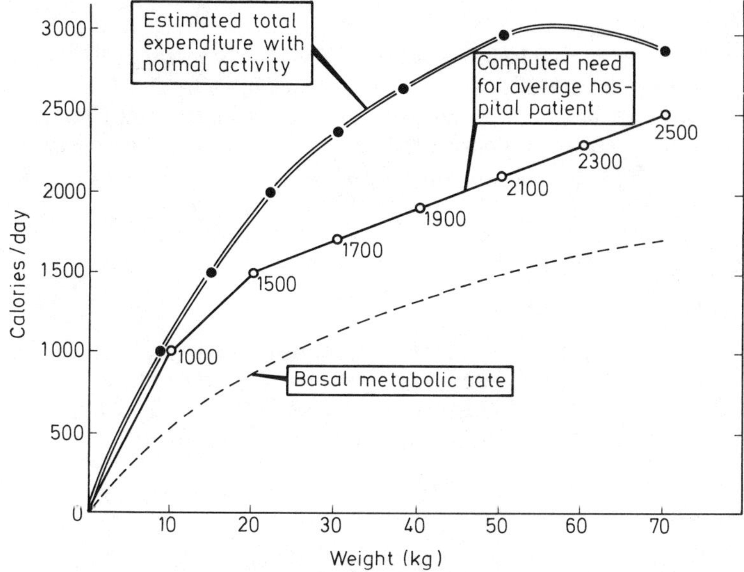

Figure A2.1. Comparison of energy expenditure in basal and ideal state. (The upper and lower lines were plotted from data of Talbot, 1949)

Weights at the 50th percentile level were selected for converting calories at various ages to calories related to weight. The computed line was derived from the following equations:

(1) 0–10 kg—100 cal/kg.
(2) 10–20 kg—1000 cal + 50 cal/kg for each kg over 10 kg
(3) 20 kg and over—1500 cal + 20 cal/kg for each kg over 20 kg

These figures compare reasonably well with those given in Table A2.I (data from Belton, 1978).

TABLE A2.I
Energy requirement for normal activity (: joules (kcalories))

Age	per 24 hours	per kg per 24 hours
0–6 months	—	462 (110)
7 months–1 year	—	420 (100)
1–3 years	5040 (1200)	378 (90)
4–6 years	6720 (1600)	336 (80)
7–10 years	8820 (2100)	294 (70)
11–14 years (girls)	10 500 (2500)	294 (70)
11–14 years (boys)	11 550 (2750)	294 (70)
Adults: males	13 600 (3000)	168–189 (40–45)

Factors which may raise or lower the energy requirement

Increased requirement.
- (a) The energy requirement increases by 12 per cent for every rise in body temperature of 1°C (approx. 2°F).
- (b) In hypermetabolic states such as thyrotoxicosis, salicylate poisoning and severe burns, the energy requirements are increased by 25 to 75 per cent; in very extensive burns (> 40 per cent surface area) the increased requirement may be as great as 100 per cent.

Decreased requirements

- (a) In hypothermia the energy requirement falls by 12 per cent for every fall of 1°C (approx. 2°F) of body temperature.
- (b) The energy requirement is presumably decreased in hypothyroidism but there do not appear to be precise figures available.

References

Belton, N. R. (1978). Biochemical and physiological tables and function tests. In *Textbook of Paediatrics*. 2nd Edn. p. 1724. Ed. J. O. Forfar and H. C. Arneil. Edinburgh and London: Churchill Livingstone

Holliday, M. A. and Segar, W. E. (1957). Water in parenteral fluid therapy. *Pediatrics* **19**, 824

Talbot, F. B. (1949). Basal metabolism in children. In *Brennemann's Practice of Paediatrics*. Ch. 22. Hagerstown, Maryland: W. F. Prior & Co. Inc.

Maintenance Water and Electrolyte Requirements

Water

This can be considered under two headings:

(a) Requirements on a normal diet

The fluid intake is normally left to the discretion of the individual but this does not apply to infants, or to other patients who are unable to obtain drinks independently. The intake of solutes (the solute load) determines the obligatory urine volume, which is the minimal volume of urine necessary to maintain homeostasis. On high solute loads both urine flow and water intake are therefore increased.

(b) Requirements on IV fluids

Excluding abnormal losses, the maintenance requirement of water is much less than on a normal diet, since the solute load is much less. Exceptions are severe burns and diabetic ketoacidosis in which there is a very high solute load and usually considerable additional water losses, especially in burns.

Water requirements according to age

Apart from the immediate postnatal period (first 7 to 10 days) the water intake is generally calculated on the basis of body weight, in a series of steps at different ages (Table A3.I). Surface area does not appear to be a very suitable basis for calculating water requirements, though a basis of 2500 ml per m^2 also may be used (Talbot, Richie and Crawford, 1959; Harris, 1972).

Electrolytes

For short-term maintenance requirements sodium and potassium only need be considered, in the absence of known depletion of other minerals

TABLE A3.I
Water requirement according to age

Age	Normal diet (ml per kg)	Maintenance IV fluids* (ml per kg)
0–7 days	up to 80–100	_1st 48 hours:_ $\frac{1}{3} \times$ 100 ml per kg (10% glucose)
		48 hours to 7 days: $\frac{2}{3} \times$ 100 ml per kg (10% glucose)
7 days to 6 months	125–150	100
6 months to 1 year	130–150	100
1–3 years	115–135	50
4–5 years	90–110	50
6–9 years	70– 90	20
10–12 years	60– 85	20
13–15 years	50– 65	20
Adult	40– 50	20

* The type of fluid depends upon the time after the operation (_see_ page 750)

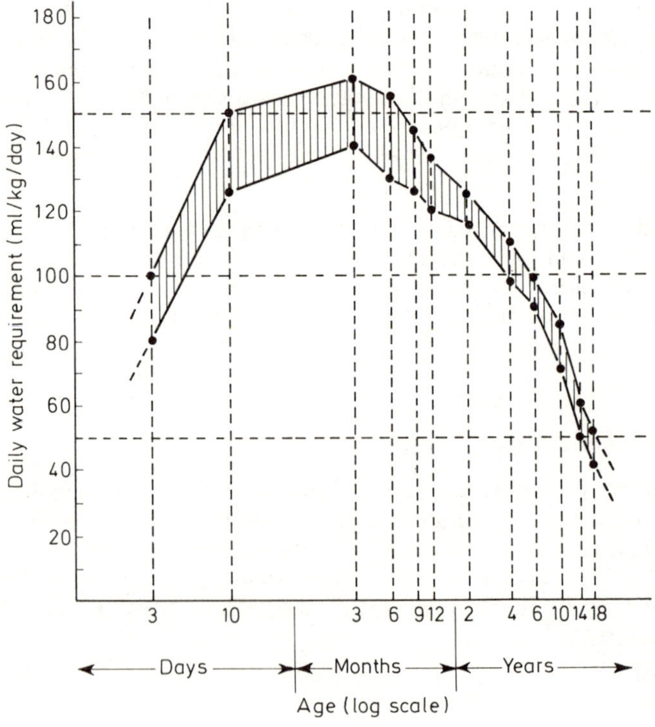

Figure A3.1. Approximate daily water intake at different ages. (Haycock, 1979. Reproduced by kind permission.)

such as magnesium (p. 147). The requirements of chloride are normally covered by the fact that electrolyte solutions are made up with sodium and potassium chloride.

Throughout the age range from infancy to 11 years it is safe to base calculations upon a requirement of:

Sodium: 2.0 mmol per kg (11 years onwards 1.5 mmol)

Potassium: 2.0 mmol per kg (11 years onwards 1.5 mmol)

Alternatively, sodium and potassium requirements can be considered as 50 mmol per m², for each cation (Harris, 1972).

Factors which may alter water and electrolyte requirements

Increased requirement

(a) Continued fluid losses by gastric suction, fistulae, vomiting, diarrhoea (water and electrolytes).
(b) Fever: the water requirement is increased by 12 per cent for every rise of 1°C (approximately 2°F).
(c) Renal disease with polyuria, (water ± sodium and potassium).
(d) Increased respiration rate (water).
(e) Phototherapy for neonatal jaundice (water) (*see* page 672).
(f) Radiant heat shields in the newborn (water).

Decreased requirements

(a) Continued postoperative antidiuresis and sodium retention (decreased requirement of water and sodium).
(b) Renal disease with oliguria.
(c) Absorption of water through the respiratory tract as droplets from a nebulizer.

References

Harris, F. (1972). *Paediatric Fluid Therapy*. p. 144. Oxford: Blackwell

Haycock, G. B. (1979). In *Paediatrics*. Ed. J. Apley. 2nd Edn. p. 416. London: Bailliere Tindall

Talbot, N. B., Richie, R. H. and Crawford, J. D. (1959). *Metabolic Homeostasis*. pp. x–xi. Harvard University Press

Water and Electrolyte Requirements in Paediatric Surgery, and Total Parenteral Nutrition

(a) REPLACEMENT AND REPAIR SOLUTIONS
These are considered in Chapter 10.

(b) INTRA-OPERATIVE FLUID REQUIREMENTS
    (i) *During the actual operation 0.18 per cent NaCl in 4 per cent glucose should be given at 3 to 7 ml per kg per hour.*
    (ii) Losses of blood or other fluids incurred during operation should be made up during the operation.

(c) POSTOPERATIVE PERIOD

(i) The immediate postoperative period of 48 to 72 hours

There is a state of antidiuresis (water retention) and sodium retention. This does not appear to be of great significance in most operations in children, but should be taken into account in the postoperative phase of cardiac surgery, and also in burns, especially small painful scalds in which water intoxication (fits) may occur (p. 130). For routine purposes there is normally no need to reduce the supply of water and sodium during this period. However, catabolism in the postoperative phase releases intracellular potassium, and there may in addition be a temporary reduction in urine flow. *Therefore additional potassium should NOT be included in the maintenance fluid until at least 48 hours after the operation.* Additional potassium may, however, be given if there is clear evidence of potassium depletion (p. 133) and the urinary output is at least 400 ml per m^2 per 24 hours. A suitable electrolyte solution for general use is 0.18 per cent NaCl in 4 per cent glucose, given at the rates shown in Table A3.I. Continued losses should be measured and replaced.

(ii) 48 hours up to 5 to 7 days

If maintenance IV fluids are required after 48 to 72 hours, additional potassium should be included in the electrolyte solution; this is safer than the intermittent addition of small amounts of potassium chloride to the intravenous system.

A suitable electrolyte solution contains:

Sodium 20 mmol per litre.

Potassium 20 mmol per litre.

Chloride 20 or 40 mmol per litre (*see below*).

Lactate 20 mmol per litre if the solution contains 20 mmol per litre of chloride.

Glucose 4 per cent or 5 per cent.

Example showing the basis for the above solution.

10-kg infant;

Water requirement at 100 ml per kg = 1000 ml = 1 litre.

Sodium requirement 2 mmol per kg = 20 mmol.

Potassium requirement 2 mmol per kg = 20 mmol.

Chloride requirement 2 mmol per kg = 20 mmol.

The addition 20 mmol of anion can be made up by chloride or lactate.

Energy requirement at 100 kcal (420 joules) per kg = 1000 kcal (4200 joules).

1 litre of 5 per cent glucose supplies 50 g of glucose = 200 kcal (840 joules). This is inadequate even to cover basal requirements but is sufficient for up to 5 to 7 days after the operation.

Such a solution should not be used as the sole source of calories for longer than 5 to 7 days after operation.

(d) TOTAL PARENTERAL NUTRITION (TPN)

Little is known about the metabolic response to TPN in the newborn and its effect upon growth and development; therefore TPN should not be embarked upon without adequate technical and biochemical facilities and without very clear indications. In neonatal surgery the usual indication is the infant which has undergone major surgery to the gastrointestinal tract.

TPN should be started in all children where IV fluids are expected to be required for longer than 7 days, or when it becomes apparent that IV fluid will be required for longer than 7 days. The following is a summary of an accepted regime.

Requirements for 24 hours.

(i) Vamin glucose[1]; 40 ml per kg.

(ii) Intralipid[2] 20 per cent; 20 ml per kg.

---

[1] Vamin Glucose (*KabiVitrum*) contains in mmol per litre, sodium 50, potassium 20, calcium 2.5, magnesium 1.5, chloride 55, with glucose 10 per cent.

[2] Intralipid (*KabiVitrum*) supplies 2000 kcal (8400 joules) per litre: *see* Appendix 6, page 763.

(iii) Glucose 10 per cent; 75 ml per kg.
Total fluid intake = 135 ml per kg.
(iv) Potassium chloride 20 per cent (2.7 mmol per ml); 0.5 ml (1.35 mmol) per kg.
 (v) Calcium gluconate 10 per cent (10 ml contains 2.3 mmol); 1.5 ml (0.3 mmol) per kg.
(vi) Multivitamin preparation to be given IV; e.g. 3 ml of Multibionta* (*Merck*).
Once or twice weekly: Plasma or Plasma-Protein Fraction 20 ml per kg.
Once weekly: Vitamin K_1 (phytomenadione) 1 mg i.m.
Every 2 weeks: Vitamin B_{12} (cyanocobalamin) 50 μg i.m. Folic acid 1 mg i.m.

INTRODUCTION OF TPN

(a) Strict aseptic technique should be used in setting up the IV drip.
(b) Peripheral veins should be used when practicable.
(c) Ideally, Vamin, Intralipid and glucose should be given simultaneously over the 24 hours using a Y-connexion for the Vamin and glucose and a further Y-connexion for Intralipid using a pump injector.
(d) Alternatively the Vamin and Intralipid can be given together over 8 hours, and the glucose and additives over the remaining 16 hours.
(e) One third of this regime should be given on the first day, the remainder of the daily requirement being supplied by 0.18 per cent NaCl in 4 per cent glucose, or the maintenance solution containing sodium and potassium (p. 751).
(f) Two thirds of this regime is given on days 2 to 4 making up the remainder of the fluid and electrolyte requirement, as in (i).
(g) Full regime on the 5th day.

ROUTINE INVESTIGATIONS

(a) Daily for 1 week, then twice weekly:
  Plasma urea and electrolytes.
  Acid-base state (Astrup).
  Plasma glucose.
(b) Twice weekly:
  Hb, WBC, Platelets.

* 3 ml contains vitamin A 3000 iu, vitamin B_1 17 mg, vitamin B_2 3 mg, nicotinamide 30 mg, pantothenyl alcohol 8 mg, vitamin B_6 5 mg, vitamin C 170 mg, vitamin E 1.7 mg.

If IV feeding is continued for longer than 1 week, biotin 0.15 to 0.2 mg and choline chloride 50 mg should be given daily IV, but suitable preparations are not easy to obtain.

Plasma calcium and magnesium.
Plasma inorganic phosphate.
(c) Weekly:
Blood culture.
Plasma bilirubin.
Liver function tests (alkaline phosphatase, transaminases).
Plasma proteins.

Reference

Harries, J. T. (1971). Intravenous feeding in infants. *Archs Dis. Childh.* **46**, 855

Urine Output in Acute Disease

Although much information can be obtained from random samples of urine, measurement of the volume passed in consecutive periods of one hour is of much greater value. *This necessitates catheterization of the bladder which should be a routine procedure in all very ill children receiving IV fluids.*

The information which can be obtained is as follows.

(*a*) *In resuscitation from states of shock or dehydration*

    (i) Has an adequate flow (i.e. > 300 ml per m² per 24 hours or 12.5 ml per m² per hour, *Figure A5.1*; Table A5.IV for rates per kg per hour) been established within 4 hours of starting IV fluids?

    (ii) If the urine flow is below that expected, the reason may be:
Inadequate resuscitation or rehydration.
Blocked catheter,
Impending renal 'shut-down'.
Persisting antidiuresis.
Extravasation of urine (rupture of bladder or kidney).

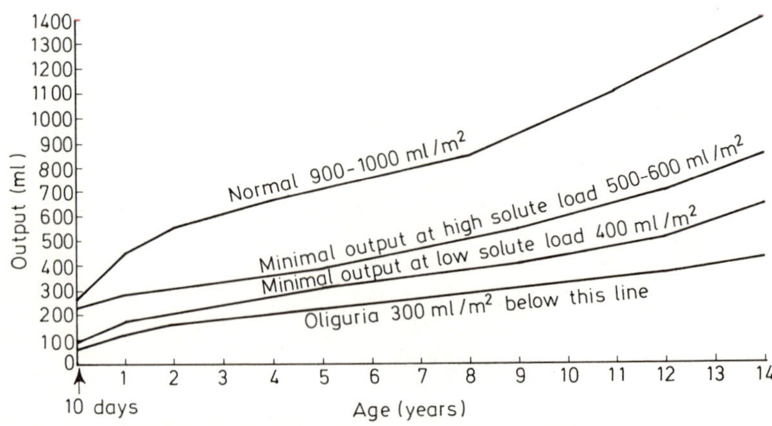

Figure A5.1. Urine output. See also Tables A5.I, II, III, IV

Bilateral obstruction to the renal tract (calculi or uric-acid nephropathy).

(b) *In cardiac conditions*

An inadequate urine flow may be due to shock or more commonly to cardiac failure with fluid retention.

(c) *In the polyuric phase of renal-tubular necrosis*

The rate of flow is very high in spite of clinical dehydration.

TABLE A5.I
Normal urine output*

Age	ml/24 h	ml/h	ml/kg/24 h	ml/kg/h	ml/m²/24 h	ml/m²/h
10 days†	250	10	70	2.5	1250	50
2 months	450	18	90	3.5	1800	75
1 year	500	20	50	2.0		
2 years	550	22	40	1.7		
4 years	650	27	40	1.7		
7 years	750	30	40	1.7	900–1000	37–40
11 years	1100	45	35	1.4		
14 years	1200	50	35	1.4		
Adult	1500	60	20	0.8		

* Midpoint figures for the ranges of age and output are given from Lafourcade and Gorin (1962) and Rubin (1969). Variations will be ± 50 per cent of the figures given.
† Output during the first 10 days depends upon the ability or desire of the infant to feed, also upon the type of milk (solute load). Thomson (1944) gives the following range for breast-fed infants. Day 1: 0–68, 2: 0–82, 3: 0–96, 4: 5–180, 6: 42–268, 8: 59–330, 10: 106–320

Standards of reference

The most convenient method of calculating urine flow is that based upon the body weight, but the same calculation cannot be used throughout the age range from infancy to adolescence. It is therefore necessary to establish standards of reference based upon surface area, and to recalculate rates of flow per kg body weight at different ages. However, even surface area is an unsatisfactory basis for the young infant, and separate calculations have been used for infants under 1 year of age.

Definitions

(a) NORMAL OUTPUT (Table A5.I, *Figure A5.1*)
This is the urinary output in a healthy individual on a diet appropriate for age. There are very large individual variations, depending upon the

type of diet (amount of water and solutes), environmental temperature, muscular activity and personal habits (e.g. amount of fluid taken with meals). The values used here are the best available from the literature (Lafourcade and Gorin, 1962; Rubin 1969) and are intended to represent average values at certain ages, without any statistical validity. It is to be expected that variations above and below these values will be of the order of about 50 per cent.

(b) OBLIGATORY URINE VOLUME (Tables A5.II and III, *Figure A5.1*) This is the minimum urine flow which is required to excrete the solute load (that proportion of solutes which is available for excretion by the kidney) in order to maintain the electrolyte content and acid-base state of the ECF within normal levels. The higher the solute load the larger the obligatory urine volume and therefore the higher the water requirement.

Obligatory urine volume is high in:
(i) Tissue catabolism (e.g. severe burns).
(ii) Increased production of solutes and acid metabolites (e.g. diabetic ketoacidosis).
(iii) Ingestion of abnormal solutes which are mainly or exclusively excreted through the kidney (e.g. salicylate poisoning).

Obligatory urine volume is low in:
(i) Maintenance IV fluids using glucose-electrolyte solution of low sodium content such as 0.18 per cent NaCl in 4 per cent glucose.
(ii) Starvation in the absence of catabolism.

Therefore it is not possible to give one obligatory urine flow for all situations, but figures are given (Tables A5.II and III) for minimal flow rates under the following conditions:
(i) High solute load (Table A5.II) (Muir and Barclay, 1974)
(ii) Low solute load (Table A5.III) (West, 1975)

TABLE A5.II

Minimal urine volumes for high solute load during resuscitation (Burns). (After Muir and Barclay, 1974)

Age	*ml/24 h*	*ml/h*	*ml/kg/24 h*	*ml/kg/h*	*ml/m²/24 h*	*ml/m²/h*
10 days	240	10	70	3.0	1200	50
2 months	240	10	50	2.0	900	37.5
1 year	290	12	30	1.2	600	25
2 years	310	13	24	1.0	600	25
4 years	360	15	21	0.9	500	20
7 years	430	18	20	0.8	500	20
11 years	625	26	19	0.8	500	20
14 years	840	35	19	0.8	500	20
Adult	840	35	12	0.5	480	20

In practice the solute load will be excreted without difficulty if the urine osmolality is maintained between 250 mosmol per kg (sp.gr. 1008) and 450 mosmol per kg (sp.gr. 1014).

(c) OLIGURIA (Table A5.IV, *Figure A5.1*)

When the urine flow is less than $\frac{1}{4}$ to $\frac{1}{3}$ of the expected normal (i.e. < 300 ml per m^2 per 24 hours or 12.5 ml per m^2 per hour) oliguria is present (*see Figure A5.1* and Table A5.IV for actual values at different ages).

Oliguria in the absence of obstruction or extravasation may be:

  (i) The physiological response of the normal kidney to dehydration, shock, hypotension, reduced blood flow, antidiuresis, or adrenocortical insufficiency.

 (ii) The pathological response (renal 'shut-down') of a kidney damaged by ischaemia, haemoglobinuria, myoglobinuria, or poisons.

TABLE A5.III

Minimal urine volumes for low solute load (maintenance IV glucose-electrolyte solutions); based on 400 ml per m^2 per 24 hours (West, 1975) except under 1 year where the figures are $\frac{2}{5}$ of the normal rate per m^2)

Age	ml/24 h	ml/h	ml/kg/24 h	ml/kg/h	ml/m²/24 h	ml/m²/h
10 days	100	4.0	28	1.2	500	20
2 months	180	7.5	36	1.5	720	30
1 year	180	7.5	18	0.75		
2 years	220	9.0	17	0.7		
4 years	280	12.0	16	0.65		
7 years	335	14.0	15	0.6	400	17
11 years	440	18.0	13	0.55		
14 years	550	20.0	12	0.5		
Adult	700	30.0	10	0.4		

Physiological oliguria cannot always be distinguished from pathological oliguria on the basis of urine flow alone, but examination of the urine (osmolality, sp.gr., urea or sodium content) in relation to the clinical state or plasma urea and electrolytes (p. 413) will usually distinguish between the two situations, as will the response to a controlled increase in the rate of infused fluid or the giving of a potent diuretic (*see also* page 415).

It should be emphasized that extreme oliguria, whether physiological or pathological, will result in a rising blood urea, a metabolic acidosis, and also electolyte disorders in certain situations.

(d) POLYURIA AND DIURESIS

The distinction between polyuria and diuresis is somewhat arbitrary;

polyuria is generally used to describe a continued state of high urine flow (e.g. uncontrolled diabetes) and a diuresis to describe a transient increase in urine flow, usually as a result of treatment. In either case the urine flow exceeds the normal value for age.

Polyuria (or diuresis) may be due to:

(i) The physiological reaction of the normal kidney to an increased intake of water or solutes, a diuretic drug, or absence of antidiuretic hormone (diabetes insipidus).

(ii) The pathological reaction of a damaged kidney in chronic renal disease, or tubular necrosis (inability of the renal tubules to modify the glomerular filtrate).

TABLE A5.IV

Oliguria: based on 300 ml per m^2 per 24 hours, except under 1 year (approximately $\frac{1}{3}$ of normal values)

Age	ml/24 h	ml/h	ml/kg/24h	ml/kg/h	ml/m^2/24 h	ml/m^2/h
10 days	80	3.5	25	1.0	400	16.5
2 months	140	6.0	28	1.25	600	25.0
1 year	140	6.0	14	0.6		
2 years	160	6.5	12	0.5		
4 years	210	8.5	12	0.5		
7 years	250	10.0	11	0.45	300	12.5
11 years	330	13.5	10	0.4		
14 years	420	17	9.5	0.4		
Adult	500	20	7.0	6.3		

Special situations

(a) BURNS

There is usually shock with diminished ECF during the first 48 to 72 hours. Antidiuresis may also be present but this is usually overcome by the high solute infusions used in most resuscitation regimes. In extensive burns there is a danger of toxic damage to the kidneys by free haemoglobin or myoglobin. In most schemes of resuscitation minimal hourly flow-rates are suggested, depending upon the type of fluids used. The antidiuretic effect is usually seen only in small painful burns or scalds in which excessive drinking of water or low-solute fluids may cause water intoxication (p. 45). After initial resuscitation has been completed a higher urine flow (up to 800 to 900 ml per m^2 per 24 hours) can be safely maintained provided there is no evidence or risk of pulmonary oedema.

(b) ACUTE POISONING

In certain poisonings, particularly with salicylate, the urinary excretion is proportional to the urine flow and treatment is by the induction of a diuresis. IV fluids must therefore be given at 2 to 3 times the normal maintenance rate in order to achieve the necessary sustained high flow of urine, which should be 2 to 3 times the normal flow (2000 to 3000 ml per m^2 per 24 hours or 5 to 6 ml per kg per hour (Mann and Sandberg, 1970). *See* Table A5.I for normal values. These high flows may be more safely achieved by an osmotic (mannitol, urea) diuresis rather than a water diuresis (Teitelbaum, 1970; Mann and Sandberg, 1970).

References

Lafourcade, J. and Gorin, R. (1962). Les Spoliations Hydro-Salines du Nourrisson et leur Traitement. p. 64. Paris: G. Doin et Compagnie

Mann, J. B. and Sandberg, D. H. (1970). Therapy of sedative overdosage. In *Poisoning in Children. Pediat. Clin. N. Am.* **17 (No. 3)**, 622

Muir, I. F. K. and Barclay, T. L. (1974). *Burns and their Treatment.* 2nd edn. p. 33 London: Lloyd-Luke

Rubin, M. I. (1969). In *Textbook of Pediatrics.* Ed. W. E. Nelson, V. C. Vaughan and R. J. McKay. p. 1106. 9th edn. Philadelphia: W. B. Saunders

Teitelbaum, D. T. (1970). Poisoning with psychoactive drugs. In *Poisoning in Children. Pediat. Clin. N. Am.* **17 (No. 3)**, 563

Thomson, J. (1944). Observation on the urine of the newborn infant. *Archs Dis. Childh.* **19**, 169

West, C. D. (1975). In *Pediatric Therapy.* Ed. H. C. Shirkey. 5th edn. p. 280. St. Louis: C. V. Mosby

Composition of Preparations and Solutions Commonly Used in Intravenous Infusions

Name	Electrolyte content (mmol/litre)				H^+ as pH^1	Glucose[2] (g/litre)	Joules[3] (kcal)/litre	Remarks
	Na	K	Cl	HCO_3 or equivalent				
Sodium chloride 0.18% in 4% glucose	31		31		3.5–4.3	40	628 (150)	Maintenance solution short-term
Sodium chloride 0.45% in 2.5% glucose	77		77		3.5–4.3	25	397 (94)	
Sodium chloride 0.9%	150		150		5.7–6.9			
Sodium chloride 0.9% in 5% glucose	154		154		3.5–4.3	50	785 (188)	
Sodium chloride 0.18%, potassium chloride 0.15% in 4% glucose	30	20	50			40	628 (150)	Maintenance solution, medium-term
Darrow's solution	121	35	103	53 (lactate)	6.7–7.1			

Hartmann's solution (= Lactate Ringer)	130	5	111	29 (lactate)		With Ca 2 mmol per litre
Plasma-Protein Fraction (PPF)	140–160	<2	100–120	15 (citrate)		400 ml contains 17–19 g protein, replaces freeze-dried pooled plasma.
Plasma from whole stored (ACD) blood, PCV 60%	150 at 0 days 148 at 7 days	3–4 at 0 days; 12 at 7 days		~103	6.9–7.0 at 0 days, 6.8 at 7 days	Expiry time 21 days. Each 495 ml contains 1.7 g sodium citrate and 0.6 g citric acid
Salt-poor albumin						25 g contains $\not>$ 17 mmol sodium & $\not>$ 1.2 mmol potassium
Dextran 40 10% (mol. weight 40 000)						
Dextran 70 6% (mol. weight 70 000)						Available in 5% glucose or 0.9% sodium chloride
Dextran 110 6% (mol. weight 110 000)						

Composition of Preparations and Solutions Commonly Used in Intravenous Infusions (*continued*)

Concentrated solutions	Electrolyte content (mmol/litre)			HCO_3 or equivalent	H^+ as pH[1]	Glucose[2] (g/litre)	Joules[3] (kcal.)/litre	Remarks
	Na	K	Cl					
Sodium bicarbonate 8.4% (1 ml = 1 mmol)	1000			1000				Store at −10 to −25°C Rapid ingestion may be harmful
Sodium bicarbonate 4.2% (2 ml = 1 mmol)	500			500				Store at −2 to −25°C
Sodium chloride 5%	855		855					
Sodium chloride 1.8%	308		308					
Sodium lactate M/6 (1.85%)	167			167 (lactate)				
Potassium chloride 0.15% in 5% Glucose		20	20			50	785 (188)	Avoid rapid infusion
Potassium chloride 0.3% in 5% Glucose		40	40			50	785 (188)	
Glucose 10%					3.7–4.2	100g	1570 (375)	

Intralipid 10%						4200 (1100)	Total Parenteral Nutrition
Intralipid 20%						8400 (2200)	p. 751
Vamin glucose	50	20	55	5.2	100	2730 (650) including 1890 (450) from glucose	Magnesium 1.5 mmol. Calcium 2.5 mmol per litre
Lignocaine 0.1% in 5% glucose					50	785 (188)	Cardiac arrhythmias
Lignocaine 0.2% in 5% glucose					50	785 (188)	p. 294

[1] Values for H' ion concentrations (pH) from Harris, F. (1972). *Paediatric Fluid Therapy.* p. 141 SI units are too cumbersome to use over such a wide range of H' concentration (*see* Table A18.II for conversion).

[2] For consistency, 'glucose' is used instead of 'dextrose', though bottles are invariably labelled in terms of dextrose content.

[3] The clinical 'Calorie'.

NOTE: IV solutions containing fructose or sorbitol should NOT be used, since they can produce fatal hypoglycaemia, with hepatic and renal damage in undiagnosed cases of fructose intolerance (*see* page 702, and Schulte and Lenz, (1977). *Lancet* (ii). 188, and a metabolic acidosis in the newborn.

APPENDIX 7

Composition of Some Oral Electrolyte Solutions

Name	Electrolyte content (mmol/litre)				Glucose (g/litre)	Joules (kcal.)[6]/litre	Remarks
	Na	K	Cl	HCO_3 or equivalent			
Sodium chloride and Dextrose (Glucose) compound powder[1] *BPC*	35	20	37	18	40	628 (150)	Mild gastroenteritis, but *see* p. 639
Darrow's solution diluted with equal parts of 5% glucose	61	18	52	26 (lactate)	25	397 (94)	For isotonic or hypertonic dehydration *see* pp. 95–100
Oral electrolyte solution for burns[2]	133	—	85	48	—	—	*See* p. 45
GE-SOL (*USP*)[3]	81	18	71	28	77	1209 (290)	For isotonic or hypertonic dehydration
Cholera solution[4]	90	20	80	30	20	314 (75)	Cholera, *see* p. 562
Nalin and Cash's solution[5]	120	25	98	48	60	942 (215)	For hypotonic dehydration or cholera, *see* pages 100, 562

[1] Sodium chloride and dextrose compound powder *BPC*; 22 g of the powder contain:
Sodium chloride 0.5 g
Sodium bicarbonate 0.75 g
Potassium chloride 0.75 g
Dextrose (Glucose) 20 g
22 g of the powder is added to 500 ml of water
(British National Formulary, p. 228, 1976–78)
[2] Sodium chloride 5 g
Sodium bicarbonate 4 g
Water 1 litre
With flavouring agent
[3] GE-SOL (*USP*)
Common salt $\frac{1}{2}$ teaspoon
Sodium bicarbonate $\frac{1}{2}$ teaspoon
Potassium chloride $\frac{1}{4}$ teaspoon
Glucose 2 tablespoons
Water 1 litre
[4] Cholera solution (H. A. Reid, p. 562)
Sodium chloride 3.5 g
Sodium bicarbonate 2.5 g
Potassium citrate 1.5 g
Glucose 20 g
Water 1 litre
[5] (a) Nalin, D. R. and Cash, R. A. (1971). Oral or nasogastric maintenance therapy in pediatric cholera patients. *J. Pediat.* **78**, 355
(b) Nalin, D. R. and Cash, R. A. (1976). Sodium content of oral therapy in diarrhoea. *Lancet* **(ii)** 957
[6] The clinical 'Calorie'.

Drug Dosage: General Principles

Use of surface area for the calculation of drug dosage in children

There are two methods of using SA for calculating drug dosage etc.

(a) When the adult dose is known. and the child's dose is to be calculated. Assuming the adult has a SA of 1.73 m², the child's dose will be:

$$\frac{\text{adult dose} \times \text{child's SA}}{1.73}$$

For less accurate purposes the fraction or percentage of adult dose can be read off a figure relating surface area at different weights (and ages) to the percentage of the adult dose required.

(b) A standard dose can be used throughout childhood (except the neonatal period) giving the dose in kg per m², ml per m², etc. This of course can be calculated from a known adult dose simply by dividing the adult dose by 1.73.

For ordinary purposes the dosage scales given in *A Paediatric Vade-Mecum* (Wood, 1977) are satisfactory and are given in the following form:

(a) First year: dose based upon body weight, from birth to 2 weeks, then from 2 weeks to one year.

(b) At ages 1 year and 7 years the dosage is based upon surface area.
At 1 year the dose is $\frac{1}{4}$ adult dose.
At 7 years the dose is $\frac{1}{2}$ adult dose.

Intermediate doses can be arrived at by extrapolation, or from *Figure A8.1* or from the simplified Table A8.I.

Difficulties in paediatric dosage

(a) Many doses after the age of 1 year in this book are, for ease of calculation, based upon body weight. It is important that unless there is some very good reason, *the maximum adult dose should not be exceeded,* so that no child should normally receive more than 4 × the dose at 1 year.

(b) When the dose must be very accurately calculated (as in

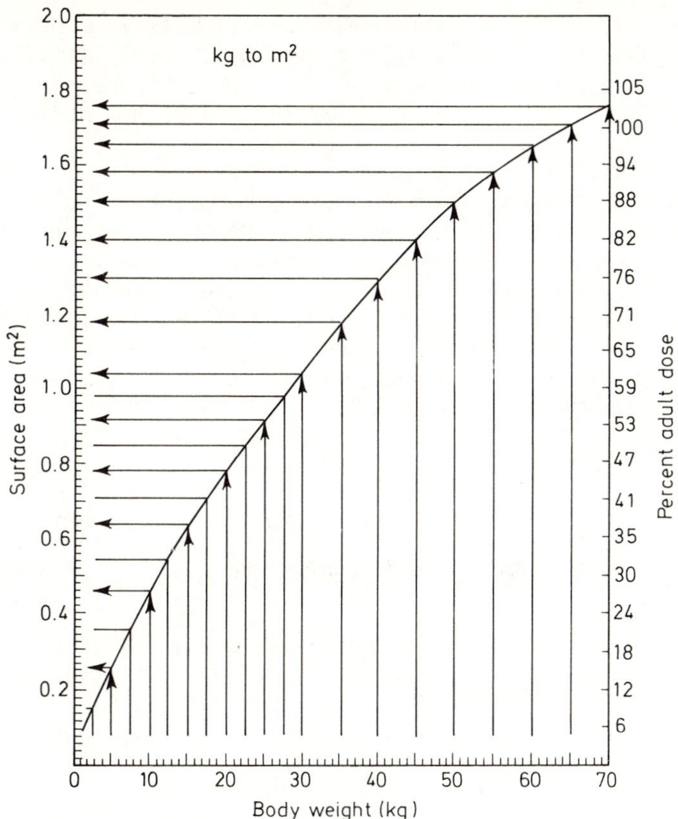

Figure A8.1.Relations between body weight (kg), body surface area and adult dosage.
(From Talbot, Richie and Crawford, 1959. Reproduced by kind permission)

TABLE A8.I
Simplified scheme for drug dosage based on surface area

Age	Average weight (kg)	Surface area (m²)	Fraction of adult dose
Birth	3–3.5	0.2	1/8
4 months	6	0.3	1/6
1 year	10	0.45	1/4
2 years	13	0.58	1/3
7 years	25	0.9	1/2
12 years	40	1.3	3/4
14 years	50	1.5	9/10
14 years +	65+	1.7	Adult

cytotoxic drugs) the initial scale should be based upon the dose per m^2, and the actual surface area of the child should be accurately determined, using a nomogram or formula.

(c) When a child has abnormal proportions the surface area should be used rather than the age or weight.

(d) Fat children: *see* pages 739–740.

(e) In renal insufficiency, the dosage of certain drugs, particularly the aminoglycosides (streptomycin, kanamycin, gentamicin, tobramycin, amikacin) antibiotics and the polymyxins (Colistin) should be reduced or the intervals between doses should be increased, published data should be consulted or the maker's literature, and serum levels should be measured at frequent intervals if this is practicable. (*See also* Appendix 10)

References

Talbot, N. B., Richie, R. H. and Crawford, J. D. (1959). *Metabolic Homeostasis.* p. i. Harvard University Press
Wood, B. (1977). *A Paediatric Vade-Mecum.* 9th Edn. London: Lloyd-Luke

Doses of Drugs

The drugs listed below are mainly those mentioned in the text. Except where otherwise indicated the figure given is for a *single dose* but the doses of antibiotics are given instead in terms of the *dose per 24 hours*. Where the method of administration is complicated and requires explanation, reference is made to the text. A route of administration indicated in brackets indicates that this route is practicable but is not recommended. When a dose is not given for a particular age group, this indicates that the drug is not normally required in that age group; but where a drug is contra-indicated, this is specifically stated.

The strength of tablets, solutions, etc., are those detailed in the *British National Formulary* (1976–1978)* and in the *Data Sheet Compendium* (1977)†; strengths and formulations in other countries may be different. The nomenclature is that of the list of Approved Names given in the *British National Formulary,* the *British Pharmacoepoeia,* or the *British Pharmaceutical Codex.* A list of American official names with the equivalent British Approved Name (when the two differ) and the commoner proprietary or alternative names is given in the Index of Drugs. pp. 839–844. The doses of antibacterial, antituberculous, antimicrobial, anthelminthic, steroid drugs, antisera and immunoglobulins are given separately. *Leukaemia*; drugs used solely for this purpose are excluded from these tables and are considered separately in Chapter 50.

---

* *British National Formulary.* (1976–78). The British Medical Association and The Pharmaceutical Society of Great Britain
† *Data Sheet Compendium.* (1977). The Association of the British Pharmaceutical Industry, London

TABLE A9.I
Dosage of commonly used drugs

Name	Routes	Doses per 24 hours	Single doses					Remarks
			0–2 weeks	2 weeks to 1 year	1 year	7 years	Adult	
Adrenaline 1:1000 (0.1%) 1 mg in 1 ml Amps. 0.5, 1 ml	s.c.	According to response	0.01 ml/kg		0.125 ml	0.25 ml	0.5 ml	Asthma, p. 253
	IV (great care)	As above	IV *see* Anaphylaxis, p. 111					
Adrenaline 1:10 000 (0.01%) 0.1 mg in 1 ml	IV (great care)	As above	Neonate 1–2 ml		Other ages 1–4 ml *see above also*			Resuscitation of newborn, p. 601 Cardiac arrest, p. 303
Adrenaline 1:1000 nebulized	Inhaled		*See* Laryngotracheobronchitis, p. 222					
Adrenaline inhaler	Inhaled		*See* Insect Stings, p. 543					
Aminocaproic acid (EACA)	Oral	4		100 mg/ kg	1.5 g	3 g	6 g	Familial Angio-oedema, p. 494
Sachet 3 g Amps 4 g in 10 ml	IV (slow)			As above	As above	As above	As above	
Aminophylline Tabs 100 mg	Oral i.m.	3–4	3 mg/kg		25 mg (oral)	50 mg (oral)	100 mg (oral)	
Amps. 250 mg in 10 ml	IV IV (slow infusion) (Rectal)	According to response	3 mg/kg		40–50 mg	80–100 mg	250–500 mg 200 mg at 12 years	Anaphylaxis, p. 111 Asthma, p. 253
Apomorphine	s.c.	Single dose				0.1 mg/kg	6 mg (max. dose)	Acute poisoning, p. 67

Drug	Route	No. of doses	Amount	Dose/kg	Dose			Indication
Ascorbic acid (vitamin C)	Oral	3–4			100 up to 500 mg			Methaemoglobinaemia, p. 646
Tabs 25 up to 500 mg, Amps 100, 500 mg	IV	1–2			As above			
Atropine Amps 1 ml containing 0.4, 0.6, 0.8 or 1 mg	(Oral) s.c. i.m. IV	As required Once		0.015 mg/kg	0.15 mg	0.3 mg	0.6 mg	Emergency anaesthesia, p. 199 Cardiac arrest, p. 303 Acute respiratory failure, p. 240
BAL (British anti-Lewisite) *See* Dimercaprol					*See* Acute Lead Poisoning, p. 371			
Bisacodyl Suppositories	Rectal	As required	$\frac{1}{4}$ supp.					Neonatal tetanus, p. 343
B$_1$ vitamin (*See* Thiamine)					*See* Infantile Beri-Beri, p. 593			
B$_6$ vitamin (*See* Pyridoxine)					*See* Neonatal Convulsion, p. 689 Tuberculous Meningitis, p. 357			
B$_{12}$ vitamin (*See* Cyanocobalamin)					*See* Total Parenteral Nutrition, p. 752			
Bentonite					*See* Acute Poisoning, (Paraquat), p. 74			
Bephenium					*See* Hookworm Infection in Newborn, p. 641			
C vitamin (*See* Ascorbic acid)								
Calcitonin					*See* Acute Hypercalcaemia, p. 145			
Calciferol Tabs 3000, 50 000 units	Oral	1–2	1000 units		3000–5000 units			Hypocalcaemia, p. 142
Calcium chloride					Use not recommended			As above
Calcium disodium versenate					*See* Acute Lead Poisoning, p. 371			

TABLE A9.I *continued*
Dosage of commonly used drugs

Name	Routes	Doses per 24 hours	Single doses					Remarks
			0–2 weeks	2 weeks to 1 year	1 year	7 years	Adult	
Calcium gluconate	Oral	4–6	Up to 1.5 g (100 mg/kg)			2 g	4 g	Hypocalcaemia, p. 143
Amps 10%, 5 or	IV	As required	0.3 ml/kg at 1 ml per minute			5 ml	10 ml	
10 ml	Not i.m.							
Calcium lactate– gluconate syrup	Oral	4–6	5 ml	5 ml	10–30 ml		20–60 ml	As above
Calcium lactate (6% suspension)	Oral	4–6	5 ml	5 ml	10–30 ml		20–60 ml	
Camphorated opium tincture (Tr. Camph. Co, Paregoric)			*See* Maternal Drug Dependence, p. 709					
Carbimazole Tabs 5 mg	Oral	3		0.3 mg/kg		5 mg	10 mg	Thyrotoxicosis, pp. 463, 464
Charcoal, activated			*See* Acute Poisoning, p. 71					
Chloral hydrate Paediatric Elixir 200 mg/5 ml	Oral (sedation)	Up to 3	7.5–30 mg/kg		300 mg	600 mg	1.5 g	For a single hypnotic dose, twice these doses can be used
Chlorpheniramine Tabs 4, 8, 12 mg Elixir 2 mg/5 ml	Oral	3–4			1 mg	2 mg	4 mg	
Parenteral 10 mg in 1 ml	s.c. i.m.	Once	0.25 mg/kg		2.5 mg	5 mg	10 mg	Anaphylaxis, p. 114

Drug / Preparation	Route	Frequency	Dose/kg				Notes
Chlorpromazine Tabs 10, 25, 50 & 100 mg.	Oral	3–6					Neonatal tetanus (by tube), p. 345 Hyperpyrexia p. 537
Elixir 25 mg/5 ml Amps 25 mg in 1 ml 50 mg in 2 ml, 50 mg in 5 ml	i.m.	As required or 4	0.5–1 mg/kg	10 mg	20–25 mg	40–50 mg	Fits in burns p. 44 Maternal drug dependence, p. 709
Chlorothiazide Tabs 500 mg	Oral	1–2	25 mg/kg	250 mg	500 mg	1 g	Cardiac Failure, p. 287
Clonazepam Tabs 0.5 mg	Oral	3–4	Initial dose 0.25 mg/kg		Initial dose 0.5 mg/kg	Initial dose 1 mg/kg	Status epilepticus. p. 319
Amps 1 mg in 1 ml	IV IV infusion	Once According to response	3 mg in 250 ml 0.9% NaCl or 5% glucose				
Cyanocobalamin (vitamin B_{12})			*See* Total Parenteral Nutrition, p. 752				
Cyclizine	Oral i.m.	1–3	1 mg/kg	12.5 mg	25 mg	50 mg	Single dose for travel sickness, p. 81
D Vitamin (*See* Calciferol)							
Desferrioxamine Vials 500 mg			*See* Acute Poisoning (Iron), p. 76				
Diazepam Tabs 2, 5, 10 mg Elixir 2 mg per 5 ml	Oral i.m.	Up to 4	0.05–0.25 mg/kg	0.5 mg	1 mg	2–5 mg	Neonatal Tetanus 2.5 mg by tube, p. 344
Amps 10 mg in 2 ml, 20 mg in 4 ml	IV (2 min)	According to response	0.25–1.0 mg/kg	2.5 mg	5 mg	10 mg	
	IV infusion	According to response	30 mg in 500 ml 0.9% NaCl or 5% glucose				

TABLE A9.I *continued*
Dosage of commonly used drugs

Name	Routes	Doses per 24 hours	Single doses					Remarks
			0–2 weeks	*2 weeks to 1 year*	*1 year*	*7 years*	*Adult*	
Diazoxide Tabs 50 mg	Oral	2–3	5–20 mg/kg/day according to response					Hypoglycaemia (Oral)
Amps 300 mg in	IV	According	Initially 5 mg/kg, up to 10 mg/kg					Hypertension, p. 415
20 ml	(Not i.m.)	to response						
Dichloralphenazone	Oral	3–4	1.25–2.5 ml		*1–5 years* 2.5–5 ml	*6–12 years* 5–10 ml	10–20 ml	For a single hypnotic
Elixir 225 mg/5 ml	(sedation)							dose twice these doses can be used.
Digoxin	Oral							
Paediatric Elixir 0.05 mg in 1 ml								
Tabs 0.0625, 0.125 and 0.25 mg			*See* Cardiac Emergencies, p. 286					
Paediatric Injection 0.1 mg per ml	i.m. IV							
Dimercaprol			*See* Acute Lead Poisoning, p. 371					
Diphenoxylate			Use in Acute Diarrhoeas not recommended					
EACA (*See* Aminocaproic acid)								
EDTA (*See* Sodium calcium-edetate)			*See* Acute Lead Poisoning, p. 371					
Edrophonium Amps 10 mg in 1 ml	i.m. } IV }	Once	0.05 mg/kg as initial test dose, then 1 mg		0.5 mg–1.0 mg as initial test dose			Myasthenia gravis, p. 240
Ephedrine Tabs 15, 30, 60 mg	Oral	4	1 mg/kg		7.5 mg	15 mg	30 mg	Stokes–Adams attacks, p. 293
Folic Acid Tabs 5 mg	Oral	1–2	0.25 mg/kg		2.5 mg	5 mg	10 mg	

Drug	Route	Frequency					Reference
Frusemide Tabs 20,40, 500 mg	Oral	Daily or alternate days	5–10 mg	20 mg	40 mg	80 mg	Cardiac Failure, p. 287 Pulmonary Oedema in Burns, p. 43
	i.m.	Once	1–1.5 mg/kg up to max of 6 mg	5–10 mg	20 mg	40 mg	Protein-Energy Malnutrition, p. 591
Amps 20 mg in 2 ml	IV (or infusion)	Once	1 mg/kg initially, then 2 mg/ kg: up to 5 mg/kg as infusion	10 mg	20 mg	40 mg	Acute Renal Failure, p. 415
Glucagon Amps containing 1 mg (1 unit) or 10 mg (10 units)	s.c. i.m. IV	1–4	0.3 mg (300 microgrammes) at all ages: 1 mg = 1 unit				Hypoglycaemia (Neonatal), p. 450 Diabetes, p. 442
Glycerol (glycerin)	Oral	4	1 g/kg at all ages				Cerebral oedema, p. 324
Heparin	_See_ Practical Procedures, p. 720, and Exchange Transfusion, p. 679						
Hydrallazine Tabs 25, 50 mg	Oral	3			12.5 mg– 25 mg	25–50 mg	
Amps 20 mg in 5 ml	IV IV by infusion	According to response	0.4–1.0 mg/kg	4–10 mg	8–20 mg	15–40 mg	Acute Renal Failure, (hypertension) p. 416
Hyoscine hydrobromide	Oral s.c.	1	0.015 mg /kg	0.15 mg	0.3 mg	0.6 mg	Travel sickness, p. 81
Imipramine Tabs 10, 25 mg	Oral (Anti- depressant)	3			10 mg	25 mg	Psychiatric Emergencies, p. 508
		Not recommended below the age of 7 years					
	Oral (Enuresis)	Once at night			25 mg	50 mg	

TABLE A9.I *continued*
Dosage of commonly used drugs

Name	Routes	Doses per 24 hours	Single doses						Remarks
			0–2 weeks	2 weeks to 1 year	1 year	7 years	Adult		
Ipecacuanna. Paediatric Emetic Draught *BPC* (Ipecac. syrup *U.S.A.*) NOT FLUID EXTRACT	Oral	Once	Do not use under 6 months		*6–18 months*, 10 ml *18 months–5 years*, 15–20 ml				Acute Poisoning, p. 67
Isoprenaline 1:1000 (0.1%) 1 mg in 1 ml	IV	Once			Stokes–Adams attacks, p. 293				
Amps 2 mg in 2 ml	IV infusion				Septic shock, p. 118				
K₁ vitamin (*See* Phytomenadione)									
Lignocaine	Slow IV infusion				Arrhythmias: Cardiac Emergencies, p. 294, Use of Sympathomimetic Agents in Shock, p. 117				
Loperamide					Use in Acute Diarrhoeas not recommended, p. 401				
Magnesium hydroxide (Milk of Magnesia) 8% suspension	Oral	3–4			1–2 ml initially		10 ml	10 ml	Hypomagnesaemia, p. 146 Protein-Energy Malnutrition, p. 590
Magnesium sulphate 50%	Oral	4	0.125–0.5 ml/kg of 50% solution; dilute to 12.5–25% in infants						
	i.m. (deep)	2	0.1–0.25 ml/kg diluted as above for infants						
Magnesium sulphate 1%	IV	As required	Not more rapidly than 1 ml per minute until relief of symptoms; use ECG control						As above

Preparation	Route	Times daily	Dose / notes				Cross-reference
Mannitol 20% (5, 10, 25% also available) 500-ml bags of 20% solution is usual preparation	IV	Once	For oliguria, test dose of 0.2 g (1 ml)/kg over 3–5 minutes. Cerebral oedema, 1–2 g (5–10 ml)/kg over 10–30 minutes				Acute renal failure, p. 415 Renal failure in burns, p. 47 Cerebral oedema, p. 323 If crystals visible heat to 60°C then cool to 37°C before infusing
Medazepam Caps 5, 10 mg	Oral	2–3	Not recommended below the age of 7 years	7.5–15 mg DAILY	15–30 mg DAILY		Psychiatric emergencies. (tranquilizer), p. 506
Mepyramine Elixir 25 mg in 5 ml Tabs 50, 100 mg	Oral	Once		2.5–5 ml (12.5–25 mg)	5–10 ml (25–50 mg)	12 years 10–15 ml (50–75 mg)	Travel sickness
Injection 50 mg in 2 ml	i.m. IV	Once		6.25–12.5 mg	12.5–25 mg	25 mg	Anaphylaxis, p. 113
Metaraminol			See Treatment of Shock with Sympathomimetic amines, p. 116 and Anaphylaxis, p. 113				
Methoxamine			See Treatment of Shock with Sympathomimetic amines, p. 116				
Methyldopa Tabs 125, 250, 500 mg Amps 50 mg in 1 ml	Oral IV	3 4	6 mg/kg	62.5 mg	125 mg	250 mg	
Methylene Blue 1%	IV	Once	1–2 mg (0.1–0.2 ml)/kg, slowly				Methaemoglobinaemia, p. 646

TABLE A9.I *continued*
Dosage of commonly used drugs

| Name | Routes | Doses per 24 hours | Single doses | | | | | Remarks |
			0–2 weeks	2 weeks to 1 year	1 year	7 years	Adult	
Morphine Amps: 1 ml containing 10, 15, 20, 30 mg	s.c. i.m.	1–2	0.15–0.2 mg/kg		2 mg	4 mg	8–15 mg	Cyanotic attacks, p. 290 Pulmonary oedema, p. 288
	IV	Once	0.1–0.2 mg/kg (max dose 15 mg)					Burns, p. 35
Nalorphine (Use Naloxone when available)	(s.c) i.m. IV	As required (usually once)	0.2 mg/kg		2 mg	5 mg	10 mg	*Note*: Adult strength amps 10 mg/1 ml Neonatal amps 1 mg/1 ml
Naloxone	(s.c.) i.m. IV	Can be repeated after 2–3 mins	Neonatal 0.01 mg/kg or standard dose of 0.04 mg	0.005–0.01 mg/kg (max dose 0.4 mg)			0.4 mg	*Note*: Adult strength amps 0.4 mg/1 ml Neonatal amps 0.02 mg/1 ml
Nandrolone decanoate Amps 25, 50 mg	i.m.	Once every 3 weeks				Adolescent 12.5–25 mg		Anorexia nervosa, p. 505
Neostigmine (Prostigmine)	Oral	3	0.35 mg/kg		3.75 mg	7.5 mg	15 mg	Myasthenia gravis, p. 240
Tabs 15 mg Amps: 1 ml containing 0.5 or 2.5 mg Nikethamide	i.m. IV	Once	0.04 mg/kg		0.625 mg	1.25 mg	2.5 mg	 Respiratory arrest p. 8

	Route						
Nitrazepam	Oral	Up to 3	0.25 mg/ kg	2.5 mg	5 mg	10 mg	
Noradrenaline	IV infusion	*See* Treatment of Shock with Sympathomimetic Amines p. 115, and Cardio respiratory Arrest, p. 5					
Opium (*See* Camphorated Opium Tincture, Paregoric)*	Oral	*See* Maternal Drug Dependence, p. 709					
Paraldehyde Amps 2, 5, 10 ml	Oral i.m. (deep)	Once or repeated as required	0.1 ml/kg	1–1.5 ml	8 ml	10 ml (over 10 years)	Status epilepticus, *Use glass syringe* p. 319
Paregoric (*See* Camphorated Opium Tincture)		*See* Maternal Drug Dependence, p. 709					
Penicillamine Tabs 125, 250 mg		*See* Acute Lead Poisoning, p. 371					
Pethidine Tabs 25, 50 mg Amps 50 mg in 1 ml	Oral s.c.	Up to 3	1 mg/kg	12.5 mg	25 mg	50 mg	
Phenelzine Tabs 15 mg	Oral	3–4		Adolescent 15 mg			Antidepressant, p. 508
Phenobarbitone Tabs 15, 30, 60, 100 mg	Oral	2–3	1.5–3.0 mg/kg	15–30 mg	30 mg	30–60 mg	Anticonvulsant
Amps 200 mg in 1 ml	i.m.	Once or repeated as required	2–6 mg/kg	60 mg	60 mg	60–120 mg	Neonatal convulsions p. 690

779

TABLE A9.I *continued*
Dosage of commonly used drugs

Name	Routes	Doses per 24 hours	Single doses					Remarks
			0–2 weeks	2 weeks to 1 year	1 year	7 years	Adult	
Phenytoin	Oral	2–3	3 mg/kg		30 mg	50 mg	100 mg	Anticonvulsant
Caps 25, 50, 100 mg		Once, or						
Tabs 50 mg	i.m.	repeated	2–5 mg/kg		50 mg	100 mg	200 mg	
Susp. 30 mg/5 ml	IV	as						
Amps 250 mg in 5 ml		required						
Phytomenadione	(Oral)							IV in Coagulation
(vitamin K$_1$)								disorders.
Oral 1 mg in 1 ml	i.m.	Once or						Newborn, p. 657
Amps 1 mg in 0.5 ml,	IV	repeated	1 mg		3 mg	5 mg	10 mg	
10 mg in 1 ml		as						
		required						
Practolol	Oral	2	2 mg/kg		25 mg	50 mg	100 mg	IV injection over
								5 min
	IV	Once	0.1–0.2 mg/kg		1 mg	2.5 mg	5 mg	
Promethazine	Oral	3		0.75 mg/kg	7.5 mg	15 mg	25 mg	For a single hypnotic
Tabs 10, 25 mg								dose twice these
Elixir 5 mg/5 ml	i.m.	Once	Half the oral dose				25–	doses can be used.
							50 mg	IV for anaphylactic
Injection 2.5%	IV	Once	Adults only: 2.5% solution diluted to 10 times its volume with water for					reactions
solution	(slow)	(emergency)	injection: maximum parenteral *adult* dose 100 mg					
Propanolol	Oral	3		1 mg/kg	10 mg	20 mg	40 mg	Neonatal
Tabs 10, 40, 80 mg								thyrotoxicosis,
Amps 1 mg in 1 ml	IV	As			0.3 mg	0.5 mg	1 mg	p. 463
		required						Arrhythmias pp. 291,
								303

Drug	Route	Doses per day	Dose				Reference
Protamine Amps. 50 mg in 5 ml, 100 mg in 10 ml	IV	As required	1 mg (0.1 ml) for each 100 units of heparin to maximum of 50 mg				
Pyridoxine (vitamin B_6) Tabs 10, 20, 50 mg	Oral		For Pyridoxine-dependent fits, 4 mg/kg For use with isoniazide, 10 mg daily				Neonatal convulsions, p. 689 Tuberculous Meningitis p. 357
Resonium A (Exchange Resin, sodium polystyrene sulphonate)	Oral Rectal		*See* Hyperkalaemia, p. 138				
Salbutamol	Oral	3–4	0.1 mg/kg	1 mg	2 mg	4 mg	Asthma, p. 253
	Inhaled	As required	0.5% solution, diluted to 0.25% under 7 years				Status Asthmaticus, p. 253
	IV	As required	4–6 μg/kg				
Sodium calcium- edetate			*See* Acute Lead Poisoning, p. 371				
Sodium bicarbonate			*See* Resuscitation of the Newborn, p. 600 Metabolic Acidosis, p. 125				
Sodium polystyrene sulphonate	Oral Rectal		*See* Hyperkalaemia, p. 138				
Spironolactone Tabs 25, 100 mg	Oral	4	0.6 mg/kg	6.25 mg	12.5 mg	25 mg	
Theophylline	Oral	1	3 mg/kg				Apnoeic attacks in newborn, p. 275
Thiamine (vitamin B_1) Amps 25 or 100 mg in 1 ml	(Oral) i.m. IV	According to response	*See* Infantile Beri-Beri, p. 593				
Thyroxine Tabs 0.05, 0.1 mg	Oral	1–2	0.0125 mg (12.5 μg)	0.025 mg (25 μg)	Over 1 year: According to requirement		Hypothyroidism (neonatal), p. 461

TABLE A9.I *continued*
Dosage of commonly used drugs

Name	Routes	Doses per 24 hours	0–2 weeks	2 weeks to 1 year	Single doses 1 year	7 years	Adult	Remarks
Trimeprazine Tabs 10 mg	Oral	3		0.25 mg/kg	2.5 mg	5 mg	10 mg	p. 713
Syrup 7.5 mg in 5 ml	i.m.	Once			*1–5 years*	*6–12 years*		
Amps 50 mg in 2 ml					0.9 mg/kg	0.6 mg/kg		
Vasopressin				*See* Acute Gastrointestinal Bleeding, p. 397				
Versenate (*See* sodium calcium edetate)				*See* Acute Lead Poisoning, p. 371				

TABLE A9.II
Antibacterial agents

(*See* pages 742–743 for modifications in dosage in pre-term infants. *See* Table A9.III for details of IV administration. For IT dose *see* Table 36.III, p. 351.)

| Name | Routes | Doses per 24 hours | Total dose per 24 hours | | | | | Remarks |
			0–2 weeks	2 weeks to 1 year	1 year	7 years	Adult	
Amikacin	i.m.	} 2	} 15 mg/kg	Total dose should not exceed 15 g: course up to 10 days.				Amps 500 mg/2 ml, 100 mg/2 ml
	IV							
Amoxycillin	Oral	3		125 mg three times daily			750 mg–4.5 g	Caps 250 mg
								Susp. 125 mg, 250 mg/5 ml
								Paed. susp. 125 mg/ 5 ml
	i.m.	3		} 50–100 mg/kg up to 10 years				Vials of powder 250,500 mg, 1 g
	IV	4						
Ampicillin	Oral	4						Tabs 125 mg.
	i.m.		} 250 mg		} 500 mg	} 1 g		} 2 g	Caps 250 mg.
	IV							Syrup 125 mg/5 ml.
								Vials 100, 250, 500 mg
Benzylpenicillin				*See* Penicillin G				
Carbenicillin	i.m.	4	200 mg/kg		2 g	4 g	8 g	Vials 1 g, 5 g
	IV							Infusion set 5 g
								Septicaemia, use four times the dose
Cephalexin*	Oral	4	25–50 mg/kg		500 mg	1 g	1–4 g	Caps 250, 500 mg
								Syrup 125, 250, 500 mg/5 ml
								Paed. drops 125 mg/ 1.25 ml

TABLE A9.II *continued*
Antibacterial agents

| Name | Routes | Doses per 24 hours | Total dose per 24 hours | | | | | Remarks |
			0–2 weeks	2 weeks to 1 year	1 year	7 years	Adult	
Cephaloridine*	i.m. IV	2 or 3	15–30 mg/kg		250 mg	500–750 mg	1–1.5 g	Vials, 100, 250, 500 mg
Cephalothin*	IV (i.m.)	4–6	80–160 mg/kg		100–300 mg/kg		Up to 12 g	Amps. 1 g, 4 g
Cephradine*	Oral	4	25–50 mg/kg		250–500 mg/kg	500 mg–1 g	1–2 g	Caps 250, 500 mg Susp. 125, 250 mg/ 5 ml
	i.m. IV	4	50–100 mg/kg				2–4 g	Vials 250, 500 mg, 1 g
Chloramphenicol	Oral i.m. IV	4	*See* page 743		500 mg	1 g	2 g	Caps 250 mg Susp. 125 mg/5 ml Vials 1.2 g succinate *Meningitis, see* p. 357
Clindamycin	Oral i.m.	3 or 4	12–25	150 mg	300 mg	600 mg	600 mg –1.8 g	Caps 75, 150 mg Susp. 75 mg/5 ml
	IV			15–40 mg/kg		600 mg	600 mg –2.7 g	Amps 150 mg/1 ml *Risk of pseudomembranous colitis*
	Infusion							
Cloxacillin	Oral i.m.	4		250 mg	500 mg	1 g	2 g	Caps 250, 500 mg Syrup 125 mg/5 ml
	IV	4 or 6		125 mg	250–375 mg	500–750 mg	1 g–1.5 g	Vials 250, 500 mg

Drug	Route						Preparations
Colistin sulphate	Oral	3	750 000 units	3.0 mega units	4.5 mega units	9.0 mega units	Tabs 1.5 mega units Syrup 250 000 units/ 5 ml *Not absorbed*
Colistin sulphomethate	i.m. IV	3	50 000 units/kg	1.5 mega units	3.0 mega units	6.0 mega units	Vials 0.5, 1.0 mega units
Cotrimoxazole Dose in terms of Trimethoprim. (Ratio of Trimethoprim to Sulphamethoxazole is 1:5 in all preparations)	Oral IV i.m.	2	Avoid during first 4 weeks 8 mg/kg avoid i.m. under 6 years	80 mg	160 mg	320 mg	Tabs 20, 80 mg, 160 mg Susp. 40, 80 mg/5 ml IV susp. 80 mg/5 ml & i.m. 160 mg/3 ml
Erythromycin	Oral	4 or 6	50 mg/kg	500 mg	1 g	2 g	Caps 250 mg Tabs 500 mg Susp. 100, 125, 250 mg/5 ml
Erythromycin ethyl succinate (i.m. preparation)	i.m. only	2 or 3	5.0–7.5 mg/kg	50–75 mg	100–150 mg	200–300 mg	50 mg/2 ml *Painful i.m.: avoid I.V. and s.c.*
Erythromycin lactobionate	IV only	3 or 6	20–30 mg/kg	225–300 mg	450–600 mg	900 mg–1.2 g	Vial 300 mg *Avoid i.m. or s.c.*
Flucloxacillin	Oral i.m. IV slow	4	*Under 2 years* 250 mg, *2–10 years* 500 mg i.m. as for oral IV as for oral or up to twice this dose			1 g	Caps 250 mg Vials 250, 500 mg
Fusidate sodium Fusidic acid (Fucidin)	Oral	3	50 mg/kg	375–500 mg	750 mg	1.5 g	Caps 250 mg Susp. 250 mg/5 ml
	IV infusion		60 mg/kg		as above	as above	Amps 500 mg

TABLE A9.II *continued*
Antibacterial agents

Name	Routes	Doses per 24 hours	Total dose per 24 hours					Remarks
			0–2 weeks	*2 weeks to 1 year*	*1 year*	*7 years*	*Adult*	
Gentamicin	i.m. IV by bolus	} 3	*12-hourly* 6 mg/ kg/24 hours	6 mg/kg	60 mg	120 mg	240 mg	Vial/Amp 40 mg/ml Paed. 10 mg/ml Course 7–10 days *Nephrotoxic, ototoxic* Blood levels if possible
Kanamycin	Oral i.m.	2–4 2	Not advised 15 mg/kg (pre-term 7.5 mg/ kg)		150 mg	300 mg	1 g 600 mg	Caps 250 mg Vial 1 g/3 ml. Paed. 75 mg/2 ml *Nephrotoxic, ototoxic*
Lincomycin	Oral	4 (under 1 year, 3)	37.5 mg (2.5 ml) 8-hourly		*1–3 years* 37.5 mg 6-hourly	*4–7 years* 75 mg 6-hourly	*8–12 years* 102.5 mg 6-hourly *Adult* 150 mg 6-hourly	Caps 75 mg Susp. 75 mg/5 ml Solution for injection 150 mg/1 ml
			Severe infection 37.5 mg 6-hourly		75 mg 6-hourly	102.5 mg 6-hourly	*8–12 years* 150 mg 6-hourly	*Risk of pseudomembranous colitis*

Drug	Route	Times per 24 h		Under 3 months	3 months–12 years		*Adult*	Preparations / notes
	i.m. IV	3–4		Over 1 month 15–25 mg/kg/24 hours *Severe infection*, up to 40 mg/kg/24 hours			300 mg 6-hourly 300 mg– 1.2 g 6-hourly Up to 2.7 g/ 24 hours	
Methicillin	i.m. only	4		*Under 3 months* 250 mg	*3 months–12 years* 100 mg/kg		4–6 g	Vials 1.0 g
Metronidazole		*See* Table A9.V						Anaerobic infections, p. 353
Nalidixic acid	Oral	4	Avoid	60–100 mg/kg	1 g	2 g	4 g	Tabs 500 mg Susp. 300 mg/5 ml
Neomycin	Oral	4		50 mg/kg	500 mg	1 g	2 g	Tabs 500 mg Elixir 100 mg/5 ml *Not absorbed*
Oxytetracycline	Oral IV	4		25 mg/kg	250 mg	500 mg	1 g	Tabs 100, 250 mg Syrup 125 mg/5 ml.
	i.m.	3		7.5 mg/kg	75 mg	150 mg	300 mg	Injection: 250 mg IV: 100 mg i.m. *Staining of teeth under 12 years*
Penicillin G (Benzylpenicillin)	i.m. IV slow	2–4		30 mg/kg	300 mg	600 mg (1 mega unit)	1200 mg (2 mega units)	1 mega unit = 600 mg. *Severe infection*: give same dose 6- hourly or IV.

TABLE A9.II *continued*
Antibacterial agents

Name	Routes	Doses per 24 hours	Total dose per 24 hours					Remarks
			0–2 weeks	2 weeks to 1 year	1 year	7 years	Adult	
Penicillin procaine	i.m. only	Once	0.05 ml/kg		0.5 ml	1 ml	2 ml	300 000 units/ml
Penicillin, prolonged injection (Triplopen)	i.m. only	Every 2–3 days	$\frac{1}{4}$ vial every 2–3 days			$\frac{1}{2}$ vial every 2–3 days	1 vial every 2–3 days	One vial contains: Benzylpenicillin 300 mg; Procaine penicillin 250 mg; Benethamine penicillin 475 mg.
Penicillin V (Phenoxymethyl penicillin)	Oral	4	250 mg		500 mg	1 g	2 g	Tabs 125, 250 mg. Syrup 125 mg/5 ml.
Penicillin eye drops			*See* Gonococcal Conjunctivitis, p. 629					25 000 units/ml or 250 000 units/l
Spectinomycin	i.m.	1	Avoid during first 4/52; otherwise 100 mg/kg				Males 2 g Females 4 g	Vial 400 mg/ml
Streptomycin			*See* Antituberculous Agents p. 794					
Sulphadimidine Sulphadiazine	Oral	4	Avoid during first 4 weeks	100 mg/kg	1 g	2 g	4 g	Tabs 500 mg. Mixt. 500 mg/5 ml. Amps 1 g in 3 ml. Severe infection; double dose
	i.m. IV	4						

Sulphafurazole	Oral	4	Avoid during first 4/52	As above	As above	As above	As above	Tabs 500 mg Syrup 500 mg in 5 ml
Tetracycline	Oral	4	25 mg/kg		250 mg	500 mg	1 g	Tabs 250 mg
	i.m.	3	10 mg/kg		100 mg	100–150 mg	200–300 mg	Syrup 125 mg/5 ml
	IV	4	As above		250 mg	500 mg	500 mg –1 g	i.m. vial 100 mg IV vials 250, 500 mg *Staining of teeth under 12 years*
Tobramycin	i.m. IV or IV infusion	3 or 4		3–5 mg/kg all ages				Vials 20, 40, 80 mg

* Contra-indicated in penicillin (group) sensitivity.

TABLE A9.III*

Antibacterial agents which can be given IV: doses are shown in Table A9.II

Name	Vehicle for dissolving or dilution	Method of administration	Stability	Remarks
Amikacin	Dilute in 0.9% NaCl, 5% glucose or lactate Ringer	Dilute to 2.5 or 5 mg/ml and infuse over 30 minutes at 12-hourly intervals	Solutions containing 2.5 or 5 mg/ml can be used within 24 hours if stored at $<25°C$	
Amoxycillin	Dissolve in water for injection: for i.m. 1.5 ml/250 mg; for IV 2.5 ml/500 mg	Infuse over $\frac{1}{2}$–1 hour	Stable in 0.9% NaCl for 6 hours, but in glucose saline for 1 hour	
Ampicillin	Dilute in 10–20 ml water for injection	IV injection over 3–4 minutes	Loses 10% of activity in glucose or glucose saline over 5–6 hours. Use immediately	Not by slow infusion
Benzylpenicillin	Dissolve 300 mg in 1 ml or 600 mg in 2 ml of water for injection	Injection over 3–4 minutes or infusion over 30–40 minutes	Use immediately after preparation	Not by continuous infusion
Carbenicillin	1-g vial: add 5 ml water for injection and shake. For 5-g vial, use 20 ml	Give every 4–6 hours by injection over 3–4 minutes, or rapid infusion over 30–40 minutes	Dry powder should be stored at 5°C. Use solutions for injection within 30 minutes	Not by slow infusion
Cephaloridine	Dissolve in 10–20 ml 0.9% NaCl or 5% glucose	Inject over 3–5 minutes or by infusion over 30–60 minutes, or by continuous infusion using fresh solution every 6 hours	Use solution immediately after preparation. Solution remains active for 24 hours at $<25°C$, or 4 days at 4°C	Warm by hand if crystallization occurs. Shake thoroughly before use

* Data mainly from the manufacturer's information in *Data Sheet Compendium* (1977), published by the Association of the British Pharmaceutical Industry, London

TABLE A9.III *continued*

Name	Vehicle for dissolving or dilution	Method of administration	Stability	Remarks
Cephalothin	Use solution of 1 g per 5 ml water for injection, or 0.9% NaCl, or 5% glucose	Inject over 3–5 minutes, or by continuous infusion at strength of 4 g per 20 ml water added to 500 ml. 0.9% NaCl or 5% glucose	Reconstituted solution (not diluted) remains active for 48 hours at 4°C. For continuous infusion replace solution every 24 hours	As above
Cephradine	Add 5 ml water for injection to 250 or 500 mg, or 10 ml to 1 g. Shake to dissolve. Dilute with 0.9% NaCl, or 5% glucose	Direct injection or by infusion	For direct injection use within 2 hours at room temperature or 24 hours at 5°C. Diluted solution remains active for 8 hours	Precipitation may occur with calcium salts
Chloramphenicol	Dilute with water for injection or 5% glucose	Inject over 3–4 minutes or infuse over 30–60 minutes		Reject cloudy solution
Clindamycin	Dilute to strength of 300 mg in 50 ml or more of 0.9% NaCl or 5% glucose. Doses and infusion times:	Infuse over 10–60 minutes or by continuous infusion		Not by bolus injection

Dose	Diluent	Time
300 mg;	50 ml;	10 minutes
600 mg;	100 ml;	30 minutes
900 mg;	150 ml;	40 minutes
1200 mg;	200 ml;	45 minutes

Not more than 1200 mg over 60 minutes

Name	Vehicle for dissolving or dilution	Method of administration	Stability	Remarks
Cloxacillin	500 mg dissolved in 10 ml water for injection	Injection over 3–4 minutes at 4–6-hourly intervals	Use within 30 minutes of preparation	
Colistin	Dissolve dose in 0.9% NaCl or 5% glucose	Infuse over 6 hours, or less	Use freshly prepared solutions	

TABLE A9.III * *continued*

Antibacterial agents which can be given IV: doses are shown in Table A9.II

Name	Vehicle for dissolving or dilution	Method of administration	Stability	Remarks
Cotrimoxazole	Dilute 5-ml ampoules in 125-ml infusion fluid (0.9% NaCl or 5% glucose) 2 amps (10 ml) in 250 ml. 3 amps (15 ml) in 500 ml	Infuse over $1-1\frac{1}{2}$ hours	Dilute immediately before use	Solution faintly yellow; shake thoroughly after dilution and reject turbid solutions
Erythromycin (lactobionate)	6 ml of water for injection or 5% glucose to vial containing 300 mg to make stock solution	Dilute stock solution with 4 times initial volume to give 1% solution, using water for injection or 5% glucose or 0.9% NaCl. Inject over 3–5 minutes or use continuous infusion over several hours	Reconstituted 5% solution is stable for 2 weeks at 4°C	Electrolyte solutions should not be used for initial dilution to make up the stock solution
Flucloxacillin	250–500 mg dissolved in 10 ml water for injection	Inject over 3–4 minutes	Use within 30 minutes of preparation	
Fusidate (sodium)	Dissolve in buffer provided. Dilute to 250–500 ml of 0.9% NaCl	Infuse over 2–4 hours	Diluted solution should be used within 24 hours	Opalescence may occur if diluted in acid solution of 5% glucose
Gentamicin	Use as in ampoule or vial, without dilution	*i.m. usually best.* If IV use bolus injection over 2–3 minutes	Very stable	Do not use continuous infusion
Kanamycin	IV injection not advised			
Lincomycin	Dilute in 250 ml or more of 5% glucose or 0.9% NaCl	Infuse over 1 hour or more (doses every 8–12 hours)	Store solution at <20°C	

TABLE A9.III *continued*

Name	Vehicle for dissolving or dilution	Method of administration	Stability	Remarks
Methicillin	1 g dissolved in 20 ml water for injection	Inject over 3–4 minutes or by continuous infusion, changing bottle every 5 hours	Use solution within 30 minutes of preparation	
Metronidazole† special preparation required	Use 0.5% solution: adult dose 500 mg	Infusions at 8-hourly intervals		*Anaerobic infections only*
Oxytetracycline	Make up stock solution with water for injection, 0.9% NaCl or 5% glucose	Dilute stock solution to 25 ml if for injection, or 250 ml for infusion		
Penicillin G *see* Benzylpenicillin				
Tetracycline	Add 5 ml water for injection to 250-mg vial, and 10 ml to 500-mg vial. Dilute to 100–1000 ml with 0.9% NaCl or 5% glucose	Infuse at not faster than 100 ml in 5 minutes. Use 12-hourly doses	Diluted solution should be used immediately	Forms precipitate with calcium compounds
Tobramycin	For infusion, dilute in 50 ml–100 ml (adult dose)	By injection or continuous infusion		

* Data mainly from the manufacturer's information in *Data Sheet Compendium* (1977), published by the Association of the British Pharmaceutical Industry. London

† *See Martindale's Extra Pharmacopoeia* for further details, pp. 1570–1573; *see* reference at foot of Table A9.V.

TABLE A9.IV
Antituberculous agents

Name	Routes	Doses per 24 hours	Dose per 24 hours					Remarks
			0–2 weeks	2 weeks– 1 year	1 year	7 years	Adult	
Ethambutol	Oral	Once	15 mg/kg in 3-drug regime					Tabs 100, 400 mg
			25 mg/kg for the first 2 months if using a 2-drug regime					
Isoniazid (INA, INAH)	Oral i.m. (IV)	3–4 4	10–20 mg/kg 100–400 mg		150 mg	300 mg	600 mg >1 year–Adult 200–800 mg	Tabs 50, 100 mg Amps 50 mg in 2 ml Add Pyridoxine 10 mg daily
Rifampicin	Oral	Once	10–20 mg/kg		200 mg	400 mg	450–600 mg	Caps 150, 300 mg
Sodium aminosalicylate (PAS)	Oral	4	300 mg/kg		3 g	5–6 g	10–20 g	Powder
Streptomycin	i.m.	2	Avoid if possible	15–25 mg/kg	250 mg	500 mg	1 g	Amps 1 g

TABLE A9.V
Antimicrobial* (excluding antibacterial) agents

Name	Routes	Doses per 24 hours	Total dose per 24 hours					Remarks
			0–2 weeks	2 weeks –1 year	1 year	7 years	Adult	
Adenine arabinoside	IV	*see* Vidarabine						
Amodiaquine	Oral	3		5 mg/kg	50 mg	100 mg	200 mg	Malaria, p. 554 Tabs 150, 200 mg
Amphotericin[1]	IV	4	Avoid if possible	Initial daily dose 0.25 mg/kg by slow IV injection over 6 hours. Increase up to 1 mg/kg/day but not more than 1.5 mg/kg			Total course should not exceed 3 g	*See* pp. 358, 643. Vials, 50 mg with deoxycholate and phosphate buffer
Chloroquine[1]	Oral i.m.	Once 1–2		5–12 mg/kg Single dose should not exceed 5 mg/kg and total dose/24 hours should not exceed 10 mg/kg. Usual single dose in newborn is 10 mg. For initial loading dose the above doses should be given twice daily.	125 mg	250–300 mg	600 mg	Malaria, p. 554 Tabs 100, 150, 200 mg. Amps 5 ml with concentration of 40 mg/1 ml
	IV	2–4	Avoid	Single dose, 5 mg/kg repeated in 6, 8 or 12 hours if necessary, *or*, 7 mg/kg by continuous drip over 24 hours Bolus doses over at least 3 minutes				
Cotrimoxazole				*See* Table A9.III				Pneumocystis, p. 476
Cytosine[1] arabinoside (cytarabine)	IV	Once or continuous infusion	Direct injection: 2 mg/kg Continuous infusion: 0.5–1 mg/kg					Herpes or CMV encephalitis. p. 627. Vials 100 mg
Emetine	s.c. i.m.	Once	} 1.5 mg/kg	} 5 mg		} 30 mg	} 60 mg	Amoebiasis, p. 570 Amps 30, 60 mg in 1 ml
Flucytosine	Oral	4	150–200 mg/kg Reduce dose in renal failure					Antifungal agents, p. 358 Tabs 500 mg

* Antiviral, antifungal, antiprotozoal

TABLE A9.V *continued*
Antimicrobial* (excluding antibacterial) agents

Name	Routes	Doses per 24 hours	Total dose per 24 hours					Remarks
			0–2 weeks	2 weeks –1 year	1 year	7 years	Adult	
Idoxuridine[1]	IV	12-hourly infusion	0.5% solution over 45–60 minutes 50–100 mg/kg for 4–5 days. Total dose should not exceed 300–400 mg/kg					Herpes or CMV encephalitis. p. 627
Metronidazole[1]	Oral: IV only for anaerobic infections	3	60 mg/kg *See* Note 1		600 mg	0.6–1.2 g	1.2–2.4 g	Amoebiasis, p. 570 Anaerobic infections: p. 353. Table A9.VI Tabs 200, 400 mg
Nifurtimox[1]	Oral	4	25 mg/kg for 15 days, then 15 mg/kg for 75 days (total course, 90 days)				Initially 5–7 mg/kg	Chagas' disease, p. 628
Pentamidine[1]	i.m. (IV)	Once or divided doses	4 mg/kg for 24 hours for 15 days: IV only in severe cases					Pneumocystis, p. 476 Amps 200 mg
Pyrimethamine	Oral	1–2	0.5–1.0 mg/kg	6.25 mg	12.5 mg		25 mg	Toxoplasmosis. (with sulphadiazine), p. 643
Quinine	Oral	3	20–30 mg/kg	300 mg	600 mg		1.2–2.4g	Malaria, p. 556 Tabs 300 mg
	(i.m.)	1–3	5 mg/kg (avoid in small children) but may be necessary in the newborn if chloroquine is unsuitable.)					Amps 600 mg in 2 ml
	IV	2–4	Average single dose 10 mg/kg but total dose/24 hours should not exceed 20 mg/kg. Avoid IV quinine in newborn. Direct IV injection: dilute in 10 times original volume and give over at least 3 minutes. Best method by slow infusion over 4–6 hours, or continuous infusion over 24 hours.					Solution containing 100 mg/3.5 ml
Spiramycin[2]	Oral	4	50 mg/kg					Toxoplasmosis in newborn p. 643

Sulphadiazine	Oral	4	150 mg/kg	Toxoplasmosis, with pyrimethamine, p. 643.
Tinidazole[1]	Oral	Once	60 mg/kg	Tabs 0.5 g Amoebiasis. p. 570
Vidarabine[3] (Vita-A) (adenine arabinoside)	IV		10–15 mg/kg/day for 10 days: each daily dose to be given by slow drip over 12 hours	Herpes simplex encephalitis. p. 631. 5-ml vials. 200 mg/ml. *See also* Table A9.VI for details of administration

---

* Antiviral, antifungal, antiprotozoal.

[1] The following pages in *Martindale's Extra Pharmacopoeia* (1977). (27th Edition) Pharmaceutical Press London give the information: Amphotericin, 637–642; Chloroquine, 344–348; Cytosine arabinoside, 141–143; Idoxuridine, 912–913; Metronidazole, 1570–1573; Nifurtimox, 1578; Tinidazole, 1574–1575; Pentamidine, 1578–1580.

[2] Davies, P. A. (1975). Antimicrobial therapy in the neonatal period. *Br. J. Hosp. Med.* **14**, 517

[3] Whitley R. J. *et al.* (1977). Adenine arabinoside therapy in biopsy-proved herpes simplex encephalitis. *New Engl. J. Med.* **297**, 289.

TABLE A9.VI
Antimicrobial* (excluding antibacterial) agents which can be given IV: (dosage shown in Table A9.V)

Name	Vehicle for dissolving or dilution	Method of administration	Stability	Remarks
Adenine arabinoside (*see* Vidarabine)				
Amphotericin[1]	Dissolve in 5% glucose solution to make a concentration of 0.1 mg/ml. Do not dilute with saline solutions	Slow infusion over 6 hours. Heparin may be used to reduce thrombophlebitis	Store vials at 2–10°C	
Chloroquine[1]	As for quinine	Direct injection, *over at least 3 minutes*, using solution diluted to 10 times. Best given by slow infusion over 6–8 hours, or continuous drip over 24 hours		
Cotrimoxazole	*See* Table A9.III			
Cytosine arabinoside (cytarabine)[1]	Dissolve powder in the accompanying ampoule containing water for injection with 0.9% benzyl alcohol. Final concentration 20 mg/ml	Direct injection or by continuous infusion over 24 hours	Reconstituted solution should be stored at room temperature and used within 24 hours	Hazy solution must be discarded
Idoxuridine[1]	To make 0.5% solution the powder is added to 5% glucose whose pH has been adjusted to 10.0 with sodium carbonate, and warmed to 37–40°C. Final pH is adjusted to	The daily dose should be given in 2 divided infusions over 45–60 minutes each	Store at 4°C for not more than 14 days	

TABLE A9.VI *continued*

Name	Vehicle for dissolving or dilution	Method of administration	Stability	Remarks
	9.0 by sodium carbonate or acid. Sterilized by membrane or candle filter			
Pentamidine[1]	Dissolve powder in water for injection	By slow IV injection	Aqueous solution should be used immediately after preparation	IV injection may cause hypotension
Quinine	For injection, dilute with at least 10 times original volume of water for injection. For infusion, dilute in up to 200 ml of 0.9% NaCl: a concentration of 0.5–1.0 mg quinine per ml should be used	Direct injection over *at least 3 minutes.* Best given by slow infusion over 4–6 hours or continuous drip over 24 hours. Rate of infusion should not exceed 50 mg per minute		
Vidarabine	Dilute 1 ml of the microcrystalline solution in 500 ml of the usual IV fluids to produce a strength of 0.4 mg per ml	Infuse over 12 hours	With good aseptic techniques a week's supply can be prepared at one time; it should *not* be stored in the refrigerator, but kept at room temperature	*See* Table A9.V for reference

Data mainly from *Data Sheet Compendium* (1977) published by the Association of British Pharmaceutical Industry, London.

* Antiviral, antifungal and antiprotozoal.

[1] *See* notes to Table A9.V.

TABLE A9.VII
Anthelminthic agents

Name	Routes	Dose	0–2 weeks	2 weeks –1 year	1 year	7 years	Adult	Remarks
Bephenium	Oral	Single dose only on one day			2.5 g	5 g		Hookworm, p. 640 Sachets, 3 g
Tetrachlorethylene	Oral	Single dose only on one day	0.2 ml per year of age				1–3 ml	Hookworm, p. 640 Caps or fluid

TABLE A9.VIII

Glucocorticoids and corticotrophins

Drug	Routes	Individual doses					Remarks
		0–2 weeks	2 weeks –1 year	1 year	7 years	Adult	
Cortisone acetate Tabs 5, 25 mg Vials of 10 ml containing 25 mg per 1 ml	Oral (i.m.)	Depends upon indication					i.m. absorption slower than by mouth; use hydrocortisone or prednisolone for parenteral route
Dexamethasone Tabs 0.5, 0.75 mg	Oral	Depends upon indication					
Solution containing 4 mg of the phosphate per 1 ml	i.m. IV	Usual dose 0.5–10 mg daily in divided doses, usually 6-hourly					
Hydrocortisone sodium succinate (hemisuccinate). Vials 100, 500 mg	i.m. IV	All ages, 100–300 mg at 6–8-hourly intervals					Use for rapid systemic effect
Hydrocortisone acetate							Unsuitable for production of systemic effects
Prednisolone Tabs 1, 5 mg Vials 32 mg in 2 ml	Oral i.m. IV	All ages: 5 up to 100 mg daily, usually given 6-, 8- or 12-hourly according to indications					
Prednisone Tabs 1 mg, 5 mg	Oral	As above					
Tetracosactrin zinc injection (corticotrophin depot injection) Amps 1 mg in 1 ml Vials 1 mg in 2 ml, 2 mg in 2 ml	i.m.	Initially every 2nd or 3rd day	Up to 2.5 mg	2.5–0.5 mg	0.25–1.0 mg	0.5–1.0 mg	
Corticotrophin gelatin injection	s.c. i.m.	Once/24 hours	1 unit/kg	10 units	20 units	40 units	Use Tetracosactrin in preference

TABLE A9.IX
Mineralocorticoids

Name	Routes	Doses per 24 hours	0–2 weeks	2 weeks –1 year	1 year	7 years	Adult	Remarks
Aldosterone Amps 0.5 mg in 1 ml	i.m. IV	4–6	0.5 mg (500 microgrammes: dose frequency depends upon response): *see* page 455					0.5 mg = ~1.0 mg DOCA but has a shorter action
Deoxycortone acetate (DOCA)	i.m.	1–3	0.75–1.0 mg			1.5 mg	3 mg	Future supply uncertain in Britain
Fludrocortisone Tabs 0.1 mg	Oral	1–2	0.05 mg			0.1 mg	0.2 mg	0.1 mg = 2.5 mg DOCA

TABLE A9.X
Anabolic steroids

Name	Route	Frequency of dose	Children	Adolescents	Remarks
Nandrolone decanoate Amps 25 mg, 50 mg in 1 ml	i.m.	Once every 3 weeks		12.5–25 mg	Anorexia nervosa, p. 505

TABLE A9.XI
Characteristics of various corticoids

Name	Equivalent dose for anti-inflammatory effect[1]	Equivalent mineralo-corticoid activity[2]	Time to achieve maximal plasma cortisol levels[2]			Biological half-life[2]
			Oral	i.m.	IV	
Deoxycortone acetate (DOCA)	No effect	1.0 mg		No effect		
Cortisone	100 mg	20 mg	2 hours	20–24 hours	—	30 minutes
Hydrocortisone sodium succinate	80 mg	20 mg	1–2 hours	$\frac{1}{2}$ 2 hours	Immediate	90 minutes
Prednisolone	20 mg	50 mg				200 minutes
Prednisone	20 mg	50 mg				60 minutes
Betamethasone	3 mg	Negligible				
Dexamethasone	3 mg	Negligible				200 minutes
Fludrocortisone		0.04 mg				

[1] Data from *British National Formulary*, (1976–78). p. 136

[2] Data from Conte, F. A., Grumbach, M. M. (1973). Endocrine emergencies: In *Pediatric Emergencies*. Eds D. J. Pascoe and M. Grossman. Philadelphia: J. B. Lipincott

TABLE A9.XII
Antisera and immunoglobulins *

Name	Route	Dose	Remarks
Diphtheria	i.m. IV		*See* Diphtheria, p. 228
Hepatitis A: Human Normal Immunoglobulin Injection	i.m.	Consult Public Health Laboratory Service or equivalent	Protects for at least 4 months after injection
Hepatitis B: Hyperimmune Gamma Globulin	i.m.	As above	For those at serious risk from Serum Hepatitis B
Measles Hyperimmune Globulin	i.m.	0.25 ml/kg	
Rabies antiserum	Wound site i.m. $\frac{1}{2}$ the dose by each route	Heterologous 40 iu./kg. Human 20 iu./kg	*See* Rabies, p. 583
Smallpox. *See* Variola			
Snake Venom	I.V.		*See* Venomous Bites and Stings, p. 549
Tetanus. Antitoxin or Human Antitetanus Immunoglobulin	i.m. IV		*See* Tetanus, pp. 337, 341
Vaccinia, Human Antivaccinia Immunoglobulin	i.m.	Consult Public Health Laboratory Service or equivalent 0.3 ml/kg	For children with eczema or immunological deficiency in whom vaccination is absolutely essential. Also provides some passive immunity to smallpox if given in the first half of the incubation period. *See* Smallpox, p. 580
Varicella. *See* Zoster			
Zoster Immune Globulin	i.m.	1 g/m²	*See* Leukaemia, p. 475

* In Britain these products, and advice on their use, can be obtained through the Public Health Laboratory Service

APPENDIX 10

Drugs in Renal Failure

The data on which the tables are based are often incomplete and their quality is varied. Furthermore, the metabolic disturbance of uraemia is complex and no two patients are alike. For these reasons the information given must be interpreted with caution and used only as a rough guide. Careful clinical judgement is necessary as well. The more toxic drugs should be used only when there is no safer alternative and when given in more than short courses their blood concentration should be monitored.

Tables A10.I and II and the accompanying text are reproduced by permission of the author and the Editor of the *British Medical Journal*. (Sharpstone, P. (1977). Prescribing for patients with renal failure. *Br. med. J.* **2**, 36)

TABLE A10.I

Dosage modification of more commonly used drugs for different degrees of renal function impairment

Drug	Dose interval (hours) in categories of impaired renal function				Dialysable		Comment (BC = measure blood concentration in severe renal failure)
	None	*Mild*	*Moderate*	*Severe*	*Haemodialysis*	*Peritoneal dialysis*	
Antibacterial agents							
Benzylpenicillin	8	8	8	12	+	?	BC in 'massive' therapy
Ampicillin	6	6	8	12	+	—	
Cloxacillin	6	6	6	6	—	?	
Carbenicillin	4	4	8	12	+	—	
Tetracycline	6	Avoid	Avoid	Avoid	—	—	Exacerbates uraemia
Doxycycline	24	24	24	24	—	—	No use for urine infection
Cephaloridine	6	12	Avoid	Avoid	+	+	Potentially nephrotoxic
Cephalexin	6	6	8–12	24–48	+	+	

TABLE A10. I *continued*

| Drug | Dose interval (hours) in categories of impaired renal function | | | | Dialysable | | Comment (BC = measure blood concentration in severe renal failure) |
	None	Mild	Moderate	Severe	Haemodialysis	Peritoneal dialysis	
Cephalothin	6	6	8	12–24	+	+	
Cephazolin	8	12	16	24	−	−	
Cephradine	6	12	24	48	?	?	
Chloramphenicol	6	6	Avoid	Avoid	−	−	Metabolites may be toxic
Co-trimoxazole	12	12	24	24–48	+	?	
Colistin	12	24	48	72	+	+	BC
Gentamicin	8	12	24	48–72	+	−	BC
Streptomycin	12	24	48	72	+	+	BC
Kanamycin	8	24	48	72	+	+	BC
Lincomycin	6	6	6	8	−	−	
Sodium fusidate	8	8	8	8	−	?	
Sulphadimidine	6	6	6	12	?	?	
Nalidixic acid	6	6	6	6	?	?	
Nitrofurantoin	6	Avoid	Avoid	Avoid	+	?	Insufficient urine concentration
Para-aminosalicylic acid	12	12	Avoid	Avoid	+	?	
Isoniazid	12	12	12	12	+	+	
Rifampicin	24	24	24	24	?	?	
Ethambutol	24	24	36	48	+	+	
Antifungal agents							
Amphotericin	24	24	24	36	−	?	Nephrotoxic
Flucytosine	6	8	12–24	24–72	+	+	BC

Hypnotics and tranquillizers							
Phenobarbitone	12	12	12	24	+	+	
Short- and medium-acting barbiturates	8	8	8	8	−	−	
Diazepam	8	8	8	8	−	?	
Chlordiazepoxide	8	8	12	24	−	?	
Phenothiazines	8	8	12	18	−	−	
Antidepressants							
Tricyclics	8	8	8	8	−	+	
Lithium carbonate	8	8	Avoid	Avoid	+	+	
Antihistamines							
Chlorpheniramine	6	6	6	6	?	?	
Diphenhydramine	6	6	8	12	−	−	
Anticonvulsants							
Diphenylhydantoin	8	8	8	8	+	?	
Primidone	8	8	12	24	+	?	
Trimethadione	8	8	12	24	?	?	
'Cardiovascular drugs and antihypertensives							
Digoxin	24	36	48	72	−	−	BC
Propranolol	8	8	8	8	−	?	
Methyldopa	8	8	12	16	+	+	
Guanethidine	24	24	36	48	?	?	
Hydrallazine	8	8	8	8	−	−	
Lignocaine	Bolus or infusion	Unchanged	Unchanged	Unchanged	?	?	
Procainamide	4	4	6	8	+	?	
Immunosuppressive agents							
Corticosteroids	Various	Unchanged	Unchanged	Unchanged	?	?	Exacerbate uraemia
Azathioprine	24	24	24	36	+	?	
Cyclophosphamide	24	24	36	48	+	?	
Antidiabetic agents							
Chlorpropamide	24	36	Avoid	Avoid	?	?	
Tolbutamide	8	8	8	12	?	?	
Phenformin	8	8	8	Avoid	?	?	
Acetohexamide	12	24	Avoid	Avoid	?	?	

+ Yes, − No.

TABLE A 10.II
Categories of impaired renal function

		None	Mild	Moderate	Severe
Creatinine clearance (ml/min)		>70	30	10	<10
Plasma creatinine	μmol/l	<114·9	265	884	>884
	mg/100 ml	<1·3	3	10	>10
Plasma urea	mmol/l	<5·8	13·3	41·5	>41·5
	mg/100 ml	<35	80	250	>250

Drug Interactions

The interactions of different combinations of drugs are extremely complex. If in any doubt, consult the hospital pharmacist as well as the manufacturer's drug literature; or the manufacturer's medical department should be consulted direct. For details of some IV drug incompatibilities *see* pages 816–817.

In Britain information on drug interactions is available in any of the following publications:

British National Formulary, published by the British Medical Association and the Pharmaceutical Society of Great Britain;

Monthly Index of Medical Specialities, (MIMS) Annual Compendium, Haymarket Publishing Ltd., London.

Drug Interaction Guide, Abbott Laboratories, Ltd., Queenborough, Kent, England.

The following list of drug interactions is reproduced from *Clinical and Resuscitative Data* by R. P. H. Dunnill and B. E. Crawley, Blackwell Scientific Publications, Oxford (1977) by kind permission of the authors and publishers.

TABLE A11.I

'Drug 1' and 'Drug 2' are the columns containing the two drugs to be mixed. Column 3 shows the effect of mixing these drugs, and Column 4 gives the possible mechanism

Drug 1	Drug 2	Effect	Mechanism
Amphetamines (ephedrine phenylephrine mephentermine)	Barbiturates	Altered CNS effect	(i.e. Purple hearts)
	MAOI	Hypertensive crises and CNS stimulation	Release of unmetabolized catecholamines in CNS
	Antihypertensives	Reversal of effect	Release of catecholamines from binding sites
Alcohol	Barbiturates Phenothiazines General anaesthetics	Potentiation of effect of Drug 2 with tolerance in chronic alcoholic	Enzyme induction especially chronic alcoholics
Anabolic steroids	Anticoagulants	Increase in anticoagulant effect	?Hepatic enzymes
Antibiotics (oral) (streptomycin neomycin colomycin kanamycin bacitracin)	Anticoagulants	Anticoagulants potentiated	Sterilization of gut thus less vitamin K
	Non-depolarizing muscle relaxants	Potentiates action of neuromuscular blockers	Curariform action of these antibiotics
Anticoagulants (warfarin dicoumarol)	Anabolic steroids	Increased anticoagulant effect	?Hepatic enzymes
	Clofibrate	As above	Unknown
	Vitamin K	Antagonism of anticoagulant	Direct antagonism
	Antibiotics (oral)	Potentiation	Sterilization of gut thus less vitamin K
	Chloral hydrate Salicylates Other acidic drugs	Increased clotting time	Release of anticoagulant from albumin binding sites
	Barbiturates Phenytoin	Potentiation of Drug 2	Inhibition of metabolism of Drug 2
	Tolbutamide	Hypoglycaemia	As above
Anticholinesterases (neostigmine dyflos ecothiopate physostigmine)	Non-depolarizing relaxants	Reversal of relaxant	Accumulation of acetyl cholinesterase swamps relaxant
	Suxamethonium	Potentiation of relaxant	Inhibition of hydrolysis of suxamethonium by cholinesterase
Antihypertensives (reserpine, methyl dopa, guanethidine)	Sympathomimetics	Reversal of effects	Release of catecholamines
	Anaesthetics	Hypotension	Potentiation of Drug 1
	Diuretics	Potentiation of hypotension	Reduced cardiac compensation

TABLE A11.I—*continued*

Drug 1	Drug 2	Effect	Mechanism
	Tricylic antidepressants	Reduced hypotensive effect of Drug 1	Sensitized receptors Release of catecholamines
Antithyroids	Benzodiazepines	Increased antithyroid effect	Drug 2 weakly antithyroid
Barbiturates (phenobarbitone hexabarbitone)	Alcohol	Potentiation of Drug 1	Synergistic reaction (i.e. Purple hearts)
	Amphetamines	Altered CNS effect	
	Phenytoin	Reduced action Drug 2	Enzyme induction
	Ketamine	Chemically incompatible	Precipitation
	Anticoagulants	Reduced Drug 2 effect	Enzyme induction
	Griseofulvin	Reduced effect	As above
Benzodiazepines (diazepam oxazepine)	Antithyroids	Increased antithyroid activity	Weak antithyroid action of Drug 1
	Halothane	MAC reduced 35%	Potentiation
Bilirubin	Sulphonamides Salicylates Pyrazolones	Raised serum bilirubin kernicterus in children	Displaced bilirubin from albumin
Beta-blockers (propanolol practolol oxprenolol)	Ether Cyclopropane Ketamine	Drug 2 potentiated	Cardiodepressant effects of Drug 2 seen due to lack of sympathetic stimulation
Chloral hydrate	Anticoagulants	Increased clotting time	Release of Drug 2 from albumin
Clofibrate	Anticoagulants	Increased clotting	Unknown
Cytotoxics (nitrogen mustards chlorambucil)	Suxamethonium	Prolonged suxamethonium activity	Inhibition of plasma cholinesterase activity
Curariform relaxants (d-Tubocurarine pancuronium gallamine alcuronium)	Streptomycin Neomycin Kanamycin	Persistent curarization	Drug 2 weakly curariform
	Thiazides	Prolongation of relaxant	K^+ depletion
	Anticholinesterases	Reversal of relaxant	Accumulation of acetyl cholinesterase
Digoxin glycosides	Calcium	Enhances dysrhythmias	High cellular Ca^{++} states
	Diuretics	Potentiation of digoxin	Low K^+ states
	Reserpines	Bradycardia	CNS depression
	Suxamethonium	Enhanced toxicity	Low K^+ in cell
Diuretics	Non-depolarizing relaxants	Prolonged relaxation	Low K^+ state
	Digoxin	Enhanced toxicity	Low K^+ state
(chlorothiazide frusemide	MAOI	Increased hypertension	Potentiation of catecholamine

TABLE A11.I—*continued*

Drug 1	Drug 2	Effect	Mechanism
ethacrynic acid)	Antihypertensive	Potentiated Drug 2	Sensitized receptors
	Ganglion blockers	As above	As above
spironolactone	Suxamethonium	Drug 1 increases K^+	With Drug 2, high K^+
Ecothiopate (phospholine eye drops)	Suxamethonium	Prolonged apnoea	Inhibition of plasma cholinesterase
Foods (cheese, Marmite, Bovril, Chianti, certain beans)	Monoamine oxidase inhibitors (MAOI)	Hypotensive crises or more usually hypertensive crises	Absorption of excess amines due to high tyramine content in foods I
Ganglion blockers (mecamylamine	Phenothiazines	Potentiation of Drug 1	α-Blockade and CNS depression
pempidine	MAOI	Hypotension	Inhibition of breakdown of Drug 1
pentolinium trimetaphan)	Tricyclic antidepressants	Reversal of hypotension	Sensitization of catecholamine receptors
	Amphetamines	As above	As above
	Antihypertensives	Potentiation hypotension	
Griseofulvin	Barbiturates	Reduced antibiotic effect	Enzyme induction
Heparin	Hydrocortisone ⎫ Penicillins ⎬	Chemically incompatible	Precipitation when mixed
	Protamine	Antagonistic	Positive and negative ions
Halothane	*d*-Tubocurarine	Potentiation hypotension	Relaxing properties of halothane
	Catecholamines	Increased tendency to dysrhythmias	Drug 2 on smooth muscle with raised CO_2 due to halothane, or hypoxia
	Carbon dioxide	More rapid induction of anaesthetic, with cardiac dysrhythmias	Hyperventilation due to raised pCO_2
Hydrocortisone	Phenytoin ⎫ Barbiturates ⎪ Glutethamide ⎬ Phenothiazines ⎭	Possible Addisonian crises in cortisone-dependent patients	Enzyme induction
	Tricyclic antidepressants ⎫ Heparin ⎬	Incompatible	Precipitation if mixed
Inhalation anaesthetics	Catecholamines ⎭	Increased tendency to dysrhythmias	Raised CO_2 and catecholamine stimulation
	Carbon dioxide	Increased depth of anaesthetic	Hyperventilation and as above

TABLE A11.I—continued

Drug 1	Drug 2	Effect	Mechanism
Insulin	Salicylates Propanolol }	Hypoglycaemia	Synergistic potentiation
Ketamine	Barbiturates	Chemically incompatible	Precipitation if mixed
Levodopa	Anaesthetics	Hypertension and vasoconstriction	Dopamine giving β and α stimulation
Local anaesthetics (lignocaine prilocaine etc.)	Vasoconstrictors	Delayed absorption and occasional necrosis	Prolongation of Drug 1 at site of action
Methotrexate	Salicylates	Potentiation Drug 1 with toxicity	Release from binding sites of Drug 1
MAOI (proniazid nialamide phenelzine isocarbazide pargyline membanazine)	Analeptics	CNS stimulation	Additive
	Antiparkinsonian drugs	Potentiation	
	Sulphonylureas	Hypoglycaemia	Sympathetic impairment
	Antihypertensives Ganglion blockers }	Increased hypotensive effects	Sympathetic system impaired
	Thiazides	Hypotension	Fluid depletion
	Foods	MAOI crises	Absorption of amines
	Narcotic analgesics	Hypo or hypertension and potentiation of Drug 2	Release of amines in CNS and delayed metabolism of Drug 2
	Tricyclic antidepressants	Potentiation and antidepressant effect	Increased CNS sensitivity
	Amphetamines	Hypertensive crises	Release of unmetabolized catecholamines
	Noradrenaline Phenylephrine }	Potentiation as above	Hypersensitivity of receptors as above
Narcotic analgesics (morphine pethidine papaveretum heroin fentanyl)	Nalorphine Levallorphan Naloxone }	Reduced and reversed effect of Drug 1	Competitive antagonism of Drug 1
	Pentazocine	As above	Nalorphine-like effect of pentazocine
	MAOI	Hypotension and coma	Delayed excretion of Drug 1 due to microsomal enzyme inhibition
Penicillin	Heparin	Chemically incompatible	Precipitation if mixed
Pentazocine	Narcotic analgesics	Reduced or reversal of effect of Drug 2	Competitive antagonism of Drug 2
Phenylephrine	MAOI	Potentiation of Drug 1	Hypersensitivity of receptors with release of catecholamines
Phenytoin	Sulphonamides	Potentiation of Drug 1	Inhibition of metabolism

TABLE A11.I—continued

Drug 1	Drug 2	Effect	Mechanism
	Pyrazolones	As above	As above
	Hydrocortisone	Increased inactivation of steroid	Converted to β-hydroxysteroid
	Barbiturate	Reduced action of Drug 1	Enzyme induction
Probenecid	Salicylate	Antagonism of uricosuric effect	Competition at renal-tubular level
Propanolol	Sulphonylureas	Hypoglycaemia	Potentiation of insulin
	Insulin	As above	
Propanidid	Suxamethonium	Prolongation of suxamethonium	Cholinesterases are used to hydrolyse Drug 1
Protamine	Heparin	Antagonism	Positive and negative ions
Salicylates (aspirin)	Anticoagulants	Increase in clotting time	Release of Drug 2 from binding sites
	Insulin	Hypoglycaemia	Unknown
	Sulphonylureas	As above	Displacement of Drug 2 from binding sites
	Methotrexate	Potentiation with toxicity	Release of Drug 2 from binding sites
	Probenecid	Antagonism of uricosuric effect	Competition at renal-tubular level
	Sulphonamides	Increased sulphonamide levels	Release of Drug 2 from binding sites
Steroids	Thiazides	Hyperglycaemia	Additive diabetogenic effect
Sulphonamides	Sulphonylureas	Hypoglycaemia	Displacement from binding sites of Drug 2
Sulphonylureas (tolbutamide)	MAOI	Hypoglycaemia	Sympathetic impairment
	Anticoagulants	As above	Inhibition of Drug 1 metabolism
	Pyrazolones	As above	Release of Drug 1 from binding sites and reduced metabolism
	Propanolol	As above	Reduced metabolism and potentiation of insulin
	Salicylates	As above	Displacement of Drug 1 from binding sites
Suxamethonium	THA	Prolonged relaxation	Inhibition of plasma cholinesterase
	Ecothiopate	As above	
	Cytotoxics	As above	As above
	Epontol Procaine	Prolonged relaxation	Cholinesterases are used to hydrolyse Drug 2

TABLE A11.I—continued

Drug 1	Drug 2	Effect	Mechanism
	Thiopentone	Shortened action of Drug 1	Rapid hydrolysis of suxamethonium due to high pH of Drug 2
	Trifluperazine	Reversed action of Drug 1	Interference at synapse
THA	Suxamethonium	Prolonged relaxation	Inhibition of plasma cholinesterase
Thiopentone	Blood	Pain and vasospasm	Precipitation of crystals
	Suxamethonium	Short action of Drug 2	High pH giving rapid hydrolysis
	Sulphafurazole	Sensitivity increased to Drug 1. Shorter action and rapid recovery of 1 if less used	Drug 2 occupies binding site on albumin
Tricylic antidepressants (imipramine amitriptyline)	MAOI	Mutual potentiation	Increased sensitivity of CNS and sympathetic receptors
	Antihypertensives	Reversal of hypotension	Sensitization of catecholamine receptors
	Sympathetic amines	Hypertension	Release of catecholamines at receptor
Trichloroethylene	Soda lime	Toxic nerve damage	Formation of dichloroacetylene and phosgene
Trifluperazine	Suxamethonium	Reversal of relaxation	Interference at synapse

Interaction of Intravenous Drugs and Other Preparations

IV drugs can be given in a number of different ways:

(a) DIRECT INJECTION
The following drugs are particularly dangerous if injected rapidly (i.e.
in <3 minutes) IV:

Aminophylline	Potassium salts
Calcium gluconate	Practolol
Chloroquine	Quinine
Digoxin	Sodium bicarbonate
Magnesium salts	

Potassium salts should NEVER be injected directly IV.

(b) DRUGS ADDED TO AN IV LINE
  (i) Avoid mixing drugs in an infusion: only one drug should be
      given at one time.
  (ii) No drugs of any sort should be added to bottles containing:

Blood	Parenteral lipid preparations
Plasma	Mannitol
Plasma-Protein Fraction	Sodium bicarbonate solution
Parenteral amino acid preparations	

  (iii) The following drugs * should NEVER be mixed with any other
        drug in an infusion:

Amphotericin	Magnesium sulphate
Barbiturates	Mannitol
Calcium gluconate	Phenothiazines (e.g. chlorpromazine)
Diazepam	Sodium bicarbonate
Frusemide	Sulphonamides
Heparin	Vitamin B complex $\pm$ Vitamin C.

* List mainly from *British National Formulary*, 1976–78, page 170

METHODS OF ADMINISTRATION INTO AN IV LINE
There are three alternative methods.

(i) Injection into the tubing followed by flushing through with infusion fluid.

Usual duration of injection: 3–4 minutes.

(ii) Addition of the drug to the drip chamber, which may contain 30 to 100 ml of fluid.

Usual duration: 30–40 minutes.

(iii) Addition to the bottle of infusion fluid: this normally involves a slow infusion over 4 to 6 hours and can only be used when the added drug is exceptionally stable under these conditions (room temperature, and in the presence of the infusion fluid) and in which a peak plasma level is not required.

For antibiotics, methods (i) or (ii) are nearly always used.

When giving more than one drug in an IV infusion always check compatibilities. Always discard any IV solution of a drug which is discoloured, or opaque, when it should be colourless or clear.

If in doubt about the best route of administration and compatibility with the infusion fluid,

(1) Check the manufacturer's instruction insert

or (2) Check with the hospital pharmacist

or (3) Check with the manufacturer by telephone.

Other Drug Effects

Information on the following can be obtained from *Pediatric Therapy*, 5th Edition, Editor H. C. Shirkey, C. V. Mosby Company, St Louis (1975)
- (a) Modification of laboratory tests caused by drugs, pp. 212–220 (T. C. Cashman).
- (b) Drugs excreted in breast milk, pp. 221–223 (J. A. Knowles); also in *Drug Information Bulletin*, Vol. 18, No. 7, Dec. 1977. Published by the Drug Information Centre.
- (c) Drugs that discolour the faeces, pp. 224–225 (H. C. Shirkey).
- (d) Drugs that discolour the urine, pp. 226–227 (H. C. Shirkey).

Normal Blood Pressure (Using the Fourth Phase Korotkoff Sound* for the Diastolic Pressure)

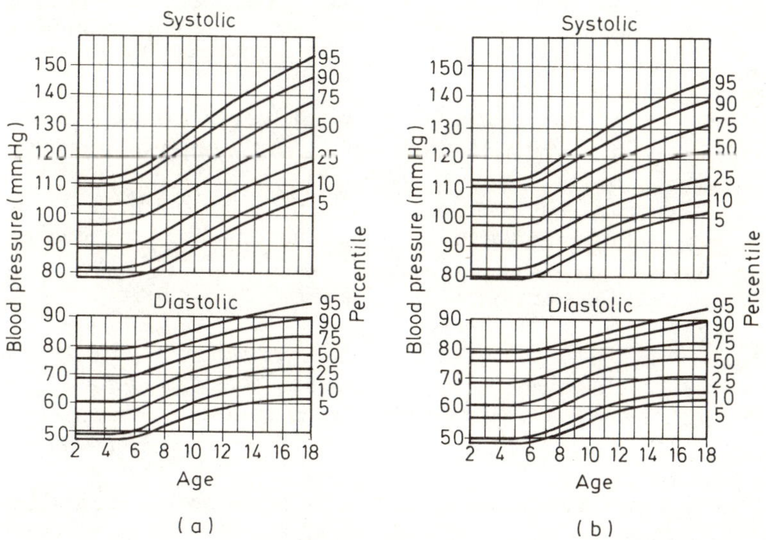

Figure A14.1. Percentiles of blood pressure measurement in (a) boys; and (b) girls. (Right arm, seated.) (Reproduced from Report of the Task Force on Blood Pressure Control in Children. (1977). Pediatrics **59**, 797, with kind permission of the Publishers and the National High Blood Pressure Education Program, Bethesda, Maryland, U.S.A.)

* Muffling of sound

Chemical Tests

FANTUS' TEST FOR CHLORIDE IN URINE
(*See* Heat Illnesses, Heat Cramps, p. 531).
10 drops of urine are placed in a wide-mouthed test tube and 1 drop of 20 per cent potassium chromate is added. A 2.9 per cent solution of silver nitrate is added drop by drop until the colour changes from yellow to brown.

The number of drops added is approximately equal to the concentration of chloride in the urine expressed as grams per litre of sodium chloride (1 g of NaCl is the equivalent of 17 mmol).

It is important that distilled water is used in the preparation of the solutions and for cleaning the test tube. The same dropper should be used for both urine and silver nitrate solutions, being rinsed with distilled water between using the urine and the silver nitrate.

TEST FOR VERDOGLOBIN IN URINE (VERDOGLOBINURIA)
(*See* Medical Emergencies with or following Burns, p. 46)
This test is used to detect the green pigment verdoglobin which is excreted in the urine in severe infections with *Pseudomonas aeruginosa*.

'Equal volumes of urine and glacial acetic acid are mixed in one tube, urine and water in the second and urine and ammonium hydroxide in the third. The three tubes are examined with ultraviolet light in the dark. Verdoglobin is present if an olive fluorescence appears in each, although the alkaline tube may be a chalky-blue. This reaction should not be confused with the yellow-green fluorescence of fluorescein, which may occur in urinary infections due to Pseudomonads.' (Monafo, 1971)

Reference

Monafo, W. W. (1971). *The Treatment of Burns*. p. 213. St Louis: Warren Green II

Temperature Conversions

TABLE A16.I
Temperature conversions

°F	°C	°C	°F
76	24.4	24	75.2
78	25.6	25	77.0
80	26.7	26	78.8
82	27.8	27	80.6
84	28.9	28	82.4
		29	84.2
86	30.0	30	86.0
88	31.1	31	87.8
90	32.2	32	89.6
92	33.3	33	91.4
94	34.4	34	93.2
		35	95.0
96	35.6	36	96.8
98	36.7	37	98.6
99	37.2		
100	37.8	38	100.4
102	38.9	39	102.2
104	40.0	40	104.0

Intermediate values

°C	0.1	0.2	0.3	0.4	0.5	0.6	0.7	0.8	0.9
°F	0.18	0.36	0.54	0.72	0.90	1.08	1.26	1.44	1.62

Needle Sizes

Gauge × length g × in	mm
$27 \times \frac{1}{2}$	12×0.4
$25 \times \frac{5}{8}$	16×0.5
$25 \times \frac{15}{16}$	24×0.5
23×1	25×0.6
$23 \times 1\frac{1}{4}$	31×0.6
22×1	25×0.7
$22 \times 1\frac{1}{2}$	38×0.7
$22 \times 1\frac{1}{2}$	38×0.7
21×1	25×0.8
$21 \times 1\frac{1}{2}$	38×0.8
$21 \times 1\frac{1}{2}$	38×0.8
20×1	25×0.9
$20 \times 1\frac{1}{2}$	38×0.9
$20 \times 1\frac{1}{2}$	38×0.9
19×1	25×1.1
$19 \times 1\frac{1}{2}$	38×1.1
$19 \times 1\frac{1}{2}$	38×1.1
$19 \times 1\frac{1}{2}$ TW	38×1.1
$19 \times 1\frac{1}{2}$ TW	38×1.1
$18 \times 1\frac{1}{2}$	38×1.2
$18 \times 1\frac{1}{2}$	38×1.2
21×2	50×0.8
20×2	50×0.9
19×2	50×1.1
$16 \times 1\frac{1}{2}$	38×1.65
1×1	25×1.65

Reproduced by permission of Monoject Division, Sherwood Medical Industries Ltd., Sherwood House, London Road, County Oak, Crawley, Sussex

Système International (SI) Units: Conversions

In view of the probable gradual acceptance of SI units, both 'old' and SI units have been given wherever possible, except for values used in pharmacology or toxicology where the use of a system based upon chemically active units has no special advantage.

MULTIPLES OF SI UNITS

The prefixes most likely to be encountered in clinical medicine are listed in Table A 18.I.

TABLE A 18.I

Factor	Name	Symbol	Factor	Name	Symbol
10^6	Mega	M	10^{-1}	deci	d
10^3	Kilo	k	10^{-2}	centi	c
10^2	hecto	h	10^{-3}	milli	m
10^1	deca	da	10^{-6}	micro	μ
			10^{-9}	nano	n

UNITS NOT PREVIOUSLY IN USE

Pressure: kilopascal (kPa). 7.5 mmHg = 1.0 kPa

Energy (Nutrition) joules (J). 1 kilocalorie 'Calorie' in clinical medicine = 4.2 J

CONVERSIONS WHICH REQUIRE NO CALCULATION

Bicarbonate
Chloride
Potassium
Sodium

mEq per litre = mmol per litre

Conversion to and from SI units

The following conversion scales are reproduced by kind permission of authors and publishers from *Clinical Chemistry*; Conversion Scales for SI Units, by A. M. Bold and P. Wilding, Blackwell Scientific Publications, Oxford (1975); (the normal adult ranges have not been included here).

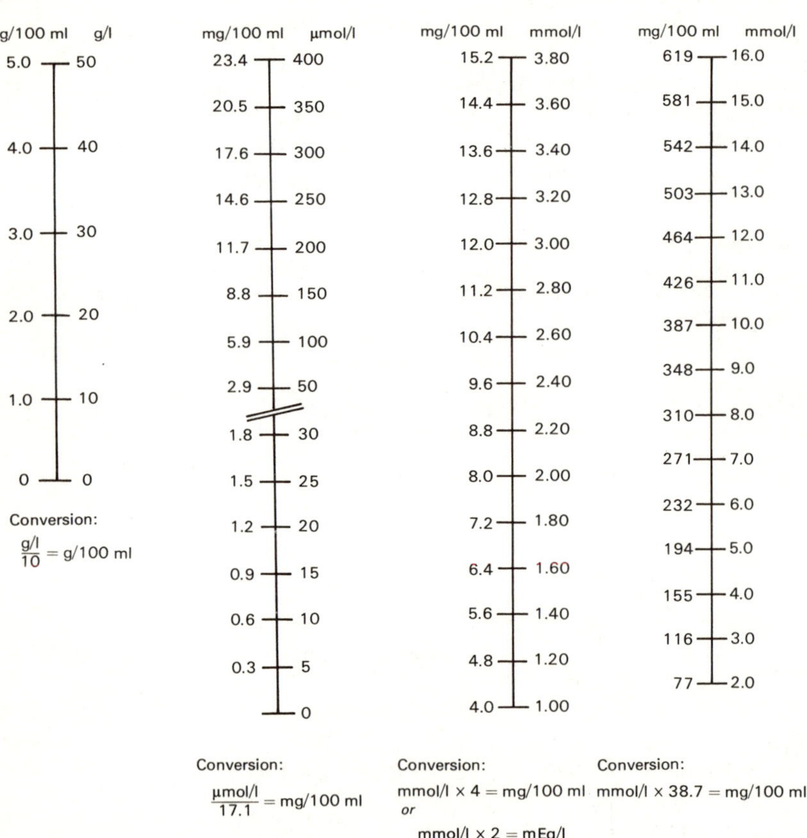

Figure A18.1. SI unit conversions: serum albumin, serum bilirubin, serum calcium, serum cholesterol

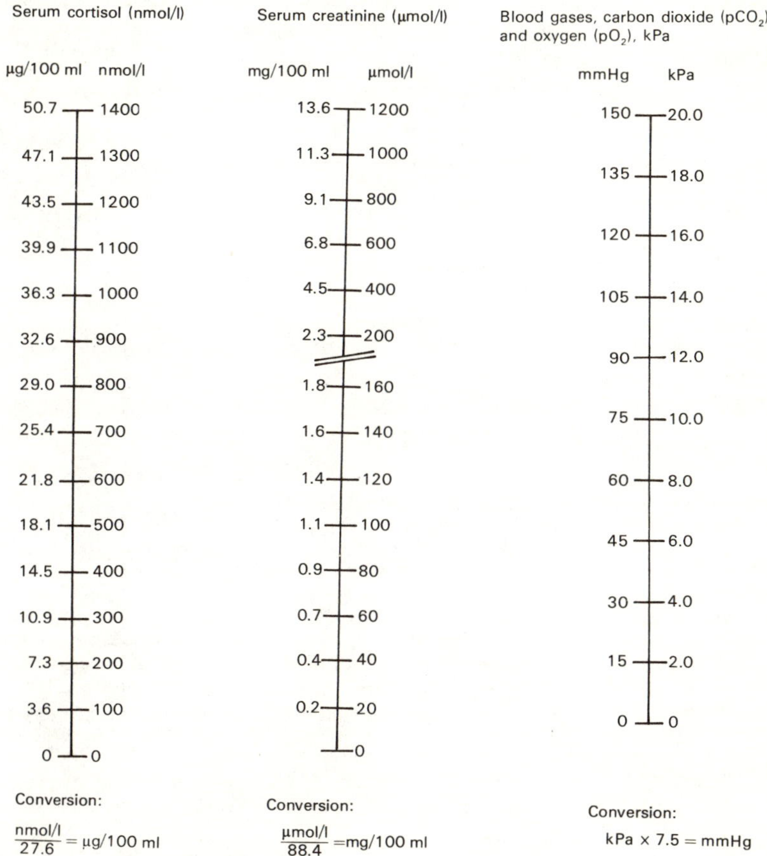

Figure A18.2. SI unit conversions: serum cortisol, serum creatinine, blood gases, carbon dioxide (pCO$_2$) and oxygen (pO$_2$)

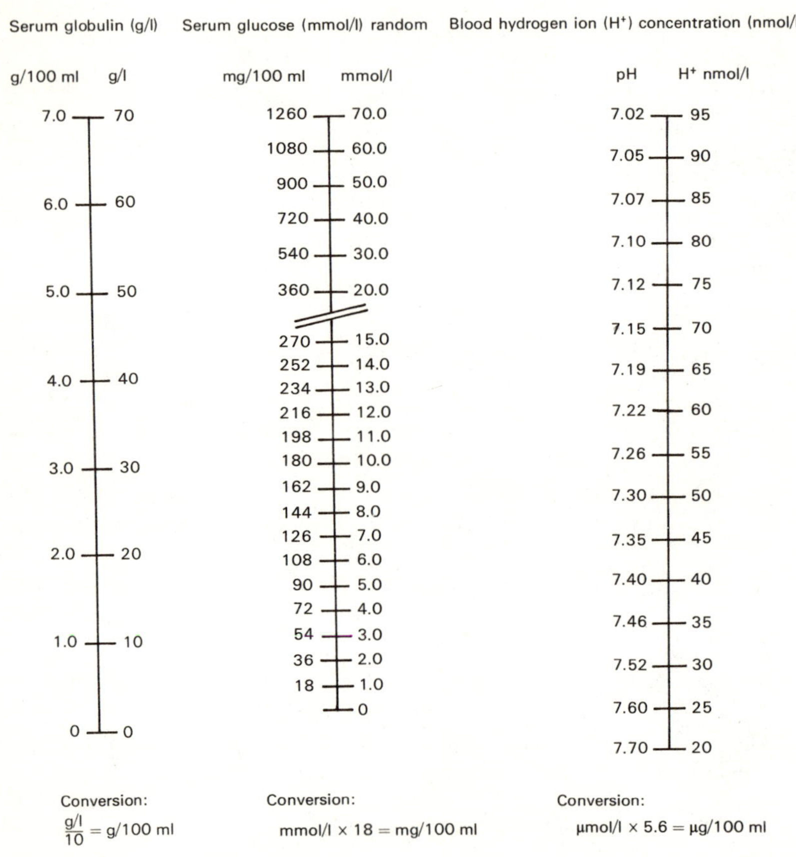

Figure A18.3. SI unit conversions: serum globulin, serum glucose, blood hydrogen ion (H+) concentration

TABLE A18.II

pH units, and their conversions to nanomoles

pH units	$[H^+]$ ion (nanomoles/l)	pH units	$[H^+]$ ion (nanomoles/l)
6.0	1000.0	7.0	100.0
6.1	794.2	7.1	79.4
6.2	630.9	7.2	63.1
6.3	501.2	7.3	50.1
6.4	398.1	7.4	39.8
6.5	316.3	7.5	31.6
6.6	251.2	7.6	25.1
6.7	199.5	7.7	19.9
6.8	158.5	7.8	15.8
6.9	125.9	7.9	12.6
		8.0	10.0

For pH's between 5.0 and 6.0, take the figures between 6.0 and 7.0 and multiply by factor of 10, i.e. pH 5.4 = 3981.0 nmol/l.

For pH's between 4.0 and 5.0, take the figures between 6.0 and 7.0 and multiply by factor of 100, i.e. pH 4.7 = 19 950.0 nmol/l.

For pH's between 3.0 and 4.0 use the same figures and multiply by 1000, i.e. pH 3.2 = 630 900 nmol/l or 630.9 mmol of H^+ ion.

For pH's between 2.0 and 3.0 use the same figures as above but multiply by 10 000.

The pH is reciprocal of the negative logarithm to base 10, of the $[H^+]$ concentration.

Table A18.II reproduced from *Clinical and Resuscitative Data* by R. P. H. Dunnill and B. E. Crawley, Blackwell Scientific Publications, Oxford, 1977, by kind permission of the authors and publishers.

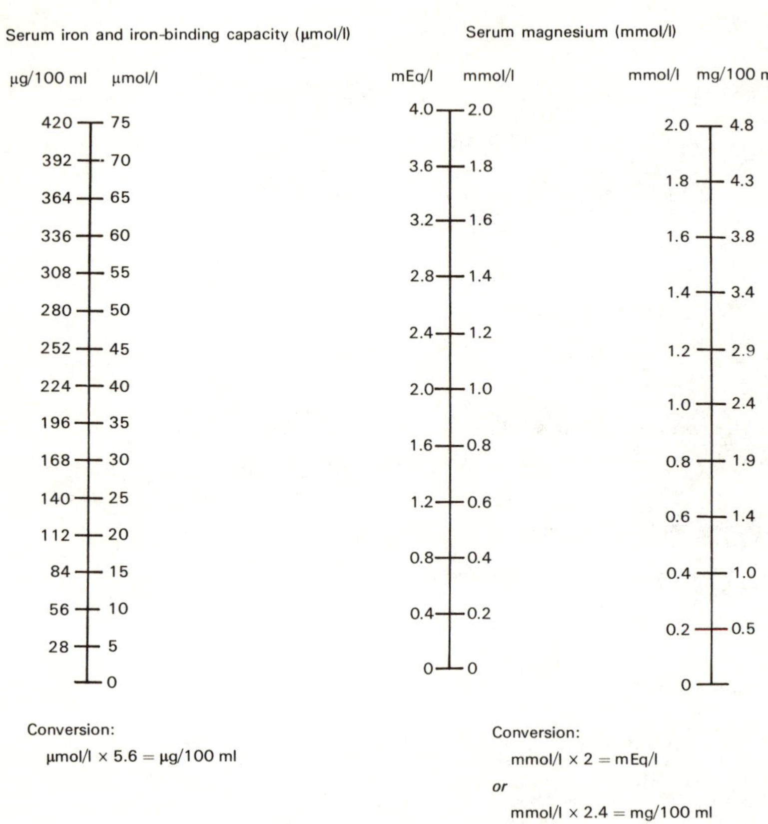

Figure A18.4. SI unit conversions: serum iron and iron-binding capacity, serum magnesium

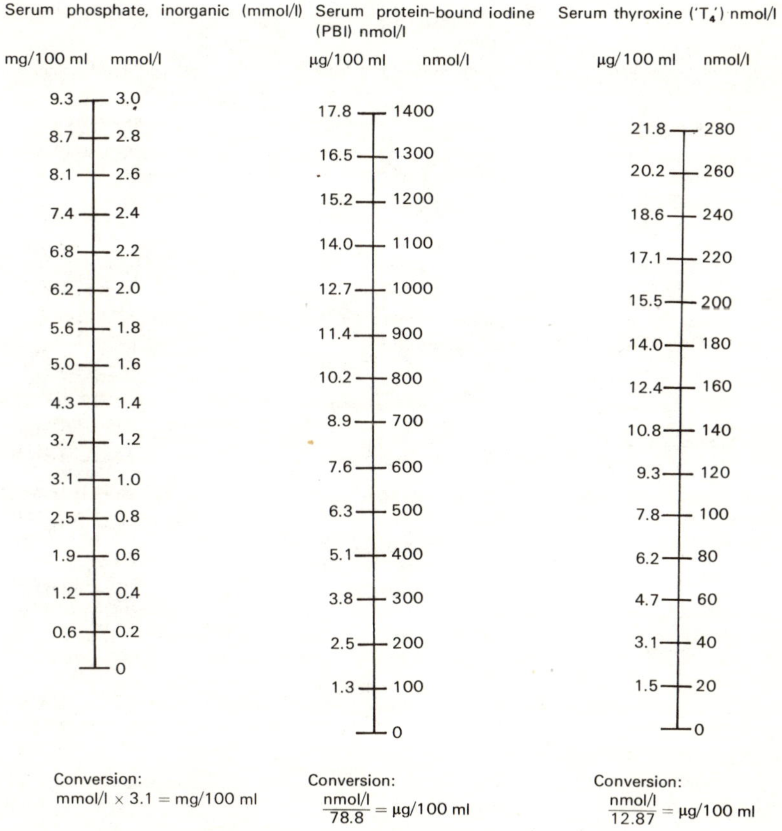

Serum phosphate, inorganic (mmol/l)   Serum protein-bound iodine (PBI) nmol/l   Serum thyroxine ('T$_4$') nmol/l

mg/100 ml   mmol/l   µg/100 ml   nmol/l   µg/100 ml   nmol/l

Serum phosphate, inorganic:

mg/100 ml	mmol/l
9.3	3.0
8.7	2.8
8.1	2.6
7.4	2.4
6.8	2.2
6.2	2.0
5.6	1.8
5.0	1.6
4.3	1.4
3.7	1.2
3.1	1.0
2.5	0.8
1.9	0.6
1.2	0.4
0.6	0.2
	0

Serum protein-bound iodine (PBI):

µg/100 ml	nmol/l
17.8	1400
16.5	1300
15.2	1200
14.0	1100
12.7	1000
11.4	900
10.2	800
8.9	700
7.6	600
6.3	500
5.1	400
3.8	300
2.5	200
1.3	100
	0

Serum thyroxine ('T$_4$'):

µg/100 ml	nmol/l
21.8	280
20.2	260
18.6	240
17.1	220
15.5	200
14.0	180
12.4	160
10.8	140
9.3	120
7.8	100
6.2	80
4.7	60
3.1	40
1.5	20
	0

Conversion:
mmol/l × 3.1 = mg/100 ml

Conversion:
$\dfrac{\text{nmol/l}}{78.8} = \text{µg/100 ml}$

Conversion:
$\dfrac{\text{nmol/l}}{12.87} = \text{µg/100 ml}$

Figure A18.5. SI unit conversions: serum phosphate (inorganic), serum protein-bound iodine (PBI), serum thyroxine ('T'$_4$)

830

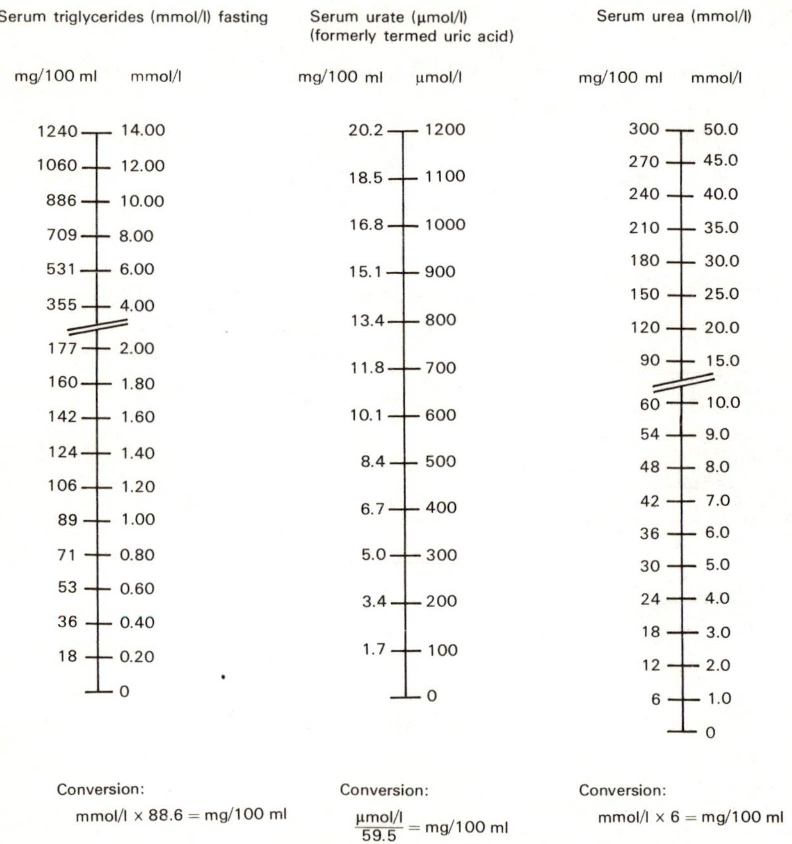

Figure A18.6. SI unit conversions: serum triglycerides (fasting), serum urate (formerly termed 'uric acid'), serum urea

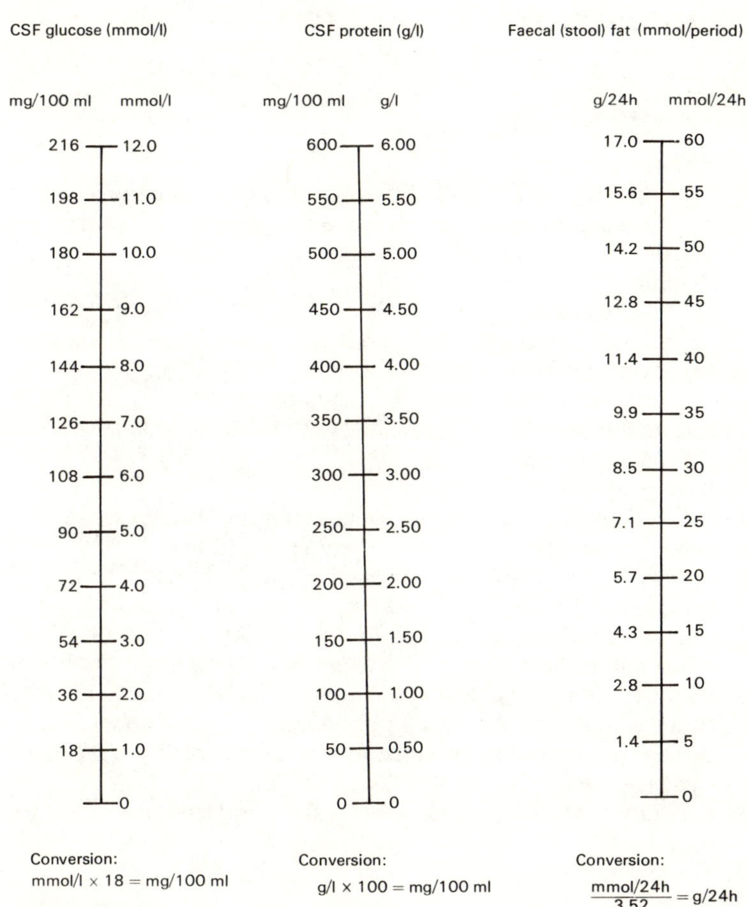

Figure A18.7. SI unit conversions: CSF glucose, CSF protein, faecal (stool) fat

Equipment for Resuscitation of the Newborn

M. F. WHITFIELD

(1) Resuscitation Trolley providing:
    (a) Facilities for O_2 IPPV by mask or endotracheal tube with a pressure-limiting blow-off valve designed to limit pressure in the circuit to 30 cm H_2O.
    (b) Suction.
    (c) Stop clock.
    (d) Sloping surface on which to place baby with head-down tilt.
    (e) Overhead heater,
        e.g. Vickers Model 60 Resuscitaire.
(2) Mucus extractors.
(3) Suction catheters
    (e.g. Argyle 5, 8 and 10).
(4) Infant bag and mask of the reinflating type which can be connected to the oxygen line, e.g. Penlon or Ambic.
(5) Infant laryngoscope with blades for the premature, and spare batteries and bulbs.
(6) Infant orotracheal tubes e.g. Warnes 8, 10, 12 and 14 Portex resuscitation sets 2.0, 2.5, 3.0 mm and open angle connecter (Cobb) to fit these tubes. (The Portex resuscitation set contains an endotracheal tube with open right angle connector and a suction catheter which passes through the constricted portion of the tube.)
(7) Oral (Guedel) airways size 0 and 00.
(8) Paediatric McGill forceps (small size) and endotracheal tube introducer.
(9) Towels.
(10) Drugs.
    10 or 20 per cent glucose: 10-ml ampoules.
    Sodium bicarbonate: 8.4 per cent 10-ml ampoules or 5 per cent.
    Naloxone (Narcan Neonatal): 2-ml ampoules (0.02 mg per ml).
    Diazepam: 2-ml ampoules (5 mg per ml).
    Adrenaline 1:1000: 1-ml ampoules.

Vitamin K_1 (phytomenadione): 0.5-ml ampoules (1 mg per 0.5 ml).

(*11*) *Syringes:* 1 ml, 2 ml, 5 ml, 10 ml, 20 ml.
Needles: 21, 23 and 25.
Butterfly needles: 23 and 25.
Alcohol swabs.
Micropore tape: $\frac{1}{2}$-inch.

NOTES

(1) It goes without saying that all resuscitation equipment must be frequently checked and be in a state of instant readiness. There must be a system for restocking as items are used, and the equipment itemized above has been deliberately restricted to be easily accommodated in a resuscitaire drawer. The more equipment the more difficult to find the item you need in a hurry.

(2) Resuscitation should be carried out in a warm draught-free room in a good light.

Equipment for Exchange Transfusion

M. F. WHITFIELD

EQUIPMENT
   (1) Resuscitation equipment (*see* Appendix 19).
   (2) Suitable environment for infant: incubator/operating table/radiant-heated intensive care crib such as Draeger Babytherm; this is most desirable, providing easy access and a warm, relatively draught-free, environment.
   (3) Drip stand with space for 2 bottles.
   (4) Oscilloscope cardiac-monitor leads, electrodes and electrode jelly.
   (5) Anglepoise light or overhead phototherapy unit.
   (6) Electronic temperature monitor with rectal and skin probes.
   (7) Clock or watch with second-hand.
   (8) 37°C (98.6°F) thermostatic water bath (if available).
  *(9) Urine-collecting bag (adult type) for collecting blood waste.
 *(10) Input/output/heart-rate record chart.

DRUGS/IV FLUIDS/CONTAINERS
   (1) Blood 1 or 2 units of semipacked cells of appropriate cross-matched group <48 hours old (on no account >5 days old).
   (2) N saline (0.9 per cent NaCl) 500 ml + 1000 units per ml heparin.
   (3) Calcium gluconate 10 per cent, 10-ml ampoules.
   (4) Sodium bicarbonate 8.4 per cent or 5 per cent 10-ml ampoules.
   (5) 1 per cent lignocaine (for umbilical cut-down, if required).
   (6) 2 sequestrene tubes.
   (7) 2 serum tubes.
   (8) 2 universal containers (sterile).
   (9) Antiseptic.
  (10) Nobecutane.

STERILE EQUIPMENT
   *2 20-ml syringes
   *1 4-way stopcock

or 2 3-way stopcocks
   2 adult blood-giving sets
   *1 extension tubing (for waste)——(e.g. tubing from a drip set)
   *2 umbilical catheters, 5 and 8 FG
   *2 sterile towels, one with central hole
      gauze swabs
   *2 gallipots
   2 gowns
      gloves sizes $6\frac{1}{2}$—8.

STERILE INSTRUMENTS
   4 pairs mosquito forceps
   1 pair dissecting forceps (fine, untoothed)
   1 pair stitch-holding forceps
   1 vascular probe
   4 towel clips
   1 scalpel and blade
   1 pair scissors
   curved needle and 2/0 catgut
   1 metal rule (centimetre graduation), unless supplied with dispos-
      able set.

Notes

(1) It is usually convenient to use a disposable exchange-transfusion
    pack which contains the items marked by an asterisk. The Pharma-
    seal set can be obtained from most medical suppliers.
(2) Exchange transfusion is a potentially hazardous procedure particu-
    larly in the hands of inexperienced operators and if the donor blood
    is more than 48 hours old. It is necessary to have a skilled assistant
    (doctor or nurse) who monitors the condition of the infant as well
    as keeping a close check on input and output. It is important to be
    as comfortable as possible but if the procedure is not carried out in
    an incubator or intensive care crib the air temperature in the room
    needs to be around 30°C (86°F) or more if the infant is not to lose
    heat.

Guide to Sizes of Tracheal Tubes

TABLE A21.I
(Table modified from D. R. G. Browne (1969). *Anaesthesia* **24**, 620)

ENDOTRACHEAL				TRACHEOSTOMY		
Magill No.		B.S. Diameter (mm)	Bronchoscope		Polyvinyl chloride	
$\dfrac{Age}{2}+1$	Age	$\dfrac{Age}{4}+4.5$ Int. Dia. (mm)	Negus	Great Ormond Street Int. Dia. (mm)	Ext. Dia. mm	PORTEX FG
000		2.5				
00		3.0				
0A	0–3 months	3.5	Suckling	3.5		
0	3–6 months	4.0		4.0		
1	6 mths–2 years	4.5	Infant	4.5	6.0	0
2	2–4 years	5.0		5.0	7.0	0
3	4–5 years	5.5	Child			
4	5–7 years	6.0		6.0	8.0	24
5	7–8 years	6.5	Adolescent			
6	8–10 years	7.0		7.0	9.0	27
7	10–12 years		Small Adult		10.0	30
8	12–14 years	8.0	Large Adult		11.0	33
9	Adult	9.0			12.0	36
10	Adult					
11	Adult	10.0			13.0	39
12	Adult	11.0			14.0	42

Useful General Data

From *Clinical and Resuscitative Data* by R. P. H. Dunnill & B. E. Crawley, Blackwell Scientific Publications, Oxford (1977), by kind permission of the authors and Publishers.

ELECTROLYTES

Milligram to millimol to milliequivalent conversion equations

$$\text{Milliequivalents/l} = \frac{\text{mg\%} \times 10 \times \text{valency}}{\text{mol. wt}} = \text{mmol/l} \times \text{valency}$$

$$\text{Milligrams\%} = \frac{\text{mEq/l} \times \text{mol. wt}}{10 \times \text{valency}} = \frac{\text{mmol/l} \times \text{mol. wt}}{10}$$

$$\text{Millimol/l} = \frac{10 \times \text{mg\%}}{\text{mol. wt}} = \frac{\text{mEq/l}}{\text{valency}}$$

MOLAR VALUES

1 g of Na^+	contains 43.5 mmol of Na^+
1 g of Na chloride	contains 17.1 mmol of Na^+
1 g of Na bicarbonate	contains 12 mmol of Na^+
1 g of Na lactate	contains 8.9 mmol of Na^+
1 g of Na citrate	contains 10.2 mmol of Na^+
1 g of K^+	contains 25.6 mmol of K^+
1 g of chloride	contains 13.5 mmol of K^+
1 g of K acetate	contains 10.2 mmol of K^+
1 g of K citrate	contains 9.3 mmol of K^+
1 g of K bicarbonate	contains 9.9 mmol of K^+
1 g of Ca^{++}	contains 25 mmol of Ca^{++}
1 g of Ca gluconate	contains 2.3 mmol of Ca^{++}
1 g of $CaCl_2 + 2H_2O$	contains 6.8 mmol of Ca^{++}
$+ 6H_2O$	contains 4.5 mmol of Ca^+
1 g of Mg^{++}	contains 42 mmol of Mg^{++}
1 g of Mg sulphate $+ 7H_2O$	contains 4 mmol of Mg^{++}

1 g of NH_4 chloride   contains 18.7 mmol of NH_4^+

i.e. 10 ml of 10 per cent calcium gluconate solution contains 1 g of calcium gluconate or 2.3 mmol Ca^{++}

CALCULATION OF PLASMA OSMOLALITY

$$1.89 \text{ (Serum } Na^+ + K^+ \text{ mmol/l)} + \frac{\text{Blood sugar in mg\%}}{18} + \frac{\text{Blood urea in mg\%}}{4}$$

INFUSION SET VOLUMES

From this list the number of drops per minute will show the amount of fluid infused using the various standard infusion sets.

Microdrop   60 drops/min = 1 ml/min i.e. Soluset type
    1 ml/h   =   1   d/min (drops/min) (microdrop)
    5 ml/h   =   5   d/min
  100 ml/day =   4   d/min
  500 ml/day =   21   d/min
1000 ml/day =   42   d/min
  500 ml/6h   =   84   d/min (2000 ml/day)

Standard   15 drops/min = 1ml/min i.e. Baxter Avon type
  20 ml/h   =   5   d/min (*standard*)
 100 ml/h   =   25   d/min
 500 ml/h   = 125   d/min
1000 ml/day = 10.5 d/min
 500 ml/6h   =   21   d/min (2000 ml/day)
1000 ml/8h   =   32   d/min (3000 ml/day)

Special   10 drops/min = 1 ml/min i.e. Hemoset type
  30 ml/h   =   5   d/min
 100 ml/h   = 16.5 d/min
 500 ml/h   =   84   d/min
1000 ml/day =   7   d/min
 500 ml/6h   =   14   d/min (2000 ml/day)
1000 ml/8h   =   21   d/min (3000 ml/day)

DOMESTIC MEASURES
1 pint   = 0.5683 litres = 20 fluid oz
1 teaspoon   = 4.5 ml
1 tablespoon   = 15 ml
1 dessertspoon = 8 ml   } Approximately
1 wine glass   = 60 ml
1 tumbler glass = 240 ml

Index of Drugs

Official and approved names of drugs with page references and commonly used proprietary names

In the left-hand column the official (US) or approved (UK) names are given. Where the two names are different both British and American names are listed. Proprietary names refer to preparations commonly used, without indication of the country of origin. The more important page references are given. For convenience a few drugs are also included which do not appear in the text.

Name	Proprietary names	Reference in text
ACTH (*see* Corticotrophin and Tetracosatrin)		Table A9.VIII
Adenine arabinoside (*see* Vidarabine)		
Adrenaline (UK) (Epinephrine US)		pp. 111, 253, 303, 543, 601
Aldosterone	Aldocorten	p. 455
Allopurinol	Zyloprim, Zyloric	p. 474
Amethopterin *now* Methotrexate	Adanon, Althose	p. 477
Aminocaproic acid (Epsilon aminocaproic acid)	Amicar, Epsikapron	p. 494
Aminophylline	Cardophylin, Phyllocontin (slow release)	pp. 111, 253
Aminosalicylic acid (US) (Sodium aminosalicylate, PAS UK)	Pamisyl, Paramisan Sodium	
Amodiaquine	Camoquin	p. 555
Amoxicillin (US) / Amoxycillin (UK)	Amoxil, Larotid	pp. 261, 407, 567, 790
Amphotericin B	Fungilin, Fungizone	pp. 358, 643
Ampicillin	Ampifen, Penbritin, Pentrezyl, Polycillin, Vidopen	pp. 261, 380, 407, 790
Amikacin	Amikin	pp. 783, 790
Apomorphine		p. 67
Ascorbic acid (Vitamin C)		p. 646
Asparaginase		pp. 111, 477
Atropine		pp. 199, 240, 303
B$_1$ vitamin (*see* Thiamine)		p. 593

Name	Proprietary names	Reference in text
B_6 vitamin (*see* Pyridoxine)		pp. 357, 689
B_{12} vitamin (*see* Cyanocobalamin)		p. 752
Bentonite		p. 74
Benzylpenicillin (Penicillin G)	Numerous names	
Bephenium	Alcopar, Alcopara	p. 641
Betamethasone	Betnelan, Celestone	
Bisacodyl	Dulcolax	p. 343
British Anti-Lewisite, BAL (*see* Dimercaprol)	Dimercaprol	p. 371
C Vitamin (*see* Ascorbic acid)		p. 646
Calciferol		p. 142
Calcitonin (Salcatonin; salmon)	Calcitaire (pork), Calsynar (salmon) Miacalcic (salmon)	p. 145
Calcium disodium versenate (US) (Sodium calcium-edetate. UK)	Edathamil Ledclair (also called Calcium EDTA)	p. 371
Calcium gluconate		p. 143
Calcium gluconogalactogluconate syrup (US) Calcium lactate gluconate syrup (UK)	Calcium Sandoz, Neo-Calglucon	p. 143
Calcium lactate		p. 143
Carbenicillin	Geopen, Pyopen	pp. 353, 475
Carbamazepine	Tegretol	
Carbimazole	Neo-Mercazole	pp. 463, 464
Camphorated opium tincture (*see* Opium, camphorated tincture)		p. 709
Cefazolin (US) Cephalozolin (UK)	Ancef, Kefzol	
Cephalexin	Ceporex, Keflex	
Cephaloridine	Ceporin, Loridine	p. 108
Cephalothin	Keflin	
Cephradine	Anspor, Eskacef, Velosef	
Charcoal, activated		p. 71
Chloral hydrate	Noctec	
Chloramphenicol	Amphicol, Chloromycetin	pp. 350, 357, 567
Chloroquine	Aralen, Avloclor, Nivaquine, Resochin, Roquine	p. 555
Chlorothiazide	Diuril, Saluric	p. 287
Chlorpheniramine	Haynon, Chlor-Trimeton, Piriton, Teldrin	p. 114
Chlorpromazine	Chloractil, Largactil, Thorazine	pp. 44, 345, 505, 537, 709
Chlortetracycline	Aureomycin	
Clindamycin	Cleocin, Dalacin C	pp. 353, 637
Clioquinol (UK) (Iodohydroxyquin US)	Entero-Vioform, Vioform	
Clonazepam	Clonopin, Rivotril	p. 319
Cloxacillin	Orbenin, Tegopen	
Colistin	Colomycin, Coly-mycin	p. 353
Cortisone acetate	Cortistab, Cortone acetate	pp. 455, 458

Name	Proprietary names	Reference in text
Corticotrophin (ACTH)	ACTH & Acthar gel	
Cotrimoxazole	Bactrim, Septra, Septrin	p. 476
Cyanocobalamin (Vitamin B_{12})	Cytacon, Cytamen	p. 752
Cyclophosphamide	Cytoxan, Endoxana	p. 477
Cyclizine	Valoid	p. 81
Cytarabine (Cytosine arabinoside)	Cytosar	p. 627
D_2 vitamin (*see* Calciferol)		p. 142
Daunorubicin (Rubidomycin)	Cerubidin	p. 474
Desferrioxamine	Desferal	p. 76
Desoxycorticosterone acetate (Doca)	Cortate, Percorten (may be unavailable in UK)	p. 457
Dexamethasone	Decadron, Deronil, Dexa-cortisyl, Oradexon, and others	pp. 109, 324, 729
Diazepam	Atensine, Tensium, Valium	pp. 318, 341, 344
Diazoxide	Eudemine, Hyperstat	p. 415
Dichloralphenazone	Welldorm	p. 225, 709
Digoxin	Lanoxin	p. 286
Dimercaprol (British Anti-Lewisite, BAL)		p. 371
Diphenylhydantoin (US) (Phenytoin UK)	Dilantin, Epanutin	p. 690
Diphenoxylate	Lomotil	p. 401
Dopamine		p. 119
Doxorubicin	Adriamycin, Vibramycin	p. 477
Edetate calcium disodium (*see* Calcium disodium versenate)		p. 371
Edrophonium	Tensilon	p. 240
Emetine		p. 570
Ephedrine		p. 293
Epinephrine (US) (Adrenaline UK)		*see* Adrenaline
Epsilon aminocaproic acid (*see* Aminocaproic acid)		p. 494
Erythromycin	Erycen, Erythrocin, Erythromid, Erythroped, Ilosone, Ilotycin, Pediamycin, Retcin	p. 261
Ethambutol	Myambutol	
Flucytosine	Alcobon, Aucobon	p. 358
Flucloxacillin	Floxapen	
Fludrocortisone	Florinef	p. 455
Folic acid	Folvite	p. 470
Frusemide (UK) Furosemide (US)	Dryptal, Frusid, Lasix	pp. 43, 287, 415, 591
Fusidate, sodium (Fusidic acid)	Fucidin	p. 637
Gentamicin	Cidomycin, Garamycin, Genticin	p. 643
Glucagon		p. 442, 450
Glutaminase		p. 111
Glutethimide	Doriden	p. 511
Glycerin (Glycerol)		p. 324
Heparin		pp. 483, 679, 720

Name	Proprietary names	Reference in text
Hydralazine (US) Hydrallazine (UK)	Apresoline	p. 416
Hydrocortisone	Cortef, Cortril, Hydrocortone, and others	p. 457
Hyoscine hydrobromide		pp. 81, 537
Idoxuridine	Dendrid, Herplex, Stoxil	p. 627
Imipramine	Imavate, Tofranil, and others	p. 508
Iodochlorhydroxyquin (US) Clioquinol (UK)	Entero-Vioform, Vioform	
Ipecacuanha		p. 67
Isoniazid (INAH, INA, INH)	Nydrazid, Rimifon	pp. 357, 628
Isoprenaline (UK) Isoproterenol (US)	Isuprel, Proterenol, Saventrine, Suscardia	pp. 118, 293
K₁ vitamin (*see* Phytomenadione)		p. 657
Kanamycin	Kannasyn, Kantrex	p. 643
Levarterenol, Norepinephrine (US) (Noradrenaline UK)	Levophed	
Levothyroxine (US) (Thyroxine, UK)	Cytoten, Eltroxin, Levoid	p. 461
Lidocaine (US) Lignocaine (UK)	Xylocaine	pp. 117, 294
Lincomycin	Lincocin, Mycivin	p. 637
Loperamide	Imodium	p. 401
Magnesium hydroxide (Milk of Magnesia)		pp. 146, 590
Magnesium sulphate		pp. 146, 590
Mannitol	Osmitrol	pp. 47, 323, 415
Medazepam	Nobrium	p. 506
Meglumine cliatrizoate (with sodium diatrizoate)	Gastrografin	p. 98
Mepyramine	Anthisan	p. 113
Meperidine (US) (Pethidine UK)	Demerol	p. 601
Mercaptopurine (6-MP)	Puri-Nethol, Purintol	p. 477
Metaraminol	Aramine	pp. 113, 116
Methadone	Amidone, Physeptone	p. 707
Methicillin	Celbenin, Dimocillin R-T, Staphcillin	
Methotrexate, formerly Amethopterin	Adanon, Althose	p. 476
Methoxamine	Vasoxine, Vasylox	p. 116
Methyldopa	Aldomet, Dopamet, Medomet	
Methylene blue		p. 646
Methylprednisolone	Depo-Medrone, Medrol, Solu-Medrone	pp. 42, 109
Metronidazole	Flagyl	pp. 353, 570
Morphine		pp. 35, 288, 290
Nalidixic acid	Negram	
Nalorphine	Lethidrone, Nalline	p. 600
Naloxone	Narcan	p. 600
Nandrolone decanoate	Deca-Durabolin	p. 505

Name	Proprietary names	Reference in text
Neomycin	Mycifradin, Neobiotic, Neomin	p. 640
Neostigmine	Prostigmin	p. 240
Nifurtimox	Lampit (Bayer)	p. 628
Nitrazepam	Mogadon, Remnos	
Opium, camphorated tincture (Paregoric)		p. 709
Oxytetracycline	Imperacin, Terramycin and others	
Paregoric (*see* Opium, camphorated tincture)		p. 709
Paraldehyde	Paral	p. 319
Paraminosalicylic acid PAS (*see* Sodium aminosalicylate)		
Penicillin G (*see* Benzylpenicillin)		
Penicillin (triple injection UK) containing benethamine penicillin, procaine penicillin and benzylpenicillin (UK)	Triplopen Bicillin all purpose (US) differs slightly from Triplopen	p. 341
Penicillamine	Cuprimine, Depamine, Distamine	p. 371
Pentamidine		
Pentazocine	Fortral	p. 707
Pethidine (Meperidine, US)		p. 601
Phenelzine	Nardil	p. 508
Phenobital (US) / Phenobarbitone (UK)	Luminal	p. 690
Phenytoin (UK) / Diphenylhydantoin (US)	Dilantin, Epanutin	p. 690
Phytomenadione (UK) / Phytonadione (US) (K_1 vitamin)	Aqua-Mephyton, Konakion	pp. 657, 664
Practol (US) / Practolol (UK)	Eraldin (restricted to arrhythmia)	
Prednisolone	Delta-Cortef, Delta-stab and others	
Prednisone	Delta-Cortone, Deltasone and others	
Prilocaine	Citanest	pp. 171, 174
Promethazine	Avomine, Phenergan	p. 114
Propanolol	Inderal	pp. 291, 303, 463
Protamine		p. 484
Pyridostigmine	Mestinon	
Pyridoxine (B_6 vitamin)	Benadon	pp. 357, 689
Pyrimethamine	Daraprim	p. 643
Quinine		p. 555
Resin, exchange, (*see* Sodium polystyrene sulphonate)		p. 138
Rifampicin	Rifadin, Rimactane	p. 357
Rubidomycin (*see* Daunorubicin)		p. 474
Salbutamol	Albuterol, Ventolin	p. 253
Salcatonin (*see* Calcitonin)		

Name	Proprietary names	Reference in text
Silver sulphadiazine	Flamazine	p. 45
Sodium calcium-edetate (UK) (*see* Calcium disodium versenate (US))		p. 371
Sodium polystyrene sulphonate	Kayexalate, Resonium A	p. 138
Spectinomycin	Trobicin	p. 630
Spiramycin	Romamycin	p. 643
Streptomycin	Orastrep, Streptaquaine	p. 357
Sulfamylon	Mafenide	p. 43
Sulphadiazine		p. 643
Tetracosatrin	Synacthen	
Tetracosatrin Zinc	Cortrosyn Depot, Synacthen Depot	
Tetracycline	Achromycin, Tetrasyn and others	p. 563
Theophylline	Elixophyllin, Theograd and others	p. 275
Theophylline ethylenediamine (*see* Aminophylline)		p. 111, 253
Thiamine (B$_1$ vitamin)	Benerva	p. 594
Thioguanine		p. 474
Thyrocalcitonin, *see* Calcitonin		p. 145
Thyroxine (UK) (Levothyroxine US)	Cytoten, Eltroxin, Levoid	p. 461
Tinidazole		p. 571
Trimethoprim— Sulfamethoxazole (*see* Cotrimoxazole)		p. 476
Trimeprazine	Temaril, Vallergan	p. 713
Triamcinolone	Aristocort, Kenocort	
Tobramycin	Nebecin, Obracin	p. 642
Urea	Ureaphil, Urevert	
Vasopressin	Pitressin	p. 397
Versenate (*see* Calcium disodium versenate)		p. 371
Vidarabine	Vira-A	p. 631
Vincristine	Oncovin	pp. 474, 477

Index

2D